THE
SKULL

VOLUME
2

THE
SKULL

VOLUME
2

Patterns of Structural and Systematic Diversity

EDITED BY

JAMES HANKEN AND BRIAN K. HALL

THE UNIVERSITY OF CHICAGO PRESS

Chicago and London

James Hanken is associate professor in the Department of Environmental, Population, and Organismic Biology at the University of Colorado, Boulder.
Brian K. Hall is Izaak Walton Killam Research Professor and professor of biology at Dalhousie University.

The University of Chicago Press, Chicago 60637
The University of Chicago Press, Ltd., London
© 1993 by The University of Chicago
All rights reserved. Published 1993
Printed in the United States of America

02 01 00 99 98 97 96 95 94 93   1 2 3 4 5

ISBN: 0-226-31568-1 (cloth)
ISBN: 0-226-31570-3 (paper)

Library of Congress Cataloging-in-Publication Data

The Skull / edited by James Hanken and Brian K. Hall.
    p.   cm.
    Includes bibliographical references and index.
    Contents: v. 1. Development—v. 2. Patterns of structural and
systematic diversity—v. 3. Functional and evolutionary
mechanisms.
    1. Skull—Anatomy.   2. Skull—Evolution.   3. Anatomy, Comparative.
I. Hanken, James.   II. Hall, Brian Keith, 1941– .
    [DNLM: 1. Skull—anatomy & histology.   2. Skull—growth &
development.   3. Skull physiology.   WE   705   S629]
QL822.S58   1993
596'.04'71—dc20
DNLM/DLC   92-49119
for Library of Congress   CIP

CONTENTS

VOLUME 2
Patterns of Structural and Systematic Diversity

Preface   *James Hanken and Brian K. Hall*   ix

1. Evolutionary Origin of the Vertebrate Skull
   Carl Gans   1
2. Segmentation, the Adult Skull, and the Problem of Homology
   Keith Stewart Thomson   36
3. Cranial Skeletal Tissues: Diversity and Evolutionary Trends
   William A. Beresford   69
4. Patterns of Diversity in the Skull of Jawless Fishes
   Philippe Janvier   131
5. Patterns of Diversity in the Skull of Jawed Fishes
   Hans-Peter Schultze   189
6. Patterns of Cranial Diversity among the Lissamphibia
   Linda Trueb   255
7. Patterns of Diversity in the Reptilian Skull
   Olivier Rieppel   344
8. Patterns of Diversity in the Avian Skull
   Richard L. Zusi   391
9. Patterns of Diversity in the Mammalian Skull
   Michael J. Novacek   438

List of Contributors   547

Index   549

VOLUME 1
Development

General Introduction   *James Hanken and Brian K. Hall*
Preface   *James Hanken and Brian K. Hall*

1. Axis Specification and Head Induction in Vertebrate Embryos
   Richard P. Elinson and Kenneth R. Kao
2. Somitomeres: Mesodermal Segments of the Head and Trunk
   Antone G. Jacobson
3. Pattern Formation and the Neural Crest
   Robert M. Langille and Brian K. Hall
4. Differentiation and Morphogenesis of Cranial Skeletal Tissues
   Peter Thorogood
5. Epigenetic and Functional Influences on Skull Growth
   Susan W. Herring
6. Genetic and Developmental Aspects of Variability in the Mammalian
   Mandible
   William R. Atchley
7. Developmental-Genetic Analysis of Skeletal Mutants
   David R. Johnson
8. Metamorphosis and the Vertebrate Skull: Ontogenetic Patterns and
   Developmental Mechanisms
   Christopher S. Rose and John O. Reiss
9. Preconception of Adult Structural Pattern in the Analysis of the
   Developing Skull
   Robert Presley
10. Bibliography of Skull Development, 1937–89
   Brian K. Hall and James Hanken

List of Contributors

Index

VOLUME 3
Functional and Evolutionary Mechanisms

Preface   *James Hanken and Brian K. Hall*

1. Mechanisms of Skull Diversity and Evolution
   James Hanken and Brian K. Hall
2. Convergent and Alternative Designs for Vertebrate Suspension Feeding
   S. Laurie Sanderson and Richard Wassersug

3. Design of Feeding Systems in Aquatic Vertebrates: Major Patterns and
   Their Evolutionary Interpretations
       George V. Lauder and H. Bradley Shaffer
4. The Form of the Feeding Apparatus in Terrestrial Vertebrates: Studies
   of Adaptation and Constraint
       Kathleen K. Smith
5. The Skull as a Locomotor Organ
       Marvalee H. Wake
6. Structural Basis of Hearing and Sound Transmission
       R. Eric Lombard and Thomas E. Hetherington
7. Beams and Machines: Modeling Approaches to the Analysis of Skull
   Form and Function
       David B. Weishampel
8. Mechanical Analysis of the Mammalian Head Skeleton
       Anthony P. Russell and Jeffrey J. Thomason
9. Scaling, Allometry, and Skull Design
       Sharon B. Emerson and Dennis M. Bramble
10. Ecomorphology of the Teleostean Skull
       Karel F. Liem

    List of Contributors

    Index

PREFACE

JAMES HANKEN AND BRIAN K. HALL

This is the second of three volumes on the vertebrate skull. Its contents complement the first volume (*Development*) in achieving several overall aims, viz., (1) to organize and present the results of recent studies of skull development and structure in such a way as to interest specialists and vertebrate morphologists generally; (2) to evaluate the implications of these results for fundamental questions in vertebrate structure and evolution; (3) to examine current studies of the functional bases and constraints of skull form; (4) to use the vertebrate skull to illustrate evolutionary patterns and processes and to test hypotheses to account for them; and (5) to promote further interest and research in these and related issues.

The main theme of this volume is cranial diversity, which is examined from two broadly different perspectives. The first three chapters consider aspects of the evolutionary origin and basic structure of the skull and its component tissues. In the first chapter, Gans discusses the initial evolution of the skull, with the principal aim of updating the "neural crest hypothesis" for head evolution developed earlier in collaboration with Glenn Northcutt. He incorporates recent findings from developmental biology, functional morphology, and paleontology, and in so doing defines a series of tests to be used in further evaluating the hypothesis.

In chapter 2, Thomson renews the discussion of head segmentation begun in volume 1 by Jacobson and extended by Gans. Thomson, however, focuses on the problem of segmentation of the adult skull and its bearing on questions of homology of dermal-bone patterns among vertebrates. These topics are very relevant to the study of patterns of skull evolution within, and especially among, major groups. They have been largely ignored in most recent studies of head segmentation, which have instead focused on early embryonic features, principally involving the brain and cranial nerves. Indeed, cranial evolution and segmentation have been of long-standing interest to students of vertebrate biology; they were the focus of some of the most famous debates in classical morphology, beginning in the eighteenth century and continuing almost unabated into the early twentieth (e.g., Appel 1987; de Beer 1937). Reexamination of these questions at this time is justified by the numerous and, in some cases, fundamental discoveries that have been made in the last few years, especially from developmental biology. A prime example is the predominant role of the embryonic neural crest in cranial development, and particularly its extensive contributions to the adult skull (see chapter 3, by Langille and Hall, in volume 1). This role went virtually unrecognized in classical treatments of cranial evolution and diversification (Hall and Hanken 1985).

In the third chapter, Beresford provides an overview of the histological building blocks of the skull—the skeletal tissues. Unlike the evolutionary origin of the skull and cranial segmentation, the diversity of cranial skeletal tissues traditionally has been underappreciated. An explicit treatment is warranted by the steadily accumulating body of knowledge that has revealed, on the one hand, an astonishing range of skeletal tissues among vertebrates, especially fishes, and, on the other, that the diversity represents variation on the two themes of cartilage and bone. Dentine and enamel, two tissues primarily associated with teeth in Recent vertebrates, also appeared very early in vertebrate history. This should serve as an effective reminder to many skeletal biologists that mammalian tissues, which are frequently offered as the paradigmatic examples in vertebrates, depict only a small fraction of the diversity that exists.

The remaining six chapters take a different tack in documenting patterns of cranial diversity within major lineages. As with other contributions in these volumes, they are not offered as encyclopedic reviews of their respective subjects. Rather, authors were asked to identify general and prominent trends of cranial evolution, illustrated with specific examples. In all chapters except the two dealing with jawless and jawed fishes by Janvier and Schultze, respectively, the primary focus is on extant forms, although fossil taxa are considered where appropriate. The differing extent of knowledge among groups, differences in the completeness of their fossil records, and, simply, differences in phylogenetic diversity and the number of component taxa, all dictated inevitable differences in the level of coverage among chapters. Schultze's assignment was especially difficult, given the tremendous diversity and number of jawed fishes, which precluded equal treatment of even only the major taxa. In view of the importance to the whole vertebrate lineage of basic structural plans established in early groups, he appropriately chose to focus his account on these forms. Recent fishes, however, are the primary subjects of three chapters in volume 3 (by Sanderson and Wassersug, Lauder and Shaffer, and Liem), illustrating important functional aspects of cranial diversification in several lineages.

These taxon-based treatments organize and synthesize existing knowledge, both as an end in itself and as a means of stimulating future research.

A predominant theme is the necessity to evaluate and document trends of cranial character evolution in the context of explicit hypotheses of phylogenetic relationship. For some groups, this represents a radical departure from the methodology employed in most previous studies. In such a phylogenetic context, features of the skull assume a dual role: as characters to be used to derive hypotheses of relationship among taxa, and as markers of trends in cranial evolution. A secondary theme is the need for better and more widespread use of ontogenetic data, both for phylogeny reconstruction and to provide a mechanistic basis for evolutionary trends.

The organization of these six chapters largely follows conventional classifications of the major groups of vertebrates, e.g., jawless fishes, amphibians, and reptiles. This organization belies the widespread conviction among contemporary systematists who favor the formal recognition of only natural (i.e., monophyletic) groups, and the general consensus that whereas some of the traditional categories of vertebrates may represent such groups (e.g., birds), many others, such as reptiles, clearly do not (Benton 1990). Indeed, in the last few years, a number of studies have proposed alternate taxonomic schemes to remove such inconsistencies (e.g., Gauthier et al. 1988a, b; Maisey 1986). At present, however, there is not widespread agreement regarding either the exact phylogenetic relationships among, or even within, all the major vertebrate groups, or the formal names that should be adopted for such groups. Primarily for this reason we have adopted the organization seen here. Phylogenetic problems pertaining to individual groups are discussed at the beginning of each chapter. Readers are advised to read this material carefully, as observed patterns of cranial diversification depend heavily on the underlying scheme of phylogenetic relationship. Indeed, as discussed by both Trueb and Zusi, the absence of a well-corroborated phylogeny may severely limit our ability to derive valid and meaningful generalizations concerning character evolution. We also urge all readers to incorporate explicit phylogenetic statements, rather than traditional groupings, into their own comparative studies.

A certain amount of overlap in chapter content both within and between volumes is unavoidable; the range of coverage of individual chapters is enormous, and there is much interdependence among many features of cranial structure and evolution. Thus, the phylogenetic distribution of secondary cartilage—and the belief that it is restricted to birds and mammals—is discussed by Beresford, Rieppel, and Novacek. Interestingly, in documenting the existence of similar tissues in fishes and reptiles, both Beresford and Rieppel illustrate the frequent, but often underappreciated, difficulty in using developmental criteria to assess homology. This problem is highlighted by Presley (volume 1) and Thomson (this volume) in other contexts, and recurs in other chapters (see also discussion in Hall 1992).

Evolution and homology of dermal-bone patterns in jawed fishes also receives multiple coverage, although different aspects are emphasized in the two principal accounts. Schultze takes a strict, phylogenetic approach, focusing on the relations among many of the complex patterns found in different groups, whereas Thomson addresses possible causal mechanisms underlying both these patterns and the likely transitions among them.

Similarly, both Gans and Beresford discuss the probable sequence of, and reasons for, evolution of the primary skeletal tissues. And while these authors agree on some points, they disagree on others; for example, the origin of vertebrate cartilage and bone from early sensory receptors (mechanoreceptors and electroreceptors, respectively). We regard these and other differences as inevitable, indeed desirable, insofar as they reflect current controversies regarding many fundamental aspects of cranial structure and evolution. Such uncertainty is perhaps no better exemplified than by the recent paper dealing with the enigmatic fossil group, the conodonts, which envisions a radically different scenario for the evolution of cartilage, bone, dentine, and enamel (Sansom et al. 1992). This scenario, published only in the last few weeks, is briefly discussed by Gans in an appendix to his chapter added as this volume is about to go to press.

Other disagreements involve differing schemes of relationship among particular groups. Thus, Thomson regards jawless and jawed vertebrates as sister groups (Agnatha and Gnathostomata, respectively) derived from an unknown craniate ancestor. Janvier, however, while conceding that the issue is far from resolved, does not accept Agnatha as a natural group, instead regarding some agnathans as more closely related to gnathostomes than others, with hagfishes as the basal out-group. Despite this disagreement over phylogeny, both authors reach the same general conclusion regarding the difficulty in deriving all but the most basic aspects of the gnathostome skull from any known agnathan condition. Indeed, this is the context for Janvier's (in many respects heretical) claim that paired visceral arches in agnathans and gnathostomes are not homologous, and that the vertebrate jaw is not derived from an ancestral anterior arch.

In view of differences in anatomical terminology among major groups, authors were asked to define explicitly their use of names that might otherwise engender confusion; e.g., the "maxilla" of birds. Similar considerations apply to terms, such as neurocranium and chondrocranium, that are widely used but used differently by different authors.

As in volume 1, it is our pleasure to thank formally and publicly the authors of volume 2, who persevered in the face of the intimidating topics we set before them. We also acknowledge the invaluable help of the editorial staff at the University of Chicago Press for their professional assistance.

REFERENCES

Appel, T. A. 1987. *The Cuvier-Geoffroy Debate: French Biology in the Decades before Darwin*. New York: Oxford University Press.

Benton, M. J. 1990. Phylogeny of the major tetrapod groups: Morphological data and divergence dates. Journal of Molecular Evolution 30: 409–424.

de Beer, G. R. 1937. *The Development of the Vertebrate Skull*. Oxford: Oxford University Press. Reprint. Chicago: University of Chicago Press, 1985.

Gauthier, J. A., A. G. Kluge, and T. Rowe. 1988a. Amniote phylogeny and the importance of fossils. Cladistics 4: 105–209.

———. 1988b. The early evolution of the Amniota. In *The Phylogeny and Classification of the Tetrapods*, vol. 1, *Amphibians, Reptiles, Birds*, M. J. Benton, ed. Systematics Association Special Volume 35A. Oxford: Clarendon Press, pp. 103–155.

Hall, B. K. 1992. *Evolutionary Developmental Biology*. London: Chapman and Hall.

Hall, B. K., and J. Hanken. 1985. Foreword to *The Development of the Vertebrate Skull*, by G. R. de Beer. Chicago: University of Chicago Press.

Maisey, J. G. 1986. Heads and tails: A chordate phylogeny. Cladistics 2: 201–256.

Sansom, I. J., M. P. Smith, H. A. Armstrong, and M. M. Smith. 1992. Presence of the earliest vertebrate hard tissues in conodonts. Science 256: 1308–1311.

1

Evolutionary Origin of the Vertebrate Skull

CARL GANS

INTRODUCTION

GAVIN DE BEER'S PATH-BREAKING BOOK, *The Development of the Vertebrate Skull* (1937), began with a series of general questions. The preamble concerns the relative fate of cartilage replacement and membrane ossifications and the implications of their distribution for issues of vertebrate evolution. However, whereas questions about the formation of bone either in membrane or by replacement of cartilage remain of substantial interest, they now must be recast in a markedly different framework.

The key confounding discovery in the interim has been the unequivocal confirmation that the development of the vertebrate anterior head skeleton proceeds by a pattern quite different from that seen in the trunk skeleton (Le Douarin 1982; Maderson 1987; Thorogood and Tickle 1988). All anterior cephalic mesenchyme derives from neural crest rather than from sclerotome and dermatome. As this portion of the head is joined to the trunk in what Lewis Wolpert (1988) refers to as a "seamless" pattern (cf. Noden 1987), it becomes of interest to establish whether the distinction of cartilage-bone precursors also reflects a head-trunk separation and whether it followed or preceded the evolution of the head.

The recognition that all derived characters of vertebrates, in cladistic terminology referred to as synapomorphies, appeared to be derivatives of, or induced by, neural crest and ectodermal neurogenic placodes, and that these embryonic tissues produce only features unique to vertebrates led to the neural crest hypothesis of vertebrate origins (Gans 1989; Gans and Northcutt 1983, 1985; Northcutt and Gans 1983). These observations suggest that the origin of these embryonic tissues (and the derivatives thereof) must have been a key step in vertebrate genesis. In turn, the neural crest hypothesis leads to the corollary that a "new head" may well have been the key apomorphy for vertebrates.

This set of hypotheses raises questions about the presumed role the

1

neural crest played in the ancestral organisms and about the roles involved in the evolutionary development of a vertebrate head. Establishment of roles requires a holistic approach. Insight into the possible options that may have been open to the transitional organisms must derive from an evaluation of transitions in many organ systems. The approach is scenario generation (Gans 1985, 1989). Questions developed during scenario generation may lead to insights and facilitate identification of significant comparisons among multiple character states.

The present chapter starts with a review of the current state of the neural crest hypothesis and its implication for the evolution of the vertebrate head. Next follow discussions of some of the scenarios developed to account for the new data, of the conclusions these lead to about the earliest skull and, of the tests they permit of conflicting views. Finally, I shall reconsider head segmentation, its origin, status, and some points required to resolve persistent questions on the basis of current information about vertebrate development.

THE NEURAL CREST HYPOTHESIS

Vertebrates differ from nonvertebrate chordates in a surprising number of synapomorphies (table 1.1). One can see that these are functionally involved in gas exchange and the procurement and use of nutrients and are developmentally associated with the neural crest and neurogenic ectodermal placodes. Development of the neural plate and of the zone immediately peripheral to it appears to be induced by the roof of the archenteron. The neural crest originates as narrow bilateral cellular strips lying immediately peripheral to the sides and anterior end of the neural plate. The cephalic portion of the crest differs from that of the trunk in its tissue-forming potential and also in its association with neurogenic ectodermal placodes (Elinson and Kao, vol. 1 of this work).

The placodal embryonic tissues apparently represent derivatives independent of and parallel to those of the neural crest (Northcutt and Gans 1983). Both arise adjacent to the developing anterior portion of the brain, which represents an outgrowth of the alar rather than the basal components of nervous tissue. Both form neuronal and associated structures far from their site of origin, often close to the integument.

Not only the cranial system can be reevaluated on the basis of new developmental information. Indeed, transplantation among segments indicated also that all of the branchiomeric musculature supplying the branchial arches, as well as the vertebrate eye muscles, derive from an anterior prolongation of epimeric myotomal tissues (Thorogood and Tickle 1988).

TABLE 1.1 Shared-derived characters of vertebrates

Vertebrate synapomorphies	Embryonic origin			Function		
Nervous system						
Sensory nerves with ganglia, cranial	NC	P		G	DI	
Sensory nerves with ganglia, trunk	NC				DI	
Peripheral motor ganglia	NC			G		P
Second- and higher-order motor neurons	NC			G		P
Forebrain	NC?				DI	P
Chromatophores	NC				DI	
Paired special sense organs						
Nose		P			DI	
Eyes (accessory organs)	NC?	(P)			DI	
Ears		P			DI	
Lateral-line mechanoreceptors		P			DI	
Lateral-line electroreceptors		P			DI	
Gustatory organs	NC?	P			DI	
Pharyngeal and alimentary modifications						
Cartilaginous bars	NC			G		
Branchiomeric muscle			ME	G	DI	P
Smooth muscle of gut			MH			P
Calcitonin cells	NC				DI	P
Chromaffin cells, adrenal cortex	NC			G	DI	P
Circulatory system						
Gill capillaries, endothelium			ME	G		
Major vessels, trunk			M	G		
Wall of aortic arches	NC			G		
Muscular heart			MH	G		
Skeletal system						
Anterior neurocranium and sensory capsules	NC				DI	P
Cephalic armor and derivatives	NC				DI	
Armor of trunk	NC??		ME?		DI	

Embryonic origin: NC, Neural crest; NC?, Mixed outgrowth, intermediate between neurectoderm and neural crest; NC??, The nature of the various trunk armors remains uncertain; P, Placodes; (P), Placodes provide lens and peripheral component, not sensory tissues; M, Mesoderm; MH, Mesoderm, hypomere; ME, Mesoderm, epimere. Function: G, Gas exchange; DI, Food, detection, and ingestion; P, Food, internal processing.

Note.—Table modified from Northcutt and Gans 1983.

The discovery that the branchiomeric muscles derive from somitomeres (Noden 1987, 1988), and not from an anterior prolongation of the hypomere (which more posteriorly forms the smooth muscle of the gut tube) conflicts with the description currently stated in all textbooks of comparative anatomy.

SCENARIOS

Approach

Why then in evolutionary time did the vertebrate head develop in a pattern
so markedly different from that of the trunk? Why do the embryological
origins of their mesenchyme differ and why are there differences in the
pattern and innervation of their striated musculature? The following historical explanation is congruent with the observations on which the neural
crest hypothesis is based.

Scenarios seem generally to postulate the transition of vertebrates from
an animal equivalent to *Branchiostoma*, or perhaps *Amphioxides,* models
of a suitable precursor. (For reasons given in earlier papers, cephalochordates make more plausible models for ancestors than do urochordates;
most of what follows requires only a minor shift from a precursor structurally parallel to a cephalochordate. See also Maisey 1986.) Such a
precursor would have displayed a larval condition in which both food
transport, in thorax and gut, and locomotion were mediated by beating
cilia. The first metamorphosis would have transformed the locomotor
system of such a larva from epithelial ciliary fields to segmented muscles acting on an elastic notochord in the second larval stage. Besides
permitting increased propulsive velocity, axial muscularization also allowed these animals to use a unidirectional propulsion. In adults (following upon a second metamorphosis associated with sexual maturation), this
established an increased selective advantage for cephalization and development of receptors capable of locating the source of signals at a
distance.

The transition from a structural pattern, such as that displayed by
Branchiostoma, to that displayed by various primitive fishes (Moy-Thomas
and Miles 1971) would have required the modification of several major
organ systems (table 1.1). In *Branchiostoma* the notochord is muscular-
ized rather than vacuolated, and the animal shows motor connections
from the axial muscles to the spinal cord rather than nerve outflow via
ventral root nerves. *Branchiostoma* lacks major, paired external sense organs and has an ependyma rather than a true forebrain. The atrium of
Branchiostoma receives the outflow of 20 or more simple and narrow pharyngeal slits rather than having only 6 to 10 slits opening directly to the
outside (some fossil agnathans had much higher numbers; Janvier, this
volume). The collagenous pharyngeal skeleton of *Branchiostoma* is invested with a mucopolysaccharide coating rather than cartilage and consists of simple unbranched rods rather than bearing lateral lamellae; the
ciliary beat of the various water pumping systems of *Branchiostoma* serves
food gathering rather than gas exchange and there is neither capillarization

of the pharyngeal slits nor endothelial lining of the vascular spaces; the neurons innervating its subpterygial muscle leave the chord dorsally, whereas the muscle lies in the atrial wall rather than within the pharyngeal one. Its excretory system lies parallel to the pharynx rather than (retroperitoneally) in the dorsal zone of the coelom. Finally, the developmental process shows some curiosities in that the pharynx starts to develop one side at a time, rather than symmetrically as does the notochordal and neuromuscular axis (Flood 1968).

Some of these aspects of *Branchiostoma* tend to be interpreted as transitional conditions between "invertebrates" and "vertebrates," others as adaptations of *Branchiostoma* to its current conditions. Such a contrast is inappropriate, because the characters of any currently surviving animal must be adequate for life in its environment, and it is quite clear that the ancestral condition will be the one from which the adequate state is derived. The attempt to decide whether the state of any animal represents either current adaptation or in contrast ancestry is flawed; the process of organic evolution assures that both aspects will always be involved.

However, the analysis deriving from the neural crest hypothesis permits various scenarios. Currently, the following transitional sequence appears to explain the largest number of characteristics.

Metamorphosis

As all postulated vertebrate ancestors and surviving members of the primitive vertebrate groups show metamorphosis, it is assumed that the transitional animals also had metamorphosis (Northcutt and Gans 1983). Several of the following steps then affect postmetamorphic animals, because it appears that the shift to predation occurred at this stage.

Gas Exchange

The initial stage appears to have been a modification of the pharynx to facilitate increased gas exchange. Such modification involved reduction of the number and widening of the diameter of the pharyngeal slits (possibly by paedomorphosis, truncating development prior to metamorphosis and thus retaining the low number of slits and not forming the atrium) and down-growth of the subpterygial musculature into the pharyngeal rather than the atrial wall. There followed addition of primary (and secondary) lamellae to the bars and vascularization (and later endothelial lining) of the increased surface of the pharyngeal slits to form a gas exchange surface. Cartilage apparently developed by spatial shift of the cupulary material of the mechanoreceptors, thus forming an elastic supportive meshwork that would regain its shape by elastic recoil after muscular deformation (Northcutt and Gans 1983). Such elastic recoil is still seen in lampreys, which show a single-stage ventilation (Rovainen and Schieber 1975; Russell 1986).

Locomotion

The facilitation of increased gas exchange was likely paralleled by more effective and protracted locomotory capacity. Locomotion was enabled by further development of the axial muscle system of the trunk. This involved a fundamental shift from synapses on the surface of the cord due to in-growing connections of the muscle cells to an out-sprouting of motor neurons with the synapse placed onto the surface of the muscle fibers, i.e., the development of the ventral root motor nerves characteristic of vertebrates. This shift may have been associated with increased size, and perhaps the extension of the musculature into more complex distal compartments. Whatever the nature of the initial adaptive basis, the shift to out-sprouting ventral root motor nerves represents a protoadaptation for further modification of the axial musculature. Also, as documented below, the innervational pattern suggests the antiquity of the fundamental difference in the architecture of head and trunk.

Predation

With the capacity for directional travel came the major shift in the evolution of vertebrates, namely the transition from filter feeding to active predation. Predation is generally discussed in terms of jaws and the implied skeletal material; however, various invertebrates and hagfish use muscular and other soft tissues to ingest and even to reduce the size of prey items. The key innovation allowing vertebrates to be effective predators, rather, required prey detection and location at a distance, using specialized distance receptors.

Distance Receptors

Once an object is contacted, recognition that it is potential prey involves chemoreception, for which sense organs already occur in *Branchiostoma* and many aquatic invertebrates, making the state plesiomorphic (Bullock and Horridge 1965). However, the initial stages of aquatic chemoreceptive organs require major modifications before they can serve distance reception. Similar major modification would be required for the use of mechanoreception and vision, because the signals to be detected must be selected from a background level normally greater than that produced by living prey. In contrast, electroreception addresses biological signals that are produced at levels and in patterns much different from background. As electroreceptors have now been demonstrated in petromyzontids, as well as in various groups of fishes, electroreception appears to represent a vertebrate synapomorphy (Bullock et al. 1983).

The neural crest hypothesis suggests that the electroreceptive cells of the transitional animals were encased by dielectric layers of hydroxyapatite that served as transduction enhancers. The differential dielectric capacity of hydroxyapatite makes this salt, rather than calcite, a preferred enhancer. The cellular sheathing next showed a multicellular variant in which the material formed a layer with parallel tubules, analogous (and presumably homologous) to dentine rather than bone. In this view, the development of a dentinous material is the earliest stage for calcification. Enameloid and enamel represent evolutionarily subsequent surface coatings that increased the dielectric effect.

In the initial presentation of this hypothesis (Northcutt and Gans 1983), reference was made to the pore canal system of fossil lungfish as containing possibly analogous electroreceptors. However, as noted later (Gans 1989), the size of the pore canals indicated that they could have housed only multicellular sense organs, rather than the unicellular ones predicated above. Now, Bemis and Northcutt (1987, 1992) have shown that the canals likely contained vascular supplies and dentinogenic organs. They note that this finding does not support the hypothesis for the origin of dentin and enameloid in association with electroreception and posit that the functional basis for the origin of these two tissues remains "one of the outstanding unsolved issues in vertebrate biology." It remains to be seen whether a careful examination of the integumentary skeleton of the earliest agnathans shows any evidence bearing on these issues.

ORIGIN OF THE SKELETON

Bone formation involves the deposition of the same hydroxyapatite salts within existing connective tissue layers. This occurred first in the dermis, but the condition also shows up internally within existing connective tissue septae. Unfortunately, various combinations of bone, dentine, and enamel appear almost simultaneously in the fossil record, which does not therefore provide unequivocal evidence for their sequence of origin (Halstead 1987; see also Smith and Hall 1990). Traditionally it has been assumed without much argument that calcification first arose in bone. However, the external armor of Paleozoic fishes tends to have a dentinelike surface texture, sometimes with a superficial coating of enamel or enameloid materials. Such sclerification covered the head and often the trunk. Deep to the thin cephalic armor there were cephalic bony tissues, and ossification often extended inward along the cranial septa outlining the sensory capsules and braincase.

The origin of bone, as the initial calcified tissue, has been associated with five possible adaptive causes. These are (1) as a barrier to osmosis

(Marshall and Smith 1930), (2) as a protective armor (Romer 1933), (3) as a site of ion storage facilitating an animal's entry into fresh waters with unpredictable concentration (Northcutt and Gans 1983; Griffith 1987), (4) as a source of buffer for the acidic by-products of the increased metabolic scope, coupled with glycolysis (the enhancement of which also seems to be a vertebrate synapomorphy; Ruben and Bennett 1987), and (5) as a device for increasing density, making organisms heavier than water.

The first of the adaptations claimed as driving the origin of bone is unlikely, because the unarmorable gill surface has an area more than 100 times that of the external surface. All of the other putative adaptations would have current utility once a substantial layer of the salt had been deposited along the external surface of the dermis. The calcium-storage function might not only have served as a reservoir of this salt, for instance in intermittent euryhaline (estuarine) conditions, but might also have been involved in buffering. However, such use would require storage of a substantial deposit of calcium before achieving adaptive value, making it unlikely that buffering represented the initial advantage. In contrast, any enhancement of an existing transductive function would incur an immediate advantage.

In the present framework, ossification represents a later shift in the use of the genetic instruction for crystallizing hydroxyapatite onto a collagenous matrix previously developed in dentine, which itself may involve stabilizing modifications. Bone represents a structural material that fixes the position of the external distance receptors relative to the axis and the mouth of the predator. Fixation would have ensured the positional integrity of the relation of distance sensors to each other (the greater the precision of angular comparison, the greater the distance within which a signal may be localized). Such structural support would require ossification of the dermal layer underlying the dentinous sensory system. Later, the central septa also mineralized, permitting maintenance of the position of the brain relative to the armored integument and also the relative positions of sense organs and buccal opening. However, once the instructions for calcification were expressed somewhere in the phenotype, most of the other putative advantages would have provided ancillary benefits; their actions would be synergistic rather than conflicting.

Digestion and Excretion

The shift from a relatively slowly moving filter feeder to a predator with a much increased metabolic scope must also have required modifications of the digestive and excretory systems (Gans 1987). The digestive system now had to deal with larger particles, and there is an emphasis on extracellular rather than intracellular digestion, and on muscular rather than ciliary transport. The excretory system shifted from the pharyngeal to the retroperitoneal position. As the absolute size of the animal increased, the relative size of the pharynx shrank; also, pharyngeal motility was required for ingestion of larger prey. The shift of the excretory system into the coelomic cavity also involved further modification of the tubular system.

The preceding argument presented in simple, defined steps does not do justice to the complexity of the transition and omits discussion of several systems and processes. Two major aspects proceeding in parallel with the above, which deserve attention, are the distributed sensory capacity and the animal's increased control over the visceral motor system of the visceral organs. In *Branchiostoma,* the neural tissues involved are diffuse, but they are centralized in vertebrates (Romer 1972), a process that also would seem to be reflected in the profound increase in neural volume occurring in the transition to vertebrates. The centralization involves both the generation of an autonomic nervous system and the several levels of endocrine function. It is possible to refer to the capture of preexisting endocrine control systems (cf. Krieger et al. 1983). However, these earlier endocrine systems also incorporated a complex history, so that the sequential details of the transition cannot now be described with any certainty.

Whereas several of the steps in the above scenario seem to deal with aspects of the trunk rather than the head, as well as with soft rather than skeletal tissues, and hence seemingly transcend questions of the vertebrate skull per se, they are interrelated. As already shown by other accounts in this work, the hard tissues do not develop in an independently selected fashion, but tend to reflect and support the adaptive needs of the remainder of the organism.

ORIGIN OF THE SKULL

It may be useful to review the origin of the cephalic skeletal elements. The skeletal system of protochordates is essentially hydrostatic (Bonik et al. 1976). It is less a matter of being liquid-filled than of being formed of gelatinous bodies, the deformation of which seems to be constrained by a collagenous meshwork. The key element in this system is the notochord, the fluid components of which incorporate contractile elements. As the notochord reaches the full length of the animal, there is opportunity for stiffening the anterior and posterior ends. Although there is no experimental proof, it has been suggested that differential stiffening of the notochord allows the animals to penetrate sands in either a forward or a backward direction (Webb 1973).

The mass of muscle plates which extends along the entire length of the animal is constrained by collagen fibers that would seem to act as tensile elements. Similar tensile arrays are seen among the other compartments of the trunk, outlining the bundles of muscles and positioning the pharynx and notochord among them. Only in the framework of the pharynx are the collagenous bundles reinforced with a coating which stiffens each rod-like element and maintains the stability of the pharyngeal framework.

Manipulation of the pharynx on living *Branchiostoma* suggests that the skeletal rods can rotate slightly about their bases, but cannot shift significantly relative to each other, as indicated also by the interbar bridges. There are two states of pharyngeal inflation or shift of the collagenous sheets. However, the bars do not seem to be exposed to much bending stress; instead, each entire sheet of pharyngeal tissue folds inward, apparently owing to the contraction of the transverse subpterygial muscles. In contrast, reinflation of the pharynx requires action of the wheel organ. In short, the configuration of the ventral portion of the anterior trunk in adult lancelets is established by the filling states of the pharynx and atrium. The network of internal collagenous fibers maintains the general shape of this portion of trunk, and also of the medial position of the notochord and pharyngeal supports relative to the skin.

The genesis of the adult vertebrate pattern was associated with a shift to more active postmetamorphic life associated with predation. It involved (1) the change of the pharynx from a filter-feeding to a gas exchange chamber that could be perfused by a muscular water pump; (2) the development of several new paired external sense organs that were capable of establishing the position of prey at a distance; key among these was electroreception. The two processes had the ancillary effects of establishing (1) development of cartilage, initially as an energy storage substance allowing pharyngeal perfusion by a one-stage muscular pump, but also as a material that permitted construction of bars bearing lateral lamellae, and (2) development of dentine and membranous bone, initially as transduction-enhancing and detector-positioning materials allowing approach to covered prey and at night.

Both the muscular pharyngeal pump and the new sense organs must have involved the addition of further nervous pathways near the tip of the dorsal nerve cord; in short, they required a new brain, most likely extending anteriorly. The special paired sense organs and new brain in turn required an expanded space anterior to the notochordal tip; this is the new head. Whereas we lack any fossils or other direct evidence representing this stage, it is likely that the support was hydrostatic, although some of the portions ventral to the elongating brain and anterior to the notochordal tip may have been stiffened by cartilaginous components associated with the pharyngeal skeleton.

The advent of mineralization, associated with metamorphosis and providing transduction enhancement and sensory positioning for the electroreceptive system, initially affected mainly the integument. Thus, there formed a boxlike enclosure holding not just the brain, but also sensory capsules and the anterior end of the pharynx. The great diversity of armor associated with different fossil "agnathans" (Moy-Thomas and Miles 1971; Halstead 1987) leaves open the question of its rigidity. However, these animals then had the capacity of transforming members of the existing collagenous framework into supportive components by the addition of proteoglycans or hydroxyapatite. Whereas the capacity initially arose in the pharynx and integument, it must soon have transcended its spatial or developmental limitations; with increasing size, at least the walls (and sometimes the contents) of the cephalic connective tissue compartments became mineralized.

Whereas other discussions (Northcutt and Gans 1983) have suggested that some cartilage is phyletically earlier than bone, it remains to be seen whether and to what extent cartilage may have been involved in the framing and filling of a head skeleton. Fossils would seem to suggest that mineralization had the primary role. The absence of juvenile fossils for most of the early species indicates that the armor may have formed after the animal had achieved its adult size; this supports Romer's argument that (in the central skeleton) cartilage (or rather cartilaginous premodeling) is secondary to ossification and represents an "embryonic adaptation" (Romer 1942).

The integumentary armor, braced internally by various septal ossifications, then represents the phyletically earliest skull. It lacks a significant postotic component, and there seems to have been an experimental radiation involving different degrees of bracing (Janvier, this volume). As the dorsal portion of the new snout would have contained minimal muscles, ossification of the spaces among the functional units would not have incurred their displacement. Furthermore, the selective factors involved with the shift to predation soon may have established advantages not only for internal bracing, but for flexibility among the several mechanical units of the skull (Gans, 1988a). The very success deriving from this stage has left us with a diversity of variants among Recent animals that apparently replaced all of the forms retaining ancestral patterns.

DEVELOPMENTAL COROLLARIES

The common denominator of the nested set of scenarios is that all of the systems involved are derivatives of, or induced by, neural crest and ectodermal neurogenic placodes. The sequence derives from an analysis that searched for the greatest number of concordances among initially unrelated observations. The decision to use developmental information was fortunate, for several of the postulated evolutionary changes appear to involve truncation of development (paedogenesis) or the addition of postadult changes. The key developmental shift leading to vertebrates apparently represents such an addition.

Theoretically there are two fundamentally distinct ways of generating a vertebrate head: by restructuring the anterior trunk, or by adding a truly new section, a neomorph organized on a distinct pattern. The latter is what we see and it is of interest to consider why. The answer appears to lie in the early life cycle of an animal such as *Branchiostoma* (Barrington 1965; Starck 1978a).

The primary developmental steps generate a freely floating ciliated larva, which is similar to larvae of urochordates, hemichordates, and echinoderms. The minimal filter-feeding (or fasting) stage then undergoes a primary metamorphosis. This shift from diffuse ciliary to directed muscular propulsion using a notochord and segmental muscles involves a major modification of the epidermal nerve plexus. Three processes are involved, namely (1) the cephalization of some sensory aspects and their concentration in the anterior end of the animal, (2) the location of effector control in a centralized rather than a peripheral and diffuse system, and (3) the retention of neuronal connections among sensors and effectors as these become displaced relative to each other.

The vertebrate head region is characterized by neurogenic ectodermal placodes, which are associated with each of the vertebrate distance receptors; their origin may reflect a phyletically earlier cephalic concentration of the initially diffuse sensory aspects of the epidermal nerve plexus. Phyletically, *Branchiostoma* represents a shift from a distributed ciliary propulsive system to a muscular one that was axially arranged, deeply placed, and controlled by a mid-dorsal concentration of motor tissues. However, centralization of the motor system has been paralleled both by the origin of new sensory cells within the central nervous system, and by continuing connection with the integumentary sensory neurons associated with the epidermal nerve plexus. Thus, the primary nerve cord of *Branchiostoma* retains connection to old organs and achieves connection to new ones. A major shift in vertebrates is the addition of the special sense organs deriving embryologically from the placodes. These may be interpreted as anterior shifts, numerical increase, and specialization of the integumentary receptors with increased cephalization and directional movement.

The development of the new motor system as a segmented axial mass in postmetamorphic *Branchiostoma* appears to begin near the anterior tip of the chordamesoderm and to extend caudad. In vertebrates, the formation of primary mesodermal somites thus proceeds by a mechanism that starts at the tip of the notochord and adds segments in antero-posterior fashion, a sequence that is significant, because the chordamesoderm itself involutes in a posterior-to-anterior direction (Gans 1987). Thus far, the developmental sequence in *Branchiostoma* appears to be retained in vertebrates; interruption of amphibian development shows a stage exactly equivalent to the level here characterized (Gerhart et al. 1986).

A second repetitive sequence in the cephalic region is the perforation of the pharynx. As noted above, the process in *Branchiostoma* differs profoundly from that shown in vertebrates. Not only is the perforation asymmetrical, so that the first set of slits forms in the ventral midline and then migrates before the second row opens, but one sees a further doubling of the slit number by the down-growth of intermediate bars at a second metamorphosis associated with sexual maturity. However, the organization of this asymmetry is secondary, because it affects perforation of the slits; furthermore, the lateral placement of the mouth may be reflected in the left-right staggering in the blocks of the axial musculature. For the moment, the functional implications of these asymmetries remain unknown.

The first major shift in vertebrate evolution appears to have been the use of the pharynx in gas exchange. We have seen that gas exchange involved muscularization, reduction in number of pharyngeal bars, addition of cartilage for energy storage, vascularization of the surfaces, and the addition of a sensory-integrative-motor component to drive the muscles. The last would have required a marked increase in the volume of the anterior end of the central nervous system, but not necessarily the development of a forebrain. However, modification of the anterior portion of the pharynx into an aperture suitable for ingestion of large food objects would have required more special restructuring of the anterior end of the animal to accommodate the associated distance receptors.

The earliest vertebrates apparently developed a set of neomorphs, modified from the outgrowth of several tissue types during development, an anterior prolongation of the alar portion of the central nervous system, and the anterior extension of the connective tissues providing a connection among the sensory capsules. The latter provides an enclosure for the brain and a connection for the initially fused elements of the pharyngeal skeleton (Marinelli and Strenger 1954, 1956).

It is interesting that the embryonic source of all of these tissues forming the new head is phylogenetically associated with the epidermal nerve plexus. The outgrowth of the central nervous system may be viewed as a secondary phase of the centralization of the nervous tissues. The anteriormost of the new connective tissues derive from the neural crest, which appears to be homologous to the embryonic source of the epidermal nerve plexus. The neural crest then produces not only neurons and associated cells, but also various connective tissues. This raises the question of whether these cells are homologous to cells of the epidermal nerve plexus proper or whether a secondary set of sustentacular cells may have been involved. Even more interesting is the origin of the smooth muscle cells of the afferent branchial vessels, which have been shown to derive from neural crest in those vertebrates for which this has been tested (Noden 1988). In contrast, recent studies show the fascinating point that the cells of the endothelia may originate from mesoderm (but not neural crest) and then migrate to line the circulatory system without retaining any relation between their place of origin and final location (Noden 1988).

The pattern of neural crest involvement in the evolutionary appearance of vertebrate synapomorphies is even clearer in the appearance of calcification. To the extent that the surface layers of early vertebrate armor were dentinous, they would seem to show equivalence to the pattern seen in the teeth of Recent forms, i.e., they are produced by odontoblasts, which are derived from the neural crest (Hall 1987; Lumsden 1987). Furthermore, formation of the thin enameloid coatings appears to arise at the "mesodermal-ectodermal" surface from cells of the neural crest. Bone, in contrast, is generally assumed to be a tissue produced by the dermatomal and sclerotomal components of mesoderm. However, the bony skeleton of the earliest vertebrates appears to have been concentrated both in the cephalic region and across the entire integument. (Vertebral ossifications—indeed, a postotic skull—appear only at the agnathan-gnathostome transition.) If the evidence that the neural crest contributes most preotic mesenchyme also applied to the transitional vertebrates, cephalic bone likely arose initially from neural crest. Also, the neural crest contributes the cells of the parathyroid system and with this affects control of calcium metabolism.

The use of cells initially instructed to be neuronal, and perhaps of their sustentacular associates, would then have generated a new source of embryonic material which permits anterior prolongation without interference with the instructions specifying development posterior to the tip of the notochord. However, such an explanation may be overly simplistic. After all, there is an outgrowth of mesoderm anterior to the notochordal tip and the start of the series of branchiomeric and true somites. These are the anterior somitomeres that give rise to the eye muscles and are followed posteriorly by those yielding the musculature and connective tissues of the otic region (Noden 1987, 1988). However, the most anterior portion of this mesodermal mesenchyme provides cells only for the anterior musculature; the preotic skeletal and connective tissues derive from neural crest. This observation once again documents that the evolution of phenotypes tends to involve unpredictability affected by potential differences in genetic and developmental pathways in the precursors.

The formation of vertebrate excretory tissues does not directly involve the neural crest. Their nephritic strip derives from the mesomeric compartment of the mesoderm; in contrast, the excretory tissues of postmetamorphic *Branchiostoma* develop in the secondary pharyngeal bars, which do not form in vertebrates. However, the excretory cells of *Branchiostoma*, once assumed to be solenocytes homologous to those in many other invertebrates, have now been shown to be cyrtopodocytes, a subclass very similar to the podocytes of vertebrates (Brandenburg and Kümmel 1961; Welsch 1975). It is interesting to note the observations of Jacobson (1987; also Jacobson and Sater 1988) that transplanted neural crest from the head region represses formation of kidney tissues in the trunk. It also is noted that trunk crest normally delays the appearance of kidney tubule formation. Trunk neural crest has been documented near the presumptive nephrons (Krotoski et al. 1988). This observation would make sense if one could find evidence that the head neural crest developed and retained the capacity of repressing the excretory tissue (and perhaps the associated secondary pharyngeal bars). In this case the observation appears to refer to a historical capacity of this tissue rather than to a present role.

The shifts in the digestive system again show a major involvement of neural crest derivatives, but also a seemingly independent process of muscularization of the gut wall. The splitting of the hypomere that forms the coelomic cavity leads to its separation into parietal (lateral) and visceral components, the latter covering the gut and proliferating into the coating of smooth muscle and connective tissues. However, the neural crest provides the complex of neurons of the enteric nervous system; it provides all second- and higher-order motor neurons in numbers rivaling those of the spinal cord (Gershon 1987). Furthermore, we see the development of several new endocrine organs. The major controlling circuits lie in the hypothalamic-pituitary axis, which itself forms near the front of the primitive brain. Another example is seen in the adrenal medulla, which derives directly from cells of the neural crest.

OTHER HYPOTHESES

The preceding account involves several components, some of which are commonplace and others variably controversial. It would seem to match much of what has become known from developmental studies to the limited data from the fossil record. However, concordance does not mean proof, and it seems useful to note additional evidence required both to confirm and perhaps to falsify much or all of the preceding account. (See also the Appendix.)

The first component of the neural crest hypothesis rests upon the discovery that the mesenchyme of the anterior portion of the head derives from neural crest. Thus, the anterior bones of the skull, as well as the associated connective tissues, are not formed from sclerotome and dermatome. This finding had been suggested on the basis of various earlier deletion studies and some labeling studies in amphibians (see review in Hall 1987), but it was absolutely confirmed on the basis of the quail-chick transplantation experiments (Le Douarin 1982; Noden 1987, 1988). Whereas more complex experiments have confirmed these results for mammals (Tan and Morris-Kay 1986), until recently we have lacked more modern observations on anamniotes. However, studies are now under way for lampreys (Langille and Hall 1988b), teleosts (Langille and Hall 1988a), and various amphibians (Sadaghiani and Thiébaud 1987). Thus far these critical analyses confirm that all vertebrates use the same pattern of neural crest derivatives to construct their skulls.

The next point concerns the nature and fate of the somitomere region. There seems to be little doubt that there is preotic mesoderm and that this is subdivided into a variable number of segments. The experiments of Noden (1987, 1988) document that we are dealing with undifferentiated mesoderm, in part with the myotomal fraction of the epimere as transplantation up and down the animal's axis produces further muscles. Noden (1987, 1988) also documented that this material produces not only the external eye muscles, but also those of the branchiomeric system. (It is tempting to speculate about the extent to which the difference in the somitomere development leading respectively to the eye muscles and to the branchiomeric system may reflect the curious contralateral-ipsilateral projection of the former; Graf and Brunken 1984.) This point needs to be confirmed for anamniotes. However, the so-called counterevidence, i.e., the concept that the branchiomeric musculature was visceral and possibly modified smooth muscle, has always been flawed. It rested to a large extent on the concept that all motor neurons left the central nervous system by a dorsal root (Gans and Northcutt 1985). The hypothesis did not provide an explanation for the fact that only the anterior, and not the posterior, "visceral" muscles lacked second-order motor neurons.

The argument was based on the fact that in the trunk, the basal region of the nerve cord has a ventro-medial somatic motor zone and a more latero-dorsal visceral one. However, the vertebrate brainstem shows three rather than two motor columns. A branchiomeric motor column (the nucleus ambiguous) lies dorsal to the somatic motor nucleus of the twelfth nerve; hence, it used to be assumed to be visceral motor. However, there is a still more dorsal column of the motor region (the nucleus dorsalis). The latter emits the true visceral motor outflow of the branchial region; hence the nucleus ambiguous is somatic rather than visceral. Whereas it remains important to characterize the developmental pattern in the two major "agnathans," only a major shift of the observed pattern would require a reevaluation.

Unless the ongoing developmental studies invalidate the neural crest origins of the many vertebrate aspects tabulated above (table 1.1), we remain with the observation that this embryonic tissue (and the ectodermal neurogenic placodes) represents the common denominator for vertebrate synapomorphies. The ubiquity of this generalization could be falsified by demonstrating that a significant fraction of the reported synapomorphies (seen for instance in agnathans) do not derive from the neural crest or placodes.

We now come to the scenario, many details of which could be falsified without affecting the validity of the preceding observations. A first argument concerns the use of *Branchiostoma* as a model for the transitional organism. The case for this has been made earlier (Northcutt and Gans 1983), and we still agree with the arguments. Indeed the most recent affinity analysis based on molecular data (Field et al. 1988; Wesley Brown, personal communication) confirms that the Recent cephalochordates would represent a sister group for vertebrates. Certainly, this deserves testing with assays utilizing further tissue systems both by cladistic and by immunological and hybridization approaches. Most important will be the inclusion of more species of urochordates and hemichordates. For that matter, the classification of cephalochordates themselves may deserve further attention, and it remains to be seen whether and how far the biological data for the species thus far sampled apply to the group as a whole.

Perhaps the most important conclusion from the neural crest hypothesis is that much of the vertebrate head is a neomorph. This disagrees with ideas such as that of Berrill (1955) that propose homologous headlike structures in tunicates. The key tests of this question should address the contribution of neural crest mesenchyme in additional species, particularly of anamniotes and in forms in which the otic region is relatively smaller. Where lies the border between neural crest and sclerotomal mesenchyme? How vagile is it among species, among families, and among orders?

One such set of tests is already in progress. The neural crest hypothesis proposes that cartilage arose as a mechanism facilitating elastic recoil during gill ventilation and that this is reflected in the neural crest contribution to the pharyngeal skeleton, connective tissues, and vasculature. If this is so, then the division of the vertebrate head into preotic and postotic zones is inappropriate. The division reflects the condition in birds in which the posterior extent of the branchial region has become reduced. However, recent studies of lampreys and teleosts (Langille and Hall 1988a, b) confirm the earlier reports on amphibians and show that the connective tissues of the entire pharyngeal region (which projects well posterior to the otic region) are neural crest–derived. Thus, the crest contribution differs in longitudinal extent in dorsal and ventral portions of the animal.

The origins of the dentine-bone-enamel system and its putative association with electroreception have attracted more arguments than any other component of the neural crest hypothesis. This perhaps reflects that skeletal materials are most of what remains in the fossil record, and hence, the enormous literature interpreting the early and late armor of fossils and its functional basis. However, those disagreeing with the hypothesis (Northcutt and Gans 1983) do not seem to agree with each other.

Several problems remain with the assumption of electroreception as the origin of calcification. The repeated and widespread occurrence of electroreception may suggest that the formation of cells with this sensory modality is part of the developmental-genetic potential of aquatic vertebrates; it represents a vertebrate synapomorphy. However, a first problem is that calcification most likely arose in association with unicellular electroreceptive organs, whereas the electroreceptive organs of gnathostomes are multicellular. A second problem is that all of the multicellular electroreceptive organs of gnathostomes use lipids rather than hydroxyapatite as a dielectric material. The electroreceptive organs of lampreys consist of single cells, but lack hydroxyapatite; thus the peripheral and central morphological patterns in petromyzontids would seem to be critical here. It would be interesting to know whether any of the earliest bits of fossil bony armor show evidence for single-celled sensory units. The argument that the transition to vertebrates involved the conflicting origin of bone and of glycolytic metabolism associated with reduced pH leading to intermittent dissolution of calcium salts is appealing (Ruben and Bennett 1980, 1981). It might provide a basis for the shift from hydroxyapatite to lipids, but unfortunately the argument is thus far based mainly on correlation.

An associated set of questions concerns the corollary that the adult products of the neural crest and placodal tissues are homologous to the cells of the epidermal nerve plexus of some other deuterostomes. It is exciting that this and the preceding hypothesis may now be testable by two approaches under current development. The first is by identification of various products using compounds now being identified as fingerprints for crest (and hopefully placodal) derivation. The second is by the techniques of monoclonal antibodies, which should show some level of affinity if the putative homology is correct. However welcome such approaches may be, we should not imply that they represent simple solutions. We know, for instance, that some enteric neural crest cell derivatives undergo chemical maturation leading to sequential reactions of the same cell line (Gershon 1987). Such aspects will have to be taken into account in unraveling acceptable from perhaps overly enthusiastic corollaries of the neural crest hypothesis.

ARGUMENTS ON SEGMENTATION

De Beer (1937) tells the story of Goethe's visit to the Jewish cemetery in Venice and reviews the subsequent history of the concept of cranial seg-

mentation. Certainly this long-unpublished (initially communicated by let-
ter) flash of insight represented an important generalization in the path to
understanding the essential similarities in the structure of organisms. The
intrinsic discovery was twofold. First, it reinforced the concept that the
cranial, indeed the general, structural pattern of animals might be expected
to be similar. This concept of a common plan was an important idea, although the causal basis of the relationship and the mechanisms that produced the similarity remained to be established. Next, and most important
in the present context, it seemed to suggest that the skull represented serial
homologues of vertebral elements. However, the idea of segmentation was
often taken further, leading to homologization such as that of jaws and
limbs. (See Russell 1916; Jollie 1984; Starck, 1987b for details of the history of the concept of segmentation).

By the middle of the nineteenth century, the hypothesis of a simple
segmentation of the cranial bones was in difficulty; Huxley's (1858)
Croonian lecture was a key to this change of paradigm. However, other
kinds of segmentation remained in the literature, namely the numbered
sequence of the cranial nerves and that of the branchial arches. Hence,
Balfour (1885), in his beautiful textbook of comparative embryology, used
the study of amphioxus to derive the conclusion that the "ancestors of the
Chordata were segmented," and that the "mesoblast of the greater part of
what is called the head of the Vertebrata proper was therefore segmented
like that of the trunk" (1885, 312). However, in the following paragraphs
he essentially dismissed the occurrence of skeletal segmentation anterior to
the pharynx. Balfour's paradigm incorporated his earlier embryological
observations that showed seemingly segmented mesoderm in the head of
sharks. The important point of these nineteenth-century studies is that discussion of head segmentation was now shifting away from anterior continuation of axial segments and segments of the branchial system to
segmentation in the developing system. Put another way, the emphasis on
segmentation as a descriptor of form was becoming a discussion of the
processes by which form was achieved.

Herrick (1899 and later) provided a further contribution by extending
forward to the brain the model of the axial nervous system furnished by
the spinal cord of lampreys (cf. Gans and Northcutt 1985). The model
allowed subdivision of the cranial nerves into ventral root nerves with
somatic motor outflow and dorsal root nerves with sensory inflow and
visceral motor outflow. This model seemed to confirm the earlier identification of the eye muscles as derivatives of preotic somites, but implied that
the branchiomeric muscles were visceral motor as their nerves left the
brain stem via a dorsal exit. It is perhaps best exemplified by figure 240 of
the Goodrich monograph (1930), which has been reprinted many times

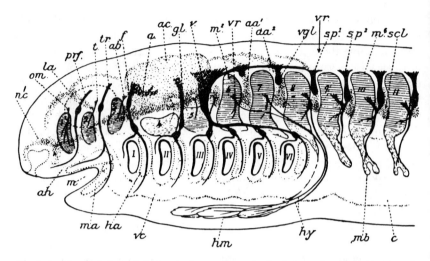

Fig. 1.1. Classical view of the head of an embryonic shark from Goodrich (1930 and earlier). This enormously influential figure has been reprinted in textbooks dozens of times. (Reprinted by permission of Macmillan Press, Ltd., London)

indeed (fig. 1.1). To the extent that the model applied to the head, it incorporated the concept of cranial segmentation.

A decade ago, it became clear that the preotic zone, which did not form classical somites, did incorporate a strip of variably segmented mesoderm, the somitomere region (Meier 1984; Jacobson and Meier 1986). Between five and nine such segments have been described, depending upon the species, but do not show a clear phylogenetic trend. In some terms these segments seemed to resurrect the concept of mesodermal segmentation as the basis for a segmented vertebrate head. However, this embryonic tissue contributes mainly muscle, namely the eye muscles and all of the branchiomeric muscles, which have quite different innervation patterns. The actual origins of skeletal structures are shown in figure 1.2.

The segmentation of the trunk apparently is induced by sclerotomal mesenchyme, for developmental studies suggest that it imposes the segmental pattern on the myotomal and external neuronal arrangement (Tosney 1987, 1988), but perhaps not on the arrangement within the column. The skeletal mesenchyme of the anterior head derives from the neural crest, providing strong developmental evidence against axial segmentation. Although such crest material is widely recognized as being involved with pattern formation, it has only recently been associated with segmentation (and then of the rhombomeres rather than the connective tissues; Lumsden and Keynes 1989; fig. 1.3). Hence, the neural crest hypothesis suggests that classical segmentation of the vertebrate head must be restricted to the branchiomeric region and the postotic axis. The connective tissues of the extreme anterior tip are likely unsegmented, because the neural crest–derived mesenchyme lacks intrinsic segmentation, but rather invests the framework established by the pharyngeal perforations (Gans and Northcutt 1983).

Clearly some of the current argument about segmentation is semantic and depends on the definition of the term. In the present context, segmentation is the repetition of portions of an animal's body that are constructed by equivalent morphogenetic processes; this implies that the components of the successive segments represent serial homologues to each other. We are used to the concept of complete segmentation or metamerism in the trunks of invertebrates. In vertebrates, indeed in chordates, segmentation in this sense is restricted to the epimeric mesoderm of the trunk and to the branchiomeric (pharyngeal) region, which lies ventral to the epimeric axis. Seemingly, there is no third segmentation, in that the cranial

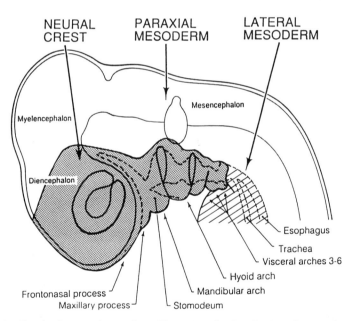

Fig. 1.2. Sketch of an amniote embryo illustrating the distribution of mesenchymal populations forming the connective and skeletal elements. The rotation of the head during development will place the neural crest component at the anteriormost sites in the adult. (After Noden 1987. Modified and reprinted by permission from *Development* 103 (suppl.): 124. Copyright, The Company of Biologists, Ltd.)

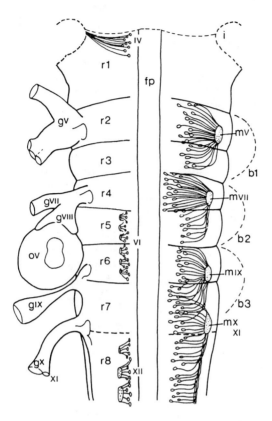

Fig. 1.3. Results of neurofilament staining and tracer injections. Schematic diagram of a stage-21 hindbrain of a chick embryo showing the distribution of the embryonic subdivisions of the brain (rhombomeres, r1–r8) and their relation to cranial sensory ganglia (g^V–g^X), branchial motor nuclei and (motor and sensory) nerves (mV–mXI), somatic motor nuclei (IV–XII), and branchial arches (b1–b3). ov, otic vesicle; fp, floor plate; i, isthmus/midbrain-hindbrain boundary. (From Lumsden and Keynes 1989. Reprinted by permission from *Nature* 337: 428. Copyright © 1989 Macmillan Magazines, Ltd.)

nerves of the special sensory organs do not represent a simply repeating series of segmented structures; nor do they correspond one to one with the rhombomeres.

Cranial nerves incorporate several quite distinct groups, and their comparison had best proceed on the basis of the kinds of connections they make, rather than a simple numerical scheme (Northcutt 1979; Bullock and Northcutt 1984). (The following represents a generalization, with the pattern in some species showing different kinds of fusion.) The terminal (O), olfactory (I), optic (II), statoaccoustic (VIII), and the anterior and posterior lateral-line nerves, as well as some of the special sensory contributions (from the epibranchial placodes) to the facial (VII), glossopharyngeal (IX), and vagal (X) nerves represent a sensory supply from the placodal receptors. These sensory nerves and components from the placodal distance receptors represent only an associated, not a sequential, series. Some of the somatic sensory input of the four last-named mixed cranial nerves derives from the integument. The oculomotor (III), trochlear (IV), and abducens (VI) nerves represent anterior somatic eye muscles, although the innervation is curious in that it is partly from contralateral nuclei. More posteriorly, the hypoglossal (XII) innervates the epibranchial and hypobranchial muscles deriving from the first somites and represents the start of a dorsal segmentation. The branchiomeric motor contributions of the trigeminal (V), facial (VII), glossopharyngeal (IX), and vagal (X), as well as of the spinal accessory (XI) nerve (where present as a cranial, rather than trunk nerve), represent an innervation of the striated epimeric muscles investing the segmented pharynx. The trigeminal, facial, glossopharyngeal, and vagal (and spinal accessory) nerves include the visceral sensory and motor components of the branchial segments. Hence, the cranial nerve pattern reflects only two primary segmentations, those of the axial and of the branchiomeric systems.

Both the axial and the branchial segmentation seem to be parallel in that the position of their anterior portion seems fixed and the posterior much more vagile. Thus, the otic region and/or notochordal tip defines the former and the mandibular arch fixes the latter. The anterior fixation of the axial system may reflect the occurrence of an anteriorly starting inductive process with the addition of posterior segments merely involving duplication. The formation of pharyngeal pouches also extends posteriorly, but at a different rate (in *Branchiostoma* the postmetamorphic addition of pharyngeal slits with growth also occurs at the end of the series). If the more anterior segments incurred such developmental fixation, additions within the anterior sequences would require major developmental reorganization.

Two important issues deserve further discussion. The first is the possible number of preotic and premandibular segments, and the second is the matching of axial and branchial segments. For both of these, the organization of the nervous system provides information that is reasonably concordant with the embryological evidence.

The number of preotic "segments" may be defined by the number of motor outflow sites (generally ventral root nerves) innervating striated muscles. Here belong the oculomotor, trochlear, and abducens nerves (reaching the eye muscles), but also the somatic motor components of the trigeminal (V), facial (VII), glossopharyngeal (IX), and vagal (X), as well as of the spinal accessory (XI) nerves ("dorsal" root nerves that supply the branchiomeric muscles of the mandibular and hyoid arches). The pattern of the eye muscles has long been assumed to reflect the presence of three preotic segments. However, the curious innervation of the six or more eye muscles (Graf and Brunken 1984) suggests that the argument for three preotic segments may deserve reexamination. The nerve supply to the mandibular segment is via the trigeminal; this sends a profundus branch to the snout, which suggests that it once may have been a separate nerve and supplied another pharyngeal segment. Hence, the innervation supports at most the idea that there has been some preotic tissue and perhaps one premandibular segment (de Beer 1937).

In amniotes we see an association of the first postmandibular arch with the otic capsule. The three "preotic somites" are referred to as hyoid, mandibular, and premandibular, with at least an implication of a degree of matching between the axial and branchiomeric regions. (It is interesting that the nucleus of the abducens is mapped in rhombomeres 5 and 6, whereas that of the facial lies in rhombomeres 4 and 5; Lumsden and Keynes 1989). However, in the chick embryo there is an evident match between branchial and midaxial (neural) segmentation at the hindbrain level. The crucially segmented system in the trunk is the sclerotome, whereas the unsegmented parachordal forms its equivalent in the preotic and metaotic regions. Presumably, the preotic mesoderm also is unsegmented. The muscular derivatives of this mesoderm depend on their patterning on the neural crest (Noden 1988), as does neuromuscular connectivity. It appears that the segmental pattern of the head is solely the province of neuromeres and branchiomeres, with the link between them being provided by the neural crest. This tissue derives from one and patterns the other; segmental or not, the neural crest is the major patterning component. However, the correlation breaks down in the more posterior postotic region in which the branchiomeric tissues underlie the independently segmented sclerotome. This is indicated by the occurrence of nerves, such as the vagus, that clearly innervate multiple branchiomeric segments, a situation that must have been even more complex in fossil vertebrates with up to 20 pharyngeal bars. Similarly, the "single" hypoglossal nerve innervates muscles deriving from multiple somites. This again documents that the two series are and remain intrinsically independent.

Perhaps one of the more promising techniques for resolving the segmentation question was only slightly over the horizon when this chapter was drafted. This is the unraveling of the genetic instructions underlying the formation of the several sets of serial structures observed. In arthropods, the coupling of multiple genetico-developmental processes required for segmentation involves so-called homeoboxes. Similar associations have been reported in vertebrates. Most recently, very exciting discoveries demonstrate their expression throughout the brain, with its major rhombomeric units corresponding to single or multiple units (Holland 1988; Kimmel et al. 1988; Lumsden and Keynes 1989). The most interesting aspect is that "brain segmentation" appears in several aspects to be distinct from that of the spinal cord, along which the connective tissues help to determine the nature of the neuronal branches (Keynes and Stern 1988; Tosney 1988); apparently the anterior neural tissues appear to have developed a distinct segmental pattern (Ross et al. 1992; Simeone et al. 1992). It remains to be seen which homeobox sequences are specific to the trunk, the pharynx, and the preotic head (Molven et al. 1990; Cho et al. 1992). Reflection of the neural segmentation in the anterior skeletal tissues would provide proof of their intrinsic segmentation, whereas the observation that seemingly sequential structures each involve distinct developmental processes would falsify it. At the moment the evidence seems to be in the direction of the latter pattern (Akam 1989; De Robertis et al. 1989; Couly and Le Douarin 1990; Lonai and Orr-Urtreger 1990; Stern 1990; Baroffio et al. 1991; Wilkinson, Hunt, et al. 1991; Hunt, Whiting et al. 1991; Xue et al. 1991; Ross et al. 1992). However, we must remember that the vertebrate head clearly arose long ago as a combination of quite separate organs (Gans 1988a). Research into its genetic and developmental patterns may improve our understanding, but the complexity which has confounded generations of scholars will inevitably remain.

ACKNOWLEDGMENTS

My concern with these issues grew during the years that I was involved in teaching various instars of comparative anatomy. It is a pleasure to express my thanks to those who taught me this discipline and to more than a generation of students and teaching assistants whose questions and arguments contributed to my changing ideas. I am particularly grateful to R. Glenn Northcutt for post-lecture discussions over innumerable cups of coffee and to Paul F. A. Maderson and Drew Noden for their patient attempts to further my education. The manuscript benefited from comments by Bob Carr, David Carrier, J.-P. Gasc, A. S. Gaunt, Andrew Lumsden, Paul F. A. Maderson, and T. S. Parsons. Professor Wesley Brown allowed me to cite his unpublished data. Preparation was supported by U.S. National Science Foundation grant G-BSR-850940 and an award from the Leo Leeser Foundation.

APPENDIX: IS THERE A CONODONT ALTERNATIVE?

One of the key questions of the vertebrate genesis remains the decision about which of the "invertebrates" might represent members of the Chordata and which might be considered sister groups thereof. Of as much interest is the argument about the most primitive vertebrates; are hagfishes a sister group to the remaining vertebrates or are they but a branch of the Recent Agnatha?

In developing the neural crest hypothesis, we naturally reviewed previous arguments and stated our reasons for selecting *Branchiostoma* and its relatives as the sister group of vertebrates that required the fewest assumptions and explanations (Gans 1989; Northcutt and Gans 1983).

(This position was, of course, rejected by Jefferies 1988, but see Gans 1989.) Whereas the evidence that hagfish were distinct and represented the earliest vertebrate offshoot did appear to have the potential of becoming accepted, it seemed premature to do so. Clearly, this group displayed enormously difficult and poorly understood phenotypic and functional differences in all of its organ systems. However, most critical in the present framework was the absence of any modern developmental material that might allow evaluation of the phenotypic states. Consequently, we based the functional developmental analyses on a *Branchiostoma*-lamprey axis, simultaneously stressing the need for new material and its analysis.

The present account appears to have been one of the earliest ones received by the editors of this volume and the editorial modifications they requested were minor. However, within weeks of presenting the definitive version to the press, the *New York Times* (29 May 1992) reported "New Evidence Shows Vertebrates to Be 40 Million Years Older," and similar reports appeared in *People* magazine and the London *Times*. All were based on a report in *Science* (Sansom et al. 1992) reporting on the histology of conodont denticles and accompanied by a "Perspective" (Briggs 1992) that placed these animals within the vertebrates, with the myxinoids representing a sister group to conodonts and all nonmyxinoid vertebrates. The implications of such global claims presumably need to be considered, and this section represents an addendum.

Conodonts, ranging back to the Cambrian, have been known for 150 years as phosphate microfossils, now very important as trace fossils for the Paleozoic and Triassic (Clark et al. 1981; Aldridge 1987; Sweet 1988; which see for many details). The tiny fossils (length 1–2 mm) consist of toothlike plates, some azygous and symmetrical and others asymmetrical, but in left- and right-handed versions; it is accepted that a series of structurally diverse elements was associated with each animal. The crowns of the teeth are formed of shiny, translucent material that has been described as layered and extends from a basal cavity often filled with a dark material of a different texture. Histological analyses have suggested a herringbone layering process which has been interpreted as growth stages (Bengtson 1976). An enormous diversity of cusp patterns has been described, mainly on geometrical bases; and a vast amount of speculation has dealt with the affinities of these fossils (Müller 1981).

Over the last decade, there have appeared a number of reports of conodont fossils in situ on remnants of a soft-bodied animal (Briggs et al. 1983; Smith et al. 1987; Aldridge et al. 1987). Most of these descriptions refer to a slender and very elongate animal (about 4 cm long) with some indication of V-shaped segmentation along part of the trunk (assumed to be myomeres) and perhaps of a longitudinal tube (assumed to be residual of a notochord). The conodonts lie far anteriorly in a region claimed to be associated with a pharynx and the largest ones are barely as long as the specimen is wide. No mouth or pharyngeal cavity is visible. Speculation refers to functions either in biting/food reduction or in support of filter-feeding structures (Sweet 1988). Two anterior lateral lobes are interpreted as sensory (Briggs 1992). Prior to the report in *Science,* there appeared to be two major views about conodont affinities, namely that they represent vertebrates (Aldridge and Briggs 1985) and that they represent a phylum by themselves (Sweet 1988).

The new report is based on histological studies (Sansom et al. 1992). It indicates that the conodont denticles are covered with a heavy calcification that appears to represent two types of acellular enamel or hyper-mineralized hard tissue, differing in the orientation of their crystallites (perpendicular or subparallel to the growth surface). The subparallel enamel type is here reported for the first time. Deep to this lies a tissue that is interpreted as bone because it contains lacunae, which presumably housed osteocytes and were connected by irregularly arranged canaliculi. There is no evidence of dentine; however, the dark aspherolytic tissue filling the bases of the conodonts is interpreted as globular calcified cartilage and reference is to its occurrence in the agnathan *Eriptychius* from the Harding sandstone. The above evidence is used to place the conodonts within the vertebrates, indeed as a sister group to all but the myxinoids (Briggs 1992). (This conclusion is similar to that of Krejsa et al. [1990], but their histological conclusions are expressly rejected.) Bone is stated to be a tissue "unique to vertebrates" (Sansom et al. 1992) and its occurrence in another group therefore forces this group into the vertebrates as well. The occurrence of enamel and cartilage is considered further evidence for craniate affinities. The absence of dentine is claimed to represent evidence for a much later origin for this tissue. We then have a group of very early "vertebrates" that had appeared in the fossil record some 40 million years before vertebrates and persists in parallel and very successfully for more than 200 million years.

What are the implications of these observations for the present account? Even if the interpretations of the histological data are correct, they provide no evidence whether the conodonts were exoskeletal or endoskeletal. Also, they do not indicate how they were placed in the animal. There is no evidence for a pharynx or pharyngeal slits or for segmented cartilages in any of the versions postulated in chordates or primitive craniates. The very interesting reconstructions of pairs of conodont elements (Aldridge et al. 1987; Nicoll 1987) indicate a strange set of curious, interlocking tiny "feeding" structures that appear to have interacted in ways substantially different from patterns seen in any vertebrates. Certainly, they are unlikely to have been directly homologous to any teeth. Consequently, there are at least three interpretations of the conodont-bearing animals. The first is that the fossils represent a group of probably carnivorous invertebrates that independently developed tissues analogous to bone and variants of hypermineralized hard tissues. A second view accepts their possession of a segmented musculature and notochord and interprets these as evidence for a status as chordates. The third accepts these animals as vertebrates but seemingly as a group with a distinct set of feeding and locomotor habits. The latter view leaves open their placement within the vertebrates, indeed, their mode of life history and that of the earliest vertebrates. (What is the meaning of the claim for immunological similarity of myxinoid keratins and enamel proteins of tetrapods [Slavkin et al. 1983]?) However, if the second and third interpretations are accepted, the fossils will pose a substantial series of additional questions.

Both dentine and enamel (and enameloid) are neural crest–associated in all vertebrates. Neural crest cells form the dentine and induce the enamel at the dermal-epidermal interface. Should we assume that the occurrence of neural crest is to be concluded from the observation of enamel-like materials in the conodonts? Does the enamel indicate the position of a dermal-epidermal interface? Could the fossil enamel have been induced directly by bone? (This hypothesis need not be rejected out of hand, because all of the connective tissues of the vertebrate head do derive from neural crest.) Does the absence of dentine represent an ancestral state or is it secondary?

Naturally, all of these histological questions have functional corollaries. The hard tissues of conodonts are supposedly homologous to two (or three) key vertebrate adaptations. There is no temporal information about the origin of cartilage, although it could be ventilation-associated, as proposed (Northcutt and Gans 1983). Still the existence of closely spaced fin rays at the end of such a long and narrow tail does not by itself support the idea of active and prolonged propulsion, requiring better gas exchange. The demonstration of both bone and enamel in Carboniferous conodonts does not imply that both arose simultaneously and even less that they arose in association with feeding. Indeed the argument that bone and enamel first appear in the fossil record after the origin of myxinoids leaves their origin wide open. (It also suggests that the myxinoids survived more than 40 million years without a fossil record!)

Many of the past arguments against amphioxus as a possible structural model for a vertebrate progenitor suggested that the cephalochordates were burrowing specialists. The shared characters were claimed to be specializations and possibly reductions. One could make a similar argument for the immensely successful conodonts; however, the new evidence does not yet bear on their life history. Their placement seems to be based mainly on the opinion that bone is unique to vertebrates (Sansom et al. 1992), without more convincing evidence about the more commonly adduced synapomorphies. The nature of possible sister groups also needs more attention. Under the circumstances, it seems best to continue watching for evidence bearing on these interesting animals rather than to accept this alternative case as proven.

References to Appendix

Aldridge, R. J., ed. 1987. *Palaeobiology of Conodonts.* Chichester: Ellis Horwood.

Aldridge, R. J., and D. E. G. Briggs. 1990. Sweet talk. Palaeobiology 16 (2): 241–246. (Book review)

Aldridge, R. J., M. P. Smith, R. D. Nordby, and D. E. G. Briggs. 1987. The architecture and function of Carboniferous polygnathacean conodont apparatuses. In *Palaeobiology of Conodonts,* vol. 4, R. J. Aldridge, ed. Chichester: Ellis Horwood, pp. 63–75.

Bengtson, S. 1976. The structure of some Middle Cambrian conodonts, and early evolution of conodont structure and function. Lethaia 9: 185–206.

Briggs, D. E. G. 1992. Conodonts: A major extinct group added to the vertebrates. Science 256 (5061): 1308–1311.

Briggs, D. E., E. N. K. Clarkson, and R. J. Aldridge. 1983. The conodont animal. Lethaia 16: 1–14.

Clark, D. L., W. C. Sweet, S. M. Bergström, G. Klapper, R. L. Austin, F. H. T. Rhodes, K. J. Müller, W. Ziegler, M. Lindström, J. F. Miller, and A. G. Harris. 1981. *Treatise on Invertebrate Paleontology,* Pt. W, suppl. 2, *Conodonta.* Lawrence, Kans.: Geological Society of America, University of Kansas.

Gans, C. 1988a. Craniofacial growth, evolutionary questions. In *Craniofacial Development,* P. Thorogood and C. Tickle, eds., Development 103 (suppl.): 3–15.

———. 1988b. Review of *The Ancestry of the Vertebrates,* by R. P. S. Jefferies. American Scientist 76 (2): 188–189.

Jefferies, R. P. S. 1988. *The Ancestry of Vertebrates.* London: British Museum.

Krejsa, R. J., P. Bringas, Jr., and H. C. Slavkin. 1990. A neontological interpretation of conodont elements based on agnathan cyclostome tooth structure, function, and development. Lethaia 23: 359–378.

Müller, K. 1981. Zoological affinities of conodonts. In *Treatise on Invertebrate Paleontology,* suppl. 2, *Conodonta.* Lawrence, Kans.: Geological Society of America and University of Kansas Press, pp. W478–W482.

Nicoll, R. S. 1987. Form and function of the Pa element in the conodont animal. In *Palaeobiology of Conodonts,* vol. 5, R. J. Aldridge, ed. Chichester: Ellis Horwood, pp. 77–90.

Sansom, I. J., M. P. Smith, H. A. Armstrong, and M. M. Smith. 1992. Presence of the earliest vertebrate hard tissues in conodonts. Science 256 (5061): 1308–1311.

Slavkin, H. C., E. Graham, M. Zeichner-David, and W. Hildemann. 1983. Enamel-like antigen in hagfish: Possible evolutionary significance. Evolution 37: 404–412.

Smith, M. P., D. E. G. Briggs, and R. J. Aldridge. 1987. A conodont animal from the lower Silurian of Wisconsin USA, and the apparatus architecture of panderodont conodonts. In *Palaeobiology of Conodonts,* vol. 6, R. J. Aldridge, ed. Chichester: Ellis Horwood, pp. 91–104.

Sweet, W. C. 1988. *The Conodonta: Morphology, Taxonomy, Paleoecology, and Evolutionary History of a Long-Extinct Animal Phylum.* Oxford: Clarendon Press.

REFERENCES

Akam, M. 1989. Hox and HOM: Homologous gene clusters in insects and vertebrates. Cell 57: 347–349.

Balfour, F. M. 1885. *A Treatise on Comparative Embryology.* 2d ed. London: Macmillan and Co.

Baroffio, A., E. Dupin, and N. M. Le Douarin. 1991. Common precursors for neural and mesectodermal derivatives in the cephalic neural crest. Development 112: 301–305.

Barrington, E. J. W. 1965. *The Biology of Hemichordata and Protochordata.* Edinburgh: Oliver and Boyd.

Bemis, W. E., and R. G. Northcutt. 1987. Pore canals of Devonian lungfishes did not house electroreceptors. American Zoologist 27: 106A.

———. 1992. Skin and blood vessels of the snout of the Australian lungfish, *Neoceratodus forsteri,* and their significance for interpreting the cosmine of Devonian lungfishes. Acta zoologica, Stockholm 73 (2): 115–139.

Berrill, N. J. 1955. *The Origin of Vertebrates.* Oxford: Clarendon Press.

Bonik, K., M. Grasshoff, and W. F. Gutmann. 1976. Die Evolution der Tierkonstructionen. III. Von Gallertoid zur Coelomhydraulik. Natur und Museum 106 (6): 178–188.

Brandenburg, J., and G. Kümmel. 1961. Die Feinstructur der Solenocyten. Journal of Ultrastructural Research 5: 437–452.

Bullock, T. H., and G. A. Horridge. 1965. *Structure and Function in the Nervous Systems of Invertebrates.* 2 vols. San Francisco: W. H. Freeman.

Bullock, T. H., D. A. Bodznick, and R. G. Northcutt. 1983. The phylogenetic distribution of electroreception: Evidence for convergent evolution of a primitive vertebrate sense modality. Brain Research Reviews 6: 25–46.

Bullock, T. H., and R. G. Northcutt. 1984. Nervus terminalis in dogfish (*Squalus acanthias,* Elasmobranchii) carries tonic efferent impulses. Neuroscience Letters 44: 155–160.

Cho, K. W. Y., B. Blumberg, H. Steinbeisser, and E. M. de Robertis. 1992. Molecular nature of Spemann's organizer: The role of the *Xenopus* homeobox gene *goosecoid* in gastrulation. Cell.·

Couly, G., and N. M. Le Douarin. 1990. Head morphogenesis in embryonic avian chimeras: Evidence for a segmental pattern in the ectoderm corresponding to the neuromeres. Development 108: 543–558.

De Beer, G. 1937. *The Development of the Vertebrate Skull.* Oxford: Clarendon Press.

De Robertis, E. M., G. Oliver, and C. V. E. Wright. 1989. Determination of axial polarity in the vertebrate embryo: Homeodomain proteins and homeogenetic induction. Cell 57: 189–191.

Field, K. G., G. J. Olsen, D. J. Lane, S. J. Giovannoni, M. T. Ghiselin, E. C. Raff, N. R. Pace, and R. A. Raff. 1986. Molecular phylogeny of the animal kingdom. Science 239: 748–753.

Flood, P. R. 1968. Structure of segmental trunk muscle in amphioxus with notes on course and endings of so-called ventral nerve fibres. Zeitschrift für Zellforschung und microskopische Anatomie 84: 389–416.

Gans, C. 1985. Scenarios: Why? In *Evolutionary Biology of Primitive Fishes*, A. Gorbman, R. Olsson, and R. E. Foreman, eds. New York: Plenum Press, pp. 1–9.

———. 1987. Concluding remarks: The neural crest; A spectacular invention. In *Developmental and Evolutionary Aspects of the Neural Crest*, P. F. A. Maderson, ed. New York: John Wiley and Sons, pp. 361–379.

———. 1988a. Craniofacial growth, evolutionary questions. In *Craniofacial Development*, P. Thorogood and C. Tickle, eds., Development 103 (suppl.): 3–15.

———. 1988b. Review of *The Ancestry of the Vertebrates*, by R. P. S. Jefferies. American Scientist 76 (2): 188–189.

———. 1989. Ecological steps in the origin of vertebrates: Analysis by means of scenarios. Biological Reviews, Cambridge 64 (3): 1–48.

Gans, C., and R. G. Northcutt. 1983. Neural crest and the origin of vertebrates: A new head. Science 220: 268–274.

———. 1985. Neural crest: The implications for comparative anatomy. In *Functional Morphology of Vertebrates*, H. R. Duncker and G. Fleischer, eds. Fortschritte der Zoologie 30. Stuttgart: Gustav Fischer Verlag, pp. 507–514.

Gerhart, J., S. Black, S. Scharf, R. Gimlich, J.-P. Vincent, M. Danilchik, B. Rowning, and J. Roberts. 1986. Amphibian early development. Research supports a stepwise view of amphibian development in which each stage builds on the previous one. Bioscience 36 (8): 541–549.

Gershon, M. 1987. Phenotypic expression by neural crest–derived precursors of enteric neurons and glia. In *Developmental and Evolutionary Aspects of the Neural Crest*, P. F. A. Maderson, ed. New York: John Wiley and Sons, pp. 181–211.

Goodrich, E. S. 1930. *Studies on the Structure and Development of Vertebrates*. London: Macmillan and Co.

Graf, W., and W. J. Brunken. 1984. Elasmobranch oculomotor organization: Anatomical and theoretical aspects of the phylogenetic development of vestibulo-oculomotor connectivity. Journal of Comparative Neurology 227: 569–581.

Griffith, R. W. 1987. Freshwater or marine origin of the vertebrates? Comparative Biochemistry and Physiology 87A: 523–531.

Hall, B. K. 1987. Tissue interactions in the development and evolution of the vertebrate head. In *Developmental and Evolutionary Aspects of the Neural Crest*, P. F. A. Maderson, ed. New York: John Wiley and Sons, pp. 215–259.

Halstead, B. T. 1987. Evolutionary aspects of neural crest–derived skeletogenic cells in the earliest vertebrates. In *Developmental and Evolutionary Aspects of the Neural Crest,* P. F. A. Maderson, ed. New York: John Wiley and Sons, pp. 339–358.

Herrick, C. J. 1899. The cranial and first spinal nerves of *Menidia:* A contribution upon the nerve components of the bony fishes. Journal of Comparative Neurology 9: 153–455.

Holland, P. W. H. 1988. Homeobox genes and the vertebrate head. In *Craniofacial Development,* P. Thorogood and C. Tickle, eds. Development 103 (suppl.): 17–24.

Hunt, P., J. Whiting, S. Nonchev, M. Sham, H. Marshall, A. Graham, R. Allemann, P. W. J. Rigby, M. Gulisano, A. Faiella, E. Boncinelli, and R. Krumlauf. 1991. The branchial *Hox* code and its implications for gene regulation, patterning of the nervous system, and head evolution. Development 2 (suppl.): 63–77.

Hunt, P., D. Wilkinson, and R. Krumlauf. 1991. Patterning the vertebrate head: Murine Hox 2 genes mark distinct subpopulations of premigratory and migrating cranial neural crest. Development 112: 43–50.

Huxley, T. H. 1858. On the theory of the vertebrate skull. Proceedings of the Royal Society of London 9: 381–457.

Jacobson, A. G. 1987. Determination and morphogenesis of axial structures: Mesodermal metamerism, shaping of the neural plate and tube, and segregation and functions of the neural crest. In *Developmental and Evolutionary Aspects of the Neural Crest,* P. F. A. Maderson, ed. New York: John Wiley and Sons, pp. 147–180.

Jacobson, A. G., and S. Meier. 1986. Somitomeres: The primordial body segments. In *Somites in Developing Embryos,* R. Bellairs, D. A. Ede, and J. W. Lash, eds. New York: Plenum Press, pp. 1–16.

Jacobson, A. G., and A. K. Sater. 1988. Features of embryonic induction. Development 104 (3): 341–359.

Jollie, M. 1984. The vertebrate head: Segmented or a single morphogenetic structure? Journal of Vertebrate Paleontology 4 (3): 320–329.

Keynes, R. J., and C. D. Stern. 1988. Somites and neural development. In *Somites in Developing Embryos,* R. Bellairs, D. A. Ede, and J. W. Lash, eds. New York: Plenum Press, pp. 189–199.

Kimmel, C. B., D. S. Sepich, and B. Trevarrow. 1988. Development of segmentation in zebrafish. Development 104 (suppl.): 197–208.

Krieger, D. T., M. J. Brownstein, and J. B. Martin, eds. *Brain Peptides.* New York: Wiley-Interscience.

Krotoski, D. M., S. E. Fraser, and M. Bronner-Fraser. 1988. Mapping of neural crest pathways in *Xenopus laevis* using inter- and intra-specific cell markers. Developmental Biology 127 (1): 119–132.

Langille, R. M., and B. K. Hall. 1988a. Role of the neural crest in development of the cartilaginous cranial and visceral skeleton of the medaka, *Oryzias latipes* (Teleostei). Anatomy and Embryology 177 (4): 297–305.

———. 1988b. Role of the neural crest in development of the trabeculae and branchial arches in embryonic sea lamprey, *Petromyzon marinus* (L.). Development 102 (2): 301–310.

Le Douarin, N. 1982. *The Neural Crest.* New York: Cambridge University Press.

Lonai, P., and A. Orr-Urtreger. 1990. Homeogenes in mammalian development and the evolution of the cranium and central nervous system. FASEB Journal 4: 1436–1443.

Lumsden, A. 1987. The neural crest contribution to tooth development in the mammalian embryo. In *Developmental and Evolutionary Aspects of the Neural Crest,* P. F. A. Maderson, ed. New York: John Wiley and Sons, pp. 261–300.

Lumsden, A., and R. Keynes. 1989. Segmental patterns of neuronal development in the chick hindbrain. Nature, London 337: 424–428.

Maderson, P. F. A., ed. 1987. *Developmental and Evolutionary Aspects of the Neural Crest.* New York: John Wiley and Sons.

Maisey, J. G. 1986. Heads and tails: A chordate phylogeny. Cladistics 2 (3): 201–256.

Marinelli, W., and A. Strenger. 1954. *Lampetra fluviatilis* (L.). Part 1 of *Vergleichende Anatomie und Morphologie der Wirbeltiere.* Vienna: Franz Deuticke, pp. 1–80.

———. 1956. *Myxine glutinosa* (L.). Part 2 of *Vergleichende Anatomie und Morphologie der Wirbeltiere.* Vienna: Franz Deuticke, pp. 81–172.

Marshall, E. K., Jr., and H. W. Smith. 1930. The glomerular development of the vertebrate kidney in relation to habitat. Biological Reviews 59 (2): 135–153.

Meier, S. 1984. Somite formation and its relationship to metameric pattern of the mesoderm. Cell Differentiation 14: 235–243.

Molven, A., C. V. E. Wright, R. Bremiller, E. M. de Robertis, and C. B. Kimmel. 1990. Expression of a homeobox gene product in normal and mutant zebrafish embryos: Evolution of the tetrapod body plan. Development 19: 279–288.

Moy-Thomas, J. A., and R. S. Miles. 1971. *Palaeozoic Fishes.* Philadelphia: W. B. Saunders Co.

Noden, D. M. 1987. Interactions between cephalic neural crest and mesodermal populations. In *Developmental and Evolutionary Aspects of the Neural Crest,* P. F. A. Maderson, ed. New York: John Wiley and Sons, pp. 89–119.

———. 1988. Interaction and fates of avian craniofacial mesenchyme. In *Craniofacial Development,* P. Thorogood and C. Tickle, eds., Development 103 (suppl.): 121–140.

Northcutt, R. G. 1979. The comparative anatomy of the nervous system and the sense organs. In *Hyman's Comparative Vertebrate Anatomy,* 3rd ed., M. H. Wake, ed. Chicago: University of Chicago Press, pp. 615–770.

Northcutt, R. G., and C. Gans. 1983. The genesis of neural crest and epidermal placodes: A reinterpretation of vertebrate origins. Quarterly Review of Biology 58 (1): 1–28.

Romer, A. S. 1933. Eurypterid influence on vertebrate history. Science 78: 114–117.

———. 1942. Cartilage: An embryonic adaptation. American Naturalist 76: 394–404.

———. 1972. The vertebrate as a dual animal—somatic and visceral. Evolutionary Biology 6: 121–156.

Ross, L. S., T. Parrett, and Stephen S. Easter, Jr. 1992. Axonogenesis and morphogenesis in the embryonic zebrafish brain. Journal of Neuroscience 12 (2): 467–482.

Rovainen, C. M., and M. H. Schieber. 1975. Ventilation of larval lampreys. Journal of Comparative Physiology 104: 185–203.

Ruben, J. A., and A. F. Bennett. 1980. Antiquity of the vertebrate pattern of activity metabolism and its possible relation to vertebrate origins. Nature, London 286: 886–888.

———. 1981. Intense exercise, bone structure, and blood calcium levels in vertebrates. Nature, London 291: 411–413.

———. 1987. The evolution of bone. Evolution 41 (6): 1187–1197.

Russell, D. F. 1986. Respiratory pattern generation in adult lampreys (*Lampetra fluviatilis*): Interneurons and burst resetting. Journal of Comparative Physiology A 158: 91–102.

Russell, E. S. 1916. *Form and Function: A Contribution to the History of Animal Morphology*. London: John Murray.

Sadaghiani, B., and C. H. Thiébaud. 1987. Neural crest development in the *Xenopus laevis* embryo, studied by interspecific transplantation and scanning electron microscopy. Developmental Biology 124 (1): 91–110.

Simeone, A., M. Gulisano, D. Acampora, M. Rambaldi, and E. Boncinelli. 1992. Two vertebrate homeobox genes related to the *Drosophila empty spiracles* gene are expressed in the embryonic cerebral cortex and a few neurectodermal locations in the head. European Molecular Biology Organization Journal 11(7):2541–2550.

Smith, M. M., and B. K. Hall. 1990. Development and evolutionary origins of vertebrate skeletogenic and odontogenic tissues. Biological Reviews 65: 277–373.

Starck, D. 1978a. *Vergleichende Anatomie der Wirbeltiere auf evolutionsbiologischer Grundlage*, vol. 1, *Theoretische Grundlage: Stammesgeschichte und Systematik unter Berücksichtigung der niederen Chordata*. Berlin: Springer Verlag.

———. 1978b. *Vergleichende Anatomie der Wirbeltiere auf evolutionsbiologischer Grundlage*, vol. 2, *Das Skeletsystem*. Berlin: Springer Verlag.

Stern, C. D. 1990. Two distinct mechanisms for segmentation? Seminars in Developmental Biology 1: 109–116.

Tan, S. S., and G. M. Morris-Kay. 1986. Analysis of cranial neural cell migration and early fates in postimplantation rat chimaeras. Journal of Embryology and Experimental Morphology 98: 21–58.

Thorogood, P., and C. Tickle, eds. 1988. *Craniofacial Development*. Development 103 (suppl.): 1–257.

Tosney, K. W. 1987. Proximal tissues and patterned neurite outgrowth at the lumbosacral level of the chick embryo: Deletion of the dermamyotome. Developmental Biology 122: 540–558.

———. 1988. Proximal tissues and patterned neurite outgrowth at the lumbosacral level of the chick embryo: Partial and complete deletion of the somite. Developmental Biology 127: 266–286.

Webb, J. E. 1973. The role of the notochord in forward and reverse swimming and burrowing in the amphioxus, *Branchiostoma lanceolatum*. Journal of Zoology, London 170: 325–338.

Welsch, U. 1975. The fine structure of the pharynx, cyrtopodocytes, and digestive caecum of amphioxus (*Branchiostoma lanceolatum*). Symposia of the Zoological Society of London 36: 17–41.

Wolpert, L. 1988. Craniofacial development: A summing up. In *Craniofacial Development*, P. Thorogood and C. Tickle, eds., Development 103 (suppl.): 245–249.

Xue, Z., W. J. Gehring, and N. M. Le Douarin. 1991. Quox-1, a quail homeobox gene expressed in the embryonic central nervous system, including the forebrain. Proceedings of the National Academy of Sciences, United States 88: 2427–2431.

2

Segmentation, the Adult Skull, and the Problem of Homology

KEITH STEWART THOMSON

The study of segmentation is comparable to study of the Apocalypse. That way leads to madness.

A. S. Romer

INTRODUCTION

MOST BIOLOGISTS CONSIDER THEMSELVES to be among the more strictly empirical of scientists—"Here is an enzyme, it is lactate dehydrogenase; here is a bone, it is the parietal." But every time a biologist works comparatively (and biology is the supremely comparative science) great assumptions have to be made, as for example in the statement "This second bone is also a parietal." Behind such simple statements lurk all the terrors of epistemology ("How do I know this is a parietal?") and of ontology ("What is a parietal?"). In order to negotiate these mine fields one needs a map, a sure guide. The purpose of this essay is to ask whether, with regard to the homology of the head skeleton of vertebrates, any part of such a map can be derived from comparative study of the adult skull.

The adult vertebrate skull was the original focus of segmental theory, by virtue of which Oken and Goethe, and then Owen, Huxley, Gegenbauer, Balfour, Goodrich, de Beer, and many others propelled comparative vertebrate morphology into a position of scientific prominence that it has never quite lost. Morphology has been an active area for such enquiry for more than two hundred years. It has been crucially important because in the empirical world skulls contain a great deal of information compared to, say, most soft organs. Because skulls are hard and fossilizable, bits of the skull are commonly the only remains that we have of many extinct taxa. In the study of vertebrate phylogeny and evolution the skull is the common denominator. If we are to be on safe ground in comparative vertebrate morphology, we had better be sure about the skull. (The reader will note that I am avoiding mentioning the dentition which, happily, falls outside my mandate.)

In this essay I will discuss some of the problems that are presented by comparative studies of the adult vertebrate skull (particularly the dermal skull), and the light (or shadow) that they cause to fall upon fundamental questions of the nature of the head and the origins of the different dermal bone patterns in gnathostomes. Those who in the past have dealt solely with the adult skull have been at a disadvantage because a lot of morphogenetic information was obviously lacking. The offsetting advantages are that functional considerations can be brought more fully into the discussion and that the lineages of skull types available in the fossil record bring in a whole new phylogenetic dimension. Now, as new morphogenetic information becomes available, we can start to combine approaches better.

HOMOLOGY

The whole matter begins and ends with homology. Paradoxically, in order to study homology ("what is the same") in evolutionary biology one must study what changes. One must study different organisms in order to decide whether two entities are different manifestations of the same thing, or two different things. And consequently, to study change (evolution) we have to know what is the same. One needs to be sure that one is dealing with the same entity changing over time, rather than with a product of convergence or parallelism. But how are we to know? To take a very simple example, one of the results from the work of Le Lièvre and Le Douarin (1975) and Noden (1983b) on the contributions of neural crest to the skeleton of the chick skull is to show that the nasal bone is formed anteriorly of neural crest cells and posteriorly from mesodermal cells. In amphibians the nasal is entirely mesodermal. What does this tell us about the bone that we call the nasal in the chick? Must we call it a compound bone because it has a double provenance in terms of tissues? Is the provenance of the mesenchyme the criterion by which we judge what the "real" bony element is? Or is the distribution of different mesenchymes to particular regions quite opportunistic, so that the real bone is the one that occupies a particular position in the skull roof, gathering mesenchyme from various sources indifferently over evolutionary time? If we are to be able truly to compare the skull of a bird with that of any other vertebrate, we have to know what we are dealing with: what is real? What seems to an outsider the dullest of activities—naming and comparing bones in the skulls of vertebrates—becomes therefore not a routine task of basic empirical science, but a difficult and challenging exercise; not merely what do we know, but how do we know?

In order to discuss anything in comparative biology we need to agree upon the criteria for sameness and difference. The problem is, however, that while homology is one of the most familiar of concepts for biologists, it is at the same time the most baffling and difficult. What may be specified in theory may be impossible to determine in practice. What may seem obvious and intuitive in practice may be impossible to defend in theory.

Let us imagine some clay pots. Two pots could readily be considered homologous if they were thrown by the same artist, even if they were different in shape and color: we would say, "These two pots are John Smith pots." Two similarly shaped pots made on different wheels by different artists in different materials could also be considered homologous if we chose the criterion that they were made to the same design pattern: "These two pots are model number 23s." What matters is the choice of a criterion that is causal. In comparative biology, because of the driving premise of evolutionary theory that all organisms are related by descent, the key criterion for homology is commonality of genetic cause.

Van Valen (1982), with his customary prescience, boils down homology to "continuity of information." Continuity of information is exactly what the working comparative morphologist has always sought in making comparisons. Information in morphology is a function of the genetic and epigenetic control of morphogenetic patterning. "Continuity" requires specification of true lines of descent and thus of relationship. However, because the morphologist can never have access to complete gene sequences, complete epigenetic pathways, or complete phylogenies for all the taxa he or she needs to compare, we have to make the best of what we have.

Unfortunately, in unraveling "continuity of information" we have first to know what it is that is being informed. Most vertebrate biologists and certainly most paleontologists act under the implicit premise that "bones"—the femur, the squamosal, or the stapes, for example—are singular "real" entities and are effectively heritable. On this basis one can freely compare the humeri or squamosals of widely divergent taxa. Implicit in this is the assumption that such elements, even if they are not coded for explicitly in the genome, will have a constant ontogenetic derivation in such matters as segmental position or source of tissue type. Taken to its extreme, this premise can be used to make extremely fine-grained analyses of evolution of structure. For instance, Jarvik (1942) argues that the posterior exterior nostril of the fish nasal sac is homologous with the nasolachrymal duct of tetrapods. This premise accords well with a "bauplan" approach to evolution because if individual structures are real, they will not appear and disappear inconsistently over time (an extension of this view is that basically nothing is ever completely lost).

An alternative view is that it is patterns of structure that are passed on within lineages and that, within the patterns, different manifestations are possible. From this it is but a small step to the premise that it is developmental pattern generating mechanisms that are real in the sense of being genetically programmed and thus heritable with modification. In this view, the individual structural elements are reduced to second-order phenomena. A dramatic example of this approach is given in Goodwin and Trainor's (1983) treatment of the morphogenesis of the pentadactyl limb, in which only the system of fields defining the limb is "real." In this case a three-digit hand might be technically homologous to a five-digit hand; digits are not lost but rather the whole system changes (their computer model does not have to be correct for the essential point to be made.) Given the conservatism of evolutionary change and the fact that each new variant structure in evolution is just that—a variant derived from a preexisting lineage, rather than a radically new entity created out of thin air—the difference between the two views is relatively unimportant for the vast majority of phylogenetic or systematic comparisons. The trouble is, where the distinction is important, it may be very important indeed, namely, where we try to deal with the disconformities in the organismal record (see examples below).

It certainly seems that when we come to compare either individual elements or patterns of elements (for example, the arrangement of the bones making up the dermal skull), we find considerable consistency *within-group*, and thus comparisons are easy to make. But there are often major inconsistencies *between or among groups* that involve all the structural elements to one degree or another. Setting aside the obvious possibility of circular reasoning in defining groups in the first place, especially where the only available evidence is anatomical, these inconsistencies become particularly interesting and important.

In practice, most comparisons of structure and estimates of homology are based on simple form: do any two given elements look alike or more alike each other than either is to a third? Comparative embryology has been the next logical place to look for help, first simply as an additional dimension, as it were, of form. Two elements (the classical case being the hyomandibular of a fish and the stapes of a mammal) could be considered homologous if they shared the same developmental origin, arising in this case from neural crest ectomesenchyme forming the dorsalmost blastema of the first visceral arch, and if this could be traced through a clade. This turns out to be surprisingly difficult to determine in practice, as witnessed by the current lack of certainty concerning the homology of the mammalian ear ossicles (Novacek, chap. 9). One problem is that, when one looks at the early blastemata in the ear region of a mammal, it is by no means simple to state that this group of cells is the epal element of the first arch, these represent the ceratal element of the second arch, and so on. Once again, by what criteria does one make the decisions?

The traditional approach has been that one gains surety by combining evolutionary transformation series (series of fossil phenotypes) with reasonable predictions concerning the transformation of ontogenies. In theory, von Baer's laws being generally correct, if one can trace the phenotypic series back, checking all along with comparative ontogeny where available, a set of trends will appear. Ear ossicle–gill arch homology is corroborated iteratively by the reptilian stapes being an epihyal, as is that of a frog and of a fish, and by assembling transformation series of adult phenotypes (usually fossils, from which no embryonic evidence can be gained) in which the change can be tracked (see Lombard and Bolt 1988 for the most penetrating of recent analyses).

All this depends in turn upon there being available an independently derived phylogeny for the phenotypic series. Not surprisingly, from time to time a voice is raised pointing out that the whole construct may be compared to a house of cards, or the emperor's new clothes.

In most cases, the comparative morphologist does not have the advantage of embryological data for the taxa under comparison. In that case, one is forced to specify (actually many merely assume) that certain key criteria are causal and consistently causal over millions of years and thus form a reliable guide to homology of elements. These criteria are chosen on the grounds that they are an available index that directly reflects the otherwise inaccessible source of continuity of information due to genetic relatedness. For example, following Allis (1898), one of the most commonly held assumptions of lower vertebrate paleontologists used to be that there is an invariate causal relationship between the lateral line system of the head and the pattern of dermal bones (see below). In this chapter I will discuss some of the criteria that have been proposed as indices of homology of elements of the vertebrate skull, concentrating on the dermal skull. Of these, historically one of the most important has been the question of segmentation.

SEGMENTATION AND THE GENERAL ORGANIZATION OF THE HEAD

Segmentation is a system of regional specification of morphogenetic information and is therefore a key to any study of homology. Segmental arrangement is as logical for bilateral, elongate organisms as the radial partitioning of the body in sessile organisms. The precise manner in which segmentation is specified in morphogenesis is in part a function of the manner of growth but also is inherent in the processes by which any tissue specification is caused in the first place. Progressive regionalization, like all other information in development, starts with the fertilized egg. Layers of new information are added at every stage of gene expression (Thomson 1988) and especially at gastrulation. In vertebrates, morphogenetic patterning in the embryo is dominated by the processes of gastrulation (or their equivalents) but significant regionalization of tissues (for example, neural crest or mesoderm) is also set up before gastrulation as a direct function of positioning along the antero-posterior axis of the elongate blastula.

Schemes of Segmentation of the Adult Head

Most of the original work on the possible segmentation of the skull was, of course, conducted as an exercise in comparative anatomy (both of embryonic and adult structures) rather than from a morphogenetic point of view. It was concerned with the data of effect, rather than the processes of cause, in the head. The work of Balfour (1876) and Goodrich (1918) on the head of *Scyllium* and *Squalus* and the somewhat generalized scheme of Goodrich (1930) were particularly influential in this regard. A basic premise (or perhaps a basic goal) of these studies was to produce a scheme combining the branchial apparatus, the mesoderm (especially the cranial musculature), the cranial nerves, and the skeleton, comparable to the pattern of segmentation of the trunk.

Goodrich's review has stood for 60 years as the foundation for discussions of cranial homology and provides the starting point for all more recent discussions. Goodrich proposed that there were a total of eight head segments: three preotic, two otic, and three postotic, each with a corresponding visceral cleft. Major attempts to apply this scheme to detailed structures of the skull were triggered by both comparative anatomy and paleontology, but particularly by the exciting results of experimental work on the neural crest by Stone (1926, 1929), and Hörstadius and Sellman (1946), and were brilliantly reviewed by Hörstadius (1950).

In 1954 Jarvik proposed a new scheme of segmental patterning of the visceral and neurocranial skeleton based on the experimental results on the range of neural crest contribution to the skull in urodeles, particularly the fascinating datum that the neural crest provides all the mesenchyme for the visceral skeleton, as well as most of the trabeculae cranii and a small portion of the lateral otic wall. Jarvik's scheme, later amplified by Bertmar (1959) and Bjerring (1967), is based upon a simple syllogism: neural crest gives rise to the visceral skeleton; parts of the neurocranium are formed from neural crest; therefore everything in the neurocranium that is derived from neural crest must represent an element that was originally part of the visceral skeleton that has subsequently become incorporated into the neurocranium.

According to this theory, portions of the nasal capsule represent epal elements of the terminal and premandibular segments, the trabeculae cranii are the transplanted infrapharyngals of the mandibular arch skeleton, and the lateral commissure is the combined infra- and suprapharyngals of the hyoid arch skeleton. If this were true, it would also follow that the vomers and parasphenoid would represent the modified dermal plates associated with the relevant visceral endocranium. There is, however, no objective justification for considering neural crest–derived components of the neurocranium as representing ancient visceral skeleton. Given the fundamental role of the trabeculae cranii in the morphogenesis of the neurocranium, for example, it is hard to image what the neurocranium would have been in the hypothetical stage before incorporation of part of the mandibular arch skeleton. That this is a plausible scheme is not sufficient; the argument needs an independent verification. Furthermore, identification of the particular segment from which the visceral element is supposed to have come requires the assumption that there was a segment or segments in that position in the first place. The dangers in this sort of argumentation are shown by the fact that by the mid-1970s, it had become clear to most workers that there is no solid evidence for the existence in any vertebrate, living or fossil, of a full premandibular branchial segment anyway, let alone a terminal arch. One of the mainstays of the "visceral origin" argument had been Stensio's identification of such a segment in the adult skull of fossil agnathan fishes, these identifications being themselves highly theory-laden. Whiting (1972, 1977) and others showed that Stensio had erred in his assignment of homologies of cranial nerves in comparison between fossil and living agnathans; his count was one segment out.

Despite this, Jarvik (1980) later expanded his views into a monumentally elaborate, entirely hypothetical scheme accounting for all the homologies of the head in terms of its origin from seven segments, not only with complete visceral pouches but also with vertebrae. In this scheme (fig. 2.1) the dermal bones of the mandible, rostrum, and cheek represent the gill covers of four gill segments (terminal, premandibular, mandibular, and hyoid); the neurocranium represents vertebral arcualia (plus visceral additions); and the dermal bones of the skull roof represent vertebral tecta that are intersegmental in position, deriving from the posterior half of one segment and the anterior half of the following one (as is the case with vertebral skeletal structures in the trunk of amniotes). One might call this "the emperor's complete new wardrobe."

The second set of discussions of head segmentation is that of Jollie (1968, 1971, 1977, 1984). Jollie reviewed the comparative embryological evidence and produced a revised scheme of fundamental head segmentation based on five and one half segments. He then turned to see what confirming evidence there was for this scheme in the patterning of the der-

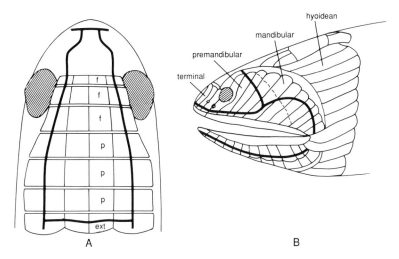

Fig. 2.1. Jarvik's hypothetical scheme of segmental relationships of the cranial dermal bones. A. Cheek and lateral head elements. B. Skull table. (After Jarvik, simplified)

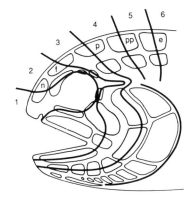

Fig. 2.2. Jollie's hypothetical scheme of segmental dermal bone relationships. (After Jollie, simplified)

mal bones of the adult head, producing the scheme shown in figure 2.2. This scheme has the great merit of attempting to find the segmental relationships only of known, rather than hypothetical, dermal elements.

Segmentation of the Skull in the Light of New Experimental Evidence

Several new studies of the developmental bases of segmentation in vertebrates in the last decade give reason either to doubt whether the vertebrate head is fundamentally segmented, or to ask, if it is segmented, how segmentation is controlled and how head segmentation differs from that of the trunk. Such studies, coupled with the general recognition of the epigenetic flexibility of developmental systems (e.g., Thomson 1988) cast a great shadow of doubt upon the worth of schemes of homology based upon an inflexible working out of some hypothetical bauplan. The challenge is then to find a more acceptable set of hypotheses.

In the vertebrate trunk, a single segment, as classically defined on the basis of adult and embryonic morphology, should include the following units: segmental mesoderm, dorsal and ventral segmental nerves and ganglia, neuromere, and neural crest (see Neal 1918; Kingsbury 1926; Romer 1977). There has also been scattered discussion concerning possible segmentation of the notochord, most of it inconclusive. The axial mesoderm classically provides segmentally arranged dermatome, sclerotome, myotome, and nephrotome, while the lateral plate mesoderm is unsegmented. Causally, the key to developmental specification of trunk segmentation is segmentation of the mesoderm. Obviously a lot of the trunk, principally those features involving the endoderm, is not segmented. Regional specification in nonsegmented portions of the trunk appears to occur much later than regional specification in the segmented parts, which is largely in place or set in process by the end of neurulation (the equivalent of the tail bud stage).

In the head, a segment is more difficult to define morphologically or morphogenetically. Most of the skeletal mesoderm is actually ectomesenchyme derived from the neural crest. The neural crest in the head seems to take on some of the functions of the lateral plate mesoderm which is otherwise missing. The question of whether the branchiomerism of the visceral apparatus represents the same causal patterning as metamerism of the mesoderm (which in turn in part at least controls patterning of the neural crest) remains unclear. The key experiments have yet to be performed. The branchial pouches are induced in the foregut of the vertebrate embryo and there is only a small amount of indirect evidence (Abercrombie and Waddington 1957) to suggest a controlling mesodermal influence in this process.

Some of the most important results concerning head segmentation have been due to the work of the late Stephen Meier and coworkers, who showed that in chick the paraxial mesoderm of the head region differentiates in a manner different from that of the trunk (see Jacobson, chap. 2, in vol. 1). Instead of the classic head somites, the paraxial mesoderm is arranged in a series of regions, starting anteriorly immediately behind, and contiguous with, the prechordal plate mesoderm. The paraxial mesoderm is arranged into a series of swirling groups of cells (Meier 1981, 1984). In amniotes the first seven of these somitomeres remain contiguous. The eighth and following units become separate and eventually differentiate in a way comparable with and serially consistent with the mesodermal somites of the trunk. Obviously great interest attaches to the relationship of the seven cranial somitomeres to the cranial segments of classical segmentation theory and historical observation.

Unfortunately, the arrangement of the axial mesoderm in the head is not consistent across vertebrates. In the chick, mouse (Tam and Meier 1982), and turtle (Meier and Packard 1984) there are equivalent numbers of cranial somitomeres. But in the newt (Jacobson and Meier 1984) the equivalent preotic and otic region of mesoderm is patterned into only four units. Results of studies of the head of sharks (Gilland, personal communication) are eagerly awaited. When the available results are compared with older work such as that of Adelman (1932) and the classical works on sharks, the obvious question arises: to what extent is it possible to distinguish between the paraxial mesoderm and the prechordal plate mesoderm at these early stages? Much work remains to be done, and for the moment the chick (through ease of experiment) remains the best known.

Work on the neural crest of chick by Le Lièvre and Le Douarin (1975), Le Lièvre (1978) and Le Douarin (1980), Noden (1982, 1983a, b, 1984), and by Anderson and Meier (1981), reveals something of the nature of the relationship between patterning of the neural crest and that of the mesoderm and cranial nerves and has, for the first time, isolated the derivatives of different regions of mesoderm and neural crest with considerable accuracy. Noden shows (1982, 1983a) that in chick all the somitomeres give rise to muscles. Therefore the classical notion that the "otic segments" (four and five) do not give rise to muscles is incorrect. A further surprise is that somitomere four gives rise to the mandibular adductor muscles, which are innervated by nerve V, and similarly the sixth and seventh somitomeres give rise to the mandibular depressor and hypobranchial musculature, innervated by cranial nerves VII and IX, respectively. This falsifies part of the classical account, which stated that nerves VII and IX had no somatic motor component.

Noden shows that somitomeres one and two (probably) give rise to the dorsal, medial, and ventral rectus and ventral oblique eye muscles innervated by nerve III, somitomere three gives the dorsal oblique (nerve IV) and somitomere five the lateral rectus muscles (nerve VI). This is in accord with the Goodrich scheme. Interestingly, Noden also shows the profundus nerve V as having no motor component, but the vagus nerve must have a somatic motor component to the muscles derived from the first somite which, together with the following segments, contributes to the musculature of the larynx and tongue. The latter is not predicted by the classical theory.

Noden (1984), following Le Lièvre's discovery that the connective tissue sheaths of the facial musculature are all of neural crest origin, used experimental extirpation of neural crest regions, coupled with knowledge of the somitomeric derivatives, to develop a map of the relationships of the cranial nerves and muscles as well.

Predictably there are some difficulties in reconciling the accounts of somitomeres given by Meier and Noden with the classic sequence of head segments of Goodrich (1930). Meier believed that the first somitomere in both the newt and the amniotes represented segment one of the Goodrich scheme, with the next six somitomeres representing in chick a doubling of segments two, three, and four. My own view is that the first mesodermal unit is the least reliable of all, owing to lack of distinction from the prechordal plate. As shown in figure 2.3, a consistent scheme can be derived if it is assumed that chick somitomeres one and two are equivalent to the first segment, three and four are equivalent to the mandibular segment, and five and six to the hyoid segment. Somitomere seven then is equivalent to the first otic segment and somite one is the second otic segment. This scheme fits the classical scheme in its alternation of targets for the dorsal and ventral root nerves, in the arrangement of three pro-otic and two otic segments, and in the requirement that the ventral root be in the anterior half of each segment and the dorsal root at the posterior end of the segment.

If, on the other hand, one follows Meier in considering the first somitomere alone to be equivalent to the first segment, this produces the fundamental difficulty (figure 2.3) that cranial nerves VII and IX (classically belonging to segments three and four) are found in the same segment. The situation cannot be resolved on present evidence.

We can extend this exercise by mapping the results of all the new experimental work by Le Douarin, le Lièvre, Noden, Meier, and their coworkers onto drawings of generalized vertebrate skulls in order to show the domains of neural crest and mesoderm. In the neurocranium there is nothing much new to add (figure 2.4). None of the new experimental evi-

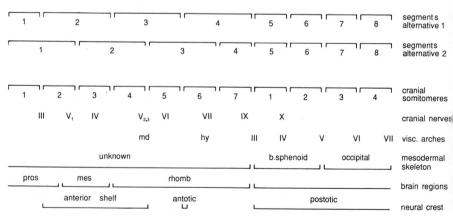

Fig. 2.3 Relations of the cranial somitomeres of the chick to the various elements of hypothetical cranial segmentation.

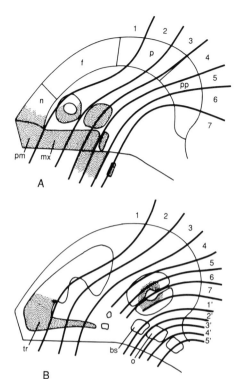

Fig. 2.4. Hypothetical patterning
of segmental domains in the
tetrapod skull. A. Dermal bones.
B. Elements of the neurocranium.
Abbreviations: bs, basisphenoid;
f, frontal; mx, maxilla; n, nasal;
o, occipital; p, parietal; pp,
postparietal; tr, trabeculae cranii.

dence has changed the observation that the visceral skeleton is formed entirely of neural crest ectomesenchyme (except for the well-known but still tantalizing fact that the second basibranchial of urodeles is mesodermal). An important question is: can we plot the domains of individual head segments or at least of somitomeres with respect to the adult dermal skull?

The results are shown in figure 2.5. The first obvious result is that, topographically at least, a large anterior portion of the dermal skull is within the domain of somitomeres one, two, and three, while almost all the rest of the skull belongs in the domain of somitomeres four through seven. The region of the premaxillary, nasal, and possibly the frontal bones all corresponds to the prechordal plate and the first somitomere. The parietal bone belongs no further back than somitomeres one, two, and three. The postparietal region corresponds to at least somitomeres four through seven, and possibly also to the first somite.

Many caveats must be appended to such analyses. In general all such tidy idealized schemes must be just as suspect as the older schemes seeking to find in the neurocranium all the "arcualial" elements of cranial vertebrae. It is much more likely that in different vertebrates a sort of developmental opportunism will partially, if not totally, obliterate any ancestral

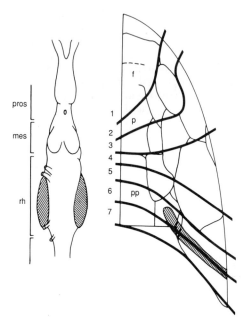

Fig. 2.5. Domains of the somitomeres in chick with respect to the skull roof of an advanced osteolepiform fish, with brain stem as a reference point. Somitomeres numbered. Abbreviations: pros, prosencephalon; mes, mesencephalon; rh, rhombencephalon; f, frontal; op, opercular; p, parietal; pm, premaxilla; pp, postparietal. Segmentation scheme after figure 2.3.

pattern. Furthermore, almost all of the evidence comes from experimental work on two species of birds—chick and quail—together with less complete work on one species each of mammal, reptile, and amphibian. Recently Langille and Hall (1988b) have added information concerning the neural crest contributions to the visceral and neurocranial skeleton of a teleost and have confirmed Newth's 1956 analysis of the lamprey (Langille and Hall 1988a). But there is nothing available on the dermal skeleton of any fish and almost nothing on any mammal. That Langille and Hall's data conform with those available for amphibians and birds gives us some confidence that we are close to seeing the basic vertebrate condition, but surprises may lie in store.

OTHER CRITERIA FOR HOMOLOGY

The bones of the dermal skull represent one of the classic central problems in homology because dermal skull patterns form the basis for comparing the vast majority of vertebrates, and particularly lower vertebrates. As already noted, systematic comparisons show that there is a remarkable consistency within groups. The difficulties of homologization of dermal elements and patterns increase with the level of group compared. Within certain taxonomic levels, differences among dermal bone patterns can be accounted for by relatively simple ad hoc hypotheses of change of relative growth, subdivision, loss, or replacement. There also appear to be common trends in the evolution of most groups toward reduction in the total number of bones in the pattern which are usually accounted for in terms of bone loss rather than fusion. But the question then arises: do the major between-group differences, like those between placoderms and osteichthyans, or lungfishes and rhipidistians, merely represent difficult examples in deciphering the working out of a single plan of dermal bone pattern control that is common to all gnathostomes? Or do they, in fact, result from qualitatively different mechanisms giving different homologies? In the following paragraphs I will attempt to analyze the value of different working criteria in assessing homology of dermal skull bones. First it is useful to set out some particularly troublesome examples from comparisons among the major early gnathostome groups (figure 2.6).

Perhaps the problem that has most resisted efforts at solution is comparison of the skull roof in placoderm fishes (fig. 2.6A) and gnathostomes (fig. 2.6, B–F). Both groups of fishes are gnathostomes, they appear at roughly the same time (late Silurian) and they diversified in parallel. Both skulls have more or less complete dermal coverings, complete with extensive lateral line systems. Yet they seem to have nothing in common (Gross 1962; cf. Graham-Smith 1978).

Within the Osteichthyes, there are consistent differences in dermal skull roof pattern between the actinopterygian condition (fig. 2.6E) and the two major lines of sarcopterygian fishes—crossopterygian and dipnoan (fig. 2.6, B–D).

Lastly, there is a vexing problem of the relationship between the dermal skulls of an early amphibian and an osteolepiform fish (fig. 2.6, D and F; cf. fig. 2.8) and there are some interesting related problems of homology of dermal bones within the tetrapods themselves (review in Borgen 1983).

Shape, Number, and Relative Position of Bones

One of the commonest practices of a paleontologist is to identify an isolated skull bone or limb bone on the basis of shape. For example, most tetrapod humeri are instantly identifiable, as are the basisphenoid of a coelacanth or the B bone of a lungfish skull. Such elements may in fact yield systematic information down to genus. But, while the shapes of individual elements of the skull are useful in homology, more useful is the pattern into which they fit. The reason for this is obvious: as all the bones are (more or less) in sutural or articulated contact with other bones, the shape of any bone is a function of the whole pattern. The dermal bone pattern grows developmentally as a whole, functions as a whole, and changes evolutionarily as a whole—all because it is created morphogenetically as a whole. It is in the patterns of arrangement of dermal elements that we find the difference between within-group and between-group com-

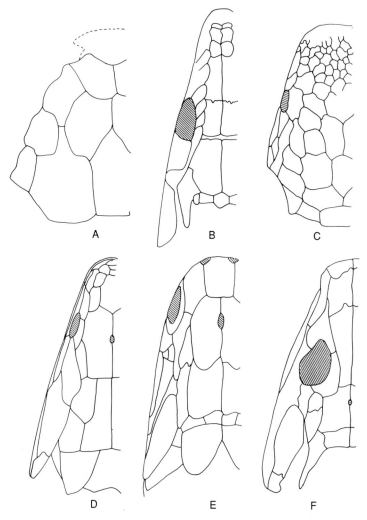

Fig. 2.6. Dorsal view of the skull in six representative gnathostome groups.
A. Placoderm. B. Coelacanth. C. Dipnoan. D. Osteolepiform, E. Actinopterygian.
F. Amphibian.

parisons. Within a group the pattern usually holds and the individual
bones are readily homologized, taxa to taxa. Some may be lost but the
general relationships are relatively clear. Between groups there are greater
differences and the homology of individual bones is less clear.

A simple example is given in figure 2.7. What is the homology of the
bone in *Holoptychius* that fills the position occupied by the postparietal
and supratemporal in *Eusthenopteron*? And what does this say about the

homologies of the laterally flanking bone series carrying the lateral line canal? This example is often used to argue two vying ad hoc theories, according to which dermal bone patterns in the skull evolve through: (a) bone fusion or (b) territorial invasion and replacement (Westoll 1941; Säve-Söderbergh 1941; Moy-Thomas 1938; Romer 1947; Parrington 1949, 1967).

Such questions cannot be settled on the basis of comparison of adult skulls alone. Fundamentally one needs to know the morphogenetic origin of each example. However, a lot can be accomplished by assembling large suites for material and looking for individual variations. Graham-Smith (1978) has reviewed this approach. But it must be pointed out that it is not legitimate to extrapolate from this and use a map of all the observed variations in a taxon as a representation of an ancestral dermal bone pattern consisting of a large number of small elements. To do so would be like analyzing all the positions that soccer or baseball players might take on the field during a season and concluding thereby that the games originally employed 35 players on each team.

Of course, if we argue from ad hoc positions concerning the morphogenesis of dermal bones (see below), then fusion or replacement becomes not a matter of evidence but of faith. A small amount of evidence might be forthcoming from the assembly of evolutionary transformation series to compare bone shapes and positions, but then we need an independent assessment of what is primitive or derived. However, the boot is usually on the other foot: the paleontologist often needs to use the dermal bone data for any analysis of evolutionary relationships.

A prime example of the use of pattern and relative position as a guide

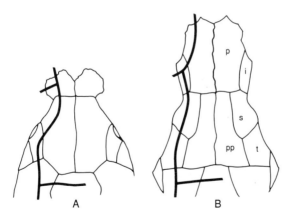

Fig. 2.7. The dermal bones of the posterior skull table in two "rhipidistian" fishes. A. *Holoptychius*. B. *Eusthenopteron*. Abbreviations: i, intertemporal; p, parietal; pp, postparietal; s, supratemporal; t, tabular.

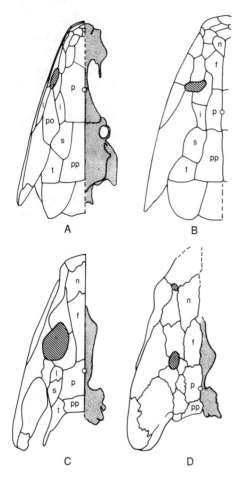

Fig. 2.8. Dermal skull of two osteolepiform fishes and two early amphibians, in dorsal aspect, showing relationship of the dermal bones to the underlying neurocranium. A. *Eusthenopteron.* B. *Panderichthys.* C. *Palaeoherpeton.* D. *Edops.* Abbreviations: f, frontal; i, intertemporal; l, lachrymal; p, parietal; pp, postparietal; s, supratemporal; t, tabular.

to bone homology is the comparison of the skull roof of *Eusthenopteron* with that of primitive tetrapods (fig. 2.8). In the long debate over this matter (Säve-Söderbergh 1941; Westoll 1943; Romer 1947; Thomson 1965; Jarvik 1967; Parrington 1967; Jarvik 1980; and for review, Borgen 1983) two basic schemes have emerged. Either (a) the two main pairs of bones in *Eusthenopteron* are the parietals (flanking the pineal) and the postparietal (in which case in tetrapods the extrascapular series has been lost from the back of the skull), or (b) the bones just mentioned are the frontal and parietal, respectively, in which case the posterior pair of bones in the tetrapod skull roof is the equivalent of the fish extrascapular series. There are parallel consequences for the homology of the flanking bone series and the position relative to the midline series. In support of the latter view Jarvik (1967; cf. Borgen 1983) uses the argument that the presence of five major paired bones (premaxillae, nasals, frontals, parietals, and postparietals) is so fundamental that they must already be represented in osteolepiform fishes such as *Eusthenopteron*. By counting back they find the five sets of bones as follows: extrascapular (= postparietal in tetrapods), parietal, rostral complex (= frontal and nasal in tetrapods), and premaxillae.

On the basis of dermal bone arrangements alone, the matter would appear to have been greatly clarified, or even settled, by the discovery that the osteolepiform fishes *Elpistostege* (Westoll 1938) and *Panderichthys* (e.g., Schultze and Arsenault 1985) show an intermediate condition between the *Eusthenopteron* and tetrapod patterns. Both have a distinct pair of "frontal" bones in addition to the rostral (fig. 2.8). The origin of a new bone pair is a predictable intermediate stage in the traditional system of bone homologies, particularly given the relative elongation of the rostral and facial region of the skull in the transition. Ironically this means that the osteolepiforms have the hypothetical five pairs of bone after all (the nasals reasonably being deriveable from the rostral complex) and that the piscine extrascapular series is not part of the skull roof, just as Westoll, Romer, and Parrington had argued.

To settle the matter, however, we have to examine two of the other major assumptions underlying the rival schemes of homology—the possibility of causal relationships of dermal bone patterns to the lateral-line system and to the neurocranium.

The Lateral-Line System

In 1898 Allis proposed a theory of skull homology according to which the lateral lines of the head play a dominant causal role in shaping dermal bone patterns. If this were true then one would expect that there would be a constant relationship between features of the lateral-line system and at least some dermal bones. Westoll (1936, 1941) used this theory in discussing dermal bone patterns and coined the term "anamestic" for those elements filling in spaces between the lateral-line-bearing elements—with the explicit notion that anamestic bones were less constant and perhaps impossible to homologize, because they lacked a constant relationship with the lateral line. Graham-Smith (1978) gives a review both of the comparative morphological evidence and of the scanty experimental and observational developmental data. After all the polemics are put aside, the answer to the question of whether there is a constant relationship between the lateral line and the dermal bones seems to be—sometimes yes and sometimes no. The "pit-line" system is even more unreliable.

A common practice (for example, Jarvik 1980) is to assume that the course of lateral lines in the head is changed by the fusion of dermal bones. It seems to me, however, that one might with profit examine the opposite—that changes in the position of the lateral lines cause changes in the pattern of the dermal bones. Similarly, while it is a reasonable argument that homologous segments of the lateral-line system should be similarly innervated, there is strong evidence (Jarvik 1980) that innervation is not a key to homology but may be more opportunistic.

In general, lateral-line relationships show considerable within-group consistency. Comparing actinopterygians and rhipidistians (figs. 2.9 and 2.10), lateral-line relationships show many basic similarities, but the Dip-

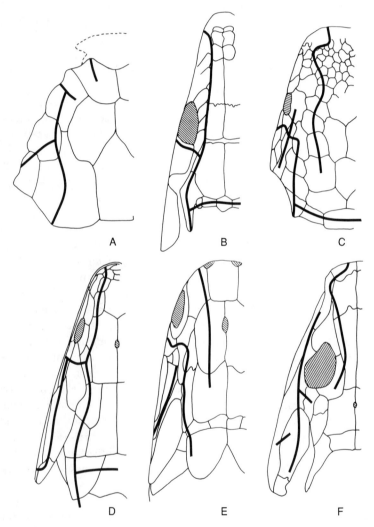

Fig. 2.9. Dermal skulls of six representative gnathostomes (see fig. 2.6), showing the major elements of the lateral-line system.

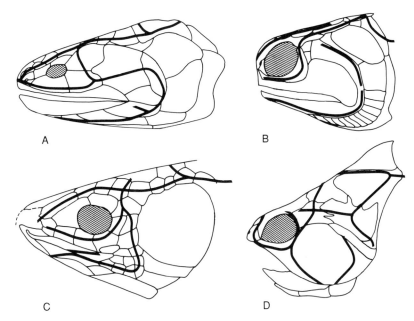

Fig. 2.10. Lateral view of the dermal bones of the head in four representative fishes, showing lateral-line canals. A. Dipnoan. B. Actinopterygian. C. Placoderm. D. Osteolepiform.

noi, with their mosaic dermal skull roof, as usual do not fit. In the case of the rhipidistian-tetrapod comparison, Allis's theory is central to the Säve-Söderbergh/Jarvik plans of bone homology, the supraoccipital commissure of the lateral line crossing the final bones in series in osteolepiforms and *Ichthyostega* (but not other tetrapods).

If the Westoll/Romer/Parrington scheme for the origin of the tetrapod skull is correct, at the fish-tetrapod transition the transverse occipital commissure between the principal lateral lines, which in fishes traverses the extrascapular series, has to become associated with the pair of bones in front (postparietals).

Graham-Smith (1978) has drawn heavily on lateral-line relationships to put together an elegant hypothetical scheme by which the dermal skull roof patterns of the placoderms and the major groups of osteichthyans can be rationalized into a single scheme (fig. 2.11) by postulating a series of intermediate stages that require some major assumptions about the lateral-line system and changes in the shape of the head (see below).

The Neurocranium and Visceral Skeleton

In most vertebrates, the skull roof is quite firmly attached to the underlying neurocranium; the cheek is directly associated functionally with the pala-

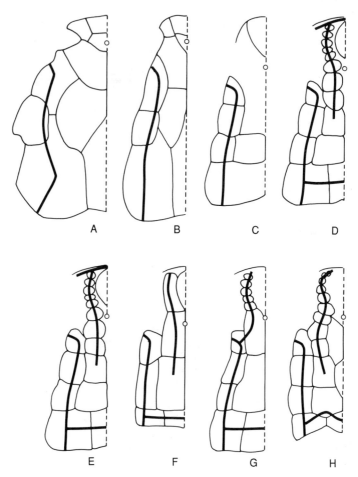

Fig. 2.11. Graham-Smith's hypothetical scheme linking the dermal bone arrangement of the head in four gnathostomes. A. Placoderm condition. F. Hypothetical early actinopterygian. G. Osteolepiform. H. Dipnoan. B, C, D, and E. Hypothetical intermediate stages.

toquadrate; and the stapes is a large, mechanically important element that integrates skull function in most fishes, "stegocephalian" amphibians, and early reptiles. Therefore one might expect to find strong relational consistencies, reflecting causal connections between dermal bone patterns and those underlying structures. This premise is central to the Westoll/Romer/Parrington scheme of osteolepiform-tetrapod dermal bone homology.

The key structures of the neurocranium as far as the dermal skull roof is concerned are clearly the pineal complex (because the pineal opening perforates the skull roof either within a single bone or between a pair of bones) and the nasal and otic capsules, both of which are sheathed dorsally by dermal bones. For the crossopterygians and the fish-tetrapod transition, the line of the intracranial joint is also useful.

In the case of placoderm-osteichthyan comparisons, Graham-Smith's scheme is consistent with the view that there is a constant relationship between the otic capsules and one pair of large posterior roofing bones in all gnathostomes (fig. 2.12). It is tempting to see this as confirmatory evidence that these elements are homologous.

In the actinopterygian-sarcopterygian comparison, the general similarity in pattern in the dermal bones alone is reinforced by the consistency in relationship to the otic capsules of the large posterior pair of median elements (called parietals in actinopterygians and either parietals or postparietals in the lobe-fins).

In the case of the *Eusthenopteron-Paleoherpeton* comparison (fig. 2.12; cf. fig. 2.8), the otic capsules and pineal relationships provide extremely useful information. The Säve-Söderbergh/Jarvik scheme of bone homology requires that the pineal opening shift from a position between the frontals and the parietals, whereas it retains its associations in the Westoll/Romer/Parrington scheme. It is worth noting that the constancy of relationship of the pineal is accomplished by the pineal developing a long anteriorly directed stalk in some tetrapods, whereas if it were to change the pair of bones with which it was associated, a small vertical passage alone would suffice. Further, there is a very constant relationship of the otic capsules and postparietals that clearly shows that the differences between the fish and tetrapod conditions reflect basic changes in the relative proportions of the head. Indeed, if one places faith in trends, the beginnings of this occur within the osteolepiforms with the origin of separate frontals. Finally, there is a hint of the old intracranial joint in *Ichthyostega* (Jarvik 1980), and its position in the neurocranium can be inferred in other early tetrapods. In every case it matches most closely with the parietal/postparietal contact (Westoll/Romer/Parrington scheme).

The neurocranial evidence, together with the evidence from the skull roof of *Panderichthys*, is sufficient to allow us to conclude that the scheme of homology shown in figure 2.8 is correct. In this case (because nomenclature is transferred backward from *Homo*) the bones customarily termed "parietals," "frontals," and "nasals" in actinopterygian fishes should be renamed "postparietals," "parietals," and "frontals," respectively, in order to bring them into line with the tetrapod system.

The dipnoan skull roof is another interesting puzzle. Dipnoans are clearly osteichthyans belonging to the Sarcopterygii group. What is the explanation of their unique dermal pattern—a mosaic of polygonal bones? One view (Westoll 1949) is that they represent the primitive skull pattern, perhaps for all osteichthyans. This accords with the more general theory

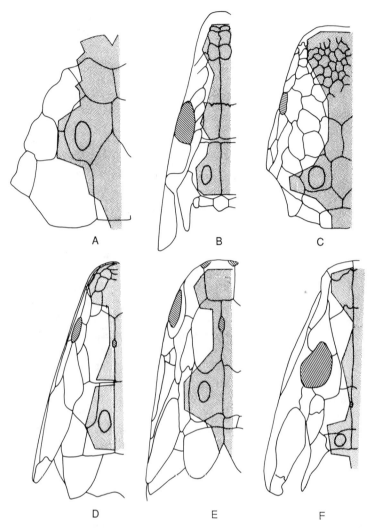

Fig. 2.12. Dorsal view of the head in six representative gnathostomes, as in figure 2.6, showing relationship to the neurocranium.

that dermal skeletal patterning in all vertebrates derives from an ancestral micromeric mosaic of multitudinous small scales, from which various dermal elements have arisen in different patterns of fusion.

A more empirical explanation derives from comparisons among sarcopterygians. It turns out that in many fishes, in regions of the skull where the dermal bones are closely fused to the underlying neurocranium, and where the dermal bones do not transfer a unique set of mechanical forces (from jaw or gill action), a mosaic arrangement appears (as in the snout of *Holoptychius*). Where the dermal bones carry strictly oriented forces, larger elements of discrete shape appear. In dipnoans the whole skull roof is closely plastered onto the neurocranium and the palatal system is also fused into this complex. A pattern of larger elements is not formed. The dipnoan mosaic may therefore be primitive in an ontogenetic sense, but not in an evolutionary one. In comparison with the patterns seen in primitive actinopterygians, or even *Eusthenopteron*, it is strictly secondary, a direct consequence of the specialized skull mechanics.

The Dipnoi are consistent with other osteichthyans in having a constant association of a large pair of bones with the otic capsules. These elements are buttressed from below by dorso-lateral flanges from the braincase. The presence of a strong medial row of bones in the dipnoan skull roof probably has a functional explanation in the totally autostylic skull and the presence of a dorso-median crest of the neurocranium separating two large muscle chambers in the back half of the skull, immediately under the dermal roof.

Soft Tissue Markers

Soft tissue markers have long been used as guides to the homology of different regions of the neurocranium. In particular, Goodrich (1930) provided an elegant summary of the use of cranial nerve, blood vessel, and notochordal markers in the unraveling of the homology of the lateral braincase wall (leaving behind one major problem in the homology of this region during the reptile-mammal transition, namely the homology of the mammalian alisphenoid). Apart from the pineal complex, and possibly the spiracle, soft tissue markers have been less useful in deciphering dermal skull roof homologies.

Dermal Bone Morphogenesis

All of the above cause us to focus attention on the mechanics of dermal bone morphogenesis. We know (review in Hall 1987) that epithelio-mesenchymal interactions are crucial in all dermal bone morphogenesis. The available data on morphogenetic pattern control in the skull has been reviewed in this work by Thorogood (vol. 1, chap. 4; cf. Thomson 1987). In general more data are needed to resolve the questions of bone homology that Allis posed. From the work of Devillers (1947) for example, we know that lateral-line neuromasts trigger (induce?) the concentration of mesenchyme around them and form the focus of dermal bone growth. So, in a sense, the neuromasts cause the pattern. But what is the cause of the prior patterning of the neuromasts? Both the neuromasts and the mesenchyme have to migrate to their target positions from elsewhere. There is every reason to expect that a layer of control resides in the generation of patterned extracellular matrices by the basal membrane of the epithelium. Is there perhaps a field phenomenon of intersecting wave fronts or lateral inhibition that causes patterns of spacing of centers relative to the whole surface of the head? Or do the neuromast precursors migrate to previously uniquely specified sites? This approach has the potential finally to give some basis for the discussion over fusion or replacement of dermal bones.

With respect to a causal role of the otic capsules vis-à-vis dermal bone patterns, one possibility is that there is a direct inductive relationship between the otic primordia and dermal bone loci. Leibel (1976) has shown that in addition the growing otic capsules provide a "substrate" guiding the growth and spreading of the dermal elements overlying them. In either case, there is reason to see a causal connection between the two systems.

FUNCTIONAL CONSIDERATIONS

Most treatments of the homology of the dermal skeleton ignore the question of the functional roles of the different elements, yet this may be highly significant. In general, homologies are easy to spot where there has been obvious continuity of function in a phylogenetic series and become difficult in proportion to the degree of functional difference, either in a single element or a complex of elements. This is no more than another way of saying that within-group comparisons are easier than between-group comparisons.

In analyzing the functional aspects of skulls, and particularly of the patterns of dermal bones, it would be highly productive if we were to try sometimes to ignore the bones themselves and to look upon the dermal skull as a series of sutures and joints. Arguably, it is the arrangement of the suture lines that is crucial in the functioning of the dermal skull.

The cheek and mandible make a good place to start (fig. 2.10), because here the shapes of the bones obviously reflect different arrangements of forces and the entirely different function of the oral-branchial apparatus (in both feeding and respiration) among placoderms, actinopterygians, crossopterygians, and dipnoans. For example, in *Moy-Thomasia* (fig. 2.6E), the role of the cheek series in anchoring to the underlying hyomandibular is quite different from that in osteolepiforms, as is shown by the principal suture line in the cheek being parallel to the orientation of the underlying hyomandibular.

The skull table is more complex. However, if we make the simplifying assumption that the sutures are arranged roughly perpendicular to the lines of force, and assume that suture patterns are arranged so as to maximize their orientation to tensile and compressive forces and to minimize their orientation to shear, we can draw some simple maps of dermal skull patterns that give us new insights into the factors underlying the bone patterns (fig. 2.13). At once we see that the arrangement of the bones is highly functional. For example, in osteichthyans, the postparietal bones play a major role as the central anchors for force transmission in the skull table. A key part of skull structure and function is the relationship between the lateral skull table and the dorsal rim of the cheek, no doubt reflecting

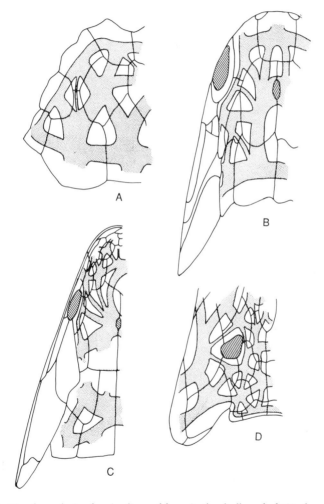

Fig. 2.13. Simple analysis of major lines of force in the skull roof of (A) placoderm, (B) actinopterygian, (C) osteolepiform, and (D) amphibian, showing lines of force transmission (in heavy line). The width of the force line is proportional to the length of the suture.

the pattern of respiratory mechanics. The whole tetrapod skull roof becomes reorganized when the cheek is no longer moveable. The differences among the major groups of fishes in terms of dermal bone arrangements clearly reflect major differences in the relative mechanical functions of the neurocranium, visceral skeleton, and dermal skeleton, particularly in feeding and respiratory movements.

NOTES TOWARD AN EXPLANATION OF DERMAL SKULL EVOLUTION AND HOMOLOGY

The above observations, despite the many gaps and difficulties, give us some clues toward an understanding of factors in the origin and evolution of gnathostome dermal bone patterns that can be tested against future comparative and experimental studies.

It is generally agreed among vertebrate paleontologists that the Gnathostomata and Agnatha are sister groups. In other words, no gnathostome is thought to be descended from any member of a known agnathan group; rather, both are descended from some common ancestor. The agnathan skull does not form the initial starting point for the evolution of the gnathostome skull, and particularly not for the dermal skull roof. We have to explain the special characters of gnathostomes as original rather than derivative.

The major gnathostome groups each deal with the major mechanical functions of the dermal skeleton (in connection with the neurocranium and primary jaws)—for the dentition, for stress transfer in connection with feeding, respiratory, and locomotory mechanics (in the sense of forming a system of fixed points and levers), as sites for muscle attachment, as passive protection—in significantly different ways. In particular, the placoderm head is constructed very differently from that of osteichthyans (dipnoans being yet a third mode). The conclusion that is forced upon us is that when true jaws first appeared there were at least three, and probably four, separate solutions to the problem of cranial architecture within the gnathostomes.

Two groups, Chondrichthyes and Acanthodii, solved the problem of inventing a new cranial mechanics by not forming a dermal skeleton of large, sutured dermal bones at all, but by having instead a flexible dermal skeleton armored with smaller, scalelike dermal units (whether this is primitive or derived is unclear). In these fishes, the dermal skeleton is not a major transmitter of mechanical forces, and especially not of compressive force, which must instead be transferred through the visceral and neurocranial skeleton. Their special condition is a flexibly articulated dermal skeleton, probably highly effective in response to tensile and shearing forces. Interestingly, some advanced acanthodians do develop a number of enlarged plates in the head region, and all acanthodians have a series of elongated scales in the gill covers. If, as seems to be the consensus view at the moment, Chondrichthyes and Acanthodii are not sister groups, then their dermal skeletons have probably evolved separately from those of the gnathostomes, in parallel.

This leaves the Placodermi and Osteichthyes, with dermal skulls made up of discrete bony elements of consistent shape. Their skull mechanics are such that these elements are major components for force transmission in the skull. While it is possible, as Graham-Smith (1978) has done, to create a hypothetical scheme linking placoderm and osteichthyan skull patterns in a linear sequence, there are in fact three possible schemes to account for placoderm-osteichthyan relationships.

The first is that the scheme proposed by Graham-Smith is generally correct, but we must add the proviso that the placoderms as we know them are not necessarily primitive. In principal any one of the "stages" in Graham-Smith's sequence could in fact be the ancestor for the rest. In this alternative we are assuming that the ancestor had an essentially complete dermal skull and that the dermal bones of any one group must be represented in some fashion by homologues in each of the others.

The second hypothesis is that placoderms and osteichthyans represent totally independent lines of evolution (as Gross 1962 concluded). The third is a compromise: that there was a common ancestor with a dermal skull skeleton but that it was incomplete and that the patterns seen in the major lines of fishes represent a mixture of transformation of the original bones in this pattern and independent evolution of other elements that are unique to their own clades.

All three hypotheses are basically testable, if at all, only in terms of the fossil record. The first predicts the eventual discovery of intermediate forms with complete skull roofs; the second predicts that no intermediates will be found (hardly a rigorous test); and the third predicts that fossils will be found with a different, incomplete, skull roof.

In addition, to discuss these hypotheses, we need to recognize the factors that may possibly be causal with respect to the patterning of the dermal skull. We may list at least the following:

1. The pattern of the lateral-line and pit-line system. This is dictated by its own functional demands, principally the lines of streamline flow of water over the head in swimming, and thus may basically depend upon the shape of the head, which is controlled in part by the other factors listed below. In any case, the eventual dermal bone pattern in part will reflect this distribution, rather than vice versa.
2. The general shape and proportions of the neurocranium and, therefore,

3. Particular neurocranial features, especially the nasal and otic capsules, the orbits, the parietal openings, and the hypophysial opening.
4. The newly evolved gnathostome jaw system, from mechanical suspensorium to jaw musculature, which is still functionally part of the branchial apparatus, especially in terms of the mechanics of expanding the orobranchial chamber. Therefore,
5. The mechanical configuration of the branchial apparatus, which reflects the basic functional patterning and adaptation of the orobranchial apparatus.
6. Morphogenetic relationships that may pre-exist among different elements (for example, the lateral line and dermal skeletogenesis) or subsequently develop (possibly the role of the otic capsule).

With respect to the first hypothesis of placoderm-osteichthyan origins, it is necessary to assume that a complete skull roof composed of a small number of discrete elements was already in existence in the gnathostome ancestor before the evolution of the different characteristic gnathostome cranial mechanism(s). The obligatory fallback position, namely that this existed in the form of a micromeric squamation continuous with that of the trunk, is a false argument because we are not discussing the existence of a dermal skeleton per se, but the origin of discrete dermal bones with a specialized function and thus a particular set of morphogenetic patterning mechanisms. The first hypothesis specifies that a single such patterning mechanism exists in all gnathostomes, while the second predicts that there were at least two independent versions. The third predicts that different versions diverged sufficiently early on from an original simple scheme that many elements of each must be independently derived.

In the light of the preceding discussion we can specify a little of what the hypothetical basal condition of hypothesis three would have looked like. There would have been a basic lateral-line system with the main trunk-line supraorbital canal, an ethmoid commissure, and at least an infraorbital, cheek, and mandibular canal loop. Small dermal ossicles may have been associated with these canals. In this early stage, a marginal dentition had not arisen, so that all the bite was borne between a dermal palatal complex and the mandibular-tongue complex. Therefore, there was probably no dermal cheek series. But in the rostral region there were already the beginnings of a premaxillary-rostral bone complex. All that is necessary to postulate in the posterior skull roof is the existence of a pair of roofing bones associated with the otic capsules of a well-ossified neurocranium. Dermal bones sheathed the mandible and possibly the gular complex. The branchial apparatus was enclosed laterally by an opercular series. Finally, it seems very likely that some sort of extrascapular bone series linked the back of the head to the shoulder girdle.

From this condition, the placoderm-osteichthyan divergence involved the origin of fundamentally different specializations of the cranial mechanics, especially with respect to the evolution of a marginal dentition, branchial function, and the jaw mechanics as indicated by, among other things, analysis of force lines in the skull and the relative position of the branchial apparatus and neurocranium. Once the patterns were set in place, their underlying morphogenetic pattern control mechanisms were highly conserved through evolution. This argument, however, does not resolve the problem of the Dipnoi: whether they are a very early divergence from the Osteichthyes, or merely a later divergence from the sarcopterygians. I am inclined to argue for the former and to conclude with Graham-Smith that the strong development of median bones in the skull roof rather than paired bones represents a unique condition in this clade.

Once each pattern had become established, it developed strong interactive constraints and from that point on the skull had to evolve as a unit, the various factors sometimes completing the relationships changing. For example, in certain cases, if the skull proportions changed too greatly in a particular direction (like lengthening of the snout) new dermal elements not in the original plan were intercalated, such as the nasals and frontals in the fish-tetrapod transition.

REFERENCES

Abercrombie, M., and C. H. Waddington. 1957. The behavior of grafts of primitive streak beneath the primitive streak of the chick. *Journal of Experimental Biology* 14: 319–326.

Adelman, H. B. 1932. The development of the prechordal plate and mesoderm of *Amblystoma punctatum*. Journal of Morphology 543: 1–53.

Allis, E. P. 1898. On the morphology of certain of the bones of the cheek and snout of *Amia*. Journal of Morphology 1: 425–466.

Anderson, C. B., and S. Meier. 1981. The influence of the metameric pattern on migration of neural crest in the chick embryo. *Developmental Biology* 85: 385–402.

Balfour, F. M. 1876. The development of elasmobranch fishes. Journal of Anatomy and Physiology 11: 128–172.

Bertmar, G. 1959. On the ontogeny of the chondral skull in Characidae, with a discussion on the chondral base and the visceral chondrocranium in fishes. Acta zoologica 40: 203–364.

Bjerring, H. C. 1967. Does a homology exist between the basicranial muscle and the polar cartilage? Colloques internationaux, Centre national de la recherche scientifique 163: 223–267.

Borgen, U. J. 1983. Homologizations of skull roofing bones between tetrapods and osteolepiform fishes. Palaeontology 26: 735–753.

Chibon, P. 1966. Analyse expérimentale de la régionalization et les capacités morphogénétiques de la crête neurale chex l'amphibien urodele *Pleurodeles waltlii* Micah. Memoires, Société Fribourgeoise des sciences naturelles, Zoologie 36: 1–107.

Devillers, C. 1947. Recherches sur la crâne dermique des téléostéens. Annales de Paleontologie 33: 1–94.

Le Douarin, N. 1980. *The Neural Crest.* Cambridge: Cambridge University Press.

Goodrich, E. S. 1918. On the development of the segments of the head in *Scyllium.* Quarterly Journal of Microscopical Science 63: 1–30.

———. 1930. *Studies on the Structure and Development of Vertebrates.* London: MacMillan.

Goodwin, B. C., and L. E. H. Trainor. 1983. The ontogeny and phylogeny of the pentadactyl limb. In *Development and Evolution,* B. C. Goodwin, N. Holder, and C. C. Wylie, eds. Cambridge: Cambridge University Press.

Graham-Smith, W. 1978. On the lateral lines and dermal bones in the parietal region of some crossopterygian and dipnoan fishes. Philosophical Transactions of the Royal Society of London, 282 B: 41–105.

Gross, W. 1962. Peut-on homologuer les os des Arthrodires et des Teleostomes? Colloques internationaux, Centre national de la recherche scientifique 104: 69–74.

Hall, B. K. 1987. Tissue interactions in the development and evolution of the vertebrate head. In *Development and Evolution of the Neural Crest,* P. F. A. Maderson, ed. New York: Wiley.

Hörstadius, S. 1950. *The Neural Crest.* Oxford: Oxford University Press.

Hörstadius, S., and S. Sellman. 1946. Experimentalle Untersuchungen uber die Determination des Knorpeligen Kopfskelettes bei Urodelen. Nova acta societatis scientiarum Uppsaliensis, ser. 4, 13: 1–170.

Jacobson, A. G., and S. Meier. 1984. Morphogenesis of the head of a newt: Mesodermal segments, neuromeres, and distribution of neural crest. Developmental Biology 106: 181–193.

Jarvik, E. 1942. On the structure of the snout of crossopterygians and lower gnathostomes in general. Zoologiska Bidrag fran Uppsala 21: 63–127.

———. 1954. On the visceral skeleton in *Eusthenopteron,* with a discussion of the parasphenoid and palatoquadrate in fishes. Kungliga Svenska Vetenskapakademiens, Handlingar 5: 1–114.

———. 1963. The composition of the intermandibular division of the head in fish and tetrapods and the diphyletic origin of the tetrapod tongue. Kungliga Svenska Vetenskapsakademiens, Handlingar 9: 1–74.

———. 1967. The homologies of the frontal and parietal bones in fishes and tetrapods. Colloques internationaux, Centre national de la recherche scientifique 163: 181–213.

———. 1980. *Basic Structure and Development of Vertebrates.* London: Academic Press.

Jollie, M. 1968. Some implications of the acceptance of a delamination principle. In *Current Problems in Lower Vertebrate Phylogeny,* T. Orvig, ed. Stockholm: Almqvist and Wiksell.

———. 1971. A theory concerning the early evolution of the visceral arches. Acta zoologica 52: 85–96.

————. 1977. Segmentation of the vertebrate head. American Zoologist 17: 323–333.

————. 1984. The vertebrate head: Segmented or a single morphogenetic structure? Journal of Vertebrate Paleontology 4: 320–329.

Kingsbury, B. F. 1926. Branchiomerism and the theory of head segmentation. Journal of Morphology 42: 83–109.

Langille, R. M., and B. K. Hall. 1988a. Development of the head skeleton of the Japanese medaka *Oryzias latipes* (Teleostei). Anatomy and Embryology 177: 297–305.

————. 1988b. Evidence for neural crest contribution to the skeleton of sea lamprey *Petromyzon marinus*. Developmental Biology 102: 301–310.

Le Lièvre, C. S. 1978. Participation of neural crest–derived cells in the genesis of the skull in birds. Journal of Embryology and Experimental Morphology 47: 17–27.

Le Lièvre, C. S., and N. M. Le Douarin. 1975. Mesenchymal derivatives of the neural crest: Analysis of chimaeric quail and chick embryos. Journal of Embryology and Experimental Morphology 47: 17–27.

Leibel, W. 1976. The influence of the otic capsule in ambystomid skull formation. Journal of Experimental Zoology 196: 85–103.

Lombard, R. E., and J. R. Bolt. 1988. Evolution of the stapes in Paleozoic tetrapods. In *The Evolution of the Amphibian Auditory System,* B. Fritsch, ed. New York: Wiley.

Meier, S. 1981. Development of the chick embryo mesoblast: Formation of the prechordal plate and cranial segment. Developmental Biology 83: 49–61.

————. 1984. Somite formation and its relation to metameric patterning of the mesoderm. Cell Differentiation 14: 235–242.

Meier, S., and D. S. Packard. 1984. Morphogenesis of the cranial segments and distribution of the neural crest in the embryos of the snapping turtle *Chelydra serpentina.* Developmental Biology 102: 309–323.

Moy-Thomas, J. A. 1938. The problem of the evolution of the dermal bones in fishes. In *Evolution: Essays on Aspects of Evolutionary Biology,* G. R. de Beer, ed. Oxford: Oxford University Press.

Neal, H. V. 1918. Neuromeres and metameres. Journal of Morphology 31: 293–315.

Newth, D. R. 1956. On the neural crest of the lamprey embryo. Journal of Embryology and Experimental Morphology 4: 358–375.

Noden, D. M. 1982. Patterns and organization of cranio-facial skeletogenic and myogenic mesenchyme: A perspective. In *Factors and Mechanisms Influencing Bone Growth,* A. D. Dixon and B. Sarnat, eds. New York: A. R. Liss.

————. 1983a. The embryonic origins of avian cranio-facial muscles and associated connective tissues. American Journal of Anatomy 168: 257–276.

————. 1983b. The role of the neural crest in patterning avian cranial skeletal, connective, and muscle tissues. Developmental Biology 96: 144–165.

————. 1984. Cranio-facial development: New views on old problems. Anatomical Record 208: 1–13.

Parrington, F. R. 1949. A theory of the relations of the lateral lines to dermal bones. Proceedings of the Zoological Society of London, pp. 119–165.

————. 1967. The identification of the dermal bones of the head. Journal of the Linnean Society, Zoology 47: 231–239.

Romer, A. S. 1947. Review of the Labyrinthodontia. Bulletin of the Museum of Comparative Zoology at Harvard 99: 1–368.

————. 1977. The vertebrate as dual animal: Somatic and visceral. Evolutionary Biology 6: 121–156.

Säve-Söderbergh, S. 1941. Notes on the dermal bones of the head of *Osteolepis macrolepidotus* Ag., and the interpretation of the lateral line system in primitive vertebrates. Zoologiska Bidrag fran Uppsala 20: 523–541.

Schultze, H.-P., and M. Arsenault. 1985. The panderichthyid fish *Elpistostege:* A close relative of tetrapods? Palaeontology 28: 293–309.

Stone, L. S. 1926. Further experiments on the extirpation and transplantation of mesectoderm in *Amblystoma punctatum.* Journal of Experimental Biology 44: 95–131.

————. 1929. Experiments showing the role of migrating neural crest (mesectoderm) in the formation of head skeleton and loose connective tissue in *Rana palustris.* Wilhelm Roux' Archiv für Entwicklungsmechanik der Organismen 118: 40–77.

Tam, P. P. L., and S. Meier. 1982. The establishment of a somitomeric pattern in the mesoderm of the gastrulating mouse embryo. American Journal of Anatomy 164: 209–225.

Thomson, K. S. 1965. The endocranium and associated structures in the Middle Devonian rhipidistian fish *Osteolepis.* Proceedings of the Linnean Society, London 176: 181–195.

————. 1987. Speculations concerning the role of the neural crest in the morphogenesis and evolution of the vertebrate skeleton. In *Development and Evolution of the Neural Crest,* P. F. A. Maderson, ed. New York: Wiley.

————. 1988. *Morphogenesis and Evolution.* New York: Oxford University Press.

van Valen, L. 1982. Homology and causes. Journal of Morphology 173: 305–315.

Westoll, T. S. 1936. On the structure of the dermal ethmoid shield of *Osteolepis.* Geological Magazine 73: 157–171.

————. 1938. Ancestry of the tetrapods. Nature 141: 127.

————. 1941. Latero-sensory canals and dermal bones. Nature 148: 168–169.

————. 1943. The origin of the tetrapods. Biological Reviews 18: 78–98.

Westoll, T. S. 1949. On the evolution of the Dipnoi. In *Genetics, Paleontology and Evolution,* G. L. Jepsen, G. G. Simpson and E. Mayr, eds. Princeton: Princeton University Press.

Whiting, H. P. 1972. Cranial anatomy of ostracoderms in relation to the organization of larval lampreys. In *Studies in Vertebrate Evolution,* K. A. Joysey and T. S. Kemp, eds. Edinburgh: Oliver and Boyd.

————. 1977. Cranial nerves in lampreys and cephalaspids. In *Problems in Vertebrate Evolution,* S. M. Andrews, ed. London: Academic Press.

3

Cranial Skeletal Tissues: Diversity and Evolutionary Trends

WILLIAM A. BERESFORD

INTRODUCTION

Context and Aims

CHESS EMBODIES SHIFTS IN THE POSITIONS of variously shaped, white or black pieces. The comparative morphology of the skull substitutes cartilage versus bone for the distinction by color, and analyzes rather than initiates the moves, but otherwise is not too fanciful a parallel. However, his or her knowledge of the game does not equip the chess player with reasoned expectations of the materials science of wood, ivory, metal, or plastic, or of the chemistry of any lacquer coating the pieces. Engineers, meanwhile, seldom are grand masters. In terms of the skull, much concerning cranial tissues is counterintuitive to the gross morphology of the skull and cranial evolution, as a few examples may show.

Bone, cartilage, and the other connective tissues in many respects are more alike than different, and extensively share materials for construction and for communication. Tissues are not absolutely stable, but sometimes turn into another type (metaplasia). The early vertebrates employed more subtypes of bone and cartilage than did later vertebrates. If range of tissue diversity is a measure of cellular powers of control, lower vertebrates appear in their cells to be more advanced than homeotherms. This paradox of light-microscopic histology has to be set against evidence that the molecular and biochemical activities of cells grow somewhat more complex during evolution (Gaill et al. 1991). Lastly, dentine, the hard core of a tooth supporting the enamel, appears well after bone in the embryology of extant vertebrates, but was probably the forerunner of bone in evolution.

Leaving aside dental tissues, it takes several skeletal tissues to construct a skull. The skull comprises an enclosing case of firm or rigid skeletal pieces held together by connective tissue, with additional pieces made more movable for respiration, sensory function, communication, and coping with food (see vol. 3 of this work). Most vertebrate classes use two principal tissues to construct the pieces and a selection of other tissues for

69

the accessory roles. Movement requires specialized tissues for inserting tendons and ligaments into the skeleton, and elsewhere for joining or capping the pieces at joints or sites of padding. Bone or cartilage can serve in the same taxon both as major pieces and in an accessory role. Also, bone or cartilage may be the main tissue in the exoskeleton, but subservient in the endoskeleton, or vice versa.

This chapter will briefly discuss the nature, locations, and diversity of the tissues individually, and seek common ground among the tissues in the behavior of cells and in the kinds of molecule that the cells make and use for these behaviors. The links revealed are among skeletal cell types and tissues, and between skeletal cells and nonskeletal cells of vertebrates and invertebrates. Looking at tissues at cellular and molecular levels serves several purposes. One goal is to understand what exactly bone- and cartilage-forming cells (osteoblasts and chondroblasts) are doing, i.e., the basis of their identities or phenotypes. A second aspect of phenotype is how these cellular activities are regulated, both in executing a selection of the instructions encoded in the genes, and in responding to the influences of other cells and tissues. A third aim is to make more sense of the distributions of microscopically defined subtypes of bone, of dentine and related hard tissues, and of cartilage, among early and extant vertebrates. Many authors have debated the evolutionary significance of the histologically discernible tissue subtypes (see Schaffer 1930; de Beer 1937; Ørvig 1951; Halstead 1969, 1973, 1974; Hall 1975, 1978, 1984; Moss 1964b, 1977; Patterson 1977; Moss and Moss-Salentijn 1983; Gans and Northcutt 1983; Maisey 1988; Francillon-Vieillot et al. 1990; and Smith and Hall 1990). My offering is to speculate in two ways on how the original skeletal cells might have come by their novel repertoires, considering first which cell behaviors were possible forerunners for skeletal cellular properties, and then possible invertebrate circumstances favoring bone or cartilage formation. These invertebrate-vertebrate transitions might also illuminate what has happened to cranial tissues during vertebrate existence, and in a roundabout way help solve critical questions, e.g., what is an osteoblast? Other questions may be more intriguing than critical, such as: Why were chondroid (cartilagelike) tissues largely abandoned after the fishes? Why are rabbits out on a limb biochemically? Why does osteodentine crop up every so often? Thus, running through this review of skeletal tissues and their diversity will be the additional threads of experimental approaches relating tissues to skeletal function, of cellular and molecular events, and of some evolutionary considerations.

Hard, Resilient, and Soft Connective Tissues

Hardness is a familiar and palpable property with which to start classifying cranial tissues (table 3.1). Into the hard category fall many kinds of

TABLE 3.1 Molecular overview of cranial skeletal tissues

Tissue	Texture	Molecular species
Bone, dentine, and cementum	Hard	Collagens I, (III), Osteopontin/Bone sialoprotein I, Bone sialoprotein II*, Osteonectin, Osteocalcin*; Decorin and Biglycan (small proteoglycans), Fibrillin; Alkaline phosphatase; Cytokines, e.g., Transforming growth factor-β
Hyaline cartilage	Resilient	Collagens II, VI, IX, XI, Aggrecan = Chondroitin sulfate/Keratan sulfate proteoglycan + Link protein*; Hyaluronic acid; Small proteoglycans: Fibromodulin, Decorin; Cartilage-matrix protein*, Fibronectin
Fibrous tissues	Soft	Collagens I, III, V, VI, XII, XIV; Proteoglycans: Decorin, Biglycan, Fibromodulin; Fibronectin, Thrombospondin, Tenascin, Fibrillin, Osteonectin
Calcified hyaline cartilage	Hard	Type X collagen*, Alkaline phosphatase + most hyaline cartilage molecules
Calcified fibrocartilage	Hard	Insufficient analyses
Chondroid bone	Hard	Disputed among sites
Chordoid tissues	Resilient	Insufficient analyses
Chondroid tissues	Resilient	Insufficient analyses
Fibrocartilage	Resilient	Collagens I, III, Thrombospondin + most hyaline-cartilage molecules
Elastic cartilage	Resilient	Elastin, Glial fibrillary acidic protein + hyaline-cartilage molecules

* Tissue-specific molecules.

bone, at least four varieties of cementum (the bone on the roots of teeth), several dentines, mineralized forms of hyaline cartilage and fibrocartilage, and intermediates between bone and cartilage—chondroid bone. Resilient tissues lack hardness, but they resist compression and are stiff. Resilient cartilages (hyaline, elastic, and fibrocartilage) participate in the skull, but the picture is clouded because of long-standing debate over the nature of numerous other resilient tissues that either resemble cartilage ("chondroid"), or are close in appearance to notochord ("chordoid"). The third category comprises the soft connective tissues. These are dense, strong, and flexible—qualities attributable to various weaves and bundles of collagen fibers—with a supporting cast of various kinds of gluing, water-binding, cell-attaching, and other molecules.

Molecular Basis of Skeletal Tissues

Before considering the cranial tissues individually, I shall briefly tabulate them against a background of the types of structural molecule employed, and of the idea of combinatorial power. A "structural molecule" is one used to construct the extracellular matrix (ECM) that confers particular biomechanical properties on each cranial skeletal tissue. There are, of course, many other types of molecule needed for tissue-specific function, for example, receptors for signals that coordinate the replacement of cartilage by bone in endochondral ossification.

Skeletal tissues are connective, requiring that the cells produce ECM. This acquires mechanical properties by the interaction of domains on a variety of protein molecules. More versatility is furnished by adding sugar groups to a core protein to create glycoproteins, or by adding sugars of a restricted class (which form unbranched, negatively charged sugar chains) to form proteoglycans. There are several classes of ECM molecule: (a) *sticky glycoproteins,* such as fibronectin and tenascin, to control cell movement and hence position, and others, e.g., cartilage matrix protein, to help stick fibrils together; (b) *proteoglycans* (Goetinck 1991; Hardingham and Fosang 1992), which, for example, create resilience by two means: binding water with their excess of negative charge; and amplifying this effect by aggregating the proteoglycans by linking them to a backbone molecule of hyaluronan/hyaluronate; (c) *collagens* of various types (table 3.2), some to build fibrils for tensile strength, others to assist in assembling the fibrils and determining their diameter; (d) other fibrillar materials, e.g., *fibrillin,* associated with *elastin;* (e) special *mineralizing* glycoproteins that, with the aid of proteoglycans and collagen, somehow cause the precipitation of calcium salts (mostly hydroxyapatite) to mineralize or calcify collagenous or cartilaginous matrices; (f) *enzymes* to destroy matrix components and enzyme inhibitors to restrain the process.

TABLE 3.2   Types of collagen and their distribution in mammals

Type	Classification	Location
I	Fibrillar	Hard and soft connective tissues, but not hyaline cartilage
II	Fibrillar	Cartilage matrix, eye's vitreous, inner ear, many embryonic sites
III	Fibrillar	Immature connective tissues, reticular tissues, and as a small supplement to type I in mature tissues
IV	Sheet-forming	Basement membranes
V	Fibrillar	Accompanies type I
VI	Filament-forming	Cartilage matrix, elastic tissue
VII	Anchoring fibrils	Anchoring basement membranes of stratified squamous epithelia to dermis/lamina propria
VIII	Sheet-forming	Endothelial basement membranes in vessels and cornea
IX	FACIT*	Accompanying type II in cartilage matrix
X	—	Hypertrophic cartilage
XI	Fibrillar	Cartilage matrix, cornea
XII	FACIT	Accompanying type I
XIV	FACIT	Accompanying type I

* FACIT: Fibril-Associated Collagens with InterrupTed helices (globular domains interrupt the helix).

Combinatorial Power

"Combinatorial power" refers to how cells and organisms deploy mechanisms to select various combinations of entities (Mayer and Baldi 1991). This combining of entities greatly enhances the usefulness of an often quite limited range of options. Cells generate extensive diversity by means of combinations of relatively few entities, be they: (1) domains or working regions in molecules; (2) molecules combined in like (homo) or unlike (hetero) dimers/pairs or trimers/triplets; (3) regulatory DNA regions for a particular gene; (4) transcription factors to bind to the gene's regulatory DNA and/or each other in order to specify which molecules are made; (5) types of collagen, proteoglycan, and glycoprotein to construct the ECMs of connective tissues; (6) peptide and other signaling molecules to allow cells to coordinate their work; (7) choices of fiber or fibril diameter and orientation; and (8) profiles of molecules in an ECM to underpin its mechanical properties. A single entity that is truly tissue- or cell-type-specific is rare. What is distinctive is the combination of entities, which has made the concept of tissues hard to grapple with.

Collagen

Collagen—the main building material of skeletal tissues—specifically illustrates combinatorial power. All collagen molecules are trimers of three helical α amino-acid chains intertwined, mostly as a robust superhelix, e.g., $[\alpha\text{-}1(II)]_3$ in cartilage, $[\alpha1(IV)_2\alpha2(IV)]$ in basement membrane—the support for epithelia. (The two-number designation gives the molecule's chain type in roman and subtype in arabic, and the subscript shows how many of that particular chain go to make a trimer.) Collagen molecules differ in their amounts of helical versus globular shapes along the molecule (fig. 1 in Burgeson 1988, 553). The ones (fibrillar) that are chopped up by enzymes to be only helical assemble into fibrils, the others (nonfibrillar) attach to and space the fibrils in scaffolds of various patterns, fibril-widths, densities, and strengths, appropriate to the mechanics of the tissue. Some of the scaffold-gluing ones are termed Fibril-Associated Collagens with InterrupTed helices, or FACIT. The types (table 3.2) are somewhat tissue-specific, but not nearly as much as once was thought. Lessons from table 3.2 are that even the more tissue-restricted collagens are still shared, e.g., collagen II between ocular and inner-ear tissues and hyaline cartilage. But one is unique: collagen type X in endothermic hypertrophic cartilage. Next, several collagens may be at work at a site, in proportions that will themselves vary during development and aging.

Limits

Turning to all the molecules that are used to construct skeletal tissues (table 3.1), we find that although tissues are recognized histologically, the molecular information is often lacking. Other points need comment. The drive for clinically relevant science skews knowledge overwhelmingly toward noncranial skeletal tissues of mammals, on which table 3.1 is based. One can cautiously extrapolate from human epiphysis to cranial base, but only direct analysis can fill the huge gaps in the table, for example, to identify the molecular types in piscine chondroid tissues. In mammalian and avian bone and cartilage, where many of the molecules are known, the pattern is that only a very few are tissue-specific. What is unique are the quantitative profiles of ECM molecules, usually the pattern of the fibrils and fibers, and certainly the profiles of cell-surface glycoproteins that receive signals, adhere to particular substrates, and attach to adjacent cells. What the table does not reveal is that certain ECM molecules may be shared not throughout the connective tissues, but among certain connective tissues and other organs. For example, bone shares several special molecules with the kidney, e.g., osteopontin.

Three distinctions that have occupied past workers are omitted from table 3.1: exoskeletal versus endoskeletal, dermal versus endochondral bone, and dentine versus bone and cementum. The first two distinctions involve mechanisms to initiate and site the tissue, but the phenotype of the tissue is essentially the same in each location, except for the differentiated cells' susceptibility to signals for local and systemic physiological integration. The conflation of bone, dentine, and cementum may surprise some readers. It is done because the molecular composition varies little among bone, cementum, and dentine, so the question becomes, how significant are the differences in cellular morphology? The short answer is that we do not know, although the evolutionary sequence of appearance of subtypes of hard tissues is known (Smith and Hall 1990), and one has an idea of relevant factors. Factors possibly influencing cellular shapes and dispositions are the direction and rate of growth, the sources of blood, the shape of the structure to be made, the future attachment of accessory tissues, and the number of generations of cells deployed (one, for dentine; successive generations for bone). Another argument for setting aside cellular morphology is that what defines bone has to be the matrix, not cellular and vascular inclusions or lamellation/layering—the properties that distinguish it from dentine—since some bone performs mechanically without internal cells, vessels, lamellae, and remodeling.

Such a reduction to the matrix could include as bone the tissue of the basal plate of certain fish scales which not only lacks cells, but is without mineral (Meunier and Huyseunne, n.d.). Although this illustrates how tissue realities evade capture by classificatory schemes, present purposes take bone to be hard. Problems of tissue classification and evolution, how combinations of basic structural elements are deployed among vertebrate hard tissues and in different taxa, and the different "levels of integration" (molecular, cellular, etc.) of tissues are topics included in the extensive review of Francillon-Vieillot et al. (1990). Their chapter defines and discusses virtually all the terms and processes related to hard skeletal tissues, proceeding level by level.

BONE, DENTINE, AND CEMENTUM

The principal bone-forming cells, osteoblasts, first synthesize and release the precursor form of collagen type I. This assembles outside the cells as densely packed fibrils (a smaller version of fibers), which vary in thickness and degree of orientation, thus offering one basis for classifying subtypes. This unmineralized matrix also includes small amounts of a variety of molecular types (table 3.1), some probably involved in fibril assembly and adhesion, others with the precipitation of fine needle-shaped crystals of calcium salts that convert the soft osteoid into hard bone. Meanwhile, the osteoblasts extend cell processes which persist within long, tiny spaces—canaliculi—in order to keep the cell alive and in indirect, metabolic communication with distant blood vessels. Dentine differs mainly in the migration of the cell body away from a single, ever-elongating, roughly unidirectional cell process. The odontoblast body is thereby not enclosed by matrix in a lacuna, but remains on the forming surface of dentine, and in consequence never has its name changed to "odontocyte." Cementum is bone that forms on the outside of the root dentine in order to anchor within it (by growth around and past them) the collagen fibers of the periodontal ligament. (Sharpey lent his name to such anchoring fibers of ligament, tendon, and the periosteal wrapping of bones.)

Thus, bone, dentine, and cementum comprise fibrous collagen of type I, combined with up to 80% by weight of small crystals of calcium-deficient hydroxyapatite, water, and small amounts of several noncollagenous proteins. Cells or cell processes are variably present in holes in the matrix. Despite the misleading "osteo" prefixes, bone and dentine both contain bone sialoprotein I (osteopontin), osteocalcin (glutamate-containing protein), osteonectin (a phosphoprotein), and bone small/type II proteoglycan. There are quantitative differences between bone and dentine in their contents of noncollagenous proteins, and mammalian dentine contains some additional kinds of sialoprotein and phosphoprotein (Butler 1984, 1991; Triffitt 1987): whether "additional" in being recent evolutionary acquisitions remains to be seen. (In both tissues, some of these proteins are apportioned very differently between the mineralized states and their soft collagenous precursors, osteoid and predentine.) There are other points of close identity between the three hard tissues. Levels of alkaline phosphatase are high in the formative cells. The fibrous matrices of woven bone and mantle dentine are similar. Varieties of bone exist that are formed by cells that retreat like odontoblasts as they deposit matrix. Vascular dentines and cementums leave bone not unique in including vessels. Actual intermediate forms, osteodentines, occur in both fishes and mammals. Finally, all three tissues are resorbed by the one kind of cell, the osteoclast.

Bone and cementum are unlike dentine in that their collagen may entirely comprise fibers made and oriented by fibroblasts as a prior soft connective tissue, which undergoes mineralization (Jones and Boyde 1972). This metaplastic ossification contributes significantly to some ectothermic bone, and in mammals participates in cementogenesis (Bosshardt and Schroeder 1991), osteogenesis at sutures, and at certain tendon and ligament insertions, and some later periosteal apposition.

Bone has been classified several times in different ways on the basis of its histology. Table 3.3 lists the many properties of bone that vary and could be used in subtyping. The goal of subtyping is to reveal what is significant for function and how the cells organize such outcomes. In the search for unifying factors hidden among the many dimensions of bony variation (table 3.3), some decisive controlling points for cell behavior stand out: whether osteocytes are included, or remain, in the bone, whether osteoclasts erode internally, and whether vessels are incorporated. As judged from their contrasting bone types, the means—epigenetic or genetic—for these controls existed in the early fishes.

Classifications of bone have changed. Extrinsic fibers of bone matrix are those made in advance as a component of a soft connective tissue adjacent to the bone. As these are incorporated into bone, osteoblasts usually add fine fibrils of collagen, as can be seen in metal-impregnated sections. The proportions of coarse and fine fibers, and the degree of fiber orientation, underlay earlier classifications of bone (e.g., Lubosch 1928; Weidenreich 1930), which paid attention to the metaplastic (tissue conversion) origin of some of the bone. More recent schemes (Enlow and Brown 1956; de Ricqlès 1974; Francillon-Vieillot et al. 1990) stressed vascularity (how many vessels are inside the bone), remodeling (destruction and replacement), and lamellation (the alternating layers of matrix with preferred and different fibrillar orientations). Polarized-light microscopy reveals the lamellation, but fidelity between lamellation and fibrillar architecture is not completely reliable (Reid 1986). As bone is partially eroded and replaced, different types can come to lie close together; and bone histology varies with the rate at which it is deposited and reworked. Thus, de Ricqlès

TABLE 3.3   Variables of bone

Aspect	Features that vary among bone types
Collagen fibers	Size, orientation, formative cells
Lamellation	Presence, site(s), prominence, orientation, lamellar width, interruption
Osteocytes	Presence, shape, orientation, spacing, size
Vessels	Presence, site(s), density, orientation
Remodeling	Extent, sites, pattern, orientation
Architecture	Porosity, cortical width and stratification, trabecular form
Chemistry	Mineral content, collagen content, amounts of noncollagenous proteins
Mechanical properties	Elasticity, ultimate tensile stress and strain, work to fracture, bending strength
Formation site	Mesenchyme, dermis, other fibrous tissue, endochondral, perichondral, on bone surfaces (external, internal dense, and internal trabecular)

(1974) termed "fibro-lamellar" the mixture of lamellar bone filling in between earlier formed, less regularly fibrillar trabeculae (internal struts). His "lamellar-zonal" type displayed prominent growth or incremental lines, reflecting repeated cessation and restarting of bone formation. De Ricqlès related fibrolamellar and lamellar-zonal types to different rates of growth and metabolism, but the anatomical distinction and the physiological connections are not entirely clear-cut and convincing (Reid 1984), and may be less relevant to the slower-growing skull than to other parts of the skeleton.

For discussing the skull, one broad comparison of vertebrate bone structure is Enlow and Brown's (1956, 1957, 1958). Moss (1961c) dealt with cranial bones of many recent teleosts. Enlow and Brown carried out extensive cranial comparisons by species, and made clear (Enlow 1969) how numerous epigenetic factors modify the histological picture, down to the level of regions of individual bones. They included and illustrated many mandibles, and sometimes mentioned other skull bones. Their classification rested heavily on vascularity and remodeling, yielding the following categories (figs. 3.1–3.8): (1) avascular, (2) primary (unremodeled) vascular, (3) secondary (remodeled) vascular, (4) special, where some other variable was dominant, e.g., the absence of cells in teleost acellular bone (fig. 3.9), or the tubules in bone of lepidosteoid fishes. Subcategories of the third main type, remodeled bone, recognized either major reconstruction, predominantly endosteal (on internal surfaces) (fig. 3.7), or the occurrence of only minor irregular Haversian/secondary replacement (fig. 3.8). The greatest variety is in primary vascular bone, with longitudinal, radial, reticular, plexiform, and laminar alignments of the vessels (figs. 3.2–3.5),

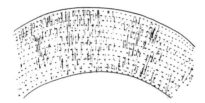

Fig. 3.1. Simple lamellar bone (nonvascular).

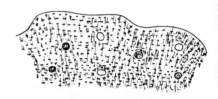

Fig. 3.2. Primary vascular bone (longitudinal).

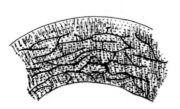

Fig. 3.3. Primary vascular bone (reticular).

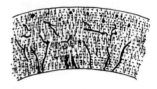

Fig. 3.4. Primary vascular bone (radial).

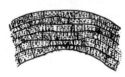

Fig. 3.5. Primary vascular bone (plexiform).

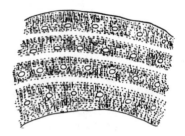

Fig. 3.6. Primary vascular bone (laminar).

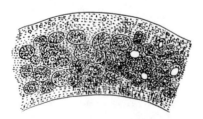

Fig. 3.7. Secondary bone tissue (dense Haversian).

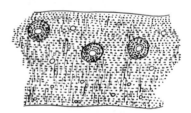

Fig. 3.8. Secondary bone tissue (irregular Haversian).

Figures 3.1–3.8 depict types of bone by drawings of transverse sections of long bones at approximately 100× magnification. They are reproduced with permission from Enlow and Brown (1956) and the Texas Academy of Sciences.

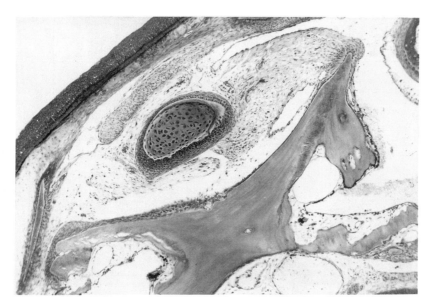

Fig. 3.9. Teleost acellular (parallel-fibered) bone in the maxillary of *Astatotilapia (Haplochromis) elegans*. Note the few vascular canals and the varying thickness of the cellular layer of the periosteum. Toluidine blue. 90× magnification. (Courtesy of A. Huysseune)

with corresponding patterns of bone around the vessels. Table 3.4 offers an interpretation of Enlow and Brown's (1958) conclusions for the mandible and skull, and follows their distinction between early and present-day forms in each vertebrate group. In general, mandibular types in tetrapods resembled those of the species' limb long bones, as expected from the limited functional parallels (English 1985). Other skull bones tend to be more cancellous/spongy or have larger marrow spaces in the compacta than did the long bones, and to be closer to rib than limb bones in the species.

A limitation of any such broad comparison is the variety of bone types present not only in one individual, but in one bone. This diversity is especially marked in large bones of old individuals, subject to modest remodeling and markedly asymmetric growth across the bone, where the location—periosteal or endosteal—greatly affects events in the bone. Such factors led Enlow (1969), when discussing reptilian bone, to introduce place in the bone as an additional element in the categorization. Three histologically different strata—superficial, middle, and basal—often are detectable where the bone is broad. Within a single layer, say, the superficial one, bone can be alternately vascular and avascular, or de Ricqlès's fibro-lamellar mixture.

TABLE 3.4 Cranial vertebrate bone types based on Enlow and Brown (1956, 1957, 1958)

	Fishes	Amphibians	Reptiles	Birds	Mammals
Early	Primary vascular, lamellar; secondary bone scarce *Exception:* acellular in heterostracan exoskeleton; tubular in Subholostei	Bone generally massive and lamellar; some endosteal or irregular remodeling	Dense, laminated bone; moderate or much remodeling *Exception:* turtles and crocodilians—mostly primary vascular	Vascular, lamellation weakly defined; some secondary systems	Laminar, with endosteal remodeling
Recent	Acellular, vascularity variable; some Sharpey-fiber regions *Exceptions:* "lower" teleosts and lungfishes—cellular, primary, vascularity variable	Delicate bones—lamellar, nonvascular Larger bones—mixed, primary vascular, and avascular	Turtles and crocodilians as earlier Snakes and lizards—avascular, lamellar	Large birds—primary vascular reticular Small birds—avascular	Primitive mammals—primary vascular Bats and insectivores—avascular or few vessels Ungulates—primary reticular or plexiform Rabbit—skull largely Haversian Carnivores—various primary forms, often widely remodeled Primates—extensive secondary bone

Any strongly preferred fiber orientation may throw light on the principal direction of tensile stress, and hence more information on the mechanical role of a bone. Moreover, fiber orientation and size, along with mineral content, likely relate to the widely varying mechanical properties of bone. For example, Currey (1987) found reptilian bone, including alligator frontal bone, to be somewhat low in calcium, but tougher than that of other tetrapods. Lauder and Lanyon (1980) were struck by the rate of development of strain in the opercular bone of sunfish during suction feeding. The value was tenfold those values registered for mammalian bones during vigorous activity.

Another mechanically relevant variable (Goldstein 1987), revealed by scanning electron microscopy, is trabecular architecture, which is patently different in human rib, femur, vertebra, sternum, and ilium (e.g., Whitehouse 1977). Since many cranial bones are porous, an understanding of their mechanical contribution to function calls for knowing their trabecular patterns.

RESILIENT CRANIAL TISSUES

Resilience is the marked ability to recover from compressive deformation. The necessary resilient storage of energy is provided either by tightly constraining turgid cells within a flexible sheath, the notochordal way, or through a firm, viscoelastic ECM produced by cells, the cartilaginous route. In hyaline cartilage, the swelling pressure arises by the avid binding of water to huge aggregations of proteoglycan molecules, and is restrained by a mesh of special collagen fibrils. The cartilage still needs a wrapping, but more for its fastening to surrounding tissues. Elastic cartilage follows a modified route to resilience by adding elastic fibers to a hyaline-like matrix. Fibrocartilage, sparse in the head, is a tough, flexible, collagenous, fibrous tissue with its resistance to compression boosted around the few cells—the chondrocytes.

Hyaline Cartilage

Hyaline refers to the glassy or translucent nature of the abundant matrix around the large ovoid cartilage cells or chondrocytes. The translucency derives from the high content of bound water, and the small size of the fine collagen fibrils that fasten the proteoglycan molecules. (Different configurations of very similar materials achieve the transparency of the eye's cornea and vitreous body.) The matrix fuses with denser fibers of the enclosing perichondrial connective tissue that fastens the piece of cartilage into biomechanical units. The matrix may also fuse with bone matrix or merge into fibrocartilage.

Under tight controls, chondrocytes can multiply in a set direction and cause crystals of hydroxyapatite to deposit in the matrix (mineralization). The mineralized matrix is then selectively destroyed in line with the established direction of growth, and bone is laid down, fused for mechanical integrity to the surviving lattice of calcified cartilage. This systematic endochondral ossification is used extensively in the development of the bony skull, especially for the bones of its base. It requires that the initial embryonic specification include the siting of numerous separate populations of chondroblasts for the individual cartilage pieces. The process of endochondral ossification also allows cartilage to join bones together (at sutures and symphyses) and to cap mobile joint surfaces, while permitting continued growth and reshaping of the skull.

Hyaline cartilage allows skulls to develop, grow, and keep working. It is stiff enough to be an independent skeletal element, but versatile enough to fuse with bone, attach to soft connective tissues, transform into fibrocartilage, mineralize and stay mineralized, or to be resorbed and replaced by bone. Are these properties common to all hyaline cartilages, and did they arise at the same time in evolution? A precise characterization of many different cartilages is needed to start to answer these questions. So far one can give a satisfactory account only for the resilient stiffness of hyaline cartilage. Sources for this information are Hall (1983), Hall and Newman (1991) and *Biology of Extracellular Matrix: A Series* (1986–91), which deal primarily with mammalian cartilage outside the skull, although avian and some cranial cartilages are covered. Moss and Moss-Salentijn (1983) described the diversity of hyaline cartilage in different species and locations, in terms of chondrocyte shape, size, and spacing, and appearance of the matrix. Fig. 3.10, from Huyseunne, displays such variety at a teleost cranial joint.

The terminology for cartilage is profoundly unsatisfactory, with nothing between the global descriptor "hyaline cartilage" and designations by species, site, and age, e.g., one-day mouse tibial-epiphysis cartilage, which even so do not do justice to the mechanical, structural, and other variables at one site. For example, one articular cartilage can in places be stiff, yet elsewhere be compliantly floppy (Silyn-Roberts and Bloom 1988). The simple tissue names in reality are rudimentary symbols for intricate, dynamic, and related cellular communities. Immunology would not have advanced if lymphocytes were still classified as large or small, mouse splenic versus human thymic: recognizable and agreed subtypes are essential to progress. What are the fundamental variables of cartilage by which to classify? Table 3.3 for bone offers a selection adaptable for cartilage.

The macromolecular chemistry of cartilage could be an element of classification, and reveals subtleties even within taxa. For instance, unlike

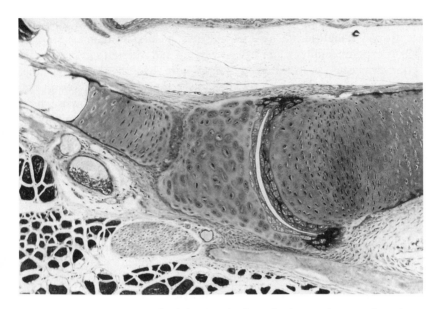

Fig. 3.10. Joints between interhyal, hyosymplectic, and palatoquadrate cartilages in *Astatotilapia elegans*. Note the different distributions of chondrocytes and the regional accumulation of ECM materials. Toluidine blue. 145× magnification. (Courtesy of A. Huysseune)

those of rat and larger mammals, mouse cartilage proteoglycans lack keratan sulfate. Why the mouse does without keratan sulfate might be another scaling effect (Moss and Moss-Salentijn 1983), reflecting the animal's small size and low loadings, or might be related to high vascular efficiency and oxygen level (Scott and Haigh 1988). How the physiology, histology, biomechanics, and biochemistry are matched with one another is the root question, still largely unanswered.

Secondary Cartilage

Schaffer (1930) defined primary cartilage as that originating early in development for the axial, appendicular, and airway skeletons. This left a large heterogeneous group of what he termed secondary cartilages to follow, including elastic cartilages, and many other formations in the head and elsewhere, arising often from periosteum. An origin in the periosteum of a membrane bone has been the hallmark of the restricted sense of "secondary cartilage" (Hall 1978; Beresford 1981), and makes it a clear instance of an accessory tissue. Secondary cartilage may occur on many developing membrane bones, and appears to provide the services of growth, articulation, and padding that primary hyaline cartilage can offer endochondral bones, since it is there from the outset. Although small and accessory, cranial secondary cartilage has a special significance: Hall (1978) experimentally demonstrated varying and intermittent pressure to be the clear cause of its differentiation in more than one site. Three other aspects are inspected here: recent characterizations of the best-known cranial example, the mandibular condylar cartilage, to show how a typical secondary cartilage is organized and how it is not a replica of epiphyseal growth cartilage; Vinkka's (1982) thorough study of cranial secondary cartilage in the rat to illustrate problems in identifying sites; and the apparent restriction of secondary cartilage to homeotherms, or the problem of finding which groups form it.

Mandibular Condyle. The load-bearing, growing condylar cartilage, attached to mandibular bone, displays appropriately specialized populations of cells disposed in layers. The layers and the cellular activities in mouse (Livne et al. 1987; Silbermann et al. 1987), rat (Shibata et al. 1991), and humans (Ben Ami et al. 1991) are from superficial to deep (fig. 3.11): (1) fibrous: fibrogenesis (type I collagen); (2) progenitor: DNA synthesis and mitosis of progenitor cells, fibrogenesis, and proteoglycan production; (3) chondroblastic: cell differentiation, but no columnar alignment (unlike growth cartilage of long bones and vertebrae), stronger synthesis of proteoglycans, and a switch to type II collagen formation; (4) hypertrophy: chondrocytic enlargement, alkaline-phosphatase production, matrix-vesicle extrusion from the cells, matrix mineralization, and synthesis of collagen types I and X; (5) erosion of cartilage and replacement ossification. Silbermann et al. interpreted the alkaline phosphatase and type I collagen in the hypertrophic, older chondrocytes as signs of an osteoblastic differentiation, bringing secondary cartilage "closer to bone than to primary cartilage." Thus, secondary cartilage differs from primary cartilage in more than its time and site of occurrence, requiring two systems of control of what is nominally hyaline cartilage. This is not a solely cranial diversity: the sternal end of the clavicle (Rönning et al. 1991) is another secondary cartilage closely resembling the mandibular condyle.

Secondary Cartilages in the Rat. That Vinkka (1982) found several new sites of secondary cartilage in an often-studied animal illustrates first what pains must be taken before one can be assured that secondary cartilage does not develop in much more poorly known groups such as amphibians and reptiles, and second how the phenomenon may involve many developing cranial bones, even if only briefly. Moreover, Vinkka observed some previously unknown secondary cartilages in soft tissues at sites close to

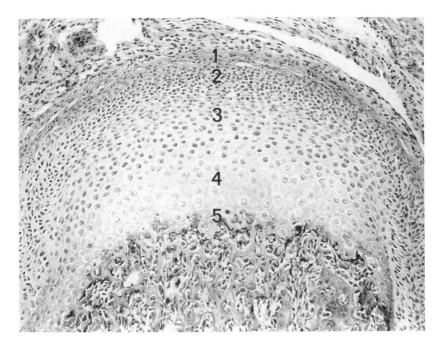

Fig. 3.11. Mandibular condyle of the 21-day rat, showing the layering of the
secondary cartilage: 1 fibroblastic, 2 progenitor, 3 chondroblastic, 4 hypertrophy,
5 erosion. Hematoxylin and Eosin (H & E). 200× magnification.

insertions, but these were not fibrocartilaginous zones typical of heavily
loaded tendons (Vogel and Koob 1989). These cartilages arose, like sesamoids, away from periosteum, and hence are secondary only in Schaffer's
looser sense. Sutural tissue and the perichondrium of Meckel's cartilage
may be other nonperiosteal origins of such secondary cartilage.

   The cartilaginous character in some instances comprised chondrocyte-
like cells in a bony matrix, i.e., chondroid bone, highlighting the question
of the exact nature(s) of secondary cartilage. After widely differing intervals, the fate of the secondary cartilages and chondroid bones was variously resorption, conversion, or persistence, thus rendering improbable
any single purpose for them. The widespread secondary chondrogenesis
(32 locations) appeared to Vinkka to occur either in an early phase to
provide a growing tissue, or at a later stage to serve as a protective or
articulating tissue reacting to mechanical stimuli. At some sites, e.g., the
alveolar bony crest of the tooth socket, a mechanical stimulation of chondrogenesis was unlikely, in her view. One aspect of phenotype is the system
of controls influencing that tissue. Secondary cartilage may isolate a grow-

ing region of a bone from one set of controls by making its cells subject to others, to produce another useful firm or even hard matrix.

Restriction to Homeotherms. Species and class differences in the distribution and presence of secondary cartilage mean less when it is doubtful that all the cartilages are known. Nonetheless, sites occupied in some mammals and birds (Murray 1963; Hall 1967) are deficient in others of the same groups. In fishes, a variety of chondroid tissues are analogous, if not homologous, to secondary cartilages, by site (on membranous bones) and function (padding and articulation), leaving amphibians and reptiles as apparently devoid of cranial secondary cartilage (Hall 1984). There are three possible exceptions: a solitary observation on the pterygoid in a lizard by Fuchs (1909), and cartilages in the stem tendon for the crocodilian jaw musculature (Busbey 1989) and in the aponeurosis of the main jaw adductor of the turtle, *Caretta caretta* (Schumacher 1956). The apparent reluctance of reptilian and amphibian cranial periosteal cells to form cartilage might be overcome experimentally by stimulation with mammalian or avian chondrogenic matrices, conditioned media, or nuclear extracts, if it is not intrinsic to genomic organization. Successful or otherwise, such experiments still could not reveal whether reptiles and amphibians have little need for secondary cartilage or solve the same requirement by other tissue arrangements.

Elastic Cartilage

Elastic cartilage closely resembles hyaline in the shape, size, and spacing of its cells, and in its perichondrium. The matrix differs in having less proteoglycan, thus making room for a dense meshwork of elastic fibers. The cartilage of the mammalian pinna and outer ear canal varies greatly in cellularity, cellular fat content, and amounts of matrix and elastin (Baecker 1928), a diversity shared with the epiglottis and some other laryngeal cartilages, and the lyssa, a rodlike support in the tongue (Schaffer 1930). According to Baecker, the large, stiff ears of ungulates have elastic cartilage, but the elephant's pendulant ear bears a hyaline kind; very small animals form a cellular cartilage, with fat filling the cells in shrew, rat, and small bats; medium-size animals have a substantial, partly elastic matrix and less fat. Glycogen content, from much to none, shows no apparent systematic variation. Electron microscopy (Sanzone and Reith 1976; Kostovic-Knezevic et al. 1986) shows more elasticlike material in the cellular cartilage of the mouse and rat ear than earlier light microscopy suggested. Although these authors saw no matrix vesicles, matrix vesicles are present in the rat's ear, but lack alkaline and acid phosphatases (Nielsen 1978). The matrix is rich in chondroitin-6-sulfated proteoglycan (Caterson et al. 1987). The auricular support thus offers a chance to relate morphology and biochemistry to mechanical properties in a relatively independent reinforcing structure.

Fibrocartilage

Fibrocartilage has been grudgingly recognized as a tissue departing from dense collagenous tissues by virtue of some larger, rounder, encapsulated cells in place of fibroblasts. Recent chemistry in mammals gives it stronger cartilaginous credentials, although the collagen is mostly thick-fibered type I. Benjamin and Evans (1990) provide the first thorough review of fibrocartilage.

Fibrocartilage arises in various ways: a hyaline secondary cartilage can become more fibrous, or a fibrous tissue, e.g., a tendon or meniscus, can turn cartilaginous, although how far the new macromolecules permeate away from the changed cells is unclear. Fibrocartilage participates in tendon insertion regions of fishes with cartilaginous skeletons, frequently in avian and piscine cranial joints, in many mental symphyses, and in the mammalian temporomandibular meniscus (Schaffer 1930, 373). As with other menisci, the temporomandibular cartilaginous regions are patchy, somewhat inconstant, and age-dependent (Kopp 1976; Fujita and Hoshino 1989). High concentrations of chondroitin-6-sulfate and keratan sulfate surround the large chondrocytes of the rabbit's meniscus or disc (Mills et al. 1988). In organ culture this disc produces proteoglycans that are cartilaginous in their hydrodynamic behavior.

Chordoid and Chondroid Tissues

Early microscopists noted that a wide range of reinforcing tissues in invertebrates and vertebrates resembled, but were not identical with, either notochord or hyaline cartilage; thus the categories of chordoid and chondroid tissues came about. The high point of this endeavor was Schaffer's (1930) compilation and classification, which drew as well on his own very wide-ranging studies. Thereafter, the approach has been piecemeal, although Person (1983) presented a modern overview of invertebrate cartilages, and work is active on the tissues in teleosts (see references to Benjamin). The chordoid and chondroid tissues are important, both as frequently deployed tissues in the skull of fishes, and as sources for tissue evolution.

Problems of Nomenclature. Schaffer (1930) used as criteria for his categories both appearance in light microscopy, including staining reactions of the matrix and the behavior of freshly isolated cells, and time of appearance in ontogeny. He set hyaline cartilage of the primary tetrapod skeleton and notochord as the reference standards. This had the effect of leaving many other tissues with diminished identities—they were only cartilage-like, or notochord-like, supporting tissues. Because the chondroid ones often stained feebly with the reagents Schaffer had available, he did indeed view them as poorly differentiated.

English-speakers have subsumed Schaffer's distinctions of German nomenclature under the already burdened term "cartilage." The result is that tissues that are very alike—bone, cementum, and dentine—have their own names, while "cartilage" labors on for what is in squid, lamprey, hagfish, teleosts, and tetrapods, despite great differences in the major structural molecular materials. The histological similarity of many of these tissues to hyaline cartilage rests alas on the absence of distinctive structure in conventionally stained hyaline-cartilage matrix: the comparison is with what is not there rather than with a positive feature. The cartilage-like tissues do in fact display recognizable ultrastructural and histochemical features.

The Tissue Types. With the above reservations in mind, Schaffer's classificatory scheme introduces the types and their distributions in the skull (table 3.5). These tissues are resilient or supporting, but are not true (hyaline) cartilage in Schaffer's sense. Thus, the chordoid tissues included notochord and a diffuse category based on either cell similarity or the cells' being restrained and turgid. Schaffer applied the name "cartilage" to cell-rich, matrix-poor tissues in lamprey and hagfish, subdividing them further, based on whether they persisted into maturity or were lost at metamorphosis. Another form of cartilage—matrix-rich, with branched/spindle cells—had cartilage-like matrix, but not the typical, rounded chondrocytes. Finally, the tissues that he would only call "chondroide" or cartilage-like were rich in either cells or matrix, with either smooth-contoured, glassy (hyaline) cells or cells bearing branched processes. His designation of the abundant matrix as mucoid reflects the imprecision of the staining at that time. True mucus contains special glycoproteins secreted by epithelial cells. Schaffer's overview demonstrated the diversity and wide use in the skull of the chondroid and chordoid tissues, but clearly needed to be extended with modern techniques and interpreted anew.

Chordoid Tissues. These can be dealt with briefly first, given the particular nature of notochord and its meager contribution to the skull in any class. The notochordal character is sheath-restrained, turgid epithelial cells. A composite notochordal sketch from various species of lamprey shows a peripheral region of chordal epithelial cells (Schwarz 1961), synthesizing a more peripheral, thick enclosing sleeve of very orderly, uniformly wide (17 nm) collagen fibrils of type II (Kimura and Kamimura 1982). These fibrils lie mostly circumferential to the chordal axis (Eikenberry et al. 1984), along with sulfated proteoglycans and small amounts of other collagens. The outer limit to the sleeve is a perforated elastic layer (Tretjakoff 1926), beyond which is a looser collagenous tissue. In contrast, the mesenchyme is the major source of the sheath in teleosts and tetrapods (Ekanayake and Hall 1991).

In deeper epithelial regions, the cells, still attached by many desmosomes, enlarge to become vacuolated chordal cells, accumulate glycogen, reduce the number of organelles, and form a broad subplasmalemmal layer of filaments (Schwarz 1961). In hagfish (Flood 1969), the filaments and desmosomes are particularly conspicuous in the central string of the notochord, emphasizing the epithelial character. It is unknown whether chordin, a glycoprotein of sturgeon notochord and central-nervous tissue, but not sturgeon cartilage (Preobrazhensky et al. 1987), is present in cyclostomian notochord.

Beyond any light-microscopic resemblance, it is difficult to assess how far other tissues may be classified as chordoid. The outer notochordal cells share properties with chondrocytes, whereas the cells of the interior are epithelial. Must a chordoid tissue engage in both sets of behaviors? Should it make chordin? Or is it enough that it reinforces by the chordoid mechanical principle? In the last circumstance, cartilage itself may operate in a chordoid manner, as proposed by Thomson (1987) for Meckel's cartilage of *Xenopus* in its early cellular phase of development.

Benjamin and Ralphs (1991) examined what Schaffer (1930) thought to be a chordoid example—the annular ligament around the fish eye. Its molecular composition from immunostaining shows no relation to cartilage, but a molecular chordoid connection has not yet been tested.

Cartilage-like Tissues in Lampreys. Schaffer (1897, 1906) compared the skeletal histologies of hagfish and lamprey. In lamprey, he carefully mapped the cranial distributions of his "soft" or mucocartilage, and of the firmer cartilage, which most superseded it at metamorphosis. Recent work shows that larval mucocartilage has narrow fibrils of a material different from lamprin, the major fibrous component of adult lamprey cartilage (Wright et al. 1983). Lamprin has some biochemical resemblance to elastin, but lacks the desmosine that makes elastin resilient. The lamprin is deposited as globules which fuse in association with a network of 20-nm diameter fibrils of an unknown composition (Armstrong et al. 1987). The mucocartilage cells of larval lamprey switch from making predominantly hyaluronan to chondroitin sulfate(s) prior to metamorphosis, whether or not the mucocartilage is to be replaced by cartilage (Mangia and Palladini 1970).

The staining of fibrils in mucoid tissues with some elastic stains, after trypsin digestion, introduced Tretjakoff (1928) to the idea of a third, nonelastic, noncollagenous fibrillar component. What binds "elastic" stains in lamprey cartilage and many other cartilage-like tissues (Schaffer 1906, 251; Wright and Youson 1982; Benjamin 1988; Wright et al. 1988; Benjamin and Sandhu 1990) is still unresolved.

TABLE 3.5 Distributions of cranial chordoid, chondroid, and atypical cartilage from Schaffer (1930)

Tissue	Taxonomic group and site	Comment
Chordoid		
Compact	Fish: notochord of lampreys, myxinoids, chimera, ganoids, and teleosts *Syngnathus* and *Lophius*	Persists in skull (de Beer 1937, 381)
	Amphibia: larval notochord	Chondrification of cranial notochord (Schaffer 1930, 28)
	Mammals: fetal notochord	
Chordoid		
Diffuse	Fish: intrameningeal reinforcement, between membranous and cartilaginous labyrinths, and external to choriocapillaris, in lampreys; Annular ligament in anterior eye of many teleosts	Brain arachnoid tissue includes pigment and fat cells, and capillaries (Schaffer 1930, 52)
		Ligament is a misnomer; cells themselves are fibrous in carp
	Mammals: whisker support in cat and rat: endoneurial cushions in facial nerve of horse and donkey; adipose tissue in lyssa and epiglottis of many species	Usually mixed with more cartilage-like tissues
Chondroid		
Cell-rich, hyaline cells	Fish: anteriorly on lip and ring cartilages, "tongue" of lampreys; "lingual" support, between eye and nasal capsule, around otic capsule, in ventral snout skin, and tendons, of *Myxine glutinosa*	Lingual support = Zungenbein
	Barbels of some teleosts, lower lip and gill support of carp, an intercalated piece in lower jaw of *Misgurnus*, premaxillary plate (*Coryodorus paleatus*), meniscus (*Trachurus*), in many species on bones as articular or marginal tissue	Literature is extensive; many sites—see table 3.6

Chondroid		
Matrix-rich, branched cells, mucoid	Fish: mucocartilage of myxine and larval lampreys, separate from and on cartilage; teleosts: anterior skin (*Misgurnus, Cobitis taenia*); on premaxilla (*Cyprinus carpio, Cobitis taenia, Cottus gobio*) Amphibia: outside membranous labyrinth (*Salamandra maculata*) Mammals: cartilage precursor in cat's epiglottis; embryonic dental pulp of pig and humans	Sites specified by Schaffer (1906, 235) and Hardisty (1981) In the first two species, with cell-rich hyaline-celled chondroid
Matrix-rich, hyaline cells, mucoid	Mammals: regions of epiglottis in cat, and lyssa of cat and lion	Very cartilage-like and becomes cartilage
Cartilage		
Permanent cell-cartilage	Fish: branchial basket, otic and nasal capsules of larval lamprey; cartilage skull of hagfishes and lampreys; gill arches of some teleosts, e.g. trout Mammals: auricle of small rodents and bats Amphibia: larval skull (*Pelobates fusca*)	Chondrocytes rich in fat—lipocartilage
Transitory cell-cartilage		Precursor to matrix-rich cartilage, and not to be confused with hypertrophic hyaline cartilage prior to mineralization
Matrix-rich, branched/spindle cells	Fish: skull regions of some selachians; sclera of *Sternoptyx, Syngnathus, Gasterosteus aculaetus*	

Hagfish Cartilage-like Tissues. Schaffer (1906, 1911) observed in the hagfish skull firm myxinoid cartilage, a soft mucocartilage, and a hyaline-celled cell-rich chondroid tissue. Although the firm cartilages of lamprey and hagfish are histologically similar (Schaffer 1906; Wright et al. 1984), the amino-acid profile of the noncollagenous fibrous residue of hagfish cartilage differs sufficiently to merit the name "myxinin" (Wright et al. 1984). This distinction supports the idea of long, separate evolutions for lamprey and hagfish (Hardisty 1981). The amino-acid composition of the flexible chondroid of the lingual posterior support in hagfish was unlike that of any cartilage.

Cartilage-like Tissues in Teleosts. Table 3.5 understates the extent of cranial chondroid tissues in fishes. Schaffer cited more instances in teleosts from major studies by Kaschkaroff, Studnicka, Petersen, and Baecker. Benjamin has recently revised Schaffer's nomenclature (Benjamin 1989b, 1990; Benjamin and Ralphs 1991), and described the histology, ultrastructure, and histochemistry at many sites in the teleost skull.

Sometimes the original German names are useful, as such or in translation; for other tissues special naming is called for. Among the teleost resilient tissues, Benjamin distinguishes as types of cartilage (figs. 3.12–3.17): cell-rich hyaline cartilage, matrix-rich hyaline cartilage (closest to human hyaline cartilage), fibro/cell-rich cartilage, elastic/cell-rich cartilage,

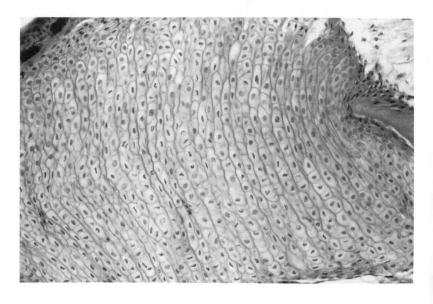

Fig. 3.12. Hyaline-cell cartilage in the rostral fold of *Labeo bicolor.* H & E. 300 × magnification. (Courtesy of M. Benjamin and Cambridge University Press)

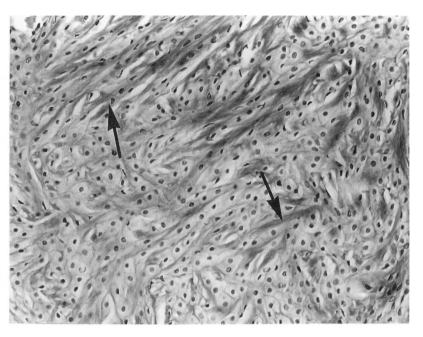

Fig. 3.13. Fibrohyaline-cell cartilage on the lateral side of the suspensorium in *Botia horae*. It contains prominent bundles of collagen fibers (arrows) interspersed with hyaline cells. Masson's trichrome. 500× magnification. (Courtesy of M. Benjamin and Cambridge University Press)

Zellknorpel, and scleral cartilage. Less like cartilage are mucochondroid, and the "chordoid" tissue of the annular ligament. Sample distributions from Benjamin's (1988, 1989b, 1990) surveys are given in table 3.6.

Secondary or Accessory Roles. Is the accessory role of secondary cartilage and other minor tissues of tetrapods mirrored among the cartilage-like tissues? For a direct secondary parallel, Benjamin (1989a) astutely noticed that the hyaline-celled chondroid on jaw bones of *Poecilia sphenops* starts to form after the membrane bone is established, and is therefore secondary. Previously, it appeared that secondary cartilage was restricted to birds and mammals (Hall 1984), experimental efforts to provoke it in amphibians and reptiles notwithstanding (Hall and Hanken 1985; Irwin and Ferguson 1986).

A broader accessory or adventitious (Murray 1963) category includes the hyaline-celled chondroid and branched-celled mucoid chondroid (mucocartilage) on the dentary and other cranial bones of teleosts (Benjamin 1986, 1988), mucocartilage on larval lamprey cartilage, e.g., nasal capsule, and hyaline-celled chondroid on myxinoid cartilage.

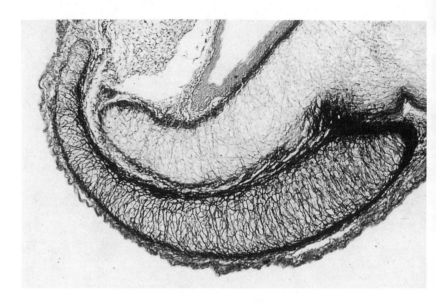

Fig. 3.14. Elastic hyaline-cell cartilage in the oral sucker of *Gyrinocheilus aymonieri* can easily be distinguished from the adjacent hyaline-cell cartilage in this Weigert's stained section. 190 × magnification. (Courtesy of M. Benjamin and Cambridge University Press)

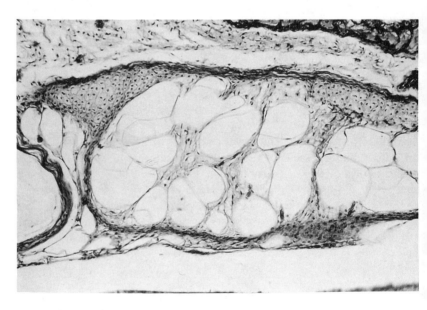

Fig. 3.15. Lipohyaline-cell cartilage, characterized by the juxtaposition of hyaline and fat cells, in the oro-mandibular region of *Pseudogastromyzon myersi*. Masson's trichrome. 190 × magnification. (Courtesy of M. Benjamin and Cambridge University Press)

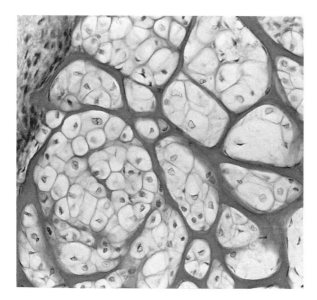

Fig. 3.16. *Zellknorpel* fills the spaces between the spicules of cancellous bone in the premaxilla of *Hypostomus* sp. H & E. 300× magnification. (Courtesy of M. Benjamin and Cambridge University Press)

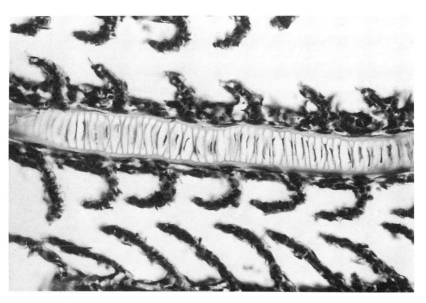

Fig. 3.17. *Zellknorpel* forming the gill filament spine in *Jordanella floridae*. The cells are greatly shrunken within lacunae and surrounded by perichondral bone. Masson's trichrome. 480× magnification. (Courtesy of M. Benjamin and Cambridge University Press)

TABLE 3.6 Sample distribution of cranial mucoid and hyaline-cellular chondroid in teleosts from Benjamin (1988, 1989b, 1990*)

Species	Bony/other site	*Cartilage type	Comment
Mucoid chondroid			
Gnathonemus petersi	lower-jaw proboscis	Fibroblastic mucoid chondroid	Thick enclosing perichondrium
Periophthalmus sp.	labial folds	Fibroblastic mucoid chondroid	—
Tinca tinca	opercular valve	Fibroblastic mucoid chondroid and hyaline-cell mucoid chondroid	Mixed with skeletal muscle and merges with hyaline-cell chondroid
Acanthopsis choirorhynchus	subcutaneous	Fibroblastic mucoid chondroid	Prominent bundles of collagen fibers
Morulius chrysophekadion	lacrimal bone	Fibroblastic mucoid chondroid	Direct tissue contact with bone, but no merging
Cellular chondroid			
Poecilia sphenops	dentary, maxilla	Hyaline-cell chondroid	Ossification precedes chondroid formation
Poecilia sphenops	lacrimal	Hyaline-cell chondroid	Cellular chondroid develops from mucoid chondroid
Morulius chrysophekadion	kinethmoid	Hyaline-cell chondroid	Chondroid common here in other species; chondroid links kinethmoid to premaxilla
Tanichthys albonubes	basihyal	Hyaline-cell chondroid	A common chondroid site; chondroid becomes hyaline cartilage
Gyrinocheilus aymonieri	oral sucker	Hyaline-cell chondroid and elastic hyaline-cell chondroid	Attached to membrane bone of jaws; chondroid is extensive and permanent
Tinca tinca	submaxillary meniscus	Hyaline-cell chondroid	Chondroid becomes cartilage

Another of Schaffer's concepts was that of substitution, meaning that the supporting tissue of an organ varies with species. Thus, a variety of tissues—chordoid, chondroid, cartilaginous, sometimes even osseous or vascular—reinforce the mammalian tongue and epiglottis, and the barbels of fishes (Baecker 1926).

Fate, Including Metaplasia. The diversity of these resilient tissues also expresses itself in their fate. Lamprey mucocartilage appears destined for destruction or dedifferentiation, according to site (Hardisty 1981; Armstrong et al. 1987). Other chondroid tissues can persist, or partly transform among each other (Schaffer 1906), become adipose tissue (Bargmann 1973), bone (Moss 1961b) or hyaline cartilage (Benjamin 1988). Some anuran larval cellular cartilage turns into a conventional matrix-rich cartilage. Especially notable is the amphibian notochordal shift to making hyaline cartilage (Schaffer 1930; Wake and Lawson 1973).

Primitiveness. Knowledgeable authors have applied the terms "primitive" and "poorly differentiated" to the chordoid and chondroid tissues. That the tissues have generally organelle-poor cells, and fewer of the macromolecules one has come to expect from cartilages, need indicate not poor differentiation, but rather a low level of those materials. Schaffer cast these tissues in a negative or deficient light by emphasizing the number of stains that bound well to parts of true cartilage, but not to chordoid or chondroid components.

Not all is negative. Glycogen-containing cells of course react with Periodic-acid-Schiff (PAS), but chondroid matrices in general are PAS-positive, react with alcian blue at some pH, and often are metachromatic. Collagen is frequently present, but is absent from the interior of the notochord and is not the major fibrous element in lamprey cartilage. Something binds "elastic" stains. The structural picture of chondroid tissues is positive in other respects. Transmission electron microscopy frequently reveals an extensive system of peripheral vesicles in chondroid (and chordoid) cells. The hyaline-cellular chondroids of some teleosts and hagfish display abundant cytoplasmic filaments (Benjamin 1986; Benjamin and Sandhu 1990; Wright et al. 1984). Among chondrocytes, only those of elastic cartilage are outstandingly filamentous (Sheldon 1983). Vessels are present in some chondroid matrices, whereas most cartilaginous matrices lack vessels.

Although one may construe an activity, such as taking nutriment from mud, as primitive, the mucous padding and supporting tissues that seem to assist the snout to do this in ammocoetes (Hardisty 1981, 343) and some teleosts (Benjamin 1988, 1990) likely are properly matched to their tasks. In this adaptive sense the tissues are not primitive (Benton 1987).

The tissues sometimes undergo metaplasia. Although some biologists regard such phenotypic conversions as a mark of immaturity or a primitive nature, the opposite interpretation is more reasonable. Since the before and after tissues are each for a period in functioning stable states, the cells are sophisticated in their ability not only to select and stabilize two active tissue phenotypes, but to manage the changeover, particularly if there is no respite in loading.

Conclusions. Resilient tissues have been treated as discrete nameable entities, but also as ill-defined regions of a supporting-tissue continuum, embraced by the one term "cartilage" (Moss and Moss-Salentijn 1983). I have sought to show that the chondroid and chordoid tissues are not unstable, primitive, or poorly differentiated variants or forerunners of the cartilages, but that they have as valid and purposeful identities as do hyaline and elastic cartilages. Moreover, a description of certain complicated skeletal structures is impossible if they are not accorded identities. For example, the "lingual" support of hagfish comprises pieces of myxinoid cartilage, joined in places by soft mucocartilage acting as a sutural tissue, and elsewhere bearing major extensions of a hyaline-celled chondroid (Schaffer 1906). The tissues need serious and separate consideration, since they are widespread, and different ones find specific uses.

The cartilage family illustrates difficulties with the concept of tissue phenotype, when it is clear that many "special" morphologies, cellular activities, and molecular species are nowhere near as special, i.e., tissue-specific, as was believed. For example, one simply cannot say that a feature is common to cartilages, but absent from chondroids. Some cartilages are as cellular (*Zellknorpel;* Schaffer 1930) as hyaline-celled chondroid; chondroids can contain glycogen or elastic fibers (Benjamin 1986), or be constructed on cartilaginous principles (Bargmann 1973); selachian chondrocytes can be stellate (Schaffer 1930), and so on.

Finally, the cartilage-like tissues are more confined to the head than are hyaline cartilage or bone, and may more accurately reflect cranial tasks. An organism's choice of cartilage or bone subtype may be based on the mechanical loading and physiological needs of the noncranial skeleton: this choice may be adequate for, but not finely matched to, cranial functions.

HARD TISSUES RELATED TO CARTILAGE

Calcified Cartilages

Calcified cartilages are fibro- or hyaline cartilages profoundly altered to be important bonding and supporting materials in embryonic, juvenile, and adult life. Mineralization takes place as a secondary step so that materials of the precursor tissue have to be reduced or modified and new molecules introduced, along with the deposition of calcium salts. Calcified cartilages are of interest with regard to whether and how their cells survive matrix calcification, how they grow, and what they do.

Universally acknowledged is the role of calcified cartilage in endochondral ossification, where it bonds growing cartilage to the bone formed in step with selective erosion of the cartilage. In birds, erosion also acts on uncalcified cartilage (Roach and Shearer 1989). Findings such as this give pause to taking the many results for the mammalian epiphysis and growth plate as givens for cranial synchondroses (Hall 1978), replacement ossifications of secondary cartilages, and cranial endochondral ossification in ectotherms.

In adults, mineralized fibrocartilage joins chondrified ligaments to bone at the mandibular symphysis in *Propithecus verreauxi* and *Hapalemur griseus* (Beecher 1977). At the same site, calcified zones unite the symphyseal fibrocartilage with bone in *Lemur fulvus* and *Lemur macaco* (Beecher 1977) and hamster (Trevisan and Scapino 1976). A layer of less fibrous mineralized cartilage constitutes the only continuous support beneath the soft cartilage of the mandibular condyle in humans until age 20 years, when the underlying bone trabeculae become confluent (Ingervall et al. 1976). A thinner layer of mineralized cartilage then persists, as in rat (Lester and Ash 1981), monkey (Luder and Schroeder 1992), and other mammals.

An inversion of these spatial relations occurs in some endocranial bones of ectotherms, particularly extant and fossil fishes (Ørvig 1951), where the skeletal element may be largely cartilaginous. Here, an outermost shell of bone is fused to a peripheral calcified layer of cartilage, or the outer calcified cartilage stands alone (Patterson 1977, 85). The mechanics may be modified by a lattice of cancellous mineralization deep within the cartilage. The selachian variation on this arrangement is to dispense with almost all the superficial bone and to keep the peripheral cartilaginous mineralizations separate as plaques or "tesserae" (Kemp and Westrin 1979). Moss (1977) and Kemp and Westrin agreed on the presence of living nonhypertrophic chondrocytes in the calcified cartilage. Cells can remain alive in other persisting mineralized cartilages, e.g., the mandibular condyle (Kopp 1978; Luder and Schroeder 1992).

Complete mineralization of the peripheral shell of a mostly cartilaginous skeletal piece halts growth. Selachian skeletal growth is allowed by separating the hard peripheral plaques (Kemp and Westrin 1979). In the placoderm *Plourdosteus canadensis* with an uninterrupted calcified shell to its cartilage, Ørvig (1951, 404) proposed that the superficial zone was resorbed before a perichondrium deposited new cartilage appositionally for another cycle of mineralization.

Moss (1977) could not endorse Ørvig's interpretation of the two patterns of crystallite deposition in cartilage—globular and prismatic—as being in phylogenetic sequence. One reason concerns the coarse dimension at which the modes of calcification have been distinguished, which is scaled substantially above that of the matrix vesicles and collagen fibrils, where mineral can first be detected in endotherms (Christofferson and Landis 1991). Kemp and Westrin (1979) could not find matrix vesicles near the deep face of selachian tesserae, but like Bargmann (1939) they saw mineralization along the collagen fibers inserting into the superficial surface. However, in the interior of the mandible of *Myliobatis aquila*, Bargmann saw the cells as having more of an orienting influence on the calcified bands than did the fibrillar architecture. All the cartilaginous mineralizations display characteristic morphologies and sizes, implicating direct or indirect cellular control.

Chondroid Bone

There are two principal categories of tissues intermediate between cartilage and bone: chondroid bone type II (Beresford 1981), the persisting mineralized cellular cartilage mentioned just above; and a type I, which consists of chondrocyte-like cells in a bony matrix, insofar as light microscopy can show. Type I arises mostly de novo from progenitor cells, although sometimes timing and layout suggest that it is an intermediary of cartilage-to-bone metaplasia. Chondroid bone I exists as part of the boundary to larger secondary cartilages; as all of some smaller mammalian secondary cartilages (Vinkka 1982); occasionally uniting superficial bone with deeper-lying calcified cartilage in placoderms (Ørvig 1951); and participating in cranial joints of modern teleosts (Schmid-Monnard 1883; Haines 1937; Huysseune and Verraes 1986). It is briefly an intermediary, while cranial chondroid experiences a bony metaplasia in teleosts (Schmid-Monnard 1883; Weisel 1967; Moss 1961b). Type I also shares some morphological characteristics with regions of antler cartilage and cementum of guinea pig.

Recent studies reveal a heterogeneity within chondroid bone type I, which might be expected, considering its diverse occurrences. Thus, the chondroid bone formed by mouse mandibular perichondrium in vitro has a bony matrix by many criteria, e.g., bone sialoprotein immunoreactivity, and ultimately no type II collagen (Silbermann et al. 1987), whereas in a persisting bone-cartilage mixed tissue of the kitten's mandibular symphysis, the pericellular region holds collagen type II (Goret-Nicaise and Dhem 1987). In general, inadequate technique may account for some apparent tissue diversity, since preparation of tissues at low temperatures is needed

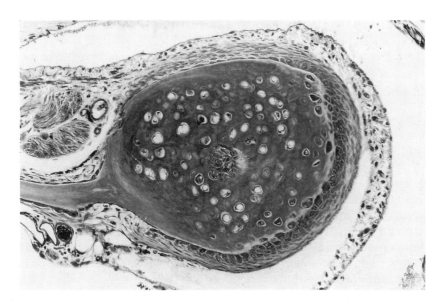

Fig. 3.18. Chondroid bone on the premaxillary of *Astatotilapia elegans*. Note the ongoing incorporation of osteoblasts into the matrix, the start of a central marrow cavity, and the merging with acellular bone. Toluidine blue. 230× magnification. (Courtesy of A. Huysseune)

to preserve ultrastructure and materials for histochemical demonstration (Hunzicker and Herrmann 1987; Huyseunne and Sire 1990).

The chondroid bone that develops late on cranial bones of the cichlid fishes, *Astatotilapia elegans* (fig. 3.18) and *Hemichromis bimaculatus,* is noteworthy in several other ways that distance it from homeothermic secondary cartilage and the acellular bone predominant in the species (Huysseune 1986; Huysseune and Verraes 1986; Huysseune and Sire 1990). It endures into adult life, but is subject to destruction by osteoclasts. It is cellular, but some cells degenerate. One of the bones on which it forms, the basioccipital, itself develops endochondrally. And the matrix is not at all cartilaginous and lacks type II collagen; only the cells display some chondrocytic characteristics. On the other hand, the tissue appears to have the role and mechanical etiology of a secondary cartilage in being subject to pressure and shear at cranial articulations.

SOFT CONNECTIVE TISSUES

The skull is an elaborate system of connective-tissue membranes and strips, some sutural, some ligamentous, in which many hard or firm reinforcing elements are imbedded, and by which these elements are shaped, sized, and moved. The connective-tissue system, in imposing mechanical constraints and freedoms, defining functional regions, and providing cellular populations to add to or subtract from more rigid tissues, is clearly a major participant in Moss's (1961a) functional matrix. Recognizable roles of the connective tissue in the biomechanics of the skull are as sutures (Jaslow 1990), fasciae (Homberger and Meyers 1989), ligament (Sanford and Lauder 1989), periosteum, etc.

Periosteum

Periosteum is the wrapping around the external surfaces of bone. It is absent at attachments of tendons and ligaments and at articular cartilage. It has an outer fibrous layer for strength and an inner cellular layer. Periosteum provides a vascular, mechanical, and cellular context, matching a bone to the changes of growth and use in its working musculature and environment. Tendinous and ligamental insertions, sutures, and the periodontal ligament serve bone very similarly.

The inner, cellular/osteogenic periosteal layer of the young rat mandible (Chong et al. 1982) displays four patterns: (1) broad and densely cellular, with elongated osteoblasts against trabecular bone; (2) cellular, up to four cells deep, with rounded osteoblasts on a compact bone surface; (3) a narrow layer of small, flattened cells appearing inactive against smooth, compact bone; (4) osteoclasts and small oval cells on an eroded surface uneven with Howship's lacunae. (Fig. 3.9 illustrates the periosteal cellular patterns in fish.) The surfaces involved in fast and slow apposition (1 and 2), or resorption (4) are visibly different at low magnification. By following the changing patterns of apposition and resorption on specific bones, one arrives at a reasonably satisfactory interpretation of how accumulated changes in, and repositioning of, craniofacial bones yield the progressively maturing mammalian face, oral cavity, and brain case (Enlow 1968; Hoyte 1971).

How inactive are the spaced-apart small cells flattened against smooth bone? This widespread covering may constitute an osteogenic source by ossifying existing fibers of the periosteum in man (Petersen 1930; Bernstein 1933) and other large mammals (Knese and Harnack 1962). Such a connective-tissue ossification (Petersen 1930) is significant for the cranium in those continuously growing ectotherms, where dermis of the skin additionally plays the role of periosteum and is incorporated into bone (Weidenreich 1930).

The outer periosteum is fibrous with bundles of collagen and smaller bundles of elastic fibers (Frankenhuis-van den Heuvel et al. 1991). Both components can be entrapped in bone in Sharpey's fibers (Petersen 1930; Tonna 1974; Knese 1979), which are numerous in piscine bone (Moss

1961c), rare in avian (Enlow and Brown 1957). Several muscle-periosteal configurations, plus an inherent periosteal lability, are needed for periosteum to mediate mechanically between muscle action and bone. Chong and Evans (1982) describe three modes of muscle attachment to the growing rat's mandibular periosteum: periosteal, endomyseal, and tendinous-insertion. They propose that the various arrangements render compatible the number of muscles and their directions of action with the available bone surface at a site, and allow relative positions to be maintained during growth. In these operations, the periosteum is viewed as the common adaptive intermediary. The periosteum also must expand and drift as its growing bone enlarges and alters its position (Enlow 1968).

Experimental work on long-bone growth indicates that periosteal growth lags behind the epiphyseal to the extent of mechanically constraining the lengthening of the enclosed bone (Harkness and Trotter 1978). Frankenhuis-van den Heuvel et al. (1991) could not determine whether such an action occurs for cranial bones, and how elastic fibers might create periosteal tension. Elastic fibers are absent from human cranial periosteum (Weidenreich 1930, 506) and 7-weeks rat mandibular periosteum (Chong and Evans 1982). Studies of longitudinal growth in the rabbit's vault after various soft-tissue excisions or transections gave no indication of a periosteal regulation of growth (Babler, Persing, Persson et al. 1982), and Rönning and Koski (1974) found a periosteal influence on mandibular condylar shape, but not overall growth.

Tendon Insertion Structures

A majority of human tendon attachments to long and other bones involve a progression from tendon to fibrocartilage, to calcified fibrocartilage, to bone (Benjamin et al. 1986; Evans et al. 1991). Becker (1971) described the ultrastructure at two mammalian sites. A similar use of cartilage as an accessory tissue for attachment in the skull is seen for certain insertions at the primate mandibular symphysis (Beecher 1977), and probably elsewhere.

Perichondrium

The perichondrium wrapping around pieces of hyaline or elastic cartilage corresponds to the fibroelastic layer of periosteum (Knese 1979, 562). It usually lacks a transitional fibrillary zone (Enlow 1968), supposedly because, during growth, movements of the cartilage and adjacent tissues remain in step. At least three regions of perichondrium take this simple story further: where cartilage and perichondrium arise secondarily from periosteum; where periosteum and perichondrium adjoin over endochondrally ossifying cartilage; and upon permanent calcified cartilages in cartilaginous fishes.

The second special perichondrial situation occurs at a circumferential ossifying annulus encircling the growth plate of tubular bones. Here lies the perichondrial ossification groove of Ranvier (*encoche d'ossification*), which contains the ring of bone bark apposed to the growth cartilage. The depth of the groove varies by species and skeletal element (Shapiro et al. 1977). The principal product of the groove cells—the bony perichondrial ring—is not specific to long bones, but is common to bones originating from a cartilaginous anlage, including the mammalian basal skull bones (Balmain et al. 1983). The fibrous, cellular, and biosynthetic patterns of the soft-tissue wrappings of the growth plate and metaphysis revealed in noncranial bones (Shapiro et al. 1977) probably apply in large part to cranial osteogenesis in cartilage.

Bargmann (1939) emphasized fiber trajectories in characterizing the perichondrium of the calcified cartilages that underlie the teeth of elasmobranchs and to which the lips attach. In batoids, the perichondrium over the peripheral mosaic of calcified plates combines deep collagen bundles uniting contiguous and nearby plates, long-ranging superficial bundles, and bundles from the base of the tooth plate penetrating to fasten into the calcified pyramids. A second instance of the internal relations of perichondrium with its enclosed tissue is the chondroid supporting rim of the sucking plate in the teleost *Echeneis naucates* (Bargmann 1973). From the perichondrium an arcade of fibers extends down internally, from which thick trabeculae of collagen, accompanied by an elastic network, run directly through the tissue to the opposite perichondrium. Thus, perichondria can be discernibly organized intermediaries uniting chondroid or cartilage internally and with local structures.

Sutures

Numerous variables describe sutural form and behavior. *Form* refers to the edges of the adjoining bones, defining butt-ended, beveled, or mortised. Also, along the line of the suture, there can be marked variation in the depth of bony interdigitation/denticulation, if present. Other *bone-surface variables* include level of osteoblastic activity, the trabecularity, or smoothness, and degrees of Sharpey-fiber inclusion, erosion, remodeling, and vascular penetration. *Fibrous orientation:* collagen fibers can cross between bones directly or obliquely; or they may fan out from a bony projection, or run parallel to the sutural margin, for example, in the pericranial-dural plane (Koskinen et al. 1974; Persson et al. 1978; Oudhof 1982). However, fibers need not be consistent in their course over even small distances along the suture. *Layering:* various authors have perceived three, four, or five layers across sutures (Pritchard et al. 1956; Ten Cate et al. 1977; Yen and Chiang 1984). The degree of layering visible histologically may reflect function at a particular time, and not be as permanent and meaningful as named layers imply (Yen and Chiang 1984). *Time of closure* has been studied most often, but still inadequately, in humans. Some sutures fuse early and almost regularly, others merge later or not at all. The consistency of fusion is variable (Kokich 1976; Furuya et al. 1984) and differs from side to side (Zivanovic 1983). *Cranial site* provides much scope for differences. One division is between facial and braincase sutures. For example, Herring (1972) compared degrees of interdigitation and times of sutural closure between pigs and peccaries, concluding that braincase sutures close earlier in pigs, palatal and facial sutures earlier in peccaries.

Another site-related grouping within a species is between sutures that contribute greatly to bone growth, e.g., rabbit's frontonasal (Babler et al. 1987), and ones where little bone is added, e.g., rabbit's anterior lambdoid (Babler, Persing, Winn et al. 1982) and temporal (Alberius and Selvik 1985). That it is position within the bony mosaic that determines growth rate perhaps is shown best, among experiments of this type, by the acceleration in an originally slow-growing sagittal graft to a "fast" coronal site (Oudhof 1982). However, the suture is not a unitary entity, since different rates of bone deposition can occur on opposite sides of a suture (Hoyte 1971; Koskinen et al. 1974), and sutures are often long enough for growth rates, interdigitation, and fiber orientation to change along their length (Herring 1972; Smith and McEown 1974; Herring and Mucci 1991). A third aspect of site related to the control and coordination of sutural growth is that sutures can join bones enclosing variously the brain, eyes, nasal and oral structures, and air sinuses.

The last comment has bearing on the hypothesis that neurocranial growth (and sutural growth, by implication) is centered on expansion of the brain, which, acting via the dura, tenses sutures and promotes marginal osteogenesis. Aside from the minor effect from cutting the mammalian dura (Babler, Persing, Persson et al. 1982), there are other objections. Brains of ectotherms may not fill their braincases for the entire period of cranial growth (van der Klaauw 1948, 6), and other cranial spaces enclose soft tissue that can expand into air sinuses (Sarnat 1980). Moreover, the sutural growth of the composite mandible, say, the reptilian, is not referrable to a restricted, internally expanding soft-tissue mass.

Sutures share developmental processes, although there is no one exact developmental plan because of the different gross forms, species-based and other variations in the eventual thickness of the bones, and the site, whether in membrane (vault) or in mesenchyme (face) (Pritchard et al. 1956; Persson and Roy 1979). Other developmental interests are the separate differentiations of fibroblastic, osteoblastic, and sometimes chondroblastic populations, the programmed death of some cells (Ten Cate et al. 1977), the initial alignment of the bones (Johansen and Hall 1982; Furtwangler et al. 1985), and the influences of compression (Sitsen 1933; Gans 1960; Prahl-Andersen 1968; Herring and Mucci 1991) as well as tension. Development also involves maturation of the soft tissue, bone morphology and bone type (Jones and Boyde 1974), and the mechanism of any fusion (Persson et al. 1978), including the role of cartilage and chondroid bone (Moss 1958; Vinkka 1982; Ghafari 1984; Hinton 1988; Manzanares et al. 1989; Alberius and Johnell 1990).

Many aspects of sutures are controversial. (1) What happens to all components after bony fusion starts (Bernstein 1933; Kokich 1976)? (2) How are sutures influenced by stress (Miyewaki and Forbes 1987; Yen et al. 1989; Wagemans et al. 1988; Herring and Mucci 1991), and which sources of force are significant—muscular actions (Moss 1961a; Koskinen 1977), cerebral expansion (Moss 1975), ocular growth (Sarnat 1980), synchondrotic growth (Rönning and Kylamärkula 1972), vascular dynamics (Oudhof and van Doorenmallen 1983), or growth at other sutures? (3) Do sutures behave only passively to accommodate the growth of primary initiators elsewhere in the skull or soft tissues, for example, interactions across interfaces between cranial base, cranial vault, and face (Babler et al. 1987; Persing et al. 1991)? (4) What is the role in cranial growth and function of sutures that stay open but hardly grow, e.g., temporal? Do they permit angular change?

Local patterns of stress can be analyzed in behavioral-anatomical terms (Gans 1960; Herring 1972) and inferred from strain measured using gauges (Oudhof and van Doorenmallen 1983; Herring and Mucci 1991). Beyond the study of individual sutural conduct (Wagemans et al. 1988), methods for identifying the sutural contributions to the skull include cephalometrics of landmarks and implanted markers, and the computed tomography of bones, sutures, and cartilages (Furuya et al. 1984).

Endosteum, Marrow, and Vasculature

The strength of periosteum and perichondrium also secures vessels of various sizes. Although there are many publications on the vessels of bone (Brookes 1971), interest has largely skipped vascular patterns of the skull (Kayanja 1970). Nevertheless, angiogenesis and vascular remodeling go hand in hand with the reworking of bone and fibrous tissues and the erosion of cartilage (Chappard et al. 1986; Caplan 1990). Even without bone resorption, it is striking how many distinct and different patterns the vessels can adopt in primary vascular bone (Enlow and Brown 1956; and figs. 3.2–3.6). What is neutral and what is adaptive about these patterns remain to be learned.

Where bone encloses marrow or blood vessels, or lies as trabeculae within marrow, a thin layer of endosteal cells covers the bone. The nature of these cells and their relations with marrow are poorly understood in light of the large endosteal expanse in cancellous and well-vascularized bone. In maturity, most endosteal surfaces are not covered by osteoclasts or blatant osteoblasts. Instead, the flat endosteal cells' (FECs) organelle-poor ultrastructure appears incompatible with making much matrix, so the cells have attracted several more or less noncommittal names (Miller and Jee 1987; Islam et al. 1990). One role collectively assigned to osteoblasts and FECs is to act as a controllable physiological barrier, important in mineral metabolism (Menton et al. 1984), which creates a compartment between cells and the bone. Whatever the physiological evidence, there is no morphological basis for an ionic barrier (Boyde et al. 1978; Miller and Jee 1987). Indeed, the extension of processes by osteoblasts probably precludes establishing the kind of barrier achieved by smooth-lateral-surfaced, columnar, epithelial cells.

FECs seem to be osteoblasts of reduced activity which have not been included in the matrix, and secondly, osteoblastic progenitors that have yet to differentiate. The progenitor role is demonstrated by mitotic figures and ^{3}H-thymidine uptake in some FECs, when endosteal osteogenesis is stimulated in male birds by estrogen (Bowman and Miller 1986). At the same time, however, marrow cells adjacent to the endosteum divide and appear to contribute to the new osteoblastic pool, raising the general issues of the cellular and humoral traffic and relations between bone and marrow.

Marrow provides a complex background for such relations (Tavassoli and Yoffey 1983): bone marrow can be predominantly (sometimes exclusively) fibrous, fatty (yellow), mucoid, hemopoietic (red), or absent, depending upon skeletal site, age, species, and vertebrate class; red marrow also occurs outside bone; and soft-tissue organs may also perform bone-marrow functions. In mammals, some fibroblast-like marrow stromal cells are osteoblast-like (Benayahu et al. 1991). Next, there is much evidence for marrow's being the source of osteoclasts, the blood-borne precursors of which must eventually lodge in the targeted bone. Third, claims have been made for a gradient of marrow phenotype based on proximity to the bone, and for a bony humoral stimulation of hemopoiesis (Tavassoli and Yoffey 1983; Felix et al. 1988).

Marrow-bone relations in ectotherms are even more fascinating. The source of osteoclasts (multinucleated or uninuclear; Sire et al. 1990) is uncertain, since almost all fishes lack red marrow and amphibians have it only transiently. The mammalian type of bone marrow is otherwise found only in ganoid fishes (Scharrer 1944; Tavassoli 1986), lying mostly in the meninges but extending into bone-lined cavities in the cranial cartilage. This tissue association brings to mind the hemopoietic tissue of cephalopod mollusks which is situated close to cranial cartilage (Cowden 1972; Claes and Morse 1991).

In general, bone and marrow are in inverse proportion. Fishes offer examples with a high proportion of marrow. In *Orthagoriscus mola* and *Lophius* some cranial bones are largely a chamber system of thin bony lamellae enclosing an almost cell-free mucoid or hyaline material (Stud-nicka 1907). Second, large quantities of lipid are stored in the bones of certain fishes. The skull of the hawkfish (*Cirrhitus rivulatus*) is one-quarter lipid by weight, which may make the head neutrally or positively bouyant and account for the head-up posture when resting on reefs (Phleger 1987).

CRANIAL SKELETAL TISSUES IN AN EVOLUTIONARY PERSPECTIVE

In what ways have skeletal tissues evolved? I find this question intriguingly hard to answer, for at least two reasons. First, one can set the classically described tissues against their distribution in extant and fossil vertebrates. What emerges displays modest temporal sequence: the early vertebrates lacked little of what is seen subsequently, and apparent reappearances puzzle more than enlighten. There is no clearcut sign of progressive change. Second, since we do not know what special benefits particular histological configurations confer, how is adaptation to be recognized? Something—the physiology and biomechanics—is missing. Therefore, the following overview merely seeks similarities and connections suggestive of possible evolutionary processes, and is conducted in the spirit that similarity only points toward homology, which must then be tested for rigor-ously (Patterson 1988).

Trends, Retentions, and Reappearances

The overall phylogenetic trends (Moss 1964b) are for cranial bone mass to lessen, the skull to employ less cartilage (de Beer 1937), the exoskeleton to diminish and disappear, and notochord, chondroid tissues, calcified car-tilage, and metaplastic bone to be used less as permanent tissues. Varieties of cartilage—hyaline, elastic, and fibrocartilage, including secondary ex-pressions—find wider deployment in the head. Mammals retain, for re-stricted adult purposes, acellular bone (cementum), calcified cartilage, and perhaps chondroid. Selachians have kept little bone, while relying heavily on calcified cartilage, which might be connected with the character of their vasculature and the lower blood pressure than in teleosts. Increasing acel-lularity is the trend in the bone of teleosts (Meunier and Huyseunne, 1992). Size of the animal is a correlate. In classes where bone is predomi-nant, small animals employ avascular bone.

There are exceptions to the trends. Denison (1963) identified certain periods when the skeletal proportion within the body held or increased. Exoskeletons reappear in a few species in all tetrapod classes except birds (Moss 1968), and, as fish scales, have undergone great change (Kemp 1984; Francillon-Vieillet et al. 1990). Extant animals bearing cellular dentine are the bowfin (*Amia calva*), whale (*Balaenoptera physalus*), and armadillo (*Dasypus novemcinctus*) (Moss 1964a). Crocodilians and mammals share a use for an acellular bone (cementum) for the attachment of dental ligaments, but the major gap in the deployment of acellular bone was between heterostracans (Ørvig 1965) and modern teleosts (Moss 1964b). Extensive Haversian remodeling is special to certain dinosaurs (Reid 1984) and primates (Enlow and Brown 1958). This aspect of the dinosaurs is conspicuous because before and after them, in early amphibians and early birds, there was but little secondary replacement.

The irregular manifestations of bone histology in evolution led Enlow and Brown (1958) to conclude that bone has not evolved morphologically, in any fashion of proceeding phylogenetically from less to better ordered. The basic bony tissue elements, including calcified cartilage (Halstead 1969, 1973), existed from bone's first detected occurrence, and have since been deployed in manifold combinations, none showing any clear superiority. "Bone is opportunistic" (Hall 1984), and each expression may be an adequate rather than ideal compromise. One persisting enigma is the utility of the Haversian system. Remodeled bone is weaker and less mineralized than primary bone (Currey 1987), however Haversian bone remodeling may redirect the grain of the bone in new mechanical circumstances (Currey 1979, 1984).

Suggestions that the variety of skeletal tissues was greatest in fishes (Moss 1964b; Moss and Moss-Salentijn 1983), and was somehow reduced and stabilized with the advent of the tetrapods, need examination. First, whether the certainly wide range of chondroid tissues in recent fishes existed in early ones is uncertain. The teleostian and cyclostomian use of chondroid to support organs for suction and microphagy (Schaffer 1930; Benjamin 1990) leads one to suspect that some heterostracans employed chondroid tissues similarly. Second, Moss (1964b) proposed that tissue phenotypes in fish are labile in some way that required subsequent evolutionary stabilization—his process of "fixation." This scenario improbably implies lax controls over cells' products in fish. Third is the difficulty of reconciling with tissue distributions the vast outnumbering by fish species of those of other classes. Thus, the seeming absence of secondary cartilage in reptiles (Hall 1984) may spring in part from the low diversity of extant species available for study. Fourth, tissue biochemistry in tetrapods may vary almost as much as does morphology in fishes. Examples are the special proteoglycan and protein profiles of lagomorph bone (Bartold 1990) and enamel, respectively; the absence of keratan sulfate from certain rodents' cartilage; and the different keratan sulfates in bovine articular and nasal-septal cartilages (Nieduszynski et al. 1990). Tetrapods make various chondroid bones, with fresh instances still being uncovered (Moury et al. 1987). The osteocalcin/osteonectin ratios in human trabecular and compact bone are quite distinct (Ninomiya et al. 1990). Lastly, trabecular bone has permitted some of the reduction in bone mass. The morphological diversity of trabecular bone could exceed that recognized by conventional histology in dense bone, variety being a function of both tissues and criteria, and trabecular patterns have so far been neglected, despite their mechanical significance (Currey 1984). The teleostian tissue diversity may be real, but overemphasized.

A factor in the marked histological diversity of early vertebrate bone and dentine may be that the cells had fewer genes, smaller gene families (Exposito and Garrone 1990), less elaborate proteins, and more often only one promoter site per gene, so that fine adaptations were created by means of cellular structural arrangements, whereas cells of endotherms deploy their greater diversity of molecules and molecular domains.

Skeletal Cell Behaviors

What activities are performed by skeletal cells and how might these be linked to the abilities of possible precursor cells in evolution?

Osteoblasts. To make skeletal matrices, the formative cells engage in numerous activities, only a few of which may be tissue-specific and therefore critically involved in the skeletal evolutionary steps. To assess the steps means knowing what behaviors and molecules had to be specially adapted, insofar as information from present cells can show. Among the formative cellular activities are proliferation, adhesion to substrates, attachment to cells, motility, extension of processes, cell polarization, synthesis of matrix materials, secretion, extracellular molecular assembly and orientation, responsiveness to mechanical forces, initial and subsequent mineralization, partial or total migration from the matrix, and limited turnover of matrix materials. There may be minor skeletal specializations in many of these processes, but the main cellular novelty, i.e., mechanical essentials, of hard tissues appears limited to shifting the collagen-type balance to type I with almost total suppression of the several other types expressed by fibroblasts (Pavlin et al. 1992); to making osteocalcin; and to controlling fibril size and direction precisely for osseous configurations. Other essentials include initiating mineralization by materials in matrix vesicles, providing more materials for a co-collagenous mineralization (Christofferson and Landis 1991), and adopting characteristic positions vis-à-vis the matrix and blood vessels.

If the ontogeny and evolution of the rostral skull are from neural crest, one anticipates the skeletal cells, as adaptations, should share behaviors, synthesized materials, and controls with ectodermal progeny such as neurons, glia, or sensory epithelia. Several such associations could be looked for. For example, one might compare the microtubule-associated proteins mediating axonal transport (Knops et al. 1991) with what moves calcium-binding proteins down the dentine-forming odontoblast process, or compare the mechanisms for polarizing the release of osteoid components and the extension of osteocyte processes (Ekanayake and Hall 1988; Watson et al. 1989; Palumbo et al. 1990) with polarization in epithelia.

Chondroblasts. These require most of the basic behaviors needed by osteoblasts, and also fibroblasts. Cartilages have little fibronectin and few vessels, but extensively share other materials with hard and soft connective tissues. However, cartilages are typified by particular fibrillar and nonfibrillar collagens, and large proteoglycans aggregated by specific core- and link-protein interactions with hyaluronan, except shark cartilage, which seems to do with hyaluronan (Michelacci and Horton 1989). Instances of microarchitectural distinction are the fibrillar layout, the pattern of deep and superficial mineralizations in selachians, and the asymmetric mineralization and columns of cells in some growth cartilages. Also, understanding the evolution and mechanics of cartilage and other skeletal tissues requires the chemistry and fine structure of the chondroid tissues—vertebrate and invertebrate. For example, that some fish chondroid is rich in microfibrils may help characterize these elusive elements, which, in vertebrates, participate in activities ranging from corneal stromal construction to dentinogenesis to reptilian dermal metaplastic ossification.

Examples exist of cartilaginous links with neural derivatives of neural crest. The conversion of quail ocular chondrogenic mesenchyme to neurogenesis (Smith-Thomas et al. 1986) demonstrates a common response between neural and chondrogenic lineages to factors controlling cellular identity. Periotic mesenchyme expresses a receptor for nerve growth factor (van Bartheld et al. 1991). Human elastic chondrocytes react positively for a glial intermediate-filament protein (Kepes and Perentes 1988).

Osteoclasts. The osteoclast fuses to bone by a seal which encircles a zone, into which enzymes and acid are released and stirred by a moving ruffled border (Jones et al. 1985; Chambers and Hall 1991). Tracing the pedigree of the various devices, mechanisms, and controls is a challenge. The forerunner of the osteoclast might have been a defensive phagocyte, although the polarized generation of acid could stem from renal epithelial behavior (Baron 1989; Blair et al. 1989). Early on, the hard matrices themselves may have taken some control over osteoclasts (Glowacki et al. 1991). A clue is the multinucleated cells appearing on bone particles implanted into dogfish (Peignoux-Deville et al. 1989). The control of osteoclastic activity with a peptide hormone again links skeleton to nervous system (and kidney) in the use of a brain-related peptide, calcitonin (Zaidi et al. 1991).

Not only can one compare the behaviors and mechanisms of vertebrate cells to gain insight into what may have been borrowed from where, one can address sharing between skeletal cells of lower vertebrates and invertebrate cells, in particular neural (Gans and Northcutt 1983), chondroid, and connective-tissue cells. How much did the first dentinoblast or osteoblast draw on invertebrate fibroblastic and/or neural abilities? How invertebrates gained the means to aggregate proteoglycans for water-binding marked steps toward cartilage; the early use of constrained turgid cells was a parallel advance toward notochord.

Evolutionary Needs or Imperatives: Superficial and Deep

What circumstances might have driven invertebrate cells to try osteoblastic and chondroblastic solutions?

Mechanical Support and Protection for the Brain. Central nervous tissue needs mechanical protection, which has to be peripheral enclosure and support, because neurons and glia cannot function with ECM between them. An early example is the neural lamella, which is a substantial sheath around the cockroach central nervous system. An early resilient skeletal manifestation was the cartilage pieces surrounding the brain and eye of cephalopods (Bairati et al. 1987; Vynios and Tsiganos 1990). Since they are not forebears of vertebrates, squid and octopus with their highly developed, cartilage-endowed eyes and brains could help with several questions of parallel or convergent evolution. These concern matrix macro-molecules, signaling systems, the role of homeodomain proteins in tissue differentiation (Mackenzie et al. 1991), and how to form "cranial" cartilage in the absence of neural crest.

Exoskeletal Armor. Imbedding calcified structures in the dermis can involve simple scales of mineralized collagen (Zylberberg and Wake 1990), or more elaborate dentinal or bony structures. A simply constructed scalelike formation could have originated vertebrate armor, and reappeared in teleosts, amphibians, and reptiles. However, an epithelial ameloblastic mineralization is another contender for first vertebrate hard tissue (Kresja et al. 1991).

Armor need not be hard: leather is effective. The squid has dermal scales consisting of its kind of cartilage (Karamanos et al. 1992), so again somewhere in the cephalopod lineage may have been the first exoskeletal use of cartilage, perhaps preceding endoskeletal neural protection.

Sensory Enhancement. Gans and Northcutt (1983) regarded the skeletal tissues as "derivatives of sensory transducers," based on two hypotheses: that the initial purpose of the enameloid and dentine of the ostracoderm exoskeleton was to insulate and boost electroreceptors, and that cartilage evolved from the gelatinous bodies of mechanoreceptors. However, the former idea requires knowledge that the soft tissues around the early electroreceptors did not meet the need for insulation, and leaves unexplained the mixture of hard tissues—insulation should have selected only the better one. The second idea conflicts with the presence of proteoglycans (Scott 1991) and many forms of cartilage (Person 1983) in invertebrates, and the likelihood that the gelatinous parts of mechanoreceptors consisted as much of glycoproteins (Sugiyama et al. 1991) as proteoglycans.

Gans's (1989) scenario that dentine and its cells originated for sensory reception or its boosting is endorsed by Smith and Hall (1990). Two reservations are that their listing of several modalities to be sensed is questionable, since transduction requires that cells make one specific chemical to respond to one class of stimulus (Shepherd 1991); and the later capping of the dentine by enameloid would have markedly altered the former's sensory competence.

Resilient Substrate. Invertebrate epithelia can secrete materials promoting mineralization, but a hard crystalline material offers more when buttressed by fusion to a still hard, but more resilient composite such as dentine or bone. Bone can itself be fastened to connective tissues for a further dissipation of energy. This is an exoskeletal requirement for a mineralized substrate matched to harder enameloid or enamel. The layering of hard tissues might be anticipated in the form of layered modifications within invertebrate calcified exoskeletons (Watabe and Pan 1984). Participation by fusion in the creation of a layered arrangement is a significant step for a tissue, involving integrated timing, direction of growth, and compatible matrices, and expressing the power of combinations. Thus from three tissues—enameloid (E), dentine (D), and bone (B)—five early vertebrate exoskeletal uses ensued: B, D, DB, ED, and EDB.

Mineral-Metabolic. A sizable, mineralized skeleton in excess of the usual mechanical demands can, by resorption and replacement, carry an animal through scarcities of exogenous calcium or phosphorus. Although hard tissues were massive in ostracoderms and showed signs of cellular resorption (Halstead 1973), the mineral-metabolic need probably appeared after much smaller, hard, collagenous structures had first met muscular, armorial, or enameloid-substrate purposes. The susceptibility to dissolution of a small calcified piece exposed to tissue fluid may have been one factor favoring the use of apatite rather than a carbonate-based crystal. Ruben and Bennett (1987) measured and discussed the comparative solubilities in a tissue milieu acidified by muscular activity. The initial metabolic need may therefore have rather been for a tissue that only intended cellular action could destroy. The secondary impulse, to extract stored mineral, brought incidental benefits such as an ability to reshape the tissue, and acted in the first instance upon the resorbing cells, and therefore needed not to show any endo- or exoskeletal preference. Key evolutionary questions center on the first recruitment, retargeting, and control of cells selectively to destroy hard tissues and to coordinate this activity with vessel ingrowth and concurrent or subsequent osteogenesis. Incidentally, since osteocytes do not lyse bone at all or to any physiologically meaningful extent (Boyde 1980; Marotti et al. 1990), the acellularity of teleostean and other bone should be unrelated to mineral and acid metabolism, perhaps being linked to a slow, indeterminate growth where matrix alone suffices. Acellularity is subtle in being not infrequent in small areas of bone in many vertebrates, and by certain teleost species' exhibiting both cellular and acellular bone (Moss 1961c; Meunier and Huyseunne, n.d.).

General Principles. Whichever of the above "imperatives" based on beneficial new relations between tissues actually took place, any one would have required tissue-tissue interactions (Hall 1991). Such instructions and responses would bring about and coordinate the growth and complementarity of the matched tissues. Previous invertebrate tissue co-operations—epithelial-stromal, muscle–connective tissue, neuron-glial, neuro-muscular—could provide a basis of inductive, adhesive, and proliferative controls for adaptation to skeletal–soft tissue interactions. Conservation of signaling molecules is demonstrated by an invertebrate (tunicate) interleukin 1-like cytokine that makes mouse thymocytes divide (Raftos et al. 1991), and by calcitonin-like peptides in invertebrates (Zaidi et al. 1991), vertebrate calcitonin being a hormone involved in controlling calcium balance.

A skeletal tissue started for one end immediately offers itself for other uses. Thus several muscles insert into the cephalopod neurocranial cartilages (Bairati et al. 1987); and scleral ossicles of the avian eye may allow intrinsic muscles to recurve and focus the cornea. Multiple uses, of course, involve structural compromise; however, some constructions can be devoted to one task and selectively specialized. For example, the bone of the whale's separate petrotympanic complex is highly mineralized to be stiff for hearing in water (Currey 1979), leaving protective strength to the skull proper.

CONCLUSIONS

The Tissues

Cranial skeletal tissue diversity expresses itself as several recognizable forms of tissue with many subtypes. This diversity signifies versatility of function, but with a difference between the two major classes of skeletal tissue, cartilage being preeminent in its range of forms and applications.

The cartilage family uses a mix of proteoglycans and glycoproteins in conjunction with a meshwork of various kinds of fibril. Cephalopods, lampreys, hagfishes, teleosts, and tetrapods have arrived at substantially different kinds of fibril in solving this need. Bone is much less variable in the properties of its matrix of mineralized collagen fibrils, but it provides diverse densities and trabecular architectures by the interplay of resorptive and formative cells, blood vessels, and bone marrow. The soft collagenous tissues are often taken for granted, but are not only essential for cranial function, as illustrated by the controversies surrounding mammalian sutures, but when interrogated appropriately across the vertebrates may be as varied as bone or cartilage.

Their visual basis gives the microscopically conceived tissue classifications of the last century a powerful hold on the mind. It is difficult to reconcile visual and tactile distinctiveness with the extensive overlap in cell activities and molecular constituents among the tissues. However, these are the elements that confer on the tissues performance and identity. Inviting our comprehension is a stupendous degree of multitiered, cellular control over numerous constituents, their assembly outside the cells, maturational change, and fusions with other tissues which are critical for biomechanical integrity.

Phylogeny

Although some very general structure-function parallels can be drawn, the fine details of histology and molecular composition have not yet been connected to differing functional demands. Secondly, the comparative evidence suggests that substantial repertoires of cell behaviors and genes for structural and coordinating molecules were available for the selection of combinations (and for mutation) very early in the vertebrate line, if not earlier. Thirdly, the trends are in the use, rather than the nature, of the tissue, but there are exceptions. Certain dinosaurs and primates, and mammals and ganoid fishes, for example, share distinctive types of bone and marrow, respectively. This is curious, and also suggests that functionally unexplained features of single tissues may be unreliable characters for phylogenetic analysis. On the other hand, learning how invertebrate cells and molecules led to the various vertebrate skeletal cell types may help explain what then happened to skeletal tissues during evolution through the vertebrates.

Approaches

Tissue identity derives from the differentiation of cells, and their continuing interactions and responses to physical stimuli, e.g., mechanical loading. Skeletal tissues acquire an additional dimension of identity through their matrices. Fundamentally important features of matrix such as the profiles of thickness and orientation of fibrils, and bone trabecularity, can be put on a more quantitative basis. One method uses laser-scanning, confocal microscopy for its three-dimensional images which can be digitally stored and analyzed with computers. Knowledge from this level lends itself to correlation with the classic biomechanical properties of strength, hardness, and elasticity, and with changes in dimensions and X-ray density (Lotz et al. 1990). With more molecular and histochemical probes available, e.g., monoclonal antibodies (James et al. 1991), the task of characterizing both matrix and cells of the many varieties of hard, resilient, and soft tissues in lower vertebrates and invertebrates should provide unifying information and meaningful classification. The chondroid or cartilage-like tissues are particularly in need of study.

The investigative tools and approaches applied to the cell and molecular biology of well-characterized cells should benefit skeletal biology. Blood cells and skeletal muscle exemplify the identification of molecules regulating cell phenotype at the transcriptional level (Olson 1991; Venutti et al. 1991). But how can several different factors regulate in unison? One particular approach has widespread application to analyzing the very common biological situation where combinations of factors operate as a cascade. Mathematical analyses of the structure of human language may clarify the informational content of cell-to-cell signaling systems (Mayer and Baldi 1991), and of combinations of transcription factors. Function derives from patterns of combinations. Even the combinations of constituents in extracellular matrix instruct skeletal cells and other tissues, and encode mechanical states. The task is to grasp simultaneously and continuously cellular phenotypes, matrix characters, and tissue interactions. The latter are especially significant in the skull with its numerous tissue boundaries, the erection and stability of which are critical to gross morphology.

ACKNOWLEDGMENTS

I thank Brian Hall and James Hanken for their very helpful criticisms of drafts of this chapter. Michael Benjamin, Donald Enlow, and Ann Huysseune very kindly gave permission for the use of their illustrations; and I appreciate the granting by Cambridge University Press of permission to reproduce figures 3.12–3.17 from articles in the *Journal of Anatomy*, and by the Texas Academy of Sciences for figures 3.1–3.8 from the *Texas Journal of Science*.

REFERENCES

Alberius, P., and O. Johnell. 1990. Immunohistochemical assessment of cranial suture development in rats. Journal of Anatomy 173: 61–68.

Alberius, P., and G. Selvik. 1985. Volumetric changes in the developing rabbit calvarium. Anatomical Record 213: 207–214.

Armstrong, L. A., G. M. Wright, and J. H. Youson. 1987. Transformation of mucocartilage to a definitive cartilage during metamorphosis in the sea lamprey, *Petromyzon marinus*. Journal of Morphology 194: 1–21.

Babler, W. J., J. A. Persing, K. M. Persson, H. R. Winn, J. A. Jane, and G. T. Rodeheaver. 1982. Skull growth after coronal suturectomy, periostectomy, and dural transection. Journal of Neurosurgery 56: 529–535.

Babler, W. J., J. A. Persing, H. R. Winn, J. A. Jane, and G. T. Rodeheaver. 1982. Compensatory growth following premature closure of the coronal suture in rabbits. Journal of Neurosurgery 57: 535–542.

Babler, W. J., J. A. Persing, H. J. Nagorsky, and J. A. Jane. 1987. Restricted growth at the frontonasal suture: Alterations in craniofacial growth in rabbits. American Journal of Anatomy 178: 90–98.

Baecker, R. 1926. Beiträge zur Histologie der Barteln der Fische. Zeitschrift für mikroskopische-anatomische Forschung 6: 489–507.

———. 1928. Zur Histologie des Ohrknorpels der Säuger. Zeitschrift für mikroskopische-anatomische Forschung 15: 274–367.

Bairati, A., S. de Baisi, F. Cheli, and A. Oggioni. 1987. The head cartilage of cephalopods. 1. Architecture and ultrastructure of the extracellular matrix. Tissue and Cell 19: 673–685.

Balmain, N., A. Moscofian, and P. Cuisinier-Gleizes. 1983. Metaphyseal pattern: Uniqueness of this structure in growing bones originating from cartilaginous anlage; A microradiographic study. Calcified Tissue International 35: 225–231.

Bargmann, W. 1939. Zur Kenntnis der Knorpelarchitekturen: Untersuchungen am Skeletsystem von Selachiern. Zeitschrift für Zellforschung 29: 404–424.

———. 1973. Zur Histologie der Säugplatte des Schiffshalters Echenesis naucrates L. Mit Bermerkungen zur Systematik der Stützgewebe. Zeitschrift für Zellforschung 139: 149–170.

Baron, R. 1989. Molecular mechanisms of bone resorption by the osteoclast. Anatomical Record 224: 317–324.

Bartold, P. M. 1990. A biochemical and immunohistochemical study of the proteoglycans of alveolar bone. Journal of Dental Research 69: 7–19.

Becker, W. 1971. Elektronenmikroskopische Untersuchung der Insertion von Sehnen am Knochen. Archiv für Orthopädie und Unfall-Chirurgie 69: 315–329.

Beecher, R. M. 1977. Function and fusion at the mandibular symphysis. American Journal of Physical Anthropology 47: 325–335.

Ben Ami, Y., K. von der Mark, A. Franzen, B. de Bernard, G. C. Lunazzi, and M. Silbermann. 1991. Immunohistochemical studies of the human fetal mandible: Collagens and noncollagenous proteins. American Journal of Anatomy 190: 157–166.

Benayahu, D., A. Fried, D. Zipori, and S. Weintroub. 1991. Subpopulations of marrow stromal cells share a variety of osteoblastic markers. Calcified Tissue International 49: 202–207.

Benjamin, M. 1986. The oral sucker of *Gyrinocheilus aymonieri* (Teleostei: Cypriniformes). Journal of Zoology, London B 1: 211–254.

————. 1988. Mucocartilage (mucous connective tissue) in the heads of teleosts. Anatomy and Embryology 178: 461–474.

————. 1989a. The development of hyaline-cell cartilage in the head of the black molly, *Poecilia sphenops:* Evidence for a secondary cartilage in a teleost. Journal of Anatomy 164: 145–154.

————. 1989b. Hyaline-cell cartilage (chondroid) in the heads of teleosts. Anatomy and Embryology 179: 285–303.

————. 1990. The cranial cartilages of teleosts and their classification. Journal of Anatomy 169: 153–172.

Benjamin, M., and E. J. Evans. 1990. Fibrocartilage. Journal of Anatomy 171: 1–15.

Benjamin, M., E. J. Evans, and L. Copp. 1986. The histology of tendon attachments to bone in man. Journal of Anatomy 149: 89–100.

Benjamin, M., and J. R. Ralphs. 1991. Extracellular matrix of connective tissues in the heads of teleosts. Journal of Anatomy 179: 137–148.

Benjamin, M., and J. S. Sandhu. 1990. The structure and ultrastructure of the rostral cartilage in the spiny eel, *Macrognathus siamensis* (Teleostei: Mastacembeloidei). Journal of Anatomy 169: 37–47.

Benton, M. J. 1987. Progress and competition in macroevolution. Biological Reviews 62: 305–338.

Beresford, W. A. 1981. *Chondroid Bone, Secondary Cartilage, and Metaplasia.* Baltimore: Urban and Schwarzenberg.

Bernstein, S. A. 1933. Über den normalen histologischen Aufbau des Schädeldaches. Zeitschrift für Anatomie und Entwickslungsgeschichte 101: 652–678.

Blair, H. C., S. L. Teitelbaum, R. Ghiselli, and S. Gluck. 1989. Osteoclastic bone resorption by a polarized vacuolar proton pump. Science 245: 855–857.

Bosshardt, D. D., and H. E. Schroeder. 1991. Establishment of acellular extrinsic fiber cementum on human teeth. Cell Tissue Research 263: 325–336.

————. 1992. Initial formation of cellular intrinsic fiber cementum in developing human teeth. Cell and Tissue Research 267: 321–335.

Bowman, B. M., and S. C. Miller. 1986. The proliferation and differentiation of the bone-lining cell in estrogen-induced osteogenesis. Bone 7: 351–357.

Boyde, A. 1980. Evidence against "osteocytic osteolysis." Metabolic Bone Disease and Related Research 2: 239–255.

Boyde, A., E. J. Reith, and S. J. Jones. 1978. Intercellular attachments between calcified collagenous tissue forming cells in the rat. Cell Tissue Research 191: 507–512.

Brookes, M. 1971. *The Blood Supply of Bone.* London: Butterworths.

Burgeson, R. E. 1988. New collagens, new concepts. Annual Review of Cell Biology 4: 551–577.

Busbey, A. B., III. 1989. Form and function of the feeding apparatus of *Alligator mississippiensis.* Journal of Morphology 202: 99–127.

Butler, W. T. 1984. Matrix macromolecules of bone and dentin. Collagen and Related Research 4: 297–307.

Butler, W. T. 1991. Sialoproteins of bone and dentin. Journal de Biologie Buccale 19: 83–89.

Caplan, A. I. 1990. Cartilage begets bone versus endochondral myelopoiesis. Clinical Orthopaedics 261: 257–267.

Caterson, B., T. Calabro, and A. Hampton. 1987. Monoclonal antibodies as probes for elucidating proteoglycan structure and function. Biology of Extracellular Matrix 2: 1–26.

Chambers, T. J., and T. J. Hall. 1991. Cellular and molecular mechanisms in the regulation and function of osteoclasts. Vitamins and Hormones 46: 41–86.

Chappard, D., C. Alexandre, and G. Riffat. 1986. Uncalcified cartilage resorption in human fetal cartilage canals. Tissue and Cell 18: 701–707.

Chong, D. A., and C. A. Evans. 1982. Histologic study of the attachment of muscles to the rat mandible. Archives of Oral Biology 27: 510–527.

Chong, D. A., C. A. Evans, and J. D. Heeley. 1982. Morphology and maturation of the rat mandible. Archives of Oral Biology 27: 777–785.

Christoffersen, J., and W. J. Landis. 1991. A contribution with review to the description of mineralization of bone and other calcified tissues in vivo. Anatomical Record 230: 435–450.

Claes, M. F., and M. P. Morse. 1991. Is the white body the blood-forming tissue in cephalopods? American Zoologist 31: 130A.

Cowden, R. R. 1972. Some cytological and cytochemical observations on the leucopoietic organs, the "white bodies" of *Octopus vulgaris*. Journal of Invertebrate Pathology 19: 113–119.

Currey, J. D. 1979. Mechanical properties of bone tissues with greatly differing functions. Journal of Biomechanics 12: 313–319.

———. 1984. Comparative mechanical properties and histology of bone. American Zoologist 24: 5–12.

———. 1987. The evolution of the mechanical properties of amniote bone. Journal of Biomechanics 20: 1035–1044.

de Beer, G. R. 1937. *The Development of the Vertebrate Skull*. London: Oxford University Press.

Denison, R. H. 1963. The early history of the vertebrate calcified skeleton. Clinical Orthopaedics 31: 141–152.

de Ricqlès, A. J. 1974. Evolution of endothermy: Histological evidence. Evolutionary Theory 1: 51–80.

Eikenberry, E. F., B. Childs, S. B. Sheren, D. A. D. Parry, A. S. Craig, and B. Brodsky. 1984. Crystalline fibril structure of type II collagen in lamprey notochord sheath. Journal of Molecular Biology 176: 261–277.

Ekanayake, S., and B. K. Hall. 1988. Ultrastructure of the osteogenesis of acellular vertebral bone in the Japanese medaka, *Oryzias Latipes* (Teleostei, Cyprinidontidae). American Journal of Anatomy 182: 241–249.

———. 1991. Development of the notochord in the Japanese medaka, *Oryzias latipes* (Teleostei; Cyprinodontidae), with special reference to desmosomal connections and functional integration with adjacent tissues. Canadian Journal of Zoology 69: 1171–1177.

English, A. W. 1985. Limbs vs. jaws: Can they be compared? American Zoologist 25: 351–363.

Enlow, D. H. 1968. *The Human Face*. New York: Harper and Row.

———. 1969. The bone of reptiles. In *Biology of the Reptilia*, vol. 1, *Morphology A*, C. Gans, A. d'A. Bellairs, and T. S. Parsons, eds. New York: Academic Press, pp. 45–80.

Enlow, D. H., and S. O. Brown. 1956. A comparative histological study of fossil and recent bone tissues. Part 1. Texas Journal of Science 8: 405–443.

———. 1957. A comparative histological study of fossil and recent bone tissues. Part II. Texas Journal of Science 9: 186–214.

———. 1958. A comparative histological study of fossil and recent bone tissues. Part III. Texas Journal of Science 10: 187–230.

Evans, E. J., M. Benjamin, and D. J. Pemberton. 1991. Variations in the amount of calcified tissue at the attachments of the quadriceps tendon and patellar ligament in man. Journal of Anatomy 174: 145–151.

Exposito, J.-Y., and R. Garrone. 1990. Characterization of a fibrillar collagen gene in sponges reveals the early evolutionary appearance of two collagen gene families. Proceedings of the National Academy of Sciences, U.S.A. 87: 6669–6673.

Felix, R., P. R. Elford, C. Stoerckle, M. Cecchini, A. Weterwald, U. Treschsel, H. Fleisch, and B. M. Stadler. 1988. Production of hemopoietic growth factors by bone tissue and bone cells in culture. Journal of Bone and Mineral Metabolism 3: 27–36.

Flood, P. R. 1969. Fine structure of the notochord of Myxine glutinosa. Journal of Ultrastructure Research 29: 573–474 P (Proceedings).

Francillon-Vieillot, H., V. de Buffrénil, J. Castenet, J. Géraudie, F. J. Meunier, J.-Y. Sire, L. Zylberberg, and A. de Ricqlès. 1990. Microstructure and mineralization of vertebrate skeletal tissues. In Skeletal Biomineralization: Patterns, Processes, and Evolutionary Trends, vol. 1, J. G. Carter, ed. New York: Van Nostrand Reinhold, pp. 471–530.

Frankenhuis-van den Heuvel, T. H. M., J. C. Maltha, and A. M. Kuijpers-Jagtman. 1991. A histological and histometric study of the periosteum in mandibular ramal and condylar areas of the rabbit. Archives of Oral Biology 36: 933–938.

Fuchs, H. 1909. Über Knorpelbildung in Deckknochen nebst Untersuchungen und Betrachtungen über Gehörknochelchen, Kiefer und Keifergelenk der Wirbeltiere. Archiv für Anatomie und Physiologie, Anatomische Ergänzungsheft: 1–256.

Fujita, S., and K. Hoshino. 1989. Histochemical and immunohistochemical studies on the articular disk of the temporomandibular joint in rats. Acta anatomica 134: 26–30.

Furtwangler, J. A., S. H. Hall, and L. K. Koskinen-Moffett. 1985. Sutural morphogenesis in the mouse calvaria: The role of apoptosis. Acta anatomica 124: 74–80.

Furuya, Y., M. S. B. Edwards, C. E. Alpers, B. M. Tress, D. K. Ousterhout, and D. Norman. 1984. Computerized tomography of cranial sutures. Part 1. Comparison of suture anatomy in children and adults. Journal of Neurosurgery 61: 53–58.

Gaill, F., H. Wiedemann, K. Mann, K. Kuhn, R. Timpl, and J. Engel. 1991. Molecular characterization of cuticle and interstitial collagens from worms collected at deep sea hydrothermal vents. Journal of Molecular Biology 221: 209–223.

Gans, C. 1960. Studies on Amphisbaenids (Amphisbaenia, Reptilia). 1. Bulletin of the American Museum of Natural History 119: 129–204.

————. 1989. Stages in the origin of vertebrates: Analysis by means of scenarios. Biological Reviews 64: 221–268.

Gans, C., and R. G. Northcutt. 1983. Neural crest and the origin of vertebrates: A new head. Science 220: 268–274.

Ghafari, J. 1984. Palatal sutural response to buccal muscular displacement in the rat. American Journal of Orthodontics 85: 351–356.

Glowacki, J., K. A. Cox, J. O'Sullivan, D. Wilkie, and L. J. Deftos. 1986. Osteoclasts can be induced in fish having an acellular bony skeleton. Proceedings of the National Academy of Sciences, U.S.A. 83: 4104–4107.

Glowacki, J., C. Rey, M. J. Glimcher, K. A. Cox, and J. Lian. 1991. A role for osteocalcin in osteoclast differentiation. Journal of Cellular Biochemistry 45: 292–302.

Goetinck, P. F. 1991. Proteoglycans in development. Current Topics in Developmental Biology 25: 111–131.

Goldstein, S. A. 1987. The mechanical properties of trabecular bone: Dependence on anatomical location and function. Journal of Biomechanics 20: 1055–1061.

Goret-Nicaise, M., and A. Dhem. 1987. Electron microscopic study of chondroid tissue in the cat mandible. Calcified Tissue International 40: 219–223.

Haines, R. W. 1937. The posterior end of Meckel's cartilage and related ossifications in bony fishes. Quarterly Journal of Microscopical Sciences 80: 1–38.

Hall, B. K. 1967. The distribution and fate of adventitious cartilage in the skull of the eastern rosella, *Platycercus eximius* (Aves: Psittaciformes). Australian Journal of Zoology 15: 685–698.

————. 1975. Evolutionary consequences of skeletal differentiation. American Zoologist 15: 329–350.

————. 1978. *Developmental and Cellular Skeletal Biology.* New York: Academic Press.

————, ed. 1983. *Cartilage.* 3 vols. Orlando: Academic Press.

————. 1984. Developmental processes underlying the evolution of bone and cartilage. Symposia of the Zoological Society of London, 52: 155–176.

————. 1991. Cellular interactions during cartilage and bone development. Journal of Craniofacial Genetics and Developmental Biology 11: 238–250.

Hall, B. K., and J. Hanken. 1985. Repair of fractured lower jaws in the spotted salamander: Do amphibians form secondary cartilage? Journal of Experimental Zoology 232: 359–368.

Hall, B. K., and S. A. Newman. 1991. *Cartilage: Molecular Aspects.* Boca Raton: CRC Press.

Halstead, L. B. 1969. Calcified tissues in the earliest vertebrates. Calcified Tissue Research 3: 107–124.

————. 1973. The heterostracan fishes. Biological Reviews 48: 279–332.

————. 1974. *Vertebrate Hard Tissues.* London: Wykeham Publications.

Hardingham, T. E., and A. J. Fosang. 1992. Proteoglycans: Many forms and many functions. FASEB Journal 6: 861–870.

Hardisty, M. W. 1981. The skeleton. In *Biology of Lampreys,* vol. 3, M. W. Hardisty, and I. C. Potter, eds. London: Academic Press, pp. 333–376.

Harkness, E. M., and W. D. Trotter. 1978. Growth of transplants of rat humerus following circumferential division of the periosteum. Journal of Anatomy 126: 275–289.

Herring, S., and R. J. Mucci. 1991. In vivo strain in cranial sutures: The zygomatic arch. Journal of Morphology 207: 225–239.

Herring, S. W. 1972. Sutures: A tool in functional cranial analysis. Acta anatomica 83: 222–247.

Hinton, D. R., L. E. Becker, K. F. Muakkassa, and H. J. Hoffman. 1984. Lambdoid synostosis. Part 1. The lambdoid suture: Normal development and pathology of "synostosis." Journal of Neurosurgery 61: 333–339.

Hinton, R. J. 1988. Response of the intermaxillary suture cartilage to alterations in masticatory function. Anatomical Record 220: 376–387.

Homberger, D. G., and R. A. Meyers. 1989. Morphology of the lingual apparatus of the domestic chicken, *Gallus gallus,* with special attention to the structure of the fasciae. American Journal of Anatomy 186: 217–257.

Hoyte, D. A. W. 1971. Mechanisms of growth in the cranial vault and base. Journal of Dental Research 50: 1447–1461.

Hunzicker, E. B., and W. Herrmann. 1987. In situ localization of cartilage extracellular matrix components by immunoelectron microscopy after cryotechnical tissue processing. Journal of Histochemistry and Cytochemistry 35: 647–655.

Huysseune, A. 1986. Late skeletal development at the articulation between upper pharyngeal jaws and neurocranial base in the fish, *Astatotilapia elegans,* with the participation of a chondroid form of bone. American Journal of Anatomy 177: 119–137.

Huysseune, A., and J. Y. Sire. 1990. Ultrastructural observations on chondroid bone in the teleost fish *Hemichromis bimaculatus.* Tissue and Cell 22: 371–383.

Huysseune, A., and W. Verraes. 1986. Chondroid bone on the upper pharyngeal jaws and neurocranial base in the adult fish *Astatotilapia elegans.* American Journal of Anatomy 177: 527–535.

Ingervall, B., G. E. Carlsson, and B. Thilander. 1976. Postnatal development of the human temporomandibular joint. II. A microradiographic study. Acta odontologica scandinavica 34: 133–139.

Irwin, C. R., and M. W. J. Ferguson. 1986. Fracture repair of reptilian dermal bones: Can reptiles form secondary cartilage? Journal of Anatomy 146: 53–64.

Islam, A., C. Glomski, and E. S. Henderson. 1990. Bone lining (endosteal) cells and hematopoiesis: A light microscopic study of normal and pathologic human bone marrow in plastic-embedded sections. Anatomical Record 227: 300–306.

James, I. E., S. Walsh, R. A. Dodds, and M. Gowen. 1991. Production and characterization of osteoclast-selective monoclonal antibodies that distinguish between mutinucleated cells derived from different human tissues. Journal of Histochemistry and Cytochemistry 39: 905–914.

Jaslow, C. R. 1990. Mechanical properties of cranial sutures. Journal of Biomechanics 23: 313–321.

Johansen, V. A., and S. H. Hall. 1982. Morphogenesis of the mouse coronal suture. Acta anatomica 114: 58–67.

Jones, S. J., and A. Boyde. 1972. A study of human root cementum surfaces as prepared for and examined in the scanning electron microscope. Zeitschrift für Zellforschung 130: 318–337.

———. 1974. The organization and gross mineralization patterns of the collagen fibres in Sharpey fibre bone. Cell and Tissue Research 148: 83–96.

Jones, S. J., A. Boyde, N. N. Ali, and E. Maconnachie. 1985. A review of bone cell and substratum interactions. Scanning 7: 5–24.

Karamanos, N. K., A. J. Aletras, T. Tsegenidis, C. P. Tsiganos, and C. A. Antonopoulos. 1992. Isolation, characterization and properties of the oversulphated chondroitin sulphate proteoglycan from squid skin with peculiar sulphation pattern. European Journal of Biochemistry 204: 553–560.

Kayanja, F. I. B. 1970. The postnatal development of the blood supply of the fronto-parietal, scapula, and mandible of the cat. Anatomischer Anzeiger 127: 369–382.

Kemp, N. E. 1984. Organic matrices and mineral crystallites in vertebrate scales, teeth, and skeletons. American Zoologist 24: 965–976.

Kemp, N. E., and S. K. Westrin. 1979. Ultrastructure of calcified cartilage in the endoskeletal tesserae of sharks. Journal of Morphology 160: 75–102.

Kepes, J. J., and F. Perentes. 1988. Glial fibrillary acidic protein in chondrocytes of elastic cartilage in the human epiglottis: An immunohistochemical study with polyvalent and monoclonal antibodies. Anatomical Record 220: 296–299.

Kimura, S., and T. Kamimura. 1982. The characterization of lamprey notochord collagen with special reference to its skin collagen. Comparative Biochemistry and Physiology 73B: 335–339.

Klaauw, C. J., van der. 1948–52. Size and position of the functional components of the skull. Archives neerlandaises de zoologie 9: 1–599.

Knese, K.-H. 1979. Stützgewebe und Skelettsystem. In Handbuch des mikroskopischen Anatomie des Menschen, vol. 2, pt. 2, W. Bargmann, ed. Berlin: Springer-Verlag.

Knese, K.-H., and M. von Harnack. 1962. Über die Faserstruktur des Knochengewebes. Zeitschrift für Zellforschung 57: 520–558.

Knops, J., K. S. Kosik, G. Lee, J. D. Pardee, L. Cohen-Gould, and L. McConlogue. 1991. Over-expression of tau in a nonneuronal cell induces long cellular processes. Journal of Cell Biology 114: 725–733.

Kokich, V. G. 1976. Age changes in the human frontozygomatic suture from 20 to 95 years. American Journal of Orthodontics 69: 411–430.

Kopp, S. 1976. Topographical distribution of sulphated glycosaminoglycans in human temporomandibular joint disks. Journal of Oral Pathology 5: 265–276.

———. 1978. Topographical distribution of glycosaminoglycans in the surface layers of the human temporomandibular joint. Journal of Oral Pathology 7: 283–294.

Koskinen, L. 1977. Adaptive sutures: Changes after unilateral masticatory muscle resection in rats; A microscopic study. Ph.D. diss., University of Turku.

Koskinen, L., K. Isotupa, and K. Koski. 1974. A note on craniofacial sutural growth. American Journal of Physical Anthropology 45: 511–516.

Kostovic-Knezevic, L., Z. Bradamante, and A. Svajger. 1986. On the ultrastructure of the developing elastic cartilage in the rat external ear. Anatomy and Embryology 173: 385–391.

Kresja, R. J., H. C. Slavkin, and P. Bringas, Jr. 1991. Hagfish Pokal cells are ameloblasts: Are conodonts the first vertebrate mineralized tissues? American Zoologist 31: 47A.

Lauder, G. V., and L. E. Lanyon. 1980. Functional anatomy of feeding in the bluegill sunfish, *Lepomis macrochirus:* In vivo measurements of bone strain. Journal of Experimental Biology 84: 33–55.

Lester, K. S., and M. M. Ash, Jr. 1981. Ossification in adult rat mandibular condyle: SEM of chondroclasia. Journal of Ultrastructure Research 74: 46–58.

Livne, E., C. Oliver, and M. Silbermann. 1987. Further characterization of the chondroprogenitor zone in mandibular condyles of suckling mice. Acta anatomica 129: 231–237.

Lotz, J. C., T. N. Gerhart, and W. C. Hayes. 1990. Mechanical properties of trabecular bone from the proximal femur. Journal of Computer Assisted Tomography 14: 107–114.

Lubosch, W. 1928. Die Osteoblasten und ihre Metamorphose. Zeitschrift für mikroskopische-anatomische Forschung 12: 280–346.

Luder, H. U., and H. E. Schroeder. 1992. Light and electron microscopic morphology of the temporomandibular joint in growing and mature crab-eating monkeys (*Macaca fascicularis*): The condylar calcified cartilage. Anatomy and Embryology 185: 189–199.

Mackenzie, A., M. W. J. Ferguson, and P. T. Sharpe. 1991. *Hox-7* expression during murine craniofacial development. Development 113: 601–611.

Maisey, J. G. 1988. Phylogeny of early vertebrate skeletal induction and ossification patterns. Evolutionary Biology 22: 1–36.

Mangia, F., and G. Palladini. 1970. Recherches histochimiques sur le mucocartilage de la lamproie pendant son ontogenèse larvaire. Archives d'anatomie microscopique 59: 283–288.

Manzanares, M. C., M. Goret-Nicaise, and A. Dehm. 1989. Metopic sutural closure in the human skull. Journal of Anatomy 161: 203–215.

Marotti, G., V. Cane, S. Palazzini, and C. Palumbo. 1990. Structure-function relationships in the osteocyte. Italian Journal of Mineral and Electrolyte Metabolism 4: 93–106.

Mayer, E. A., and J. P. Baldi. 1991. Can regulatory peptides be regarded as words of a biological language? American Journal of Physiology 251: G171–G184.

Menton, D. N., D. J. Simmons, S.-L. Chang, and B. Y. Orr. 1984. From bone lining cell to osteocyte: An SEM study. Anatomical Record 209: 29–39.

Meunier, F. J., and A. Huyseunne. 1992. The concept of bone tissue in osteichthyes. Netherlands Journal of Zoology. Forthcoming.

Michelacci, Y. M., and D. S. P. Q. Horton. 1989. Proteoglycans from the cartilage of young hammerhead shark *Sphyrna lewini*. Comparative Biochemistry and Physiology 92B: 651–658.

Miller, S. C., and W. S. S. Jee. 1987. The bone lining cells: A distinct phenotype? Calcified Tissue International 41: 1–5.

Mills, D. K., J. C. Daniel, and R. Scapino. 1988. Histological features and *in-vitro* proteoglycan synthesis in the rabbit craniomandibular joint disc. Archives of Oral Biology 33: 195–202.

Miyawaki, S., and D. P. Forbes. 1987. The morphologic and biochemical effects of tensile force application to the interparietal suture of the Sprague-Dawley rat. American Journal of Orthodontics and Dentofacial Orthopedics 92: 123–133.

Moss, M. L. 1958. Fusion of the frontal suture in the rat. American Journal of Anatomy 102: 141–165.

———. 1961a. Extrinsic determination of sutural area morphology in the rat calvaria. Acta anatomica 44: 263–272.

———. 1961b. Osteogenesis of acellular teleost fish bone. American Journal of Anatomy 108: 99–109.

———. 1961c. Studies of the acellular bone of teleost fish. 1. Morphological and systematic variations. Acta anatomica 46: 343–362.

———. 1964a. Development of cellular dentin and lepidosteal tubules in the bowfin, Amia calva. Acta anatomica 58: 333–354.

———. 1964b. The phylogeny of mineralized tissues. International Review of General and Experimental Zoology 1: 297–331.

———. 1968. Comparative anatomy of vertebrate dermal bone and teeth. Acta anatomica 71: 178–208.

———. 1975. Functional anatomy of cranial synostosis. Child's Brain 1: 22–33.

———. 1977. Skeletal tissues in sharks. American Zoologist 17: 335–342.

Moss, M. L., and L. Moss-Salentijn. 1983. Vertebrate cartilages. In Cartilage, vol. 1, B. K. Hall, ed. New York: Academic Press, pp. 1–30.

Moury, J. D., S. K. Curtis, and D. I. Pav. 1987. Structural heterogeneity in the basal regions of the teeth of the red-backed salamander, Plethodon cinereus (Amphibia, Plethodontidae). Journal of Morphology 194: 111–127.

Murray, P. D. F. 1963. Adventitious (secondary) cartilage in the chick embryo, and the development of certain bones and articulations in the chick skull. Australian Journal of Zoology 11: 368–430.

Nash, S. B., and V. G. Kokich. 1985. Evaluation of cranial bone suture autotransplants in the growing rabbit. Acta anatomica 123: 39–44.

Nieduszynski, I. A., T. N. Huckerby, J. M. Dickenson, G. M. Brown, G.-H. Tai, H. G. Morris, and S. Eady. 1990. There are two major types of skeletal keratan sulphate. Biochemical Journal 271: 243–245.

Nielsen, E. H. 1978. Ultrahistochemistry of matrix vesicles in elastic cartilage. Acta anatomica 100: 268–272.

Ninomiya, J. T., R. P. Tacy, J. D. Calore, M. A. Gendrea, R. J. Kelm, and K. G. Mann. 1990. Heterogeneity of human bone. Journal of Bone and Mineral Research 5: 933–938.

Olson, E. N. 1991. MyoD family: A paradigm for development? Genes and Development 4: 1454–1461.

Ørvig, T. 1951. Histological studies of placoderm and fossil elasmobranchs. I. The endoskeleton with remarks on the hard tissues of lower vertebrates in general. Arkiv för Zoologi 2: 321–456.

———. 1965. Palaeohistological notes. 2. Certain comments on the phyletic significance of acellular bone tissue in early lower vertebrates. Arkiv för Zoologi 16: 551–556.

Oudhof, H. A. J. 1982. Sutural growth. Acta anatomica 112: 58–68.

Oudhof, H. A. J., and W. J. van Doorenmaalen. 1983. Skull morphogenesis and growth: Hemodynamic influences. Acta anatomica 117: 181–186.

Palumbo, C., S. Palazzini, D. Zaffe, and G. Marotti. 1990. Osteocyte differentiation in the tibia of newborn rabbit: An ultrastructural study of the formation of cytoplasmic processes. Acta anatomica 137: 350–358.

Patterson, C. 1977. Cartilage bones, dermal bones, and membrane bones, or the exoskeleton versus the endoskeleton. In Problems in Vertebrate Evolution, S. M. Andrews, R. S. Miles, and A. D. Walker, eds. London: Academic Press, pp. 77–121.

———. 1988. Homology in classical and molecular biology. Molecular Biology and Evolution 5: 603–625.

Pavlin, D., A. C. Lichtler, A. Bedalov, B. E. Kream, H. R. Harrison, H. F. Thomas, G. A. Gronowicz, S. H. Clark, C. O. Woody, and D. W. Rowe. 1992. Differential utilization of regulatory domains within the $\alpha 1(I)$ collagen promoter in osseous and fibroblastic cells. Journal of Cell Biology 116: 227–236.

Peignoux-Deville, J., C. Bordat, and B. Vidal. 1989. Demonstration of bone resorbing cells in elasmobranchs: Comparison with osteoclasts. Tissue and Cell 21: 925–933.

Persing, P. A., J. T. Lettieri, A. J. Cronin, W. P. Wolcott, V. Singh, and E. Morgan. 1991. Craniofacial suture stenosis: Morphologic effects. Plastic and Reconstructive Surgery 88: 563–571.

Person, P. 1983. Invertebrate Cartilages. In Cartilage, vol. 1, B. K. Hall, ed. Orlando: Academic Press, pp. 31–53.

Persson, M., B. C. Magnusson, and B. Thilander. 1978. Sutural closure in rabbit and man: A morphological histochemical study. Journal of Anatomy 125: 313–321.

Persson, M., and W. Roy. 1979. Suture development and bony fusion in the fetal rabbit palate. Archives of Oral Biology 24: 283–291.

Petersen, H. 1930. Die Organe des Skeletsystems. In Handbuch der mikroskopischen Anatomie des menschen, vol. 2, pt. 2, W. von Möllendorff, ed. Berlin: J. Springer, pp. 521–678.

Phleger, C. F. 1987. Bone lipids of tropical reef fishes. Comparative Biochemistry and Physiology 86B: 509–512.

Prahl-Andersen, B. 1968. Sutural growth: Investigations on the growth mechanism of the coronal suture and its relation to growth in the rat. Ph.D. diss., University of Nijmegen.

Preobrazhensky, A. A., A. I. Rodionova, I. N. Trakht, and V. S. Rukosuev. 1987. Monoclonal antibodies against chordin. FEBS Letters 224: 23–28.

Pritchard, J. J., J. H. Scott, and F. G. Girgis. 1956. The structure and development of cranial and facial sutures. Journal of Anatomy 90: 73–86.

Raftos, D. A., E. L. Cooper, G. S. Habicht, and G. Beck. 1991. Invertebrate cytokines: Tunicate cell proliferation stimulated by an interleukin 1-like molecule. Proceedings of the National Academy of Sciences, U.S.A. 88: 9518–9522.

Reid, R. E. H. 1984. The histology of dinosaurian bone, and its possible bearing on dinosaurian physiology. Symposia of the Zoological Society, London 52: 629–663.

Reid, S. A. 1986. A study of lamellar organization in juvenile and adult bone. Anatomy and Embryology 174: 329–338.

Reid, S. A., and A. Boyde. 1987. Changes in the mineral density distribution in human bone with age: Image analysis using backscattered electrons in the SEM. Journal of Bone and Mineral Research 2: 13–22.

Roach, H. I., and Shearer, J. R. 1989. Cartilage resorption and endochondral bone formation during the development of long bones in chick embryos. Bone and Mineral 6: 289–309.

Rönning, O., and K. Koski. 1974. The effect of periostomy on the growth of the condylar process in the rat. Proceedings of the Finnish Dental Society 70: 28–29.

Rönning, O., and S. Kylamärkula. 1982. Morphogenetic potential of rat growth cartilages as isogeneic transplants in the interparietal sutural area. Archives of Oral Biology 27: 581–588.

Rönning, O., M. Rintala, and T. Kantomaa. 1991. Growth potential of the rat clavicle. Journal of Oral and Maxillofacial Surgery 49: 1176–1180.

Ruben, J. A., and A. F. Bennett. 1987. The evolution of bone. Evolution 41: 1187–1197.

Sanford, C. P., and G. V. Lauder. 1989. Functional morphology of the "tongue-bite" in the osteoglossomorph fish *Notopterus*. Journal of Morphology 202: 379–408.

Sanzone, C. F., and E. J. Reith. 1976. The development of the elastic cartilage of the mouse pinna. American Journal of Anatomy 146: 31–72.

Sarnat, B. G. 1980. Orbital volume in young and adult rabbits. Anatomy and Embryology 159: 211–221.

Schaffer, J. 1897. Bemerkungen über die Histologie und Histogenese des Knorpels der Cyclostomen. Archiv für mikroskopische Anatomie 50: 170–188.

———. 1906. Über den feineren Bau und die Entwicklung des Knorpelgewebes und über verwandte Formen der Stützsubstanz. II. Das Knorpelgewebe und das knorpelähnliche, blasige Stützgewebe von *Myxine glutinosa*, nebst Bemerkungen zur Morphologie des Schädelskelettes dieses Tieres und einem Nachtrage über das harte Knorpelgewebe der Petromyzonten. Zeitschrift für wissenschaftliche Zoologie 80: 155–258.

———. 1911. Über den feineren Bau und die Entwicklung des Knorpelgewebes und über verwandte Formen der Stützsubstanz. III. Zeitschrift für wissenschaftliche Zoologie 97: 1–90.

———. 1930. Die Stützgewebe. In *Handbuch der mikroskopischen Anatomie des Menschen*, vol. 2, pt. 2, W. von Möllendorff, ed. Berlin: J. Springer, pp. 1–390.

Scharrer, E. 1944. The histology of the ganoids Amia and Lepisosteus. Anatomical Record 88: 291–310.

Schmid-Monnard, C. 1883. Die Histogenese des Knochens der Teleostier. Zeitschrift für wissenschaftliche Zoologie 39: 97–136.

Schumacher, G. H. 1956. Morphologische Studie zum Gleitmechanismus des

M. adductor mandibularis externus bei Schildkröten. Anatomischer Anzeiger 103: 1–12.

Schwarz, W. 1961. Elektronenmikroskopische Untersuchungen an den Chorda-zellen von Petromyzon. Zeitschrift für Zellforschung 55: 597–609.

Scott, J. E. 1991. Proteoglycan:collagen interactions in tissues: Ultrastructural, biochemical, functional, and evolutionary aspects. International Journal of Biological Macromolecules 13: 147–151.

Scott, J. E., and M. Haigh. 1988. Keratan sulphate and the ultrastructure of cornea and cartilage: A "stand-in" for chondroitin sulphate in conditions of oxygen lack? Journal of Anatomy 158: 95–108.

Shapiro, F., M. E. Holtrop, and M. J. Glimcher. 1977. Organization and cellular biology of the perichondrial ossification groove of Ranvier. Journal of Bone and Joint Surgery 59-A: 703–723.

Sheldon, H. 1983. Transmission electron microscopy of cartilage. In Cartilage, vol. 1, B. K. Hall, ed. New York: Academic Press, pp. 87–104.

Shepherd, G. M. 1991. Sensory transduction: Entering the mainstream of membrane signalling. Cell 67: 845–851.

Shibata, S., O. Baba, M. Ohsako, S. Suzuki, Y. Yamashita, and T. Ichijo. 1991. Ultrastructural observation on matrix fibers in the condylar cartilage of the adult rat mandible. Bulletin of the Tokyo Medical and Dental University 38: 53–61.

Silbermann, M., A. H. Reddi, A. R. Hand, R. Leapman, K. von der Mark, and A. Franzen. 1987. Chondroid bone arises from mesenchymal stem cells in organ culture of mandibular condyles. Journal of Craniofacial Genetics 7: 59–79.

Silbermann, M., K. von der Mark, and D. Heinegard. 1990. An immunohisto-chemical study of the distribution of matrical proteins in the mandibular condyle of neonatal mice. II. Non-collagenous proteins. Journal of Anatomy 170: 23–31.

Silyn-Roberts, H., and N. D. Bloom. 1988. A biomechanical profile across the patellar groove articular cartilage: Implications for defining matrix health. Journal of Anatomy 160: 175–188.

Sire, J.-Y., A. Huyseunne, and F. J. Meunier. 1990. Osteoclasts in teleost fish: Light- and electron-microscopical observations. Cell and Tissue Research 260: 85–94.

Sitsen, A. E. 1933. Zur Entwicklung der Nähte des Schädeldachs. Zeitschrift für die gesammte Anatomie und Entwicklungsgeschichte 101: 121–152.

Smith, H. G., and M. McKeown. 1974. Experimental alteration of the coronal sutural area: A histological and quantitative microscopic assessment. Journal of Anatomy 118: 543–559.

Smith, M. M., and B. K. Hall. 1990. Development and evolutionary origins of vertebrate skeletogenic and odontogenic tissues. Biological Reviews 65: 277–373.

Smith-Thomas, L. C., J. P. Davis, and M. L. Epstein. 1986. The gut supports neu-rogenic differentiation of periocular mesenchyme, a chondrogenic neural crest–derived cell population. Developmental Biology 115: 293–300.

Studnicka, F. K. 1907. Über einige Grundsubstanzgewebe. Anatomischer Anzeiger 31: 497–522.

———. 1911. Das Gewebe der Chorda dorsalis und die Klassifikation der sogenannten "Stützgewebe." Anatomischer Anzeiger 38: 497–504.

Stutzmann, J., T. J. Yoo, A. Petrovic, and T. Ishibe. 1987. Immunofluorescent localization of type II and type X collagens in "primary" and "secondary" growth cartilages. Calcified Tissue International 36 (suppl.): 37A.

Sugiyama, S., S. S. Spicer, P. D. Munyer, and B. A. Schulte. 1991. Histochemical analysis of glycoconjugates in gelatinous membranes of the gerbil's inner ear. Hearing Research 55: 263–272.

Tavassoli, M. 1986. Bone marrow in boneless fish: Lessons of evolution. Medical Hypotheses 20: 9–15.

Tavassoli, M., and J. M. Yoffey. 1983. Bone Marrow: Structure and Function. New York: Alan R. Liss.

Ten Cate, A. R., E. Freeman, and J. B. Dickinson. 1977. Sutural development: Structure and its response to rapid expansion. American Journal of Orthodontics 71: 622–636.

Thomson, D. A. R. 1987. A quantitative analysis of cellular and matrix changes in Meckel's cartilage in Xenopus laevis. Journal of Anatomy 151: 249–254.

Tonna, E. A. 1974. Electron microscopy of aging skeletal cells. III. The periosteum. Laboratory Investigation 31: 609–632.

Tretjakoff, D. 1926. Die funktionelle Struktur der Chordascheiden und der Wirbel bei Zyklostomen und Fischen. Zeitschrift für Zellforschung 4: 266–312.

———. 1928. Das basophile Gallertgewebe. Zeitschrift für mikroskopische-anatomische Forschung 12: 29–60.

Trevisan, R. A., and R. P. Scapino. 1976. The symphyseal cartilage and growth of the symphysis menti in the hamster. Acta anatomica 96: 335–355.

Triffitt, J. T. 1987. The special proteins of bone tissue. Clinical Science 72: 399–408.

Venutti, J. M., L. Goldberg, T. Chakraborty, E. N. Olson, and W. H. Klein. 1991. A myogenic factor from sea urchin capable of programming muscle differentiation in mammalian cells. Proceedings of the National Academy of Sciences, U.S.A. 88: 6219–6223.

Vinkka, H. 1982. Secondary cartilages in the facial skeleton of the rat. Proceedings of the Finnish Dental Society 78 (suppl. 7).

Vogel, K. G., and T. J. Koob. 1989. Structural specialization in tendons under compression. International Review of Cytology 115: 267–293.

von Bartheld, C. S., S. L. Patterson, J. G. Heuer, E. F. Wheeler, M. Bothwell, and E. W. Rubel. 1991. Expression of nerve growth factor (NGF) in the developing inner ear of chick and rat. Development 113: 455–470.

Vynios, D. H., and C. P. Tsiganos. 1990. Squid proteoglycans: Isolation and characterization of three populations from cranial cartilage. Biochimica et biophysica acta 1033: 139–147.

Wagemans, P. A. H. M., J.-P. van de Velde, and A. M. Kuijpers-Jagtman. 1988. Sutures and forces: A review. American Journal of Orthodontics 94: 129–141.

Wake, D. B., and R. Lawson. 1973. Developmental and adult morphology of the vertebral column in the plethodontid salamander *Eurycea bislineata*, with comments on vertebral evolution in the amphibia. Journal of Morphology 139: 251–300.

Watabe, N., and C.-M., Pan. 1984. Phosphatic shell formation in atremate brachiopods. American Zoologist 24: 977–985.

Watson, L. P., Y.-H. Kang, and M. C. Falk. 1989. Cytochemical properties of osteoblast cell membrane domains. Journal of Histochemistry and Cytochemistry 37: 1235–1246.

Weidenreich, F. 1930. Das Knochengewebe. In *Handbuch der mikroskopischen Anatomie des Menschen*, vol. 2, pt. 2, W. von Möllendorff, ed. Berlin: J. Springer, pp. 391–520.

Weisel, G. F. 1967. Early ossification in the skeleton of the sucker (*Catostomus macrocheilus*) and the guppy (*Poecilia reticulata*). Journal of Morphology 121: 1–18.

Whitehouse, W. J. 1977. Cancellous bone in the anterior part of the iliac crest. Calcified Tissue Research 23: 67–76.

Wright, G. M., L. A. Armstrong, A. M. Jacques, and J. H. Youson. 1988. Trabecular, nasal, branchial, and pericardial cartilages in the sea lamprey, *Petromyzon marinus*. American Journal of Anatomy 182: 1–15.

Wright, G. M., F. W. Keeley, and J. H. Youson. 1983. Lamprin: A new vertebrate protein comprising the major structural protein of adult lamprey cartilage. Experientia 39: 495–497.

Wright, G. M., F. W. Keeley, J. H. Youson, and D. L. Babineau. 1984. Cartilage in the Atlantic hagfish, *Myxine glutinosa*. American Journal of Anatomy 169: 407–424.

Wright, G. M., and J. H. Youson. 1982. Ultrastructure of mucocartilage in the larval anadromous sea lamprey, *Petromyzon marinus* L. American Journal of Anatomy 165: 39–51.

Yen, E. H. K., and S. K. T. Chiang. 1984. A radioautographic study of the effect of age on the protein-synthetic and bone-deposition activity in the interparietal sutures of male white mice. Archives of Oral Biology 29: 1041–1047.

Yen, E. H. K., C. S. Yue, and D. M. Suga. 1989. The effect of sutural growth rate on collagen phenotype synthesis. Journal of Dental Research 68: 1058–1063.

Zaidi, M., B. S. Moonga, P. J. R. Bevis, A. S. M. Towhidul Alam, S. Legon, S. Wimalawaansa, I. MacIntyre, and L. H. Breimer. 1991. Expression and function of the calcitonin gene products. Vitamins and Hormones 46: 87–164.

Zivanovic, S. 1983. A note on the effect of asymmetry in suture closure in mature human skulls. American Journal of Physical Anthropology 60: 431–435.

Zylberberg, L., and M. H. Wake. 1990. Structure of the scales of *Dermophis* and *Microaecilia* (Amphibia: Gymnophiona), and a comparison to dermal ossifications of other vertebrates. Journal of Morphology 206: 25–43.

4

Patterns of Diversity in the Skull of Jawless Fishes

INTRODUCTION

THERE ARE ONLY TWO GROUPS of Recent jawless vertebrates: the Hyperotreti (Myxinoidea or hagfishes), and the Hyperoartia (Petromyzontida or lampreys). Each of these two groups is homogeneous in morphology and behavior but, despite some overall resemblances, their relationships, either to each other or to the jawed fishes (Gnathostomata), are still the subject of heated discussions. Briefly, there are two competing theories about this three-taxon problem: either lampreys and hagfishes form a monophyletic group, the Cyclostomi, or only lampreys and gnathostomes are closely related, hagfishes being the sister group of both (fig 4.1). In the latter case, the cyclostomes would be a paraphyletic group. Moreover, hagfishes, being devoid of any arcualia or vertebral element, may be excluded from the Vertebrata, a taxon which would include the lampreys and gnathostomes only. This question of monophyly versus paraphyly of the jawless vertebrates (or jawless craniates, if hagfishes are excluded from the vertebrates) will be discussed in this chapter, with particular reference to the problem of cranial homologies.

The pattern of jawless vertebrate morphology and phylogeny is further complicated by the existence of highly diversified fossil taxa: the Heterostraci, Galeaspida, Osteostraci, Anaspida, Pituriaspida, and Thelodonti. Most of these fossil jawless vertebrates lived during the Silurian and the Devonian, that is from 438 to 365 million years ago, but some of them occur earlier, in Ordovician and perhaps Cambrian rocks (up to 510 million years ago). The earliest undisputed jawless vertebrate (which is also the earliest known vertebrate) is from the Lower Ordovician (470 million years ago). For unknown reasons, all these heavily ossified, jawless vertebrate groups were already rare in the Middle Devonian and became extinct by the end of the Devonian, more precisely in the Frasnian (365 million years ago). Thus, the golden age of these groups is the Upper Silurian and the Lower Devonian.

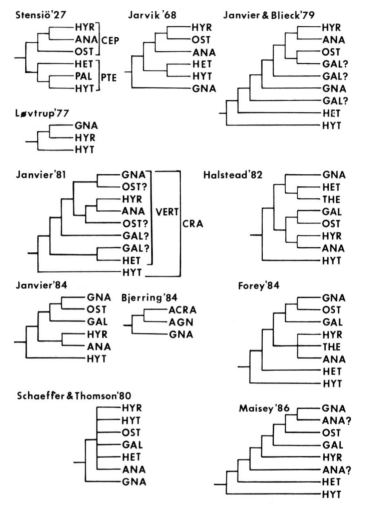

Fig. 4.1. Major theories of agnathan or craniate relationships proposed since Stensiö (1927). The reader is referred to the original publications for information on the characters used to support the respective theories. AGN, Agnatha; ANA, Anaspida; ACRA, Acrania; CEP, Cephalaspidomorphi; CRA, Craniata; GAL, Galeaspida; GNA, Gnathostomata; HET, Heterostraci; HYR, Hyperoartia (lampreys); HYT, Hyperotreti (hagfishes); OST, Osteostraci; PAL, *Palaeospondylus* (no longer regarded as an agnathan); PTE, Pteraspidomorphi; THE, Thelodonti; VERT, Vertebrata. Question marks indicate uncertain positions of groups.

A preliminary phylogenetic framework is certainly useful—yet not indispensable—to the understanding of this chapter. Therefore, I shall briefly depict the various hypotheses of craniate or vertebrate interrelationships which have been proposed over the past 60 years. Then, readers may forge their own opinions on the basis of the data in this volume and elsewhere. Any topic of comparative biology is almost senseless without a phylogenetic goal, and the search for diversity patterns of the vertebrate skull should also be aimed at contributing to understanding phylogenetic patterns.

PHYLOGENY OF CRANIATES

First regarded by Linnaeus as "intestinal worms," hagfishes were grouped together with lampreys by Duméril (1806) into the taxon Cyclostomi. Since then, and despite tremendous difficulties in finding reliable structural homologies between the two groups, most authors have regarded the cyclostomes as a natural group of equal rank with the gnathostomes. In 1889, Cope erected the taxon Agnatha for the extant cyclostomes and the newly discovered fossil jawless vertebrate groups, thereby increasing the importance of the jawless vertebrates in the history of the vertebrates in general. Thus, from a pre-evolutionary classification, one can trace a progressive shift toward an evolutionary classification where the Agnatha represent a historically natural group, characterized by the lack of gnathostome characters. In the search for characters to support this view, anatomists and paleontologists found some apparently unique agnathan features, such as the endodermal origin of the gills (e.g., Sewertzoff 1917; see however reservations in Goodrich 1930, 505) or spermatozoids shed directly into the coelom. The characters which contradict this monophyly were either omitted or regarded as reversions (in hagfishes) and convergences (in lampreys and gnathostomes). Stensiö (1927), in his master work on the Spitsbergen osteostracans, proposed the first phylogeny of the Agnatha and tried to determine the relationships between the two Recent and the fossil groups (fig. 4.1). This phylogeny has been later defended by, among others, Jarvik (1980), who, however, rejected a close relationship between lampreys and anaspids. In contrast, Holmgren (1943), Romer (1944), and, to some extent, Säve-Söderbergh (1941) suggested that the Agnatha was a grade, and that the gnathostomes arose from some agnathan ancestor. Thus, one of the known extant or fossil jawless vertebrate groups may be more closely related to the gnathostomes than to other jawless groups. In this early search for agnathan paraphyly, the Heterostraci were chosen as the most probable gnathostome relative, possibly as a consequence of early statements that their oral plates could bite against the ventral side of the rostrum in the same way as gnathostome jaws. This opinion is still defended by Halstead (1973) and Novitskaya (1983). However, as to the origin and relationships of lampreys and hagfishes to the fossil groups, the ideas were, until recently, of two kinds: either lampreys and hagfishes arose independently from two different groups of fossil armored agnathans, the osteostracans (or anaspids) and heterostracans respectively, or they diverged from a more recent, possibly Mesozoic, and naked ancestor. The recency of this common cyclostome ancestor was refuted by the discovery of typical lampreys and hagfish-like forms as early as the Carboniferous (Bardack and Zangerl 1971; Bardack 1991). Similarly, the diphyly of the cyclostomes as seen by Stensiö (1927) has been more and more widely rejected, in particular the relationships between heterostracans and hagfishes.

In 1977, Løvtrup, for the first time, clearly proposed that the cyclostomes were paraphyletic, lampreys being more closely related to the gnathostomes than to hagfishes. Apparently, this idea was ripe and ready to burst in the late seventies, since Løvtrup's proposal was immediately followed by biologists and paleontologists (Dingerkus 1979; Janvier 1978; Jefferies and Lewis 1978; Hardisty 1982; Mallatt 1984). As a consequence of a pendulum effect, this sudden—and perhaps overenthusiastic—consensus has been moderately criticized (e.g., Schaeffer and Thomson 1980; Yalden 1985; Jollie 1984). Although I consider that the synamorphies shared by lampreys and gnathostomes largely outnumber the characters shared by hagfishes and lampreys (including some molecular characters), I admit that the question is far from settled. Some of the apparent cyclostome synapomorphies, such as the "lingual" apparatus, are in fact possibly homologous structures, but the question remains as to whether they are synapomorphies or symplesiomorphies, that is, general primitive craniate features, lost in the gnathostomes. The profound morphological divergence between lampreys and the gnathostomes should not be an obstacle to the derivation of the latter from a common ancestor which may have resembled a larval lamprey or certain fossil jawless forms such as thelodonts. In fact, despite these apparent skeletal differences, others organs of lampreys and gnathostomes, such as gill structure and kidneys, are strikingly similar (Mallatt 1984). In sum, the problem of cranial homologies and phylogenetic patterns among hagfishes, lampreys, and gnathostomes can be compared to what would be the search for the phylogenetic pattern of the gnathostomes if the only known taxa were one shark family, one actinopterygian genus, and the amniotes.

These modern ideas on extant vertebrate phylogeny have clear bearings on the interrelationships of the fossil jawless groups. On the basis of synapomorphy distribution, some of them (e.g., osteostracans) are now seen as being even more closely related to the gnathostomes than are lampreys (fig. 4.21). I give here a review of the current vertebrate—or craniate—phylogenies, expressed in the form of cladograms (fig. 4.1). The reader is referred to the respective authors for the synapomorphies which support the dichotomies. This diversity of opinions is enough to show that the debate is far from settled.

HYPEROTRETI (MYXINOIDEA, HAGFISHES)

The Hyperotreti, or hagfishes, are represented by four extant genera: *Myxine, Neomyxine, Paramyxine,* and *Eptatretus,* and a fossil, Carboniferous form, *Myxinikela siroka* Bardack (1991). The extant genera differ from each other mainly by the arrangement of their external branchial openings and other minor anatomical traits. The morphology of the skull, which is solely cartilaginous and the only chondrified skeletal element besides the median fin rays, is homogeneous throughout the entire group. The example chosen here is the Atlantic hagfish, *Myxine glutinosa,* which is by far the best-known species as to the anatomy of the adult, thanks to the superb monograph by Marinelli and Strenger (1956). In contrast, the early stages of hagfish ontogeny are known almost exclusively from the Pacific hagfish *Eptratretus (Bdellostoma)* (Dean 1899; Neumayer 1938; see also the excellent review by Gorbman and Tamarin 1985).

The skull of hagfishes is made up of sinuous cartilaginous arches and plates onto which muscles attach, and which strengthen the wall of ducts (fig. 4.2B). As in lampreys, it acts mainly as an elastic antagonist to muscles. Since the embryology of hagfishes is poorly known and the various skull components fused together, it is difficult to separate the neurocranium from the visceral skeleton. Therefore, the components described here separately are merely major recognizable functional units.

The Braincase and Nasal Basket: The "Axocranium"

The brain and spinal cord of hagfishes are protected mainly by a thick fibrous sheath of connective tissue, the thela perimeningealis (tp, fig. 4.2B), which lies on the dorsal surface of the notochord, and represents most of the braincase or "axocranium" (Marinelli and Strenger 1956). Anteriorly, this perimeningeal sheath is prolonged by the corbiculum nasale (corbn, fig. 4.2B, C), or nasal basket, which contains the olfactory organ and is made up of parallel, longitudinal cartilaginous rods. The latter are fused anteriorly to the series of ring-like cartilages which strengthen the wall of the prenasal sinus of the naso-pharyngeal duct (prns, fig. 4.2B, C). This series of axocranial component rests on a series of more ventrally situated cartilaginous elements, the rearmost of which bears the ovoid otic capsules (otc, fig. 4.2B, D). This ventral series of cartilages is referred to here as the basicranial series.

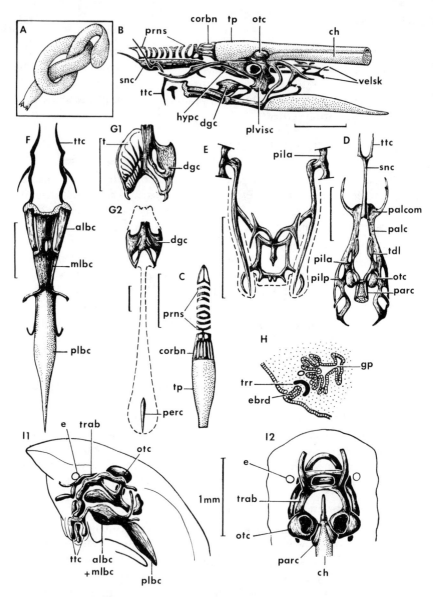

Fig. 4.2. The skull of the Hyperotreti (hagfishes). A. General aspect of *Myxine glutinosa* L., showing the head tentacles. B. Skull of *Myxine glutinosa* in lateral view (cartilages in black). C. Axocranium in dorsal view. D. Basicranial series in dorsal view. E. Velar skeleton in dorsal view. F. Basal cartilages of the "lingual" apparatus in ventral view. G. Dentigerous cartilage of the lingual apparatus in dorsal view (G1), with the horny teeth of the left side, and in ventral view (G2), with the cartilage of the perpendicular muscle and the outline of the clavatus muscle. H. Section of embryo of *Eptatretus,* showing the small cartilage associated with the branchial ducts. I. Skull of an embryo of *Myxine glutinosa* in lateral (I1) and dorsal (I2) views. Scale: 10 mm, unless indicated otherwise. See abbreviations list. (B–G, redrawn from Marinelli and Strenger 1956; H, from Stockard 1906 in Schaeffer and Thomson 1980; I, from Holmgren 1946)

The Basicranial Series

This series comprises, from rear to front: (1) Paired rods flanking the tip of the notochord (parc, fig. 4.2D), united by a short transverse commissure and contacting laterally the otic capsules; (2) The taenia dorsolateralis (tdl, fig. 4.2D), a paired anterior process of the large visceral plate complex, on which rests the anterior part of the thela perimeningealis and the nasal basket. This taenia dorsolateralis is prolonged anteriorly by the palatine cartilage (palc, fig. 4.2D), and the cornual cartilage; and (3) The median subnasal cartilage (snc, fig. 4.2B, D), which is a thick element underlying the prenasal sinus and extending anteriorly into a tentacular cartilage (ttc, fig. 4.2D). Posteriorly, the subnasal cartilage is followed by the thin hypophysial cartilage (hypc, fig. 4.2B), which strengthens the floor of the naso-pharyngeal duct. The palatine cartilages (palc, fig. 4.2D) of both sides fuse anteriorly into a palatine commissure (palcom, fig. 4.2D) which passes ventrally to the subnasal cartilage.

The Hypotic Arch Complex

Ventro-lateral to the otic capsules, a large cartilaginous structure extends around the pharynx. This hypotic arch complex descends from the taenia dorsolateralis and consists of two large pilae, the pila anterior (pila, fig. 4.2D) and the pila posterior (pilp, fig. 4.2D), which fuse ventrally into a large plate, the planum viscerale (plvisc, fig. 4.2B). Posteriorly to the latter, there are slender and sinuous arches which support the "lingual" skeleton (fig. 4.2B).

The Velar Skeleton

Hagfishes possess a particular water-pumping device, the velum, which consists of a trifid and posteriorly directed lamina arising from the roof of the pharynx, just behind the posterior end of the naso-pharyngeal duct. The velum possesses a complex skeleton, which consists of thin cartilaginous rods and arches (fig. 4.2E), and is attached to the internal surface of the planum viscerale near the root of the anterior pila. On each side, the "root" of the velar skeleton branches off posteriorly into a lateral rod, which arms the lateral horn of the velum, and a medial branch, which fuses with its opposite member by two commissures and strengthens the median flap of the velum.

The "Lingual" Skeleton

The mouth of hagfishes is provided with protractile and retractile horny teeth, which, by analogy with the condition in lampreys, have been often referred to as a "rasping tongue." Although the "tongue" in both hagfishes and lampreys probably has nothing to do with that of the gnathostomes, the term "lingual apparatus" to designate it has now become widespread and useful. The skeleton of the lingual apparatus of hagfishes consists of a series of three median ventral elements—the posterior, middle, and anterior basal cartilages (plbc, mlbc, albc, fig. 4.2F)—situated below the wall of the pharynx, and a relatively mobile dentigerous cartilage (dgc, fig. 4.2G), which bears the two paired rows of horny teeth (t, fig. 4.2G) and rotates around the anterior tip of the anterior basal cartilage (fig. 4.2C). The latter has a trifid structure (fig. 4.2F), and its median part itself displays a median fissure suggesting a paired origin.

The movements of the lingual apparatus are effected by two major sets of muscles: the protractor dentis muscle (mprotr, fig. 4.3C1), which pulls the dentigerous cartilage forward and outward, the clavatus and hyocopuloglossus muscles (mcl, mhyc, fig. 4.3C1), which draw the dentigerous cartilage backward. The clavatus muscle is a huge, club-shaped muscle, which reaches back to the branchial region and is aided in its retraction function by a surrounding tubular muscle. The latter acts like fingers pressing a lemon seed, forcing the club-shaped muscle backward. In the posterior part of the club-shaped muscle, a small median cartilaginous element, the cartilage of the perpendicular muscle (perc, fig. 4.2G2) serves for the attachment of a small median vertical muscle.

Structure of the Teeth

The horny teeth of hagfishes have long been an enigma as to their mode of growth or replacement. Contrary to those of lampreys, which always show in cross section an underlying replacement tooth (fig. 4.5B), no replacement tooth has been observed in hagfishes until recently (Krejsa et al. 1989) (fig. 4.3B). The "pulp cavity" of these horny teeth is occupied by several layers of various soft tissues, in particular a massive plug of so-called pokal-cells (pkc, fig. 4.3B), that is, large and spindle-shaped cells of poorly known function (Dawson 1963). Having first been regarded by early anatomists as a possible replacement tooth in process of formation, the pokal cell cone was considered to be a particular type of supporting tissue which strengthens and buffers the overlying tooth but is again believed to be linked with tooth replacement. The teeth of myxinoids seem thus to exhibit a replacement, yet probably slower than lampreys.

The Skeleton of the Tentacles

Hagfishes possess four pairs of tentacles: two on each side of the opening of the prenasal sinus, and two on each side of the mouth (fig. 4.2A). Each of these tentacles is strengthened by cartilaginous rods. The skeleton of the medial pair of nasal tentacles arises from the tip of the subnasal cartilage (ttc, fig. 4.2D), whereas that of the lateral pair is a dorsal branch of the cartilaginous rod which also supports the lateral oral tentacle of the same side. Both are attached by a thin pedicle to the lateral element of the ante-

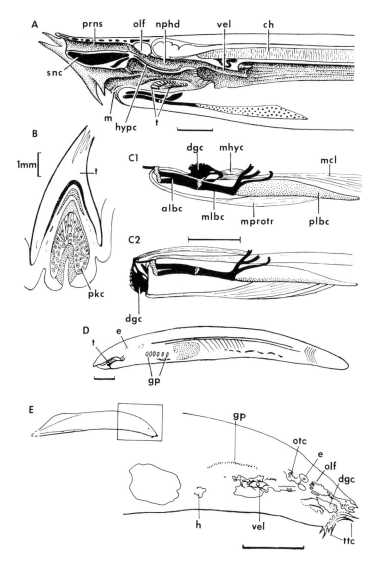

Fig. 4.3. A–C. *Myxine glutinosa* L. A. Longitudinal section of the head, showing the
position of the velum and naso-pharyngeal duct. B. Section of a horny tooth.
C. Lateral view of the skeleton of the lingual apparatus and some associated muscles,
with teeth inside the mouth (C1) and everted (C2). D. *Gilpichthys greeni* Bardack &
Richardson, Upper Carboniferous of the United States, a possible fossil myxinoid,
reconstruction in lateral view. E. *Myxinikela siroka* Bardack, Upper Carboniferous of
the United States, outline of the body and detail of head skeletal structures in lateral
view. Scale: 10 mm, unless indicated otherwise. (A, redrawn and simplified from
Marinelli and Strenger 1956; B, from Dawson 1963; C, from Yalden 1985; D, from
Bardack and Richardson 1977; E, from Bardack 1991)

rior lingual basal cartilage (fig. 4.2F). Finally, the small medial oral tentacle contains an independant cartilaginous core.

Branchial Skeleton

In *Myxine,* there is no skeleton associated with the gill pouches, thus no branchial skeleton proper. However, in the embryo of *Eptatretus,* small cartilaginous ring-like elements (trr, fig. 4.2H) are associated with the extrabranchial ducts (ebrd, fig. 4.2H) (Stockard 1906). Whether these small and often elusive elements are homologous to the trematic rings of lampreys cannot be decided.

Ontogeny

Very little is known of the ontogeny of hagfishes. Besides the works of Kupffer (1899; see reinterpretation in Gorbman and Tamarin 1985), Dean (1899), Stockard (1906), and Neumayer (1938) on relatively late embryos of *Eptatretus,* the best description of the skull in the early *Myxine* embryo was made by Holmgren (1946). Contrary to Neumayer, Holmgren has carefully recorded all the areas of the skull which are still in the state of procartilage, thus giving a much more complete account of its structure (fig. 4.2I). Despite the very strong ventral flexure which characterizes the head of all myxinoid embryos, nearly all the components of the adult skull are already visible, except perhaps the nasal basket and the rings of the prenasal sinus. The otic capsules (otc, fig. 4.2I) are disproportionately large and seem to be the center chondrification of the skull. The massive plates of the lingual apparatus, in particular the anterior and posterior basal lingual cartilages, are clearly visible (albc, plbc, fig. 4.2I1). Holmgren (1946), with some reservations, called a pair of large rods "trabecles" (trab, fig. 4.2I), which may be fused in the adult with the more ventrally placed taenia dorsolateralis, unless it is the same element.

Despite Holmgren's attempts at finding homologies between the myxinoid skull and that of other craniates, one must recognize that neither his nor other myxinoid embryos are of any help in solving this problem (see below). However, the embryo of *Myxine* clearly shows that separate external branchial openings are a plesiomorphous character state for the myxinoids in general. The early development of the myxinoid head seems to be radically different from that of both lampreys and gnathostomes; in particular, the entire naso-pharyngeal duct, including the anlage of what is regarded as a very simple adenohypophysis, would be of endodermal origin, deriving from a dorsal gut process (Gorbman and Tamarin 1985).

Fossil Hagfishes

A fossil hagfish, *Myxinikela siroka,* has been described from the Upper Carboniferous of Illinois (Bardack 1991, fig. 3E). It shows a remarkable resemblance to the Recent members of the group, in particular by the presence of tentacles and prenasal sinus. The only difference rests perhaps on the size of the tentacles, which are shorter in the fossil form, and the less slender shape of the body. The gill pouches, although difficult to locate, seem to have been situated closer to the braincase. The lingual apparatus may have been shorter than in extant forms. Moreover, there are good reasons to believe that an enigmatic jawless craniate, *Gilpichthys greeni* (Bardack and Richardson 1977) also from the Carboniferous of Illinois, is a close relative of hagfishes (fig. 4.3D). Its general shape and peculiar row of unmineralized teeth are strongly suggestive of myxinoids. If *Gilpichthys* is a myxinoid—or a close relative to that group—it would suggest, as do *Myxinikela* and the development of extant myxinoid embryos, that the elongation of the body and the backward migration of the branchial apparatus are derived features of modern forms.

HYPEROARTIA (PETROMYZONTIDA, LAMPREYS)

The Hyperoartia, or lampreys, are represented by nine extant genera or subgenera (*Ichthyomyzon, Petromyzon, Caspiomyzon, Eudontomyzon, Tetrapleurodon, Okkelbergia, Lampetra, Geotria,* and *Mordacia*) and three fossil genera (*Mayomyzon, Hardistiella,* and, with some reservations, *Pipiscius*) from the Carboniferous of the United States (Bardack and Zangerl 1971; Bardack and Richardson 1977, Janvier and Lund 1983). The extant genera differ from each other by the arrangement of the horny teeth of the "tongue" and oral disc, the shape of the unpaired fins, and the mode of life. However, the overall morphology of lampreys is very homogeneous. Most of them have an ectoparasitic mode of life, but many species have gained nonparasitic habits. *Ichthyomyzon* is generally regarded as the most primitive extant genus (Hubbs and Potter 1971). If the haematophagous ectoparasitic mode of life of lampreys is a much-derived and specialized condition, it has probably existed at least since the Upper Carboniferous, as evidenced by the presence of a piston cartilage—hence a rasping-sucking tongue device—in *Mayomyzon* (pistc, fig. 4.7A), and a sucker armed with horny plates in *Pipiscius*.

The skull of lampreys has been abundantly described, mainly on the basis of the brook lamprey *Lampetra fluviatilis* and the sea lamprey *Petromyzon marinus*. Among these anatomical descriptions, those of Sewertzoff (1916–17), Tretjakoff (1926), and in particular Marinelli and Strenger (1954) are by far the most extensive. As in hagfishes, the skull of the adult lampreys consists of sinuous cartilaginous arches and plates. There is a well-developed branchial skeleton which surrounds the series of gill pouches and is therefore referred to as the branchial basket (brbsk,

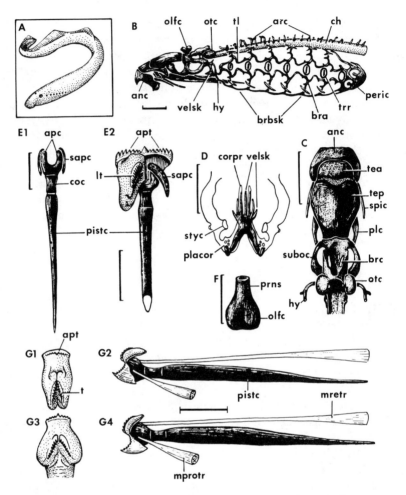

Fig. 4.4. The skull of adult Hyperoartia (lampreys). A. General aspect of *Lampetra fluviatilis* L. B. Skull of *Lampetra fluviatilis* in lateral view, with part of the axial skeleton (cartilages in black). C. Anterior part of the skull in dorsal view. D. Velar skeleton in dorsal view; underlying planum cornuale and styliform cartilage in white. E. Skeleton of the lingual apparatus in ventral view (E1), and dorsal view of its anterior part (E2) with horny teeth added. F. Olfactory capsule in dorsal view. G. Skeleton of the lingual apparatus and some associated muscles in lateral view, with the apical tooth protracted (G4) and retracted (G2), and corresponding positions of the paired teeth in dorsal view (G3, G1). Scale: 10 mm. (B–F, redrawn from Marinelli and Strenger 1954; G, from Yalden 1985)

fig. 4.4B). Moreover, there is an orbital cavity into which are attached the extrinsic eye muscles. The mouth is surrounded by a large sucker, or oral disc, which is strengthened by an annular cartilage, and the snout is armed by large cartilaginous plates which overlap like tiles and give the snout relative mobility (fig. 4.4C). The skull of adult lampreys is generally regarded as entirely cartilaginous or fibrous, but Bardack and Zangerl (1971) have recorded some calcified areas on the basis of radiographs.

Unlike hagfishes, lampreys pass through a larval stage and metamorphosis, during which the skeleton and the musculature are considerably reworked. Consequently, the nature of the various skeletal elements of the adult skull is obscured and it is sometimes difficult to decide what is neurocranial or visceral in origin. The following description is of the skull of the adult lamprey, but I shall add some final comments on larval stages and metamorphosis.

The Braincase

The braincase of lampreys is a roughly cylindrical structure (brc, fig. 4.4C), not completely closed dorsally and bearing on each side the ovoid otic capsules (otc, fig. 4.4B, C). Its floor is derived from the parachordals and trabecles (see discussion on the trabecles below), and lies above the foremost part of the notochord. Anterior to the tip of the notochord, the braincase is hollowed by a pit which accommodates the hypophysial tube, the latter passing ventrally to the braincase and entering into contact with the dorsal wall of the pharynx (hyt, fig. 4.5A). The lateral walls of the braincase are made up of orbital cartilages pierced by large fenestrations through which pass the cranial nerves. Posteriorly, there is a large foramen magnum, but no occipital region proper, and the series of arcualia (arc, fig. 4.4B) which straddle the notochord begins just behind the otic capsules.

The olfactory organ is enclosed in a pear-shaped cartilaginous olfactory capsule (olfc, fig. 4.4B, F) which is prolonged antero-dorsally by the tubular prenasal sinus (prns, fig. 4.4F) and pierced ventrally by a large opening for the hypophysial tube.

The Prebranchial Visceral Skeleton

The foremost cartilaginous arch of the branchial skeleton is regarded, based on embryological evidence, as belonging to the hyoid arch (be it a branchial arch proper or an extrabranchial component) (hy, fig. 4.4B). All the complex structures which extend anteriorly to it, and form the prebranchial skeleton, are supposed to be mandibular (or even premandibular) somite derivatives or neomorphs of visceral derivation.

Four major anatomical units can be distinguished in this prebranchial

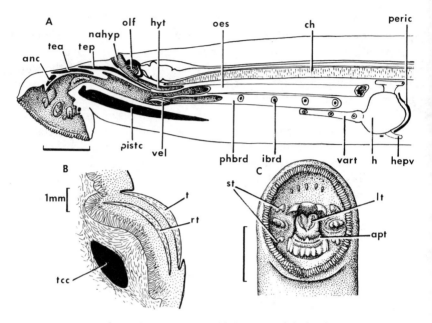

Fig. 4.5. *Lampetra fluviatilis* L. A. Longitudinal section of the head, showing the position of the naso-hypophysial complex. B. Section of a horny tooth of the oral sucker, showing the replacement tooth. C. Oral sucker and mouth in ventral view. Scale: 10 mm unless indicated otherwise. (Redrawn and simplified from Marinelli and Strenger 1954)

skeleton: the lateral arches, the snout plates, the velar skeleton, and the lingual apparatus.

The lateral arches consist of two large and coalescent cartilaginous arches, the rearmost of which is fused to the braincase: the subocular arch (suboc, fig. 4.4C), which lines ventrally the orbital cavity, and the posterior lateral cartilage (plc, fig. 4.4C).

The snout plates comprise the large median anterior and posterior tectal plates (tea, tep, figs. 4.4C, 4.5A), the paired anterior lateral cartilage, the paired spiniform cartilages (spic, fig. 4.4C), and the annular cartilage (anc, figs. 4.4B, C, 4.5A).

The velar skeleton is undoubtedly derived from the mandibular segment. Lampreys, like hagfishes, possess a water pumping device, or velum, but it is uncertain whether this organ is homologous in both groups. The skeleton of the velum in adult lampreys is a small hand-shaped cartilage (velsk, fig. 4.4B, D) which lies free upon the dorsal wall of the pharyngo-branchial duct, between the latter and the entrance to the esophagus (vel, fig. 4.5A). However, it is linked by musculature to a cartilaginous process, the styliform cartilage (styc, fig. 4.4D), which descends from the subocular arch, and its ventral branches, the planum cornuale (placor, fig. 4.4D) and the cornual process (corpr, fig. 4.4D). The styliform cartilage passes laterally to the pharyngeal musculature and expands ventrally to the pharyngobranchial duct into a planum cornuale which, in turn, is produced anteriorly into a paired cornual process (placor, corpr, fig. 4.4D). The movements of the velar skeleton proper are effected by small muscles which unite it to the styliform cartilage and the cornual plate. In the adult lamprey, the function of the velum is restricted to the sucking mechanism of the mouth; it plays no major role in circulation of the respiratory water current.

The lingual apparatus comprises the large piston cartilage (pistc, fig. 4.4E, G), the copular cartilage (coc, fig. 4.4E), the apical cartilage (apc, fig. 4.4E1), and the paired supra-apical cartilages (sapc, fig. 4.4E) on which rest a pair of horny teeth (lt, fig. 4.4E2). The apical cartilage is capped anteriorly by a large median beaklike horny tooth which has a rasping function (apt, fig. 4.4E2). The lingual skeleton is associated with a very complex musculature (for detailed description, see Hardisty and Rovainen 1982), the general effect of which is to protract and retract the entire "tongue," and to rotate the apical cartilage in a vertical plane (fig. 4.4G2, 4). During the latter movement, the supra-apical cartilages and their teeth move in a horizontal plane, coming into close contact when the tongue is retracted (fig. 4.4G1, 3).

Structure of the Teeth

The horny teeth of lampreys extend over the internal surface of the oral disc as well as on the tip of the tongue. They show a replacement process and are always strengthened by a small cartilaginous core (tcc, fig. 4.5B).

The Branchial Skeleton

The branchial skeleton is united to the skull by a small cartilaginous bar which meets the subocular arch on each side, below the otic capsule (fig. 4.4B). It consists of a series of seven roughly vertical and sinuous bars, which are connected to each other by two lateral and one median ventral horizontal and similarly sinuous bars, the taenia longitudinalis (tl, fig. 4.4B). Whether the vertical bars can be called branchial or extrabranchial arches depends on the homology between the agnathan and gnathostome visceral arches supporting the gills (Balabai 1937). There is now relatively convincing evidence that such a homology does not exist, since the structure of the gill lamellae in lampreys and gnathostomes is similar, which implies, therefore, a homology of the gills in both groups. Since the position of the gills relative to the skeletal arches is different in lampreys and gnathostomes, it is far more parsimonious to consider the gills homologous and the arches as nonhomologous (Jollie 1968; Mallatt 1984).

For the sake of simplicity I refer to these agnathan arches as "branchial arches."

Both the branchial arches and the longitudinal teniae bear spiniform processes which serve for attachment of the musculature. Laterally, there is a series of free cartilaginous rings, the trematic rings (trr, fig. 4.4B), which surround the external branchial openings. Posteriorly, the branchial basket is terminated by a more or less bowl-shaped structure, the pericardiac cartilage (peric, fig. 4.4B), which lies posteriorly to the heart. It is pierced ventrally by a broad slit for the hepatic vein and a large dorsal opening for the passage of the sinus venosus of the heart.

Ontogeny and Development

Development of lamprey head skeleton has been the subject of very detailed descriptions since the mid-nineteenth century. Among these studies, the works of Kupffer (1898), Koltzoff (1901), Sewertzoff (1916–17), Tretjakoff (1929), Balabai (1935), Damas (1942, 1944), and Johnels (1948) are by far the most accurate; the reader should refer to them for further information. During embryonic and larval development of lampreys, the skeleton of the head is made up of three different types of tissues: fibrous tissue, cartilage, and mucocartilage. Fibrous connective tissue fills the gaps in the braincase, in particular dorsally, surrounds the olfactory organ, and lines the orbital cavity. Cartilaginous elements form the basal part of the braincase, the olfactory and otic capsules, the prebranchial elements, and the branchial basket (fig. 4.6C–E).

Mucocartilage (Schneider 1879) is a peculiar and unique type of chondroid tissue which appears during larval stages of lampreys and disappears during metamorphosis. It consists of large, undifferentiated cells with long processes in a homogeneous matrix. In later stages, it contains chondroitin sulfate, a substance generally associated with true cartilage. Mucocartilage develops at the 12 mm stage, increasing in larger larvae, where it is associated with a particular musculature which works as its antagonist. During metamorphosis the mucocartilage breaks down or differentiates into true cartilage or muscles. Johnels (1948) illustrated this particular case with the formation of the piston cartilage of the tongue within the median ventral longitudinal of mucocartilage (mvlb, fig. 4.6D). The breaking down of the mucocartilage is a complex process which has been described in detail by

Fig. 4.6. (*opposite*) Development of the lamprey skull: *Lampetra planeri* (Bloch). A, B. Lateral view of the embryonic skull at 317 hours (A) and 410 hours (B) (cartilages in black). C. Skull of 8 mm larva in lateral (C1) and ventral (C2) views. D. Distribution of the mucocartilage in 128 mm larva, lateral view (cartilage in black, mucocartilage stippled, section of mucocartilage obliquely hatched). E. Larval skull at metamorphic stage 12. (Redrawn from Johnels 1948)

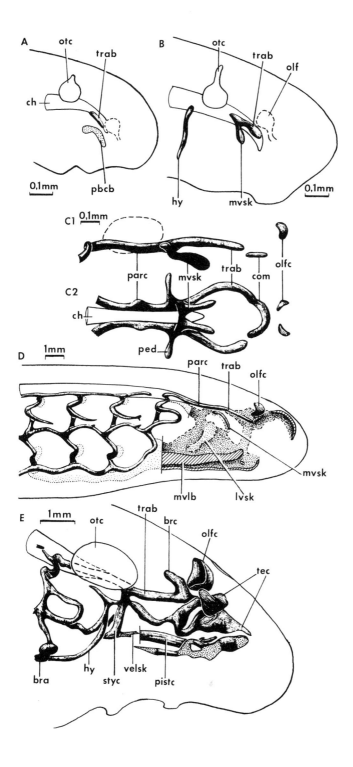

Damas (1958) and more recently by Wright and Youson (1982). In places where no new structure is formed, the intercellular substance disappears first and mucocartilage is replaced by large vascular and lymphatic spaces which probably play a major role in elimination of this larval tissue.

Mucocartilage was long regarded as derived from the mesectoderm and, thus, a neural crest derivative like the splanchnocranial cartilages, olfactory capsules, and part of the trabecles. However, recent experimental works do not confirm this statement (Langille and Hall 1986, 1988). Sewertzoff (1916−17), Tretjakoff (1929), and de Beer (1937), among others, have looked for homologies and metamery in mucocartilage, but none of their speculations is satisfactory. Stensiö suggested that mucocartilage may be derived from, or at least compared to, the endoskeletal shield of fossil osteostracans (see below), but now mucocartilage is regarded as a specialized larval tissue, linked with the burrowing mode of life of ammocoetes larvae (Hardisty 1981).

In its maximum extension, as in a 128 mm larva, mucocartilage largely pervades the dorsal and ventral parts of the head (fig. 4.6D). It forms a large plate in the snout and an even larger ventral plate extending beneath the branchial basket. These two plates are connected laterally by two commissures. Moreover, mucocartilage processes extend into the larval velum (mvsk, lvsk, fig. 4.6D), and a thick median longitudinal bar (mvlb, fig. 4.6D) extends ventrally to the pharynx in the median crest which will later give rise to the tongue.

In the course of embryonic development of the skull, the first skeletal primordia to appear are those of the trabecles (trab, fig. 4.6A, B) and the "parabuccal cell band" (pbcb, fig. 4.6A) which will later give rise to the median velar skeleton (mvsk, fig. 4.6B). At the 410-hours stage the trabecles and median velar skeleton chondrify, the parabuccal cell band disappears, and the vertical bars of the branchial arch primordia appear (hy, fig. 4.6B). Later, the parachordals (parc, fig. 4.6C) extend medially to the otic capsules and the branchial skeleton is almost achieved.

There is a controversy as to the homology between the trabecles (or anterior trabeculae) of lampreys and gnathostomes. In gnathostomes, the trabecles are neural crest derivatives and, therefore, have been regarded by some anatomists as parts of the mandibular or premandibular visceral arches, incorporated into the neurocranium. Sewertzoff (1916−17) and de Beer (1937) considered that the trabecles of lampreys were not true trabecles but mere anterior prolongations of parachordals. In contrast, Damas (1944) regarded them as true trabecles, and Newth (1956) demonstrated experimentally that they were, at least in part, neural crest derivatives, as in gnathostomes. This has received further confirmation by Langille and Hall (1988).

In an 8 mm larva, the parachordals are in contact posteriorly with the branchial skeleton, there is a clear anterior commissure between the trabeculae (com, fig. 4.6C), and a paired primordium of the olfactory capsule is visible (olfc, fig. 4.6C). At this stage, the trabecles develop a short, lateral rod, the pedicel (ped, fig. 4.6C2), which will later join the blastema of the hyoid arch and form, in the adult, the root of the subocular arch.

Early in metamorphosis, the branchial skeleton is present (although somewhat different in shape than in the adult), as are the trabecles, parachordals, otic and olfactory capsules, median velar skeleton, and the blastemas of the hyoid arch, styliform cartilage, lateral mouth plate, subocular arch, and posterior lateral cartilage (fig. 4.6E). All these blastemas are surrounded by mucocartilage plates. The median ventral longitudinal bar of mucocartilage contains a blastema of the piston, copular, and apical cartilages (pistc, fig. 4.6E). In later stages, the descending processes of the dorsal mesenchymatous or mucocartilage plate become isolated into small islets, within which form the primordia of the anterior lateral cartilages. During the latest stages of metamorphosis the styliform cartilage (styc, fig. 4.6E) and its ventral cornual processes appear. The velar skeleton becomes independent from the rest of the skull, and the large cartilaginous plates of the snout (tec, fig. 4.6E) develop from their respective blastemas in the mouth plate. The walls of the braincase form from a dorsal process of the trabecles (brc, fig. 4.6E). Finally, the small cartilaginous elements associated with the lingual apparatus chondrify.

In sum, development of the lamprey skull involves the following phases: (1) embryonic development of the trabeculae, velar skeleton, otic and olfactory capsules, and branchial arches; (2) larval development of prebranchial blastemas and the large mucocartilage plates; (3) metamorphic stages, where some cartilaginous elements begin to form within the mucocartilage; and (4) breakdown of mucocartilage and formation of the adult skull.

Fossil Lampreys

The best preserved of the two fossil lampreys yet recorded (all of Carboniferous age) is *Mayomyzon* (fig. 4.7A), in which tectal, annular, and piston cartilages are clearly visible (tea, anc, pistc, fig. 4.7A). It shows that the structure of the skull of lampreys was already achieved in Late Carboniferous times (330 million years ago). However, one can note a difference between the skull of all Carboniferous lampreys and that of Recent lampreys: the branchial apparatus is much shorter and concentrated in the former (gp, fig. 4.7A, C2) than in the latter (fig. 4.7C1). In both *Mayomyzon* and *Hardistiella* (which is slightly older), the length of the branchial apparatus is equal to the preotic length of the head, whereas in Recent lampreys, it is more than twice as long as the preotic length. The number of gill pouches in Carboniferous lampreys seems to be only six,

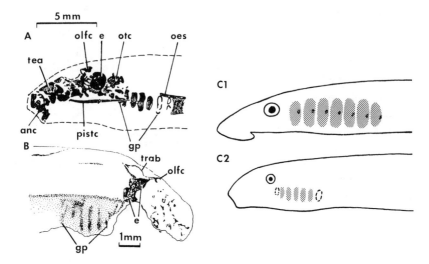

Fig. 4.7. Fossil lampreys. A. *Mayomyzon pieckoensis* Bardack & Zangerl, Upper Carboniferous of Illinois, U.S.A., head in lateral view, showing impression of the skull. B. ?*Hardistiella montanensis* Janvier & Lund, Early Carboniferous of Montana, U.S.A., head of a possibly larval individual. C. Relative position of the gill pouches (stippled) in a Recent (C1) and Carboniferous (C2) lamprey. (A, redrawn from Bardack and Zangerl 1971; B, C, from Lund and Janvier 1985)

instead of seven in Recent forms. In *Hardistiella* there are vague indications of spiniform processes on the branchial arches. The small size of the apparently adult Carboniferous lampreys suggests that these early forms underwent neither larval development nor metamorphosis. However, a specimen of *Hardistiella* from the Lower Carboniferous of Montana seems to show impressions of the trabecles and olfactory capsule (trab, olfc, fig. 4.7B) which are strongly suggestive of the condition in extant larval lampreys (Lund and Janvier 1986), *Pipiscius* is a badly preserved form from the Upper Carboniferous of Illinois which Bardack and Richardson (1977) regarded as being not closely related to lampreys. Nevertheless, it possesses an oral sucker strengthened by horny plates, the arrangement of which recalls those of the extant primitive genus *Ichthyomyzon*.

SKULL HOMOLOGIES IN RECENT JAWLESS CRANIATES

There are two ways of considering homologies among elements in the skull of Recent jawless craniates, depending on whether they are regarded as a monophyletic taxon or not. As mentioned above, paraphyly of the cyclostomes (hagfishes and lampreys) is largely based on nonskeletal characteristics (i.e., soft-tissue anatomy, physiology, biochemistry), with the exception of the arcualia shared by lampreys and gnathostomes. In contrast, the skull, and in particular the skeleton of the lingual apparatus, has often been claimed to support cyclostome monophyly (e.g., Yalden 1985). Clearly, the cartilaginous arch structure of the skull of these jawless craniates has been an early source of intuitive or inductive homologizations, but when considering the various attempts at homologizing the components of the hagfish and lamprey skull one can only arrive at the conclusion put by Johnels (1948, 141): "In the comprehensive literature on this subject, practically all conceivable views have been expressed." The same applies to comparisons between these two groups and the gnathostomes (for detailed discussions, the reader is referred to Johnels 1948 and Hardisty 1981).

As early as 1936, Holmgren and Stensiö arrived at the same pessimistic conclusion, that besides the otic capsule, the parachordals, the trabecles, and the olfactory capsule, no structure of hagfish and lamprey skull could be reasonably homologized. This statement still prevails, yet one may add that trematic rings (if any exist in myxinoids) can be homologous in both groups. The skeleton of the lingual apparatus in hagfishes and lampreys is perhaps the most striking structural resemblance, which can lead to a hypothesis of homology. Yalden (1985) suggested a homology between the three basal cartilages of hagfishes and the piston, copular, and apical cartilages of lampreys. From this admittedly striking similarity, as well as from the functional anatomy of the lingual musculature in both groups, he concluded that the cyclostomes are a monophyletic group. In contrast, Janvier (1981) considered that, if the lingual apparatus of hagfishes and lampreys is inherited from a common ancestor, it is from an ancestral craniate. In fact, the in-and-out movement of the horny teeth of hagfishes, which persists in the apical teeth of lampreys, may well be the primitive masticatory device of craniates. It may have arisen from a simple evagination-invagination movement of the skin of the lips.

The velum, which in hagfishes and lampreys is a mandibular-segment derivative, may also be homologous in both groups, although there is not a single muscular or skeletal element which convincingly supports such a hypothesis, besides the fact that both are innervated by the mandibular ramus of the trigeminal nerve.

In sum, the search for cranial homologies between hagfishes and lampreys seems to be an endless quest paved with hopeful wishes. There, we encounter the same problem as when trying to find homologies between the various chordate or even metzoan groups: one never knows where homology becomes a mere impressionistic view, hence a desperate appeal to molecular characteristics. Patterson (1982) wrote that homologies need not be weighted; they weight themselves by congruence which is beyond the bounds of chance. In the hagfish-lamprey-gnathostome problem, the

self-weighting of homologies is clearly in favor of monophyly of the vertebrata (lampreys and gnathostomes), but cranial features alone have virtually no bearing on this conclusion. Thus, their interpretation should be
made in light of other homologies.

SKULL OF EXCLUSIVELY FOSSIL JAWLESS CRANIATES

During the Ordovician, Silurian, and Devonian (i.e., over a period of
nearly 120 million years), six jawless craniate groups diversified in a near-
shore marine and possibly freshwater environment: the Heterostraci, Anaspida, Galeaspida, Pituriaspida, Osteostraci, and Thelodonti. All these
groups became extinct in the Upper Frasnian, by the end of the Devonian,
with a possible exception of the anaspids, which are regarded by some
paleontologists as closely related or even ancestral to lampreys. Heterostracans, galeaspids, pituriaspids, and osteostracans are surely monophyletic, but anaspids are paraphyletic if ancestral to lampreys, and the
thelodonts are not united by any clear synapomorphy and may well be a
paraphyletic ensemble of primitive craniates, some being related to heterostracans, galeaspids, osteostracans, anaspids, and gnathostomes, respectively (Janvier 1981; see however Turner 1991).

Practically all these fossil jawless craniates have a well-developed
dermal skeleton, be it micromeric (i.e., made up of small scales as in thelodonts), or macromeric (i.e., made up of larger bony plates as in heterostracans), but only the galeaspids, pituriaspids, and osteostracans display a
well ossified endoskeleton. Thanks to this perichondrally ossified endoskeleton, we have now a relatively good knowledge of their internal anatomy, in particular the brain cavity, otic capsules, and cranial nerves.

These fossil jawless craniates will be described here briefly, regardless
of their respective phylogenetic position, which will be discussed later.
However, I begin this review with a section on the Ordovician and Cambrian craniate remains (i.e., the earliest known records of the group) which
were classically regarded as belonging to the Heterostraci, on the basis of
characteristics now considered to be symplesiomorphies.

Cambrian and Ordovician Craniates: Earliest Known Skulls

The Cambrian craniate records are mere fragments of exoskeleton made
up of apparently acellular bone and dentine, but which are interpreted by
some paleontologists as fragments of the carapace of aglaspid arthropods.
The earliest undoubted records of larger craniate skeletons are from the
Late Lower Ordovician (Llanvirnian, 470 million years ago), with the recent discovery of *Sacabambaspis* (fig. 4.8A) from Bolivia (Gagnier et al.
1986; Gagnier 1989a, b). Slightly younger forms, from the early Upper

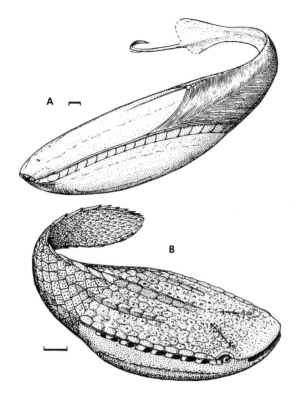

Fig. 4.8. Dermal skeleton of the earliest known craniates. A. *Sacabambaspis janvieri* Gagnier, Blieck & Rodrigo, Ordovician of Bolivia. B. *Astraspis desiderata* Walcott, Ordovician of the U.S.A. Scale: 10 mm. (A, based on Gagnier 1989a; B, on Elliott 1987)

Ordovician (Caradocian, 450 million years ago), are known from Australia and North America: *Arandaspis, Astraspis*, and *Eriptychius*. The two arandaspids, *Sacabambaspis* and *Arandaspis* (Ritchie and Gilbert-Tomlinson 1977), are by far the best documented forms; they possess an elongated dermal head shield and slender scales. They seem to have numerous (up to 10) pairs of gill pouches which open to the exterior by separate openings probably situated between lateral dermal platelets. The eyeballs and, possibly, paired nostrils are situated in a notch of the anterior margin of the shield. The mouth is lined ventrally by numerous rows of minute dermal elements. *Astraspis* (fig. 4.8B) possessed nearly the same type of head shield, but its scales are larger and more massive than in arandaspids. It did possess a series of at least eight distinct external branchial openings extending in a horizontal row behind the orbit (Elliott 1987). *Eriptychius*, although poorly known, has yielded evidence of endoskeletal calcified cartilage with some vascular canals (Denison 1967).

In all these Ordovician forms, the exoskeleton consists of aspidin, a type of acellular bone quite similar to that of the Heterostraci (see below). Aspidin is variously regarded as either a derived (Ørvig 1965, 1989) or primitive (Denison 1963; Halstead 1973, 1987; Maisey 1988) condition, relatively to cellular bone. For various reasons, the latter solution is more acceptable. Smith and Hall (1990), too, consider aspidine as close either to dentine or cement, but not derived from bone. The general aspect of the head shield of these Ordovician craniates is homogeneous: a relatively flat dorsal surface, a strongly convex ventral surface, and straight longitudinal ridges in particular on the dorsal surface. These early craniates do not tell us much of the primitive structure of the vertebrate head, except that minute eyes, lateral-line system, and pineal organ did exist as early as 470 million years ago. A peculiarity observed in these forms is the paired pineal foramen of *Sacabambaspis* (Gagnier 1989a). The relationships between them and the later Silurian and Devonian taxa are still obscure. The shield shape and superficial ornamentation of *Arandaspis* and *Sacabambaspis* are suggestive of primitive heterostracans, but their scales rather recall those of anaspids.

The Heterostraci

The Heterostraci, often referred to as "pteraspids," are characterized by a dermal head armor which consists chiefly of large dorsal and ventral plates pierced laterally by a single common external branchial opening (ebro, fig. 4.9B1, 3). They lived from the Lower Silurian to Upper Devonian (438–367 million years ago). A typical heterostracan is the now classic *Errivaspis waynensis* ("*Pteraspis rostrata*"), which belongs to the relatively derived group Pteraspidiformes (fig. 4.9A, B). In this form, the dorsal side of the head is covered by the dorsal disc (dd, fig. 4.9B1), which bears a dorsal spinal plate (sppl, fig. 4.9B1), the pineal plate (pipl, fig. 4.9B1), the paired orbital plates (orbpl, fig. 4.9B1) pierced by the orbit (orb, fig. 4.9B1), and the rostral plate (rpl, fig. 4.9B1). Ventrally, the head is covered by the ventral disc (vd, fig. 4.9B2); anteriorly, some postoral and elongated oral plates (popl, opl, fig. 4.9B2, 3) protected the lower lip and may have served in feeding to grab in the sand or mud. In fact, there are good reasons to believe that these thin oral plates could expand in a fan like manner (fig. 4.9C) if the mucosa oris was everted more or less in the same way as in myxinoids. Laterally, the head was covered by elongate branchial plates (brpl, fig. 4.9B1, 2) and the common external branchial openings were lined posteriorly by the cornual plates (cpl, fig. 4.9B1, 2). Most of these dermal plates enclosed a more or less complex network of sensory-line canals which opened to the exterior by pores or thin slits.

One of the most debated questions of heterostracan anatomy is

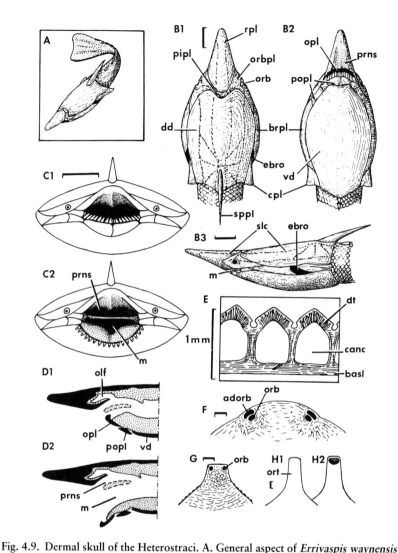

Fig. 4.9. Dermal skull of the Heterostraci. A. General aspect of *Errivaspis waynensis* (White) (Lower Devonian). B. Head shield of *Errivaspis* in dorsal (B1), ventral (B2), and lateral (B3) views; C. Pteraspidiform head in anterior view, showing the position of the oral plates when the mouth was closed (C1) and open (C2). D. The same in longitudinal section, showing the possible outline of the endoskeleton and soft parts (stippled). E. Microstructure of heterostracan armor, showing basal and cancellar layers. F. Anterior part of the head shield of an amphiaspid (*Gabreyaspis*), showing the adorbital opening. G–H. Two amphiaspids with elongated oral tube: *Empedaspis* (G) and *Eglonaspis* in dorsal (H1) and ventral (H2) views. Scale: 10 mm unless indicated otherwise. (B, redrawn from White 1935; C, from Janvier 1981; E–H, from Novitskaya 1971)

whether the oral plates could bite against the rostral plate in the same way as gnathostome jaws, or if they did not reach the ventral side of the rostrum, leaving a free passage for the intake of the respiratory water (Halstead 1973; Janvier 1974, 1981). Since the presumed "upper oral plates" recorded in some heterostracans have turned out to be mere pathological outgrowth of the exoskeleton, I consider that the two broad furrows on the ventral side of the rostrum (prns, fig. 4.9B2) correspond to the passage of an inhalent prenasal sinus which may possibly have been completely separated from the mouth as in hagfishes (fig. 4.9C, D). In some heterostracans, this prenasal sinus forms a distinct paired notch (fig. 4.10C).

Histologically the exoskeleton of heterostracans consists of aspidin (fig. 4.9E), which bears a superficial layer of dentine, forming ridges or tubercles (dt, fig. 4.9E). In the middle part of the exoskeleton there is in most heterostracans a typical honeycomb-shaped cancellar layer (canc, fig. 4.9E). The aspidin was generated by a single cell front which lined the basal layer and the inside of the cancellae. This mode of production of a mineralized hard tissue is now generally regarded as primitive and comparable to that of dentine (Halstead 1987; Smith and Hall 1990).

In no known typical heterostracan is the endoskeleton preserved, but the pattern of the internal organs of the head is partly known from the impressions on internal surfaces of exoskeletal plates. These impressions are often beautifully displayed on the natural cast of the shield (fig. 4.10A, B, D), and one may easily recognize those left by the brain, the two dorsal semicircular canals (asc, psc, fig. 4.10A), the eyeballs (e, fig. 4.10A), the pineal organ (pi, fig. 4.10A), the olfactory organ (olf, fig. 4.10A), and the gill pouches with individual gill lamellae (gp, fig. 4.10A, B). Between the gill pouch impressions, Janvier and Blieck (1979) identified possible impressions of branchial arches connected with the enigmatic Y-shaped impressions (y, fig. 4.10A). The ventral disc also shows gill pouch impressions and a peculiar median groove which may correspond to some structure of the oral mechanism ("lingual" apparatus?). Some particularly well preserved specimens show rare features, such as the various division of the brain impressions (mes, met, myc, fig. 4.10A), some faint impressions of the arcualia of the vertebral column (arc, fig. 4.10A), or extrabranchial blood vessels (ebrv, fig. 4.10D).

As is often the case with incomplete fossils, the heterostracans gave rise to fanciful interpretations, being reconstructed on the basis of either a myxinoid (Stensiö 1927, 1964; Janvier 1974, 1975b) or a gnathostome pattern (Halstead 1973; Novitskaya 1983). Most of their internal anatomy will be unavailable as long as no endoskeleton is known. However, some inferences can be made from the observed data; e.g., the absence of a horizontal semicircular canal, which is inferred from the fact that the third gill

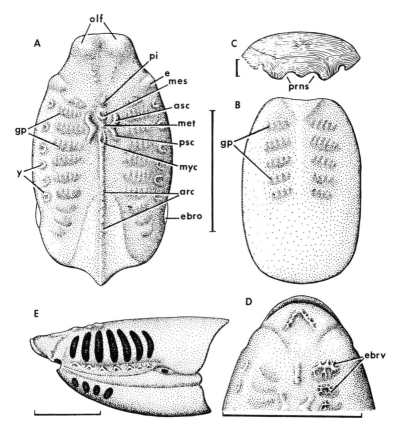

Fig. 4.10. Internal anatomy of the heterostracan head. A, B. Natural internal cast of the shield of a cyathaspidiform heterostracan, showing impressions on the dorsal (A) and ventral (B) shields. C. External opening of the prenasal sinus in the cyathaspidiform *Dikenaspis*, anterior view. D. Impressions of blood vessels in the shield of the cyathaspidiform *Poraspis*. E. Attempted reconstruction of the cartilaginous endoskeleton (if any) of a cyathaspidiform, lateral view. Scale: 10 mm. (A, B, combined from various sources, e.g., Stensiö 1964, and Novitskaya 1983; C, from Denison 1964; D, E, from Novitskaya 1983)

pouch impression penetrates deeply between the two vertical semicircular canal impressions (fig. 4.10A). Some features of heterostracans remain unexplained, such as the adorbital opening of some Lower Devonian amphiaspids from Siberia (adorb, fig. 4.9F), which has been regarded as either a displaced opening of the prenasal sinus, a spiraculum, or even a prespiraculum (Halstead 1973; Janvier 1974; Novitskaya 1983). Finally, the common external branchial openings have been interpreted as a jet propulsion device (Bendix-Almgreen 1986).

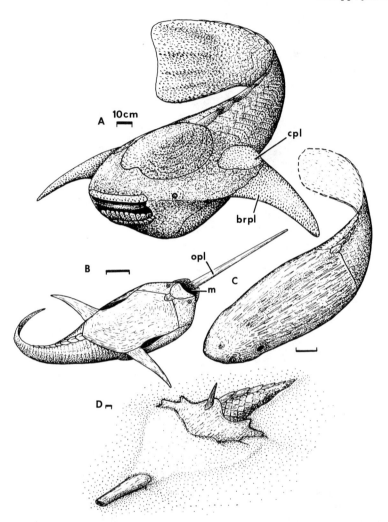

Fig. 4.11. Diversity of dermal head armors in Devonian heterostracans. A. *Pycnosteus* (Upper Devonian). B. *Doryaspis* (Lower Devonian). C. *Traquairaspis* (Lower Devonian). D. *Eglonaspis* (Lower Devonian). Scale: 10 mm, unless indicated otherwise. (A, based on Obruchev and Mark-Kurik 1965; B, on Heintz 1968; C, on Dineley and Loeffler 1976; D, on Novitskaya 1971)

Heterostracans display a large variety of shield shape, here illustrated by four extreme types: the psammosteid *Pycnosteus* (fig. 4.11A), one of the largest and latest known heterostracans, with largely expanded branchial plates and which reached over 1 m in breadth; the protopteraspid *Doryaspis* from the Lower Devonian of Spitsbergen (fig. 4.11B), with a peculiar rostrumlike oral plate and a dorsal mouth; the traquairaspidiform

Traquairaspis (fig. 4.11C), which may be among the most primitive heterostracans; and the amphiaspid *Eglonaspis* (fig. 4.11D), in which all the shield plates are fused into a single unit, and the head produced anteriorly into a long oral tube, suggesting burrowing habits. *Eglonaspis* was blind and represents the most derived form of a group of amphiaspids in which the oral tube became progressively elongated (fig. 4.9G, H).

Anaspida

Relative to heterostracans, Anaspida are slender-bodied, jawless craniates covered with a micromeric to mesomeric exoskeleton—hence their name ("without shield"). Typical anaspids are characterized by a strongly hypocercal tail and a triradiate postbranchial spine (fig. 4.12A). They lived during the Silurian (438–408 million years ago). However, some poorly ossified forms of uncertain affinities, e.g., *Jamoytius* (Lower Silurian), and *Endeiolepis* or *Euphanerops* (Upper Devonian) (fig. 4.12E, F), are traditionally referred to as anaspids.

Virtually nothing is known of the cranial endoskeleton of anaspids, since no internal impressions are visible. Their skull is known essentially from the exoskeleton, which consists of variously associated scales and platelets. In a few forms (e.g., *Pterygolepis*) relatively large plates occur on the ventral side of the head (fig. 4.12D). In *Pharyngolepis* (fig. 4.12B), one of the best-known anaspids, from the Silurian of Norway, the dorsal surface of the head is covered with a dermal roof of medium-sized plates which enclose sensory-line canals (slc, fig. 4.12B2) and circumscribe four openings: the two orbits, the pineal foramen (pi, fig. 4.12B2), and a possible naso-hypophysial opening (?nahyp, fig. 4.12B2). Ventro-laterally, a series of 15 external branchial openings (ebro, fig. 4.12B1) pierce a single elongated dermal plate, the branchial plate (brpl, fig. 4.12B1). These are followed posteriorly by a large, triradiate postbranchial spine (psp, fig. 4.12B1). Ventral to the mouth there is a median oral plate (opl, fig. 4.12B3, D) which bears a pair of deep internal impressions (fig. 4.12C2), presumably for attachment of some muscles. This oral plate probably could bite against the anterior margin (?bs, fig. 4.12C1) of the dorsal head plates or the rostral plates, thus acting like the jaws of gnathostomes.

The dermal bones of anaspids are acellular and histologically resemble the aspidin of heterostracans, yet there is no cancellar layer and no dentine (fig. 4.12E); the scales and dermal plates are thus essentially laminar in structure.

Some tarry impressions of the endoskeleton are visible in forms questionably referred to the Anaspida: *Jamoytius* and *Euphanerops*. In a specimen of the Upper Devonian *Euphanerops* there seems to be a very elongated branchial basket with over 25 branchial arches ("?brbsk," fig. 4.12F2), and corresponding impressions of possible external branchial

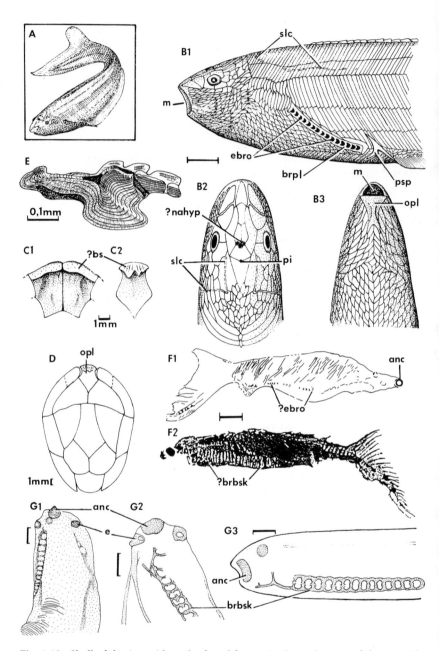

Fig. 4.12. Skull of the Anaspida and referred forms. A. General aspect of the anaspid *Pharyngolepis* (Upper Silurian). B. *Pharyngolepis oblongus* Kiaer, dermal head skeleton in lateral (B1), dorsal (B2), and ventral (B3) views. C. Isolated rostral (C1) and oral (C2) plates of *Rhyncholepis* in internal view, showing possible biting

openings are visible in the type specimen (?ebro, fig. 4.12F1). Also in this form, a possible annular cartilage has been observed around the mouth (anc, fig. 4.12F1) (Arsenault and Janvier 1991).

In the Lower Silurian *Jamoytius,* which has been regarded by Forey and Gardiner (1981) as a true lamprey, there is a clear branchial skeleton (brbsk, fig. 4.12G) with a series of 14 (and perhaps more) ringlike structures which may be compared to the trematic rings of lampreys. Again, there seems to be a large annular cartilage (anc, fig. 4.12G).

Since Kiaer's (1924) suggestion that the anaspids possess a dorsal naso-hypophysial opening, this group has been regarded as closely related or even ancestral to lampreys, a hypothesis further supported by the similarly elongated body shape, annular cartilage, hypocercal tail, and branchial openings arranged in a slanting line. However, this relationship is far from demonstrated, and it is by no means certain that anaspids did possess a naso-hypophysial complex of petromyzontid type, since no endoskeletal structure supports this interpretation of the median dorsal opening referred to as a naso-hypophysial opening.

The Anaspida appear to have been rather similar in shape. Their diversification bears on the extension of the dermal plates over the head, the size of the paired fin, the number of external branchial openings (from 8 to 15, or perhaps more if *Jamoytius* and *Euphanerops* are included in the group), and the degree of reduction of the body scales.

The Osteostraci

The Osteostraci, or "cephalaspids," are by far the best known of all fossil jawless vertebrates. This is primarily because the cartilaginous endoskeleton of their head shield was lined with a thin lamella of perichondral bone which favored preserving the shape of all internal cavities and canals occupied by the nerves, blood vessels, and other soft structures. They are characterized by peculiar median and lateral fields (see below) on the dorsal surface of the head. They lived from the Lower Silurian to Upper Devonian (425–467 million years ago).

The head shield of osteostracans is primitively horseshoe-shaped in

---

surfaces. D. *Rhyncholepis* (Upper Silurian), ventral dermal cover of the head.
E. Section of an anaspid scale, showing the laminar and acellular structure.
F. *Euphanerops* (Upper Devonian), complete specimens in lateral view, showing possible external branchial openings (F1) and branchial basket (F2). G. *Jamoytius* (Lower Silurian), two heads showing some skeletal impressions (G1, G2) and attempted reconstruction of the skull (G3). Scale: 10 mm, unless indicated otherwise. (B, redrawn and combined from Stensiö 1964 and Ritchie 1964; C, D, from Ritchie 1980; E, from Gross 1958; F, from Arsenault and Janvier 1991; G, from Ritchie 1968 and Forey and Gardiner 1981)

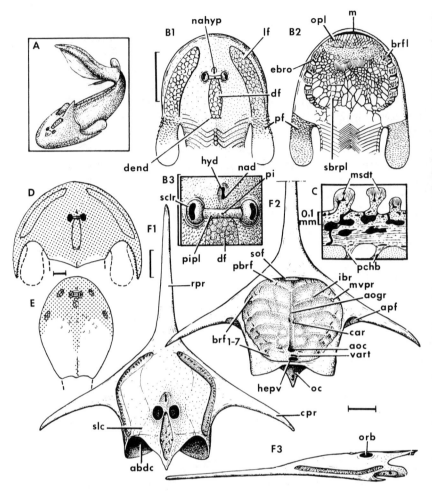

Fig. 4.13. Skull of the Osteostraci. A. General aspect of the osteostracan *Zenaspis* (Lower Devonian). B. Head shield of the primitive osteostracan *Hirella* (Upper Silurian) in dorsal (B1) and ventral (B2) views, and detail of the orbito-pineal region (B3). C. Microstructure of the dermal and endoskeletal shield of an osteostracan (cartilage stippled). D, E. Relative extension of the endoskeleton (stippled) in the shield of two osteostracans: a primitive (D), and a very derived cornuate (E) in dorsal view. F. Head shield of a derived benneviaspidian osteostracan, *Boreaspis,* in dorsal (F1), ventral (F2), and lateral (F3) views, showing the roof of the orobranchial cavity. Scale: 10 mm, unless indicated otherwise. (B, from Heintz 1939; C, from Wängsjö 1952; D–F, from Janvier 1985)

dorsal view (fig. 4.13A, B, D), but may develop various cornual or rostral processes in some derived forms (figs. 4.13F, 4.16B). Since the paired fins are attached on the shield (pf, fig. 4.13B), one may infer that it actually includes endo- and exoskeletal components of the shoulder girdle. The eyes are closely set (fig. 4.13B3) and separated in primitive forms by a small free dermal element, the pineal plate (pipl, fig. 4.13B3) pierced by the pineal foramen (pi, fig. 4.13B3). Anterior to it there is a keyhole-shaped naso-hypophysial opening (nahyp, fig. 4.13B1), which comprises an anterior hypophysial division (hyd, fig. 4.13B3), by which the hypophysial tube opened to the exterior, and a nasal division (nad, fig. 4.13B3), through which the water entered the olfactory organ. The eyeballs were often covered with a dermal slerotic ring (sclr, fig. 4.13B3) pierced by an elliptic optic window which probably enabled partial stereoscopic vision. In rare instances, the sclera itself was lined with perichondral bone (fig. 4.15D).

On the dorsal surface, the shield displays variously developed areas where the exoskeleton is not attached to the underlying endoskeleton, and where the endoskeleton is hollowed by a shallow depression: the lateral and dorsal cephalic fields (df, lf, fig. 4.13B1). These fields are unique to osteostracans but remain unexplained. They are linked to the labyrinth cavity by large and ramified canals (sel, fig. 4.15C) which suggest that they housed either sensory or electric organs. Behind the median dorsal field there is a paired opening for the endolymphatic ducts (dend, fig. 4.13B1).

In ventral aspect, the shield was covered by a soft membrane armed with polygonal dermal plates (sbrpl, fig. 4.13B2). This membrane closed a vast orobranchial fenestra, along the rim of which opened the mouth (m, fig. 4.13B2), lined posteriorly by oral plates (opl, fig. 4.13B2), and 8 to 10 external branchial openings (ebro, fig. 4.13B2), each protected by a small skin flap (brfl, fig. 4.13B2).

The head shield of osteostracans consists of a single mass of cartilaginous endoskeleton lined with perichondral bone (pchb, fig. 4.13C) and covered externally with cellular exoskeleton. The latter bears tubercles of mesodentine (msdt, fig. 4.13C) and contains sensory line canals (slc, fig. 4.13F1). In most osteostracans, the exoskeleton of the head shield covers almost exactly the surface of the endoskeleton (fig. 4.13D), but in some derived forms, the exoskeletal shield extends posteriorly beyond the endoskeletal shield (fig. 4.13E).

The endoskeletal shield is hollowed ventrally by a large, roughly hemispherical or spoon-shaped cavity, the orobranchial cavity (fig. 4.13F2), which contains gill pouches, velum, esophagus, and structures associated with the mouth. Posteriorly, it is separated from the abdominal cavity (abdc, fig. 4.14A1) by a complex postbranchial wall pierced by three large median foramina (aoc, vart, hepv, fig. 4.13F2).

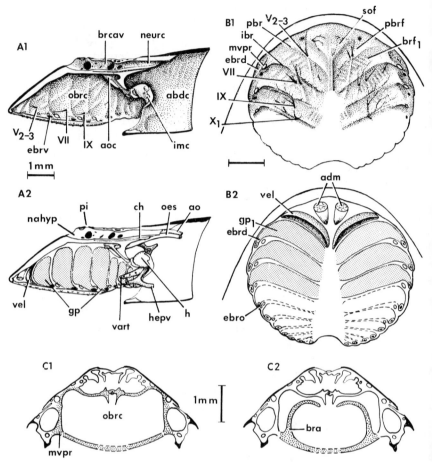

Fig. 4.14. Organization of the orobranchial cavity of the osteostracan shield.
A. Sagittal section of the shield of *Norselaspis* (Lower Devonian) (A1), and attempted
reconstruction of the gill pouches (stippled), velum, esophagus, heart, and major blood
vessels (A2) (section of endoskeleton in white and exoskeleton in black). B. Ventral
view of the orobranchial cavity of *Scolenaspis* (Lower Devonian) (B1) and attempted
reconstruction of the gill pouches (stippled) and velum (B2). C. Transverse section of
the shield of *Norselaspis,* showing two possible interpretations of the visceral arches in
osteostracans (stippled), being either incorporated to the shield (C1) or separated from
the roof of the oralobranchial cavity (C2). Scale: 10 mm unless indicated otherwise.
(A, from Janvier 1985, simplified; B, from Wängsjö 1952; C, from Janvier 1985)

The orobranchial cavity displays some constant features which have received various interpretations. These structures are described here succinctly:

—The median aortic groove (aogr, fig. 4.13F2) is a large median and slightly elevated groove which housed the dorsal aorta, esophagus, and possibly the anterior cardinal veins.
—The supraoral field (sof, figs. 4.13F2, 4.14B1) is a triangular area which formed the roof of the mouth cavity. It is often hollowed by a pair of deep depressions for attachment of possible adductor muscles (adm, fig. 4.14B2).
—The prebranchial fossae (pbrf, figs. 4.13F2, 4.14B1) probably housed a velum (vel, fig. 4.14A2, B2) which resembled that of larval lampreys.
—The branchial fossae (brf$_{1-7}$, figs. 4.13F2–4.14B1), which housed the gill pouches, sometimes show impressions of the individual gill lamellae or efferent arterioles (fig. 4.14B1). Laterally the branchial fossae communicate with extrabranchial areas and extrabranchial ducts (ebrd, fig. 4.14B1). The branchial fossae are separated by interbranchial ridges (ibr, figs. 4.13F2, 4.14B1) which bear a groove, probably for an extrabranchial artery. Each interbranchial ridge ends laterally by a short process, the medial ventral process (mvpr, figs. 4.13F2, 4.14C1), to which was attached a cartilaginous component of the branchial arch (fig. 4.14C1) or the entire branchial arch (fig. 4.14C2).

The roof of the orobranchial cavity is pierced by numerous foramina, namely for the carotid arteries (car, fig. 4.13F2), the visceromotor and viscerosensory nerves (V$_{2-3}$, VII, IX, X, fig. 4.14B1), and, laterally, the extrabranchial veins (ebrv, figs. 4.14A1, 4.15C).

Finally, the postbranchial wall is pierced by three large median foramina: a dorsal one for the esophagus and dorsal aorta (aoc, figs. 4.13F2, 4.14A), a central one for the ventral arterial trunk (vart, figs. 4.13F2, 4.14A2), and a ventral one for the hepatic vein (hepv, figs. 4.13F2, 4.14A2) opening toward a cavity which houses the heart (h, fig. 4.14A2). This cavity is divided by a ridge which marks the limit between the ventricle and atrium of the heart, and suggests a heart morphology and function quite similar to that of larval lampreys (Janvier et al. 1991).

Posterior to the orobranchial cavity, the abdominal cavity contained the anterior part of the liver, the gonads, and large blood sinuses. It is limited laterally by the endoskeletal scapular component of the shield and dorsally by the occipital region, which contains the median chordal (ch, fig. 4.14A2) and neural canals (neurc, fig. 4.14A1).

Above the orobranchial and abdominal cavities, the endoskeletal shield is hollowed by complex cavities and canals which housed the brain (figs.

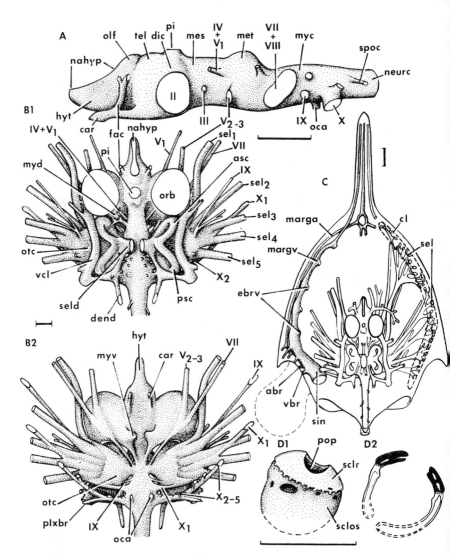

Fig. 4.15. Internal anatomy of the osteostracan head shield. A. Internal cast of the brain cavity of *Norselaspis* (Lower Devonian) in lateral view. B. Internal cast of the cavities and canals of the central part of the shield of *Benneviaspis* (Lower Devonian) in dorsal (B1) and ventral (B2) views. C. Internal cast of the cavities and canals of the shield of the boreaspid *Belonaspis* (Lower Devonian), with marginal blood vascular canals of the left side (stippled), dorsal view. D. Sclerotic ring (black) and scleral ossification (white) of the eyeball of the tremataspid *Tremataspis* (Upper Silurian) in posterior view (D1) and transverse section (D2). Scale: 1 mm. (From Janvier 1985)

4.14A, C, 4.15A, B), cranial nerves (fig. 4.15B, C), cephalic blood vessels (fig. 4.15C), and sensory capsules.

The elongated axial brain cavity (brcav, figs. 4.14A1, 4.14A) communicates anteriorly with the ethmoid cavity (olf, hyt, fig. 4.15A). Its walls were close enough to the brain to reproduce its major external features: the rhombencephalon and myelencephalon (myc, fig. 4.15A), metencephalon (met, fig. 4.15A), mesencephalon (mes, fig. 4.15A), and telencephalon (tel, fig. 4.15A). Laterally, it is pierced by canals or fenestrae for the cranial nerves (II, III, IV, V, VII + VIII, IX, X, fig. 4.15A).

The ethmoid cavity enclosed the olfactory organ (olf, fig. 4.15A) in a small, dorsal piriform division, and the hypophysial tube (hyt, fig. 4.15A, B2) in a more ventral part, which met posteriorly the diencephalic part of the brain cavity.

The labyrinth cavity has a large, olive-shaped vestibular division, and two vertical semicircular canals (asc, psc, fig. 4.15B1), each possessing a large ampullar space. These canals meet in a crus commune from which arises a posteriorly directed endolymphatic duct (dend, fig. 4.15B1). One large dorsal and five lateral canals arise from the vestibular division (seld, sel_{1-5}, fig. 4.15B, C) and ramify distally before opening into the dorsal and lateral fields. These peculiar canals have been interpreted as housing either expansions of the membranous labyrinth or electric nerves.

The orbital cavities (orb, fig. 4.15B1) are large and hollowed by some well-marked myodomes for the eye muscles (myd, myv, fig. 4.15B). In most primitive osteostracans, the eyeball possessed a dermal sclerotic ring (sclr, fig. 4.15D1); in some forms, the sclera is perichondrally ossified (sclos, fig. 4.15D).

The cranial nerves passed through relatively thin canals, which can be identified according to their area of exit from the brain cavity or their destination. The most clearly visible of these canals are those for the oculomotor (III), trochlear (IV), trigeminal (V_{1-3}), facial (VII), glossopharyngeal (IX), and vagus (X_{1-5}) nerves (fig. 4.15A, B). There has been much discussion as to the possible region innervated by the two foremost visceral nerves in osteostracans (see review in Janvier 1985). However, since the canals for the vagus, glossopharyngeal, and facial nerves are now clearly identified, there remains only one nerve canal leading to the orobranchial cavity in front of the facial. This implies either that the two visceromotor branches of the trigeminal passed in the same canal (V_{2-3}, figs. 4.14B1, 4.15B), or that the mandibular branch accompanied the facial nerve.

The major blood vessels of the head shield are those for the carotid artery (car, figs. 4.13F2, 4.15A, B2) and its offshoots, the facial and adorbital arteries, and the lateral head vein, or dorsal jugular (vcl, fig. 4.15B1), which passes dorsally to the otic capsule and all cranial nerve roots. Strangely, the posterior part of the brain cavity was irrigated by the occipital cranial arteries, a pair of small arteries arising from the dorsal aorta, which were probably modified vertebromedullar arteries (oca, fig. 4.15A, B2).

In the lateral part of the shield, there is a unique complex of large vessels, the marginal artery and vein (marga, margv, fig. 4.15C) to which were connected the branchial blood vessels of the paired fins (abr, vbr, fig. 4.15C). The large marginal veins, which obviously drained the orobranchial cavity via the extrabranchial veins (ebrv, figs. 4.14A1, 4.15C), played the same role as the anterior cardinal veins, and may actually be the cardinal veins in an aberrant position (Janvier et al. 1991). Finally, the occipital region, on each side of which opened the lateral head vein, and the foramina for the brachial nerve plexus (plxbr, fig. 4.15B2), contained the neural canal (neurc, fig. 4.14A1) and underlying chordal canal. The latter is thin and ends anteriorly just behind the hypophysial division of the ethmoid cavity.

The nature of the endoskeletal shield of osteostracans has been the subject of various interpretations. Its vague resemblance to the dorsal mucocartilage plate of larval lampreys gave rise to the idea that these two structures are homologous (Stensiö 1927). Later, Johnels (1950) suggested that the two-layered dermis of the lamprey head may correspond to the former extension of a head shield of osteostracan type. This author also suggested that the endoskeletal shield of osteostracans is more comparable to the ectomesoderm of larval lampreys than to mucocartilage. These comparisons are now spurious, since mucocartilage is regarded as a specialization of lampreys.

Another important question is whether this endoskeletal mass of the osteostracan shield is uniquely of neurocranial origin, or comprises visceral components. Stensiö (1927, 1964) regarded the interbranchial ridges as epitrematic divisions of the branchial arches fused to the neurocranial shield (fig. 4.14C1). In contrast, Janvier (1985) suggested that the neurocranial shield has expanded over the branchial apparatus (including branchial arches), and made a sort of cast of its dorsal surface (fig. 4.14C2). The latter interpretation is supported by the study of the extrabranchial blood vascular canals of the shield. The same tendency occurs on some flat-headed gnathostomes (e.g., Arthrodires).

The diversity of the Osteostraci has approximately the same morphological range as the Heterostraci. Most osteostracans have a more or less horseshoe-shaped head shield, the most primitive forms being devoid of cornual processes (fig. 4.13B). Figure 4.16 illustrates three very derived types: the kiaeraspid *Gustavaspis* (Lower Devonian) with secondarily reduced cornual processes and lateral fields and a dorsally placed mouth; the

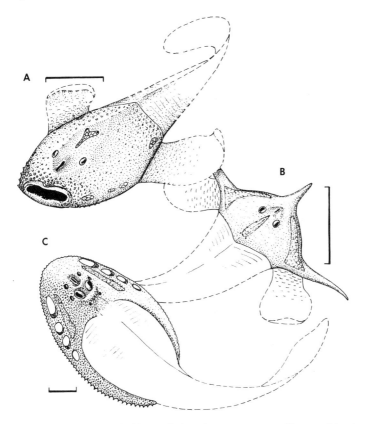

Fig. 4.16. Diversity of head shield morphology in osteostracans, illustrated by three extremely derived forms. A, B. *Gustavaspis* and *Hoelaspis,* both from the Lower Devonian of Spitsbergen. C. *Sclerodus,* from the Upper Silurian and Lower Devonian of Europe. Scale: 10mm. (A, B, based on Janvier 1985; C, based on Forey 1986)

benneviaspid *Hoelaspis* (Lower Devonian), with a short rostral process and anteriorly projected cornual processes; and the tremataspid *Sclerodus* (Uppermost Silurian–Lower Devonian), which has lost the paired fins and possessed peculiar fenestrations in the shield margin.

The Galeaspida

The Galeaspida are known exclusively from the Silurian and Devonian of China and Vietnam. They were thus probably endemic to East Asia, a relatively isolated area at that time. The overall shape of the head vaguely recalls that of osteostracans (fig. 4.17A, B), yet they lack paired fins. This is mainly because the head consists of a single endoskeletal mass lined with perichondral bone and covered with exoskeleton. However, a more ana-

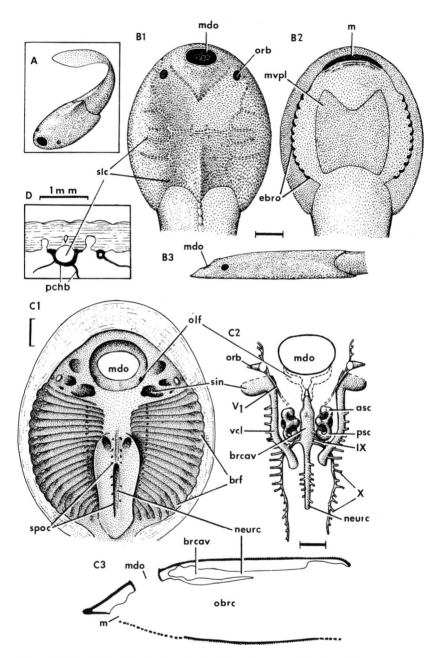

Fig. 4.17. The skull of the Galeaspida. A. General aspect of *Polybranchiaspis liaojaoshanensis* Liu (Lower Devonian). B. The head of *Polybranchiaspis* in dorsal (B1), ventral (B2), and lateral (B3) views. C. *Duyunolepis* (Lower Devonian), ventral

lytic examination reveals many differences: the eyes are widely separated (orb, fig. 4.17B1), and in front of them there is a large bean- or slit-shaped median opening (mdo, fig. 4.17) which communicated ventrally with the underlying orobranchial cavity (fig. 4.17C3). Contrary to the naso-hypophysial opening of osteostracans, this median dorsal opening probably served as an intake for respiratory water, yet Belles-Isles (1986) regards it as an excurrent opening. As in osteostracans, however, the orobranchial cavity was closed ventrally by teguments covered with minute scales and a large median ventral plate (mvpl, fig. 4.17B2). The numerous external branchial openings (up to 24 pairs) were situated along the lateral margin of the orobranchial fenestra (ebro, fig. 4.17B2), and the mouth along the anterior margin (m, fig. 4.17B2). The orobranchial cavity is not separated from the abdominal cavity (obrc, fig. 4.17C3), and its roof is marked with narrow and closely set branchial fossae (brf, fig. 4.17C1). The exoskeleton consists of small, polygonal units of laminar, probably acellular bone and bears no dentine tubercle (Janvier 1990). Basally, it is hollowed by small cavities (fig. 4.17D). The lateral sensory-line canals (slc, fig. 4.17B1) have a typical festooned pattern and are completely closed, lying below the exoskeleton (fig. 4.17D).

The internal anatomy of the head is not fully known, but we have relatively good data on its major features (fig. 4.17C2). The brain cavity (brcav, fig. 4.17C2) is strikingly similar to that of osteostracans and also the brain impression of heterostracans. The labyrinth cavity has a small vestibular division of two vertical semicircular canals (asc, psc, fig. 4.17C2) with a crus commune. The orbital cavities are poorly known but seem to have been small and conical in shape (orb, fig. 4.17C2).

Like osteostracans and gnathostomes, the brain cavity is flanked on each side by a large canal for the dorsal jugular or lateral head vein (vcl, fig. 4.17C2) which opens anteriorly into vast sinuses (sin, fig. 4.17C). This large vein seems to have received numerous lateral extrabranchial veins, a condition which may be explained by the lack of a marginal vein.

The prebranchial part of the roof of the orobranchial cavity is hollowed by several recesses of unknown function (fig. 4.17C1). They may have accommodated some mouth musculature. The olfactory organ was paired and opened into the posterior part of the duct leading to the median

---

view of the orobranchial cavity (C1), dorsal view of the internal cast of the cavities and canals of the head shield (C2), and sagittal section of the head shield (C3) (exoskeleton in black, endoskeleton in white). D. Structure of the exoskeletal shield of *Polybranchiaspis*. Scale: 10 mm unless indicated otherwise. (A, B, based on various data, e.g., Liu 1975 and Janvier 1975a; C, based on P'an and Wang 1978 and Janvier 1984; D, original)

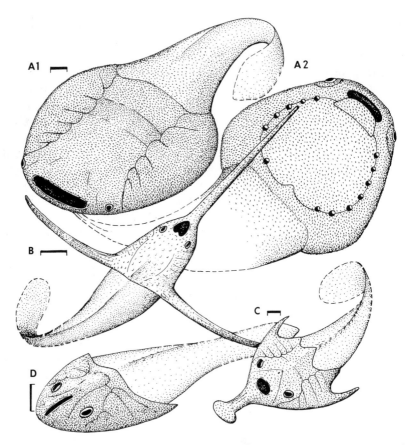

Fig. 4.18. Diversity of head shield morphology in galeaspids. A. *Hanyangaspis* (Upper Silurian–Lower Devonian) in dorsal (A1) and ventral (A2) views. B. *Lungmenshanaspis* (Lower Devonian). C. *Sanchaspis* (Lower Devonian). D. *Eugaleaspis* (Lower Devonian). Scale: 10 mm. (Based on P'an 1984; P'an et al. 1975; Wang 1986; P'an and Wang 1978)

dorsal opening (Wang 1991; olf, fig. 4.17C). The position of the hypophysis is still unknown, and this important point of cranial anatomy is crucial to the question of whether the median dorsal opening is homologous and similar in structure to the naso-pharyngeal duct of hagfishes, as suggested by Janvier (1981, 1984).

The morphological diversity of galeaspids is comparable to that of osteostracans. The most primitive (e.g., the Silurian *Hanyangaspis* (fig. 4.18A) have a broad and flattened shield, a transversely elongated and almost terminal median dorsal opening, laterally placed eyes, and seven external branchial openings (fig. 4.18A2). In most other galeaspids the number of branchial openings is considerably increased (up to 24 pairs). In the Hua-nanaspidiformes, such as *Lungmenshanaspis* (fig. 4.18B), lateral processes and rostral processes may occur, the latter being sometimes spatulate in shape distally as in *Sanchaspis* (fig. 4.18C). Finally, in such Eugaleaspidi-formes as *Eugaleaspis* (fig. 4.18D), the median dorsal opening becomes pear-shaped or even slit-shaped, and the shield is considerably shortened and horseshoe-shaped, superficially resembling that of osteostracans.

The Pituriaspida

The Pituriaspida is a poorly known group, represented by two genera from the Early Devonian of Australia, *Pituriaspis* and *Neeyambaspis* (Young 1991). *Pituriaspis,* by far the best-known genus, possessed an elongated shield which resembles somewhat that of the Osteostraci, with a long ros-tral process, a pair of cornual processes, an orobranchial chamber (obrc, fig. 4.19A), and paired insertion areas for the paired fins (apf, fig. 4.19A). However, it differs from osteostracans in having no dorsal and lateral fields, and no dorsal naso-hypophysial opening. Some evidence of endo-skeleton (possibly lined with perichondral bone, as in osteostracans and galeaspids) suggests the presence of two separate olfactory tracts leading

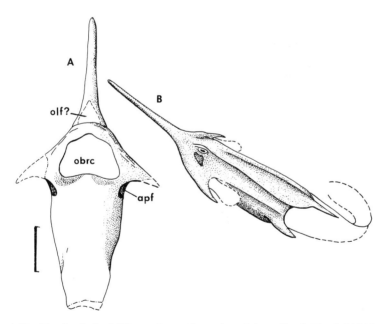

Fig. 4.19. *Pituriaspis doylei* Young, Lower Devonian of Australia. A. Head shield in ventral view. B. Attempted reconstruction. Scale: 10 mm. (Based on Young 1991)

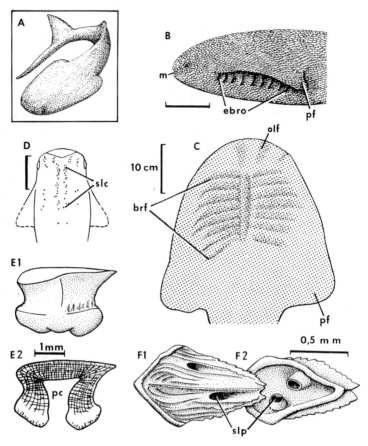

Fig. 4.20. Dermal head skeleton of the "Thelodonti." A. General aspect of *Loganellia scotica* (Upper Silurian). B. Reconstruction of the head of *Loganellia* in lateral view. C. Schematic representation of the head of a specimen of *Turinia pagei* (Lower Devonian) showing impressions of branchial fossae or gill pouches, dorsal view. D. Reconstruction of the head of *Phlebolepis* (Upper Silurian), showing the distribution of the sensory lines. E. Scale of *Thelodus* type in lateral view (E1) and vertical section (E2). F. Scale of *Phlebolepis*, showing sensory-line pores, external (F1) and internal (F2) views. Scale: 10 mm unless indicated otherwise. (A, B, from Turner 1970; C, from Stensiö 1964, simplified; D, from Märss 1979; E, from Karatayute-Talimaa 1978; F, from Gross 1968)

to olfactory organs situated on the ventral side of the shield, in front of the mouth (olf?, fig. 4.19A). A peculiar pit opening ventrally to each orbit may have housed some sensory organ, but is unlikely to be homologous with the lateral fields of osteostracans. Young (1991) suggested that the Pituriaspida may belong to a monophyletic group including the Galeaspida, Osteostraci, and Gnathostomata.

The "Thelodonti"

The "Thelodonti" are poorly known Silurian and Devonian craniates, the exoskeleton of which consists exclusively of small placoidlike scales. Since there is no clear derived characteristic shared uniquely by the thelodonts, this group is probably paraphyletic, that is, they may be ancestral to some of the monophyletic groups described above, and even to the gnathostomes. However, Turner (1991) has expressed a totally different viewpoint, suggesting that the Thelodonti are monophyletic and characterized by particular processes and anchoring devices on the root of the scales.

Articulated thelodonts are rare, but the most accurate reconstructions (fig. 4.20A) show a relatively depressed head flanked by paired flaps or fins (pf, fig. 4.20B, C), which expand over the series of 8 to 10 slitlike branchial openings. The eyes are small and surrounded by two larger and crescentiform scales. Detailed structure of the mouth and rostral region are unknown. Almost nothing is known of the endoskeleton. However, a single specimen of *Turinia* displays vague impressions of gill pouches or branchial fossae (brf, fig. 4.20C) and olfactory organ (olf, fig. 4.20C).

Thelodont scales are very small and their shape varies according to the taxon and position on the body (fig. 4.20E, F). They bear a crown of dentine or mesodentine, and a root of acellular bone similar to aspidin (fig. 4.20E2). However, the earliest known forms (achanolepids) possess a peculiar type of dentine referred to by Turner (1991) as "primitive dentine." They are hollowed by a variously developed pulp cavity (pc, fig. 4.20E2), except in the earliest forms (Turner 1991). The canals of the lateral sensory-line system (slc, fig. 4.20D) open to the exterior by small pores piercing the scale crowns (slp, fig. 4.20F).

Thelodonts are quite similar in aspect, but this is probably due to their shared primitive state. Despite the fact that their internal anatomy is unknown, I predict that it may be very similar to that of primitive galeaspids, but with a terminal median inhalent opening. In fact, primitive galeaspids (e.g., *Hanyangaspis,* fig. 4.18A) are quite similar to a thelodont with a consolidated head shield. Minute scales recalling those of the thelodonts are found here and there in most monophyletic jawless craniate groups: on the subbranchial membrane of primitive osteostracans, on the ventral side of the head of primitive anaspids, on the body of galeaspids, and in primitive heterostracans. This is an indication that all these groups may have been derived from thelodont-like forms.

CONCLUSIONS

The diversity of cranial morphology among extant and fossil jawless craniates is so great that it is extremely difficult to make sense out of these often strongly divergent patterns. The profound difference between the skull of a lamprey and that of an osteostracan, for instance, makes their morphology almost irreconcilable; besides the sensory capsules or the dorsal naso-hypophysial opening, there is not a single endoskeletal element which could be homologized between the two groups with fairly good reliability. In contrast, the massive endoskeletal shield (?neurocranium) of osteostracans rather resembles the relatively broad neurocranium of some gnathostomes, such as placoderms.

The distribution of some probably homologous cranial features of these primitive craniates given here (fig. 4.21) is the only basis on which one can try to identify evolutionary trends. Instead of trying once more to build up a scenario of the early craniate evolution, I prefer, as a conclusion, to stress some still unanswered questions of skull morphology in Recent and fossil jawless craniates.

Agnathan-Gnathostome Homologies and the Origin of Jaws

The question of skull homologies between jawless and jawed craniates (gnathostomes) bears the same kind of uncertainties as that of the hagfish-lamprey homologies discussed above. There have been many attempts at defining homologies between hagfish or lampreys and gnathostomes (e.g., Holmgren 1946; Johnels 1948; review in Hardisty 1981), but none of them is convincing in detail, besides obvious homologizations of the otic capsules, parachordals, and trabecles. This task is even more frustrating when fossil forms are taken into consideration. In fact, the head of most fossil jawless craniates displays a large number of generalized primitive craniate or vertebrate internal features (elongated brain, labyrinth with two vertical semicircular canals, subcephalic gill pouches, etc.) and some particular derived features, but very few shared features which can be used for constructing a structural hierarchy. The distribution of some of these features (fig. 4.21) shows a possible hierarchic pattern. For example, the broad and perichondrally ossified head skeleton of galeaspids and osteostracans is more suggestive of the gnathostome braincase than of that of lampreys and hagfishes. The same applies to the distribution of the jugular vein, morphology of brain cavity, and sclerotic ossification (fig. 4.21). These and other noncranial characteristics tend to support the idea that agnathans are a paraphyletic taxon, and that the gnathostomes are more closely related to one particular agnathan group (osteostracans). This point of view is totally different from the long-prevailing theory, that agnathans and gnathostomes were two monophyletic groups with separate evolutionary histories.

The theory that gnathostomes descended from an unknown agnathan implies that there is some structural continuity between their respective skull structures. Is there anything in the skull of Recent and fossil agna-

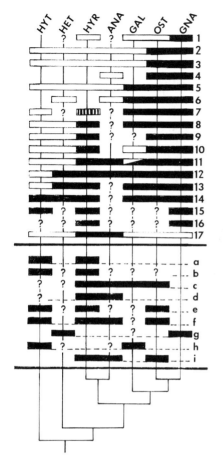

Fig. 4.21. Distribution of some major anatomical characteristics of the head among the monophyletic groups of craniates (thelodonts and pituriaspids omitted. For abbreviation of taxa, see caption to fig. 4.1). 1–17. Hierarchical distribution of cranial characteristics consistent with the relationships based on both cranial and noncranial characteristics, and indicated in the lower part of the diagram (plesiomorphous character state in white; apomorphous character state in black; apomorphous character state occurring only in larva vertically hatched). a–i. Distribution of characters which are inconsistent with the pattern of relationships in the lower part of the diagram (presumed homoplasies, reversions or symplesiomorphies regarded by other authors as synapomorphies).

List of synamorphies (apomorphous state cited first): 1. Gill arches medial to gills/lateral to gills. 2. Externally open endolymphatic duct/closed (an open endolymphatic duct is now claimed to be present in galeaspids). 3. Dermal sclerotic ring/no sclerotic ring. 4. Paired fins concentrated in a postbranchial or epibranchial position/very elongate in shape and broad-based. 5. Perichondral bone in endocranium/no perichondral bone. 6. Exoskeleton made up of cellular bone/acellular bone (aspidin) (still uncertain in galeaspids). 7. Large lateral head vein (dorsal jugular vein)/no large lateral head vein. 8. Cartilaginous or bony braincase/braincase made up of fibrous tissue. 9. Extrinsic eye musculature/no extrinsic eye musculature (presumed in heterostracans on the basis of the very small eye size). 10. Blind hypophysial tube or bucco-hypophysial duct/naso-pharyngeal duct opening into pharynx. 11. Pineal foramen and photosensory pineal organ/no photosensory pineal organ and pineal foramen. 12. Lateral sensory-line system present/absent. 13. At least two vertical semicircular canals/a single canal. 14. Otic capsule present/absent. 15. Parachordals present/absent. 16. True trabecles deriving from neural crest/no true trabecles. 17. Annular cartilage present/absent. a. Lingual apparatus. b. Horny teeth. c. External branchial arches. d. Trematic rings. e. Velum. f. Apparently unpaired olfactory organ (now known to be paired in galeaspids). g. Apparently paired olfactory organ. h. Naso-pharyngeal duct. i. Dorsal opening of naso-hypophysial complex.

thans which may have given rise to one of the major gnathostome apomorphies: the jaws? If, as admitted here, agnathan visceral arches are not homologous to that of gnathostomes, the latter being a neomorph in the medial part of the branchial septa, there is no hope of finding any precursor of jaws in agnathans. However, in lampreys, the velar skeleton, which develops from the mandibular somitomere, possesses a medial component, hence the suggestion that the velum may be a precursor of jaws. Consequently, one has to admit that jaws have never been branchial arches, but developed primarily as a biting device (possibly from a velumlike organ?), and that the internal hyoid and branchial arches were formed later along the same basic model as jaws, in order to supply the pharynx with a biting function. This theory, foreshadowed by Jollie (1971) and Maisey (1989), is, thus, radically different from the view that jaws are modified branchial arches, and that the pregnathostomes had only medial gill arches. However, it presents the advantage of explaining why, in Recent jawless craniates, in particular in lampreys, the mandibular segment is the only one which produces a medial visceral skeletal component (strengthening the velum), a condition which is a prerequisite to the formation of jaws.

History of Naso-Hypophysial Complex and Monophyly of the Cephalaspidomorphi

One of the most diversified areas of the skull of primitive craniates is the naso-hypophysial complex which arises during ontogeny from the nasal placode and Rathke's pouch (except in hagfishes). It comprises in the adult the olfactory organ and its surrounding capsule, the prenasal sinus, the hypophysial duct (or blind hypophysial tube) and the naso-pharyngeal duct. The condition in hagfishes (e.g., with a terminal prenasal sinus and naso-pharyngeal duct which communicates with the pharynx; nphd, fig. 4.3A) is for various reasons regarded as primitive for craniates (Janvier 1981). It was possibly also present in heterostracans, thelodonts, and galeaspids, yet in the latter the opening of the prenasal sinus has migrated onto the dorsal surface of the head. In these forms, the primary function of the prenasal sinus and nasopharyngeal duct was the intake of respiratory water.

In contrast, there is no longer any naso-pharyngeal duct in lampreys and osteostracans (the condition in anaspids is unknown), and the prenasal sinus is followed posteriorly by a blind hypophysial tube (hyt, figs. 4.5A, 15A). In these forms, the intake of respiratory water takes place directly through the mouth or the external branchial openings. Moreover, the entire nasohypophysial complex (olfactory organ + hypophysial tube) migrates dorsally during ontogeny. This condition has long been regarded as the autapomorphy of a group, the Cephalaspidomorphi, including the lampreys, osteostracans, and possible anaspids. However, more recently it has been stressed that osteostracans may be more closely related to gnathostomes than to lampreys (Janvier 1984; Maisey 1986) and, consequently, that this dorsal position of the naso-hypophysial complex is either a convergence (Schaeffer and Thomson 1980) or a plesiomorphous condition for the gnathostomes (that is, they descend from a form with a dorsal, or at least terminal, naso-hypophysial opening).

In all known gnathostomes, there is no naso-hypophysial complex, the nasal placode becoming separated from Rathke's pouch (primordium of the hypophysial tube), which remains in the roof of the mouth during early ontogeny. Whether or not this important event played a role in the rise of jaws is unknown.

Paired and well-separated nasal sacs occur with certainty in the gnathostomes and galeaspids, and probably also in the heterostracans and thelodonts. In hagfishes, there is an apparently single, median olfactory organ showing, however, a slight indication of parity. In lampreys, the olfactory organ, though arising from a single placode, displays a median septum and can be regarded as paired. This condition could match the olfactory cavity in osteostracans, yet the structure of the olfactory organ proper remains unknown. The condition in anaspids is unknown. The phylogeny of the craniates shown in figure 4.21 is based on many cranial and postcranial characteristics and implies that hagfishes are the sister group of all other craniates, that is, the Vertebrata. Being the out-group of the vertebrates, the condition of its olfactory organ may be regarded the plesiomorphous state. Two separate nasal sacs opening in a median naso-pharyngheal duct are thus a synapomorphy of the vertebrates, although a secondary fusion along-side these sacs occurs in lampreys and, perhaps, osteostracans. The loss of the median naso-pharyngeal duct and gain of two separate external nasal openings are a synapomorphy of the gnathostomes.

The Contribution of Fossil Jawless Craniates to the Understanding of the Skull

After an early period of enthusiasm, when fossils were thought to explain all of evolution, we are now passing through a time of disillusion, and fossils are regarded as having poor explanatory power as to the origin of major structural characteristics. In fact, the fossil jawless craniates tell us very little of the evolutionary story of this group (e.g., the origin of the labyrinth, paired fins, jaws), but, by their diversity, they display structures or associations of structures which could never have been predicted on the basis of only Recent forms. For example, the cartilaginous endoskeleton of chondrichthyans has long been regarded as primitive for the gnathostomes relative to that of hagfishes and lampreys, until perichondral bone was shown to be widely distributed among fossil jawless craniates (galeaspids, osteostracans). The same applies to other features such as the jugular vein or paired fins. Thus, it is clear that without the fossil jawless craniates our conception of Recent craniate phylogeny would possibly be the same as now, but our way of looking at and interpreting it would certainly be different. Moreover, the discovery of shield-headed agnathans, such as galeaspids or osteostracans, has shredded most attempts at finding homologies between the cartilaginous arches of the hagfish and lamprey skull and that of gnathostomes.

LIST OF ABBREVIATIONS

(Note: the same abbreviation can designate a canal or cavity and the soft structure it contains.)

abdc	abdominal cavity	corbn	corbiculum nasale (nasal basket)
abr	brachial artery	corpr	cornual process of velar apparatus
adm	adductor muscle		
adorb	adorbital opening	cpl	cornual plate
albc	anterior lingual basal cartilage	cpr	cornual process of head shield
anc	annular cartilage	dd	dorsal disc
ao	dorsal aorta	dend	endolymphatic duct
aoc	canal for the dorsal aorta and esophagus	df	dorsal field
aogr	aortic groove	dgc	dentigerous cartilage
apc	apical cartilage	dic	diencephalon
apf	area for attachment of paired fins	dt	dentine
		e	eyeball
apt	apical tooth	ebrd	external branchial duct
arc	arcualia	ebro	external branchial opening
asc	anterior semicircular canal	ebrv	extrabranchial vessel
basl	basal layer	fac	facial artery
bra	branchial arch	gp	gill pouch or branchial compartment
brbsk	branchial basket		
brc	braincase	h	heart
brcav	brain cavity	hepv	hepatic vein
brf	branchial fossae	hy	hyoid arch
brfl	branchial flap	hyd	hypophysial division of naso-hypophysial opening
brpl	branchial plate		
?bs	possible biting area	hypc	hypophysial cartilage
canc	cancellar layer	hyt	hypophysial tube
car	carotid artery	ibr	interbranchial ridge
ch	notochord	ibrd	internal branchial duct
cl	contour of lateral field	imc	intramural cavity for the heart
coc	copular cartilage		
com	trabecular commissure	lf	lateral field

lt	lateral lingual teeth	ped	pedicel
lvsk	lateral velar skeleton	perc	perpendicular muscle
m	mouth		cartilage
marga, v	marginal artery and vein	peric	pericardic cartilage
mcl	clavatus muscle	pf	pectoral fin
mdo	median dorsal opening	phbrd	pharyngobranchial duct
mes	mesencephalon	pi	pineal organ or pineal
met	metencephalon		foramen
mhyc	hyocopuloglossus muscle	pila	pila anterior
mlbc	middle lingual basal cartilage	pilp	pila posterior
mprotr	protractor dentis muscle	pipl	pineal plate
mretr	retractor dentis muscle	pistc	piston cartilage
msdt	mesodentine	pkc	pokal cell cone
mvlb	median ventral longitudinal	placor	planum cornuale
	bar of mucocartilage	plbc	posterior lingual basal
mvpr	medial ventral process for at-		cartilage
	tachment of branchial arch	plc	posterior lateral cartilage
	element	plvisc	planum viscerale
mvpl	median ventral plate	plxbr	brachial plexus
mvsk	medial velar skeleton	pop	pupilar opening
myc	myelencephalon	popl	postoral plates
myd, v	dorsal and ventral	prns	prenasal sinus
	myodomes	psc	posterior semicircular canal
nad	nasal division of naso-hypo-	psp	postbranchial spine
	physial opening	rpl	rostral plate
nahyp	naso-hypophysial opening	rpr	rostral process
neurc	neural canal	rt	replacement tooth
nphd	naso-pharyngeal duct	sapc	supra-apical cartilage
obrc	orobranchial cavity	sbrpl	sub-branchial platelets
oc	occipital region	sclr	sclerotic ring
oca	occipital cranial artery	sclos	scleral ossification
oes	esophagus	sel	canals linking lateral fields to
olf	olfactory organ or its cavity		labyrinth cavity
olfc	olfactory capsule	seld	canal linking dorsal field to
opl	oral plates		labyrinth cavity
orb	orbit	sin	cavity for venous sinus
orbpl	orbital plate	slc	sensory-line canals
ort	oral tube	slp	sensory-line pore
otc	otic capsule	snc	subnasal cartilage
palc	palatine cartilage	sof	supra-oral field
palcom	palatine commissure	spic	spiniform cartilage
parc	parachordals	sppl	spinal plate
pbcb	parabuccal cell band	spoc	spino-occipital nerves
pbr	prebranchial ridge	st	tooth on oral sucker
pbrf	prebranchial fossa	styc	styliform cartilage
pc	pulp cavity	suboc	subocular arch
pchb	perichondral bone	t	horny teeth

tcc	cartilaginous core of horny tooth	vart	ventral arterial trunk
tdl	taenia dorsalis	vbr	branchial vein
tea	anterior tectal cartilage	vcl	lateral head vein, or dorsal jugular
tec	tectal cartilages	vd	ventral disc
tel	telencephalon	vel	velum
tep	posterior tectal cartilage	velsk	velar skeleton
tl	taenia longitudinalis	y	y- or v-shaped impressions of unknown nature
tp	thela perimeningealis		
trab	trabecles	I, II, III, IV, V $_{1,2,3}$, VII, VIII, X$_{1-5}$ cranial nerves.	
trr	trematic rings		
ttc	tentacle cartilages		

REFERENCES

Arsenault, M., and P. Janvier. 1991. The anaspid-like craniates of the Escuminac Formation (Upper Devonian) from Miguasha (Québec, Canada), with remarks on anaspid-petromyzontid relationships. In *Early Vertebrates and Related Problems of Evolutionary Biology*, M. M. Chang, Y. H. Liu, and G. R. Zhang, eds. Beijing: Science Press, pp. 19–40.

Balabai, P. 1935. Zur morphologischen Charakteristik des präbranchialen Teiles des viscerales Apparates bei den Petromizonten. Bulletin de l'Académie des sciences d'Ukraine, Travaux de l'Institut de zoologie 3: 131–168.

———. 1937. Zur Frage über die Homologie der visceralen Bogen der Cyclostomen und Gnathostomen. Travaux sur la morphologie des animaux, Kiev 4: 45–78.

Bardack, D. 1991. First fossil hagfish (Myxinoidea): A record from the Pennsylvanian of Illinois. Science: 701–703.

Bardack, D., and E. S. Richardson. 1977. New agnathous fishes from the Pennsylvanian of Illinois. Fieldiana: Geology 33 (26): 489–510.

Bardack, D., and R. Zangerl. 1971. Lampreys in the fossil record. In *The Biology of Lampreys*, M. W. Hardisty and I. C. Potter, eds., vol. 1. London: Academic Press, pp. 67–84.

Belles-Isles, M. 1986. Nouvelle interprétation de l'orifice médio-dorsal des Galéaspidomorphes ("Agnatha," Dévonien, Chine). Neues Jahrbuch für Geologie und Paläontologie Monatshefte H7: 385–394.

Bendix-Almgreen, S. E. 1986. Silurian ostracoderms from Washington Land (North Greenland), with comments on cyathaspid structure, systematics, and phyletic position. Rapport fra Grønlands geologiske Undersøgelser 132: 89–123.

Bjerring, H. 1984. Major anatomical steps toward craniotedness: A heterodox view based largely on embryological data. Journal of Vertebrate Paleontology 4: 17–29.

Cope, E. D. 1889. Synopsis of the families of Vertebrata. American Naturalist 23 (2): 1–29.

Damas, H. 1942. Le dévoloppement de la tête de la lamproie (*Lampetra fluviatilis* L.). Annales de la Société royale de Belgique 73: 201–211.

————. 1944. Recherches sur le développement de *Lampetra fluviatilis* L. Archives de biologie 55: 1–284.

————. 1958. Crâne des Agnathes. In *Traité de Zoologie*, P. P. Grassé, ed., vol. 13. Paris: Masson, 22–39.

Dawson, J. A. 1963. The oral cavity, the "jaws," and the horny teeth of *Myxine glutinosa*. In *Biology of Myxine*, A. Brodal and R. Fänge, eds. Oslo: Universitetsforlaget, pp. 235–255.

Dean, B. 1899. On the embryology of *Bdellostoma stouti:* A general account of myxinoid development from the egg and segmentation to hatching. In *Festschrift C. F. v. Kuppfer*. Jena: G. Fischer, pp. 221–276.

de Beer, G. R. 1937. *The Development of the Vertebrate Skull*. Oxford: Oxford University Press.

Denison, R. H. 1963. The early history of the vertebrate calcified skeleton. Clinical Orthopaedics 31: 141–152.

————. 1964. The Cyathaspididae, a family of Silurian and Devonian jawless vertebrates. Fieldiana: Geology 13 (5): 311–473.

————. 1967. Ordovician vertebrates from Western United States. Fieldiana: Geology 16 (6): 131–192.

Dineley, D., and E. J. Loeffler. 1976. Ostracoderm faunas of the Delorme and associated Siluro-Devonian formations, North-West Territories, Canada. Special Papers in Palaeontology 18: 1–214.

Dingerkus, G. 1979. Chordate cytogenetic studies: An analysis of their phylogenetic implications with particular reference to fishes and the living coelacanth. Occasional Papers of the California Academy of Sciences 134: 111–127.

Duméril, A. 1806. *Dissertation sur les Poissons Cyclostomes*. Paris, pp. 1–20.

Elliott, D. 1987. A reassessment of *Astraspis desiderata,* the oldest North American vertebrate. Science 237: 190–192.

Forey, P. L. 1984. Yet more reflections on agnathan-gnathostome relationships. Journal of Vertebrate Paleontology 4 (3): 330–343.

————. 1986. The Downtonian ostracoderm *Sclerodus* Agassiz (Osteostraci: Tremataspididae). Bulletin of the British Museum (Natural History), Geology series 41 (1): 1–30.

Forey, P., and B. Gardiner. 1981. J. A. Moy-Thomas and his association with the British Museum (Natural History). Bulletin of the British Museum (Natural History), Geology 35 (3): 131–144.

Gagnier, P. Y. 1989a. Analyses anatomiques et phylogénétiques de quelques Vertébrés paléozoïques américains. 1. Les Vertébrés ordoviciens de Bolivie. Thesis, University Paris VII.

————. 1989b. A new image of *Sacabambaspis janvieri,* an early Ordovician jawless vertebrate from Bolivia. National Geographic Research 5: 250–253.

Gagnier, P. Y., A. Blieck, and G. Rodrigo. 1986. First Ordovician vertebrate of South America. Géobios 19 (5): 629–634.

Goodrich, E. S. 1930. *Studies on the Structure and Development of Vertebrates*. London: MacMillan and Co.

Gorbman, A., and A. Tamarin. 1985. Early development of oral, olfactory, and adenohypophyseal structures of agnathans and its evolutionary implications. In *Evolutionary Biology of Primitive Fishes*, R. E. Foreman, A. Gorbman,

J. M. Dodd, and R. Olsson, eds., NATO ASI series, A, Life Sciences 103: 165–185.

Gross, W. 1958. Anaspiden-Schuppen aus dem Ludlow des Ostseegebiets. Paläontologische Zeitschrift 32: 24–37.

———. 1968. Porenschuppen und Sinneslinien des Thelodontiers *Phlebolepsis elegans* Pander. Paläontologische Zeitschrift 42: 131–146.

Halstead, L. B. 1973. The heterostracan fishes. Biological Review 48: 279–332.

———. 1982. Evolutionary trends and the phylogeny of the Agnatha. In *Problems of Phylogenetic Reconstruction*, K. A. Joysey and A. Friday, eds., Systematic Association Special Papers, vol. 21. London: Academic Press, pp. 159–196.

———. 1987. Evolutionary aspects of neural crest–derived skeletogenic cells in the earliest vertebrates. In *Developmental and Evolutionary Aspects of the Neural Crest*, P. Maderson, ed. New York: J. Wiley and Sons, pp. 339–358.

Hardisty, M. W. 1981. The skeleton. In *The Biology of Lampreys*, M. W. Hardisty and I. C. Potter, eds., vol. 3. New York: Academic Press, pp. 333–376.

———. 1982. Lampreys and hagfishes: Analysis of cyclostome relationships. In *The Biology of Lampreys*, M. W. Hardisty and I. C. Potter, eds., vol. 4B. London: Academic Press, pp. 165–260.

Hardisty, M. W., and C. M. Rovainen. 1982. Morphological and functional aspects of the muscular system. In *The Biology of Lampreys*, M. W. Hardisty and I. C. Potter, eds., vol. 4A. New York: Academic Press, pp. 137–228.

Heintz, A. 1939. Cephalaspids from the Downtonian of Norway. Norske Videnskapsakademiens Skrifter (Matematiske-naturvetenskapslige Klasse) 5: 1–119.

Heintz, N. 1968. The pteraspid *Lyktaspis* n.g. from the Devonian of Vestspitsbergen. In *Current Problems of Lower Vertebrate Phylogeny*, T. Ørvig, ed. Stockholm: Almquist and Wiksell, pp. 73–80.

Holmgren, N. 1943. Agnather och Gnathostomer. Kungliga svenska Vetenskapsakademiens arsbok 41: 337–351.

———. 1946. On two embryos of *Myxine glutinosa*. Acta zoologica 27: 1–90.

Holmgren, N., and E. Stensiö. 1936. Kranium und Visceralskelett der Akranier, Cyclostomen und Fische. In *Handbuch der Vergleichenden Anatomie und Morphologie der Wirbeltiere*, L. Bolk, E. Göppert, E. Kallius, and W. Lubosch, eds., vol. 4. Berlin: Urban and Schwarzenberg, pp. 233–500.

Hubbs, C. L., and I. C. Potter. 1971. Distribution, phylogeny, and taxonomy. In *The Biology of Lampreys*, M. W. Hardisty and I. C. Potter, eds., vol. 1. London: Academic Press, pp. 1–66.

Janvier, P. 1974. The structure of the naso-hypophysial complex and the mouth in fossil and extant cyclostomes, with remarks on amphiaspiforms. Zoologica scripta 3: 193–200.

———. 1975a. Anatomie et position systématique des Galéaspides (Vertebrata, Cyclostomata), Céphalaspidomorphes du Dévonien inférieur du Yunnan (Chine). Bulletin du Muséum national d'histoire naturelle, Paris 278: 1–16.

———. 1975b. Les yeux des cyclostomes fossiles et le problème de l'origine des Myxinoïdes. Acta zoologica 56: 1–9.

———. 1978. Les nageoires paires des Ostéostracés et la position systématique des Céphalaspidomorphes. Annales de paléontologie (Vertébrés) 64 (2): 113–142.

———. 1981. The phylogeny of the Craniata, with particular reference to the significance of fossil "agnathans." Journal of Vertebrate Paleontology 1 (2): 121–159.

———. 1984. The relationships of the Osteostraci and Galeaspida. Journal of Vertebrate Paleontology 4 (3): 344–358.

———. 1985. *Les Céphalaspides du Spitsberg.* Cahiers de paléontologie (Vertébrés). Paris: Éditions du CNRS.

———. 1990. La structure de l'exosquelette des Galéaspides (Vertebrata). Comptes rendus de l'Académie des sciences, Paris 310: 655–659.

Janvier, P., and A. Blieck. 1979. New data on the internal anatomy of the Heterostraci (Agnatha), with general remarks on the phylogeny of the craniata. Zoologica scripta 8: 287–296.

Janvier, P., and R. Lund. 1983. *Hardistiella montanensis* n.gen. et sp. (Petromyzontida) from the Lower Carboniferous of Montana, with remarks on the affinities of the lampreys. Journal of Vertebrate Paleontology 2 (4): 407–413.

Janvier, P., the late Lord R. Percy, and I. C. Potter. 1991. The arrangement of the heart chambers and associated blood vessels in the Devonian osteostracan *Norselaspis glacialis:* A reinterpretation based on recent studies of the circulatory system in lampreys. Journal of Zoology, London 223: 567–576.

Jarvik, E. 1968. Aspects of vertebrate phylogeny. In *Current Problems of Lower Vertebrate Phylogeny,* T. Ørvig, ed., Nobel Symposium 4. Stockholm: Almqvist and Wiksell, pp. 497–527.

———. 1980. *Basic Structure and Evolution of Vertebrates.* 2 vols. London: Academic Press.

Jefferies, R. P. S., and D. N. Lewis. 1978. The English Silurian fossil *Placocystites forbesianus* and the ancestry of the vertebrates. Philosophical Transactions of the Royal Society of London B 382: 205–323.

Johnels, A. 1948. On the development and morphology of the skeleton of the head of *Petromyzon.* Acta zoologica 29: 139–179.

———. 1950. On the dermal connective tissue of the head of *Petromyzon.* Acta zoologica 31: 177–185.

Jollie, M. 1968. Some implications of the acceptance of a delamination principle. In *Current Problems of Lower Vertebrate Phylogeny,* T. Ørvig, ed. Stockholm: Almqvist and Wiksell, pp. 89–107.

———. 1971. A theory concerning the early evolution of the visceral arches. Acta zoologica 52: 85–96.

———. 1984. The vertebrate head: Segmented or a single morphogenetic structure? Journal of Vertebrate Paleontology 4 (3): 320–329.

Karatayute-Talimaa, V. N. 1978. Silurian and Devonian thelodonts of U.R.S.S. and Spitsbergen. Vilnius: Mokslas. (In Russian)

Kiaer, J. 1924. The Downtonian fauna of Norway. 1. Anaspida. Norske Videnskapsakademiens Skrifter (Matematiske-naturvetenskapslige Klasse) 6: 1–139.

Koltzoff, N. K. 1901. Entwicklungsgeschichte des Kopfes von *Petromyzon planeri.* Bulletin de la Société des naturalistes, Moscow 15: 259–589.

Krejsa, R. J., P. Bringas, M. Nakamura, C. Bessem, M. L. Snead, and H. C. Slavkin.

1989. Epithelial cytodifferentiation during hagfish (*Eptatretus stoutii* and *Myxine glutinosa* L.) embryonic and early postnatal tooth morphogenesis. Journal of Dental Research, special issue 67: 392.

Kupffer, C. W. von. 1894–1900. *Studien zur vergleichenden Entwicklungsgeschichte des Kopfes der Kranioten.* Munich: Lehmann.

Langille, R. M., and B. K. Hall. 1986. Evidence of cranial neural crest contribution to the skeleton of the sea lamprey, *Petromyzon marinus.* Progress in Developmental Biology B: 263–266.

————. 1988. Role of the neural crest in the development of the trabeculae and branchial skeleton in embryonic sea lamprey, *Petromyzon marinus* (L.). Development 102: 301–310.

Liu, Y. H. 1975. [Lower Devonian agnathans from Yunnan and Sichuan]. Vertebrata palasiatica 13 (4): 202–216. (In Chinese with English summary)

Løvtrup, S. 1977. The phylogeny of the Vertebrata. London: Wiley and Sons.

Lund, R., and P. Janvier. 1986. A second lamprey from the Lower Carboniferous (Namurian) of Bear Gulch, Montana (U.S.A.). Géobios 19 (5): 647–652.

Maisey, J. G. 1986. Heads and tails: A chordate phylogeny. Cladistics 2 (3): 201–256.

————. 1988. Phylogeny of early vertebrate skeletal induction and ossification patterns. Evolutionary Biology 22: 1–36.

————. 1989. Visceral skeleton and musculature of a Late Devonian shark. Journal of Vertebrate Paleontology 9 (2): 174–190.

Mallatt, J. 1984. Early vertebrate evolution: Pharyngeal structure and the origin of gnathostomes. Journal of the Zoological Society, London 204: 169–183.

Marinelli, W., and A. Strenger. 1954. *Vergleichende Anatomie und Morphologie der Wirbeltiere.* 1. *Lampetra fluviatilis* (L.). Vienna: Franz Deuticke, pp. 1–80.

————. 1956. *Vergleichende Anatomie und Morphologie der Wirbeltiere,* vol. 2, *Myxine glutinosa* L. Vienna: Franz Deuticke, pp. 82–272.

Märss, T. 1979. [Lateral-line sensory system of the Ludlovian thelodont *Phlebolepis elegans* Pander]. Eesti NSV Teaduste Akadeemia Toimetised, Geoloogia 28: 108–111. (In Russian with English and Estonian summaries)

Neumayer, L. 1938. Die Entwicklung des Kopfskelettes von *Bdellostoma stoutii.* Archivio italiano de anatomia e embriologia, suppl. 40: 1–122.

Newth, D. R. 1956. On the neural crest of lamprey embryos. Journal of Embryology and Experimental Morphology 4: 358–375.

Novitskaya, L. 1971. Les Amphiaspides (Heterostraci) du Dévonien de la Sibérie. Cahiers de paléontologie, Éditions du CNRS, Paris 130: 1–325.

————. 1983. [*Evolutionary Morphology of Agnathans*]. Moscow: Trudy paleontologicheskogo instituta, Nauka. (In Russian)

Obruchev, D. V., and E. Mark-Kurik. 1965. [*The psammosteids (Agnatha, Psammosteidae) from the Devonian of U.S.R.R.*]. Tallinn: Izd-Vo, Akademia Nauka. (In Russian)

Orvig, T. 1965. Paleohistological notes. 2. Certain comments on the phyletic significance of acellular bone tissue in early lower vertebrates. Arkiv för Zoologi (2) 16 (29): 551–556.

————. 1989. Histologic studies of ostracoderms, placoderms, and fossil elasmobranchs. 6. Hard tissues of Ordovician vertebrates. Zoologica scripta 18 (3): 427–446.

Pan Jiang (P'an Kiang). 1984. The phylogenetic position of the Eugaleaspida in China. Proceedings of the Linnean Society of New South Wales 107 (3): 309–319.

P'an, K., and S. T. Wang. 1978. [Devonian agnatha and Pisces of South China]. Symposium on the Devonian system of South China. Peking: Geological Press, pp. 240–269. (In Chinese)

P'an, K., S. T. Wang, and Y. P. Liu. 1975. [The Lower Devonian Agnatha and Pisces from South China]. Professional Papers of Stratigraphy and Paleontology, vol. 1. Peking: Geological Press, pp. 153–169. (In Chinese)

Patterson, C. 1982. Morphological characters and homology. In *Problems of Phylogenetic Reconstruction*, K. A. Joysey and A. E. Friday, eds. London: Academic Press, pp. 21–74.

Ritchie, A. 1964. New lights on the morphology of the Norwegian Anaspida. Norske Videnskapsakademiens Skrifter (Matematiske-naturvidenskapslige Klasse): 1–22.

———. 1968. New evidence on *Jamoytius kerwoodi* White, an important ostracoderm from the Silurian of Lanarkshire, Scotland. Palaeontology 11: 21–39.

———. 1980. The Late Silurian anaspid genus *Rhyncholepis* from Oesel, Estonia, and Ringerike, Norway. American Museum Novitates 2699: 1–18.

———. 1984. Conflicting interpretations of the Silurian agnathan, *Jamoytius*. Scottish Journal of Geology 20 (2): 249–256.

Ritchie, A., and J. Gilbert-Tomlinson. 1977. First Ordovician vertebrate from the Southern Hemisphere. Alcheringa 1: 351–368.

Romer, A. S. 1944. *Vertebrate Paleontology*. 1st ed. Chicago: University of Chicago Press.

Säve-Söderbergh, G. 1941. Notes on the dermal bones of the head in *Osteolepis macrolepidotus* Ag., and the interpretation of the lateral-line system in certain primitive vertebrates. Zoologiska Bidrag Uppsala 20: 523–541.

Schaeffer, B., and K. S. Thomson. 1980. Reflections on the Agnathan-Gnathostome relationships. In *Aspects of Vertebrate History*, L. L. Jacobs, ed. Flagstaff: Museum of Northern Arizona Press, pp. 19–33.

Schneider, A. 1879. Anatomie und Entwicklungsgeschichte von *Petromyzon* und Ammocoetes. In *Beiträge zur vergleichende Entwicklungsgeschichte der Wirbeltiere*. Berlin: Reimer, pp. 85–92.

Sewertzoff, A. N. 1916–17. Études sur l'évolution des Vertébrés inférieurs. 1. Morphologie du squelette et de la musculature de la tête des Cyclostomes. 2. Organisation des ancêtres des Vertébrés actuels. Archives russes d'anatomie, d'histologie et d'embryologie, 1: 1–104 and 425–572.

Smith, M. M., and B. K. Hall. 1990. Development and evolutionary origins of vertebrate skeletogenic and odontogenic tissues. Biological Review 65: 277–373.

Stensiö, E. A. 1927. The Devonian and Downtonian vertebrates of Spitsbergen. 1. Family Cephalaspidae. Skifter om Svalbard og Ishavet 12: 1–391.

————. 1964. Les cyclostomes fossiles ou Ostracodermes. In *Traité de paléontologie,* J. Piveteau, ed. Paris: Masson, pp. 96–382.

Stockard, C. R. 1906. The development of the mouth and gills in *Bdellostoma stoutii.* American Journal of Anatomy 5: 482–517.

Tretjakoff, D. 1926. Das skelett und die Muskulatur im Kopfe des Flüssneunauges. Zeitschrift für Wissenschaftliche Zoologie 128: 267–304.

————. 1929. Die Schleimknorpeligen Bestandteile im Kopfskelett von Ammocoetes. Zeitschrift für Wissenschaftliche Zoologie 133: 470–516.

Turner, S. 1970. Fish help to trace continental movements. Spectrum 79: 8–10.

————. 1991. Monophyly and interrelationships of the Thelodonti. In *Early Vertebrates and Related Problems of Evolutionary Biology,* M. M. Chang, Y. H. Liu, and G. R. Zhang, eds. Beijing: Science Press, pp. 87–119.

Wang, N. Z. 1986. Notes on two genera of Middle Silurian Agnatha (*Hanyangaspis* and *Latirostraspis*) of China. In *Fourteenth Annual Convention of the Palaeontological Society of China.* Peking: Palaeontological Society of China, pp. 49–57. (In Chinese with English summary)

————. 1991. Two new Silurian galeaspids (jawless craniates) from Zhejiang Province, China, with a discussion of galeaspid-Gnathostome relationships. In *Early Vertebrates and Related Problems of Evolutionary Biology,* M. M. Chang, Y. H. Liu, and G. R. Zhang, eds. Beijing: Science Press, pp. 41–65.

Wängsjö, G. 1952. The Downtonian and Devonian vertebrates of Spitsbergen. 9. Morphologic and systematic studies of the Spitsbergen cephalaspids: Results of Th. Vogt's expedition 1928 and the English-Norwegian-Swedish expedition in 1939. Norsk Polarinstitutt Skrifter 97: 1–611.

White, E. I. 1935. The ostracoderm *Pteraspis* Kner, and the relationships of agnathous vertebrates. Philosophical Transactions of the Royal Society B 225: 381–457.

Wright, G. M., and J. H. Youson. 1982. Ultrastructure of mucocartilage in the larval anadromous sea lamprey, *Petromyzon marinus.* Journal of Anatomy 165: 39–51.

Yalden, D. W. 1985. Feeding mechanisms as evidence for cyclostome monophyly. Zoological Journal of the Linnean Society, London 84: 291–300.

Young, G. C. 1991. The first armoured agnathan vertebrates from the Devonian of Australia. In *Early Vertebrates and Related Problems of Evolutionary Biology,* M. M. Chang, Y. H. Liu, and G. R. Zhang, eds. Beijing: Science Press, pp. 67–85.

5

Patterns of Diversity in the Skulls of Jawed Fishes

HANS-PETER SCHULTZE

INTRODUCTION

SINCE THE DEVONIAN (355–410 million years ago [mya]) fishes with jaws have formed the majority of aquatic vertebrates. They appeared more than 430 mya in the Silurian, and reached their greatest diversity for major taxonomic groups in the Devonian. All basal bauplans were represented; representatives of some bauplans have become extinct since the Devonian. Today a minor part of that diversity, especially the most advanced actinopterygians, the teleosts, form more than 96% of all species of fishes, followed by 3.5% of cartilaginous elasmobranch fishes (calculated from data in Nelson 1984). The remaining few families are survivors of once flourishing groups (six holocephalan genera, eleven primitive actinopterygian genera, three lungfish genera, and one actinistian genus). Devonian groups such as placoderms and acanthodians are completely extinct. Therefore to present the diversity of jawed fishes, one has to include fossil forms, preferably from the Devonian, because they represent the basal structure of all major groups. Fortunately, Devonian jawed fishes were strongly ossified so that exo- and endocranial structures are very well preserved. They have been studied extensively (see Jarvik 1980). In addition, the last major group of vertebrates, the tetrapods, evolved from jawed fishes at the end of the Devonian.

Jawed fishes (jawed fishes + tetrapods = Gnathostomata) possess biting jaws that, together with the presence of trabeculae cranii, external gills, three semicircular canals in the labyrinths, and paired pectoral and pelvic fins supported by endoskeletal girdles, distinguish gnathostomes from agnathans (Schaeffer and Thomson 1980; Janvier 1981; Maisey 1986). The jaws are formed by the palatoquadrate dorsally and Meckel's cartilage ventrally. Teeth are located either in connective tissue above and lingual to the palatoquadrate and Meckel's cartilage, or on dermal bones that cover them. If the jaws are ossified, ossification occurs first at the articulation between the upper and lower jaws; thus, the articular ossifies at the pos-

189

terior end of Meckel's cartilage and the quadrate at the postero-ventral end of the palatoquadrate. In this primary jaw articulation the head of the quadrate reaches into the glenoid fossa of the articular.

The palatoquadrate ossifies primitively as one unit (Arratia and Schultze 1991); two or three ossification centers occur independently in different groups—e.g., ptyctodontid and some arthrodiran placoderms, acanthodid acanthodians, halecostome actinopterygians, actinistians, and tetrapods. The two or three centers of palatoquadrate ossification give rise to the autopalatine anteriorly, the metapterygoid dorsally, and the quadrate postero-ventrally, independently in the cited groups. The anterior end of Meckel's cartilage may ossify to form the anterior mentomeckelian in addition to the posterior articular. The palatoquadrate and Meckel's cartilages may be homologous with the first arch of agnathans, which supports the velum (Moy-Thomas and Miles 1971; Whiting 1972). There is no evidence of the existence of premandibular arches as suggested by Jarvik (1981). Primitively, there is a dorsal half of a gill slit between the mandibular and hyoid arches; the existence of a complete gill slit as proposed by Watson (1937), Zangerl and Williams (1975), and Zangerl and Case (1976) generally is not accepted (Maisey 1986). All branchial arches, including the hyoid arch, are composed of paired ventral (hypohyal, ceratohyal/hypobranchial, ceratobranchial) and dorsal (epihyal = hypobranchial, pharyngohyal/epibranchial, pharyngobranchial) elements; the unpaired basihyal and basibranchials unite each side of the branchial skeleton in the midline. Because the gills are located externally on the gill arches, the internal surfaces of the arches may bear teeth or dental plates as does the mandibular arch.

Paired trabeculae cranii appear early in ontogeny below the ethmo-sphenoidal region. Although the initial orientation of the trabeculae is antero-ventral, during development, they gradually become oriented parallel to the plane of the ventral otico-occipital region as the forebrain moves upward. In the labyrinth a third horizontal semicircular canal develops in addition to the two vertical canals present in agnathans. A utricular recess also is present in gnathostomes.

Jawed fishes comprise three monophyletic groups—the Placodermi, the Chondrichthyes, and the Teleostomi. The Chondrichthyes and the Teleostomi are extant, but the Placodermi are more or less limited to the Devonian. The relationship of placoderms to chondrichthyans and teleostomes is unresolved (Schaeffer 1975; Miles and Young 1977; Denison 1978; Forey 1980; Goujet 1982; Gardiner 1984a; Young 1986). The dermal bone covers in placoderms and teleostomes developed independently from a micromeric stage (Gross 1962; Young 1986); hence, there is no commonality among gnathostomes in the arrangement of bony plates. In the cases of both placoderms and teleostomes, the bone arrangements developed from tessellate forms (Stensioellida and Pseudopetalichthyida in placoderms, and Acanthodii in teleostomes). Chondrichthyans, having never passed beyond a micromeric stage, lack bony plates; however, perichondral bone does occur in chondrichthyans (Peignoux-Deville et al. 1982). Because bone can form in all three groups, its presence is not a feature uniting placoderms and osteichthyans.

The endocranium of adult chondrichthyans represents a single unit (fig. 5.1C), whereas that of placoderms is bipartite, having a very small anterior portion, and a larger posterior portion. The teleostome endocranium is divided by fissures. In all gnathostomes, the anterior floor of the endocranium is formed by the prechordal trabeculae cranii. The so-called trabeculae of agnathans lie lateral to the anterior notochord (Jollie 1962). The endocranium is open antero-dorsally (precerebral fontanelle) in chondrichthyans.

There is no evidence that a common exocranial bauplan exists for all gnathostomes (Gross 1962 contra Stensiö 1945). Osteological nomenclature was developed in tetrapods, especially in humans, and subsequently applied to fishes. The tetrapod skull-roof pattern, consisting of paired, medial postparietals, parietals, and frontals, is found only in panderichthyid fishes (Schultze and Arsenault 1985) among osteichthyans. Although primitive crossopterygians possess paired postparietals and parietals, the mosaic pattern of the snout region has not been replaced by paired frontals. The postparietals cover the otic region of tetrapods (Westoll 1938, 1943; Shishkin 1973) and crossopytergians (fig. 5.1E). The postparietals cover only the posterior part of the otic region of actinopterygians; the anterior part of the otic region is covered by the posterior parts of the parietals (fig. 5.1B). Because of the postparietal and parietal of actinopterygians may not be homologous with the two bones of the same name in crossopterygians, the pattern in this group might be called "tetrapod-like" rather than "tetrapod," as in crossopterygians. In actinopterygians, the parietal covers the anterior part of the otic region and the orbitotemporal region including the pineal organ. However, in tetrapods and crossopterygians, the parietal covers only the orbitotemporal region; thus, the external opening of the pineal organ lies between the parietals in all osteichthyans. In primitive crossopterygians in which the parietal does not incorporate the anterior bone mosaic, the pineal opening is located farther anteriorly (fig. 5.1E). In dipnoans (fig. 5.1D), the otic region is covered primarily by three elements—the unpaired B-bone and the paired I- and J-bones. In addition, the posterior part of the C-bones (i.e., A-, B-, C-pattern as introduced by Forster-Cooper 1937) contributes to the otic roof.

A direct comparison of the dipnoan skull-roof pattern with the tetrapod pattern is not possible. Because acanthodians lack a stabilized skull-roof pattern, it is possible that the three skull-roof patterns in osteichthyans

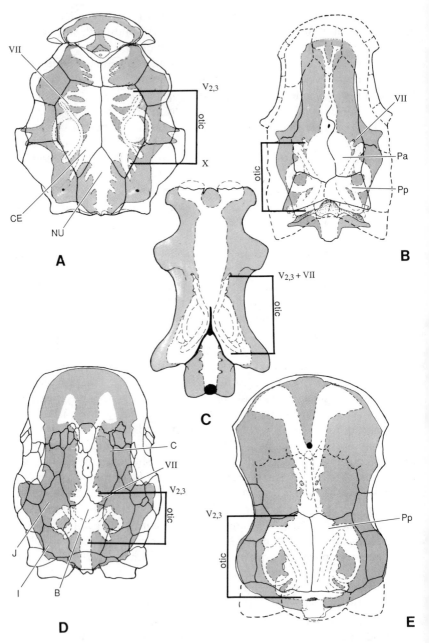

Fig. 5.1. Relationship among dermal skull roof, endocranium (shaded), and brain cavity (clear) in gnathostomes. A. Arthrodiran placoderm *Dicksonosteus arcticus* Goujet (combination of Goujet 1984b, fig. 31, with figs. 4 and 26). B. Palaeonisciform

originated independently from a micromeric, mosaic pattern. The skull-roof pattern of placoderms (fig. 5.1A) is completely different from that of osteichthyans (Jarvik 1980; Young 1986). It may have arisen independently from a micromeric stage as in Stensioellida or Pseudopetalichthyida in which only a few bones of the placoderm pattern are present (Denison 1983). The main paired bones (centrals) of placoderms lie above the otic region (fig. 5.1A), as do the postparietals in crossopterygians (fig. 5.1E) and the parietals and postparietals in actinopterygians (fig. 5.1B). One median bone (nuchal) lies posteriorly adjacent to the centrals, and the paired paranuchals lie lateral to the nuchal in placoderms. In addition, the surrounding bones have a completely different pattern from that of osteichthyans.

The dermal cover of the visceral skeleton is as variable as the skull roof. Crossopterygians (fig. 5.2E) possess the tetrapod pattern; thus, the upper jaw and palate are composed of the premaxillae, maxillae, dermopalatines, ecto- and endopterygoids, and vomers and a median parasphenoid. The lower jaw consists of the dentary, four infradentaries (i.e., splenial, postsplenial, angular, and surangular carrying the mandibular canal), coronoids, prearticular, and Meckel's cartilage. The composition of the dermal cover of the palatoquadrate and Meckel's cartilage in actinopterygians (fig. 5.2C) is consistent with that in crossopterygians and tetrapods, except that the dentary (dentalosplenial) includes the splenial and postsplenial with the anterior portion of the mandibular canal in actinopterygians. Dipnoans (fig. 5.2D) differ greatly from other osteichthyans. They lack a premaxilla and maxilla, and the homologies of the palatal bones are uncertain (Campbell and Barwick 1984a). Except for the prearticular medial to Meckel's cartilage, the dermal cover of the lower jaw is unique. Jarvik (1967) designated the dermal bones of the lower jaw by letters in the same way Forster-Cooper (1937) labeled elements of the skull roof. Some acanthodians are unique in possessing dentigerous bones on the palatoquadrate and Meckel's cartilage, in addition to a bone (mandibular bone of Denison 1978) below Meckel's cartilage. These bones are dissimilar in shape, arrangement, and position to the dermal elements of osteichthyans. Similarly, the dermal bones on the palatoquadrate and Meckel's cartilage in placoderms are different from those of osteichthyans. Primitively, placoderms possess small denticles (Stensioellida) or denticulate plates (Pseu-

---

actinopterygian *Kansasiella eatoni* Poplin (combination of Poplin 1974, fig. 4, with figs. 12 and 22). C. Xenacanth elasmobranch *Xenacanthus* sp. (after Schaeffer 1981, fig. 14b). D. Dipnoan *Chirodipterus australis* Miles (combination of Miles 1977, fig. 116, with figs. 34 and 47). E. Porolepiform crossopterygian *Youngolepis praecursor* Zhang and Yu (combination of Chang 1982, figs. 5C, E, 6A, with figs. 9 and 17).

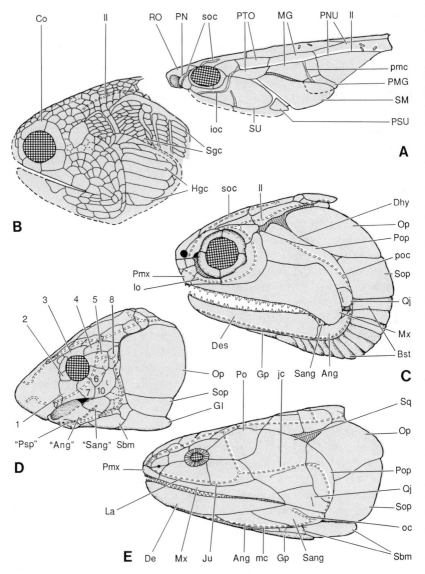

Fig. 5.2. Dermal skull of gnathostomes in lateral view. A. Arthrodiran placoderm *Dicksonosteus arcticus* Goujet (after Goujet 1975, fig. 6B). B. Acanthodian *Brachyacanthus scutiger* Egerton (after Watson 1937, fig. 5). C. Palaeonisciform actinopterygian *Moythomasia durgaringa* Gardiner and Bartram (after Gardiner 1984b, fig. 103). D. Dipnoan *Chirodipterus australis* Miles (after Miles 1977, fig. 117). E. Osteolepiform crossopterygian *Eusthenopteron foordi* Whiteaves (after Moy-Thomas and Miles 1971, fig. 6.6).

dopetalichthyida, Rhenanida). In more advanced placoderms, a single pair of supra- (two pairs in arthrodires) and infragnathals occur; the biting edge of these bones is serrated.

In order to characterize the three major gnathostome groups and the groups within them, it would be ideal to know the anatomy of the most primitive member of the group (i.e., the plesiomorphic or basal taxon; Schultze 1987) so that one could recognize convergent structures (i.e., homoplasies). As an approximation of this ideal, I designated a basal taxon for each group from fossil Devonian taxa. The diversity within each group then can be expressed by describing deviations from the pattern of the basal taxon.

Herein, cranial descriptions are divided into descriptions of the exocranium, endocranium, and visceral skeleton. The exocranium or dermatocranium consists of the dermal bones that cover the endocranium dorsally to form the skull roof and laterally to form the cheek region; ventrally, the exocranium is composed of the vomer and parasphenoid. The endo- or chondrocranium encloses the brain. The visceral skeleton or splanchnocranium lies ventral to the exo- and endocrania and is composed of endoskeletal arches (i.e., endoskeletal splanchnocranium). These endoskeletal arches are covered by dermal plates, mainly on the mandibular arch (i.e., exoskeletal splanchnocranium). Where known, the development of skull features are described in general for each group. Demonstration of monophyly and relationship to other groups are given for each major group and features of the skull are emphasized. Not presented here are functional aspects because these are mostly unknown for the basal forms of all major groups and can only be deduced from extant forms.

PLACODERMI

Monophyly and Relationship to Other Groups

The Placodermi (table 5.1; comprehensive presentation of the group in Denison 1978; for monophyly see Goujet 1982, 1984a; Young 1986) are diagnosed by possession of the following characters: (1) a unique pattern of bony plates on the head and shoulder girdle; (2) a double cervical articu-

TABLE 5.1   Classification of Placodermi (after Denison 1978)

Order Stensioellida	Order Petalichthyida
Order Pseudopetalichthyida	Dolichothoraci:
Order Ptyctodontida	Order Phyllolepida
Order Acanthothoraci	Order Antiarcha
Order Rhenanida	Order Arthodira
(Position of Ptyctodontida and Antiarcha in question)	

lation between the endoskeletal occipital region of the endocranium and the synarcual, and between the exoskeletal plates of the skull (paranuchal) and shoulder girdle (anterior dorso-lateral); (3) semidentine in bone tubercles and teeth; (4) omega-shaped palatoquadrate closely associated with cheek plates and with internal (lingual) attachment of adductor muscles; and (5) close association between dorsal hyoid arch (epihyal after Goujet 1984b or opercular cartilage after Young 1986) and opercle (submarginal).

Placoderms have one of three possible relationships with chondrichthyans and osteichthyans. They may be the sister group of (1) all other gnathostomes (Schaeffer 1975, 1981; Denison 1978), (2) chondrichthyans (Stensiö 1959, 1963b; Moy-Thomas and Miles 1971; Jarvik 1980; Goujet 1982), or (3) osteichthyans (Forey 1980; Gardiner 1984a). Aside from general features that also occur in some agnathans, there are no synapomorphies of cranial structure shared by placoderms and osteichthyans (Young 1986). Some features in the skull (eyestalk, "loss" of occipital and ventral fissures in neurocranium, extensive subocular shelves), together with the presence of pelvic claspers, seem to support a sister group relationship of placoderms with some chondrichthyans. The "loss" of neurocranial fissures assumes that formation of the neurocranium as a single unit is not a plesiomorphic feature of gnathostomes, whereas the proper statement, "absence" of neurocranial fissures, signifies the primitive feature of gnathostomes. Eyestalk (Goujet 1984b) and pelvic claspers (Goujet 1984a) are morphologically different in representatives of placoderms and chondrichthyans, and therefore do not pass the first condition of homology, the similarity test. Among the features that distinguish placoderms from all other gnathostomes are the following: (1) unique bone (i.e., skull-roof) pattern, (2) articulation between skull and trunk armor, (3) omega-shaped palatoquadrate fused to the cheek bones, (4) fusion of the epihyal (or opercular cartilage) to the submarginal, and (5) rigid dermal shoulder girdle. Four of the many synapomorphies that unite gnathostomes exclusive of placoderms (Young 1986) are cited here: (1) fusion of ethmoid region to endocranium, (2) postorbital connection between palatoquadrate and endocranium, (3) presence of a dental lamina and true dentine (ortho- and osteodentine), and (4) position of internal rectus and superior oblique eye muscles. The arrangement dictates parallel development of an eyestalk, and subocular shelves and claspers in those placoderms and chondrichthyans that possess these structures as indicated by their morphological differences.

Exocranium

The basic bauplan of placoderms (fig. 5.1A) was derived from a primitive micromeric stage by Gross (1962) and Denison (1975, 1978, 1983) or a macromeric stage by Goujet (1982, 1984a), Gardiner (1984a), and Forey

(1980). Yet none of these authors proposed a pattern in common for placoderms and osteichthyans contrary to Stensiö (1945) and Graham-Smith (1978). The placoderm skull roof (fig. 5.3A) is composed of a median nuchal, paired centrals, paired preorbitals, median postpineal, and pineal, and the rostral plate. A single postnuchal or a pair of postnuchals ("extrascapulars") covers the gap between the nuchal and the shoulder girdle. Lateral to the nuchal, the paranuchals form the dermal articulation with the shoulder girdle. The main lateral line extends from the body onto the skull roof in the region of the dermal shoulder girdle articulation and continues anteriorly over the marginal and postorbital. It continues as the infraorbital line postero-ventrally and beneath the orbit over the suborbital. The lateral lines, supraoccipital canal, central canal, and posterior "pit-line" converge toward the midpoint of the skull and meet either on the postpineal (Ptyctodontida and Acanthothoraci), the centrals (Arthrodira), or the nuchal (Petalichthyida, Phyllolepida, Antiarcha). Primitive placoderms lack a full set of skull-roof bones; only centrals and one or the other plate are recognizable (Stensioellida, Pseudopetalichthyida, Rhenanida) between tesserae or small bone plates.

In the Acanthothoraci, a diverse group of Early Devonian placoderms, the skull roof may be tesserate, or have a recognizable pattern; some members of this group have two pairs of centrals. In the Ptyctodontida, the nuchal is small or missing, a suborbital is missing, and the dermal cover of the snout is not ossified. Petalichthyids have an elongate nuchal separating the centrals that border the orbits. The pineal and rostral plate are fused. Phyllolepids are distinguished by possession of a large, wide nuchal, and loss of the rostral plate; all other skull-roof bones are marginal plates of the nuchal. The bone arrangement in arthrodires, which are the most common placoderms and which lack a postpineal plate, usually is accepted as the standard from which all other patterns are interpreted. Among placoderms, the pattern of antiarchs is the most divergent from that of arthrodires. Although the posterior exocranium is composed of nuchal, paranuchal, postmarginal, postpineal, and pineal and is comparable to that of other placoderms, the anterior and antero-lateral exocranium is different. It is composed of a median bone—the premedian plate—and a pair of lateral plates; centrals, preorbitals, postorbitals, and suborbitals are recognizable as separate bones. Owing to the substantial variation in arrangements of skull roofing bones among placoderms, the homologies of some of the elements are uncertain.

The cheek (fig. 5.2A) of placoderms is composed of the suborbital, postsuborbital, and the submarginal; the submarginal is the functional equivalent of the osteichthyan opercle. Primitively, the submarginal is free (e.g., Ptyctodontida and primitive Arthrodira), but in advanced arthrodires, it is enclosed in the cheek and sutured with surrounding bones. In

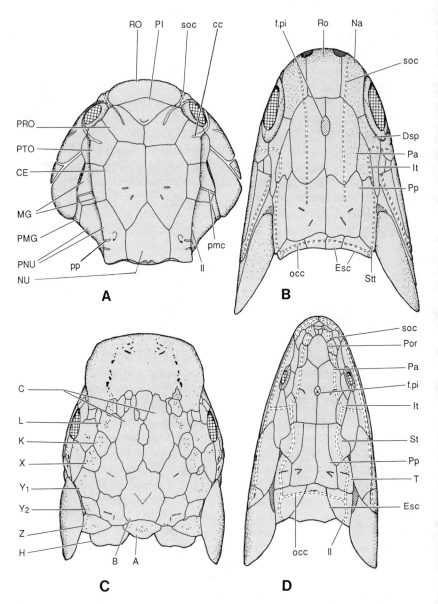

Fig. 5.3. Dermal skull roof of gnathostomes. A. Arthrodiran placoderm *Dicksonosteus arcticus* Goujet (after Goujet 1975, fig. 6A). B. Palaeonisciform actinopterygian *Moythomasia nitida* Gross (after Jessen 1968, fig. 1B). C. Dipnoan *Chirodipterus australis* Miles (after Miles 1977, fig. 116). D. Osteolepiform crossopterygian *Eusthenopteron foordi* Whiteaves (after Moy-Thomas and Miles 1971, fig. 6.6).

advanced arthrodires, the postorbital, marginal, postmarginal, and even the paranuchal form large portions of the cheek region.

In some placoderms, there is a broad bone surrounding the bucco-hypophysial opening on the ventral side of the endocranium. Owing to the shape of the bone and its lack of association with adjacent elements, its homology with the parasphenoid in osteichthyans cannot be determined (Jarvik 1980; Young 1986).

Endocranium

The endocranium is well known in many placoderms (Stensiö 1963a, 1969; Goujet 1984b). Although the orbitotemporal, otic, and occipital regions form a single unit in all placoderms, there is a separate anterior portion in some placoderms (rhinocapsular bone of Stensiö representing at least part of ethmoidal region; figs. 5.4A, 5.5A). Miles and Young (1977) described three ossifications—ethmoidal, orbital, and occipital—in the endocranium of ptyctodonts. The occipital ossification surrounds the foramen magnum ventrally and laterally, whereas the orbital ossification forms the posterior wall of the orbit; the position of the ethmoidal ossification is unknown.

Visceral Skeleton

Only the mandibular arch of placoderms is well known. In most taxa, the omega-shaped palatoquadrate is fused (fig. 5.6A) to the exoskeletal cheek plates (suborbital, postsuborbital). Thus, the adductor muscles attach on the medial side in contrast to all other gnathostomes, in which they attach on the lateral side (Schaeffer 1975). The lower jaw articulates medially on a condyle at the postero-ventral corner of the palatoquadrate. The palato-quadrate may ossify in one, two, or three units—the placoderm autopala-tine, quadrate, and metapterygoid, respectively. The connection of the palatoquadrate with the endocranium is variable. In ptyctodonts, the palatoquadrate is firmly attached to the endocranium; this seems to be correlated with the presence of crushing dentition in this group. In arthro-dires, the palatoquadrate bears orbital and palatobasal connections with the endocranium; in some taxa, both are double articulations. Meckel's cartilage may ossify in two parts—the anterior mentomeckelian bone and the posterior articular. The glenoid fossa usually is located on the lateral (i.e., external) surface of the articular, and receives the condyle of the palatoquadrate; in some taxa, however, the articular bone bears the con-dyle and palatoquadrate the glenoid fossa.

Primitively, Meckel's cartilage and the palatoquadrate bear denticles or small plates (Stensioellida, Pseudopetalichthyida, Rhenanida). Com-monly, one identifies placoderms with fishes (arthrodires and antiarchs) having jaw bones with cutting edges on the ventral margin of autopalatine (supragnathal) and on the dorsal margin of Meckel's cartilage (infragna-

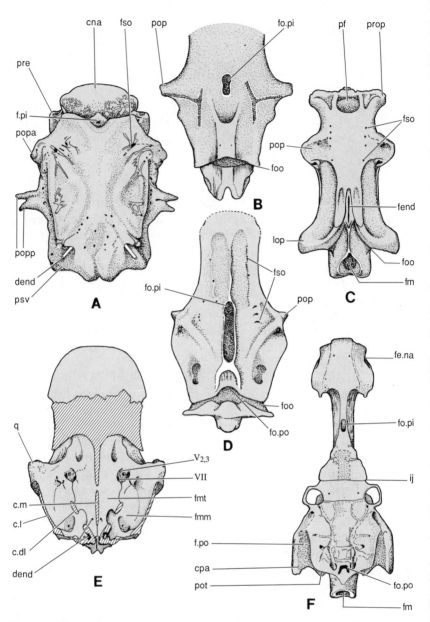

Fig. 5.4. Endocranium of gnathostomes in dorsal view. A. Arthrodiran placoderm *Dicksonosteus arcticus* Goujet (after Goujet 1984b, fig. 4). B. Acanthodian *Acanthodes bronni* Kner (combination of Jarvik 1977, fig. 12; and Miles 1973b, fig. 3). C. Xenacanth elasmobranch *Xenacanthus* sp. (after Schaeffer 1981, fig. 6). D. Palaeonisciform actinopterygian *Kansasiella eatoni* Poplin (after Poplin 1974, fig. 12). E. Dipnoan *Chirodipterus australis* Miles (after Miles 1977, fig. 34). F. Osteolepiform crossopterygian *Eusthenopteron foordi* Whiteaves (after Jarvik 1980, fig. 88A).

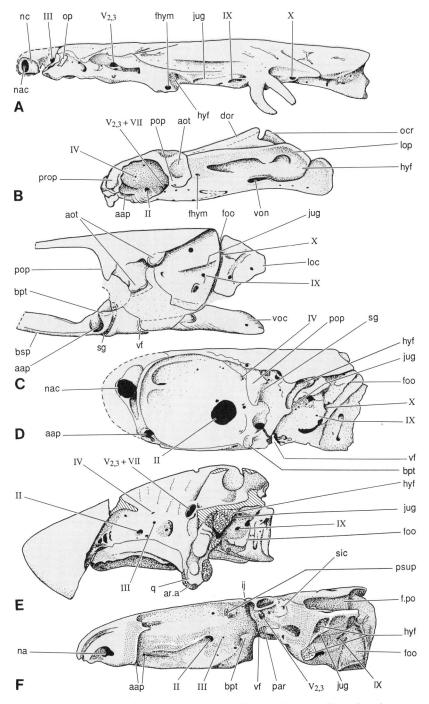

Fig. 5.5. Endocranium of gnathostomes in lateral view. A. Arthrodiran placoderm *Kujdanowiaspis* sp. (combination of Stensiö 1969, figs. 13A, 13B, and Goujet 1984b, fig. 13). B. Xenacanth elasmobranch *Xenacanthus* sp. (after Schaeffer 1981, fig. 6). C. Acanthodian *Acanthodes bronni* Kner (after Miles 1973, fig. 2). D. Palaeonisciform actinopterygian *Mimia toombis* Gardiner and Bartram (after Gardiner 1984b, fig. 13). E. Dipnoan *Chirodipterus australis* Miles (after 1977, fig. 35). F. Osteolepiform crossopterygian *Eusthenopteron foordi* Whiteaves (after Jarvik 1980, fig. 86A).

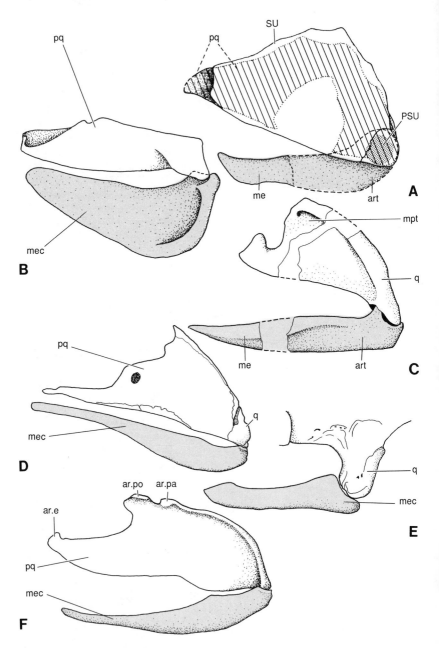

Fig. 5.6. Endoskeletal mandibular arch (upper and lower jaw) of gnathostomes in lateral view. A. Arthrodiran placoderm *Holonema westolli* Miles (combination of Miles 1971, figs. 33A, B, and 63). B. Hybodont elasmobranch *Hybodus basanus* Egerton (after Maisey 1982, fig. 7A). C. Acanthodian *Acanthodes bronni* Kner (after Miles 1973b, fig. 12). D. Palaeonisciform actinopterygian *Mimia toombsi* Gardiner and Bartram (combination of Gardiner 1984b, figs. 55 and 91). E. Dipnoan *Neoceratodus forsteri* (Krefft) (combination of Jarvik 1980, figs. 313A and 325A). F. Osteolepiform crossopterygian *Eusthenopteron foordi* Whiteaves (combination of Jarvik 1954, fig. 23B, with Jarvik 1980, fig. 125).

thal). Because the lower jaw articulates in a fixed fashion with the palato-quadrate via a condyle on the inside of the palatoquadrate, there is a precise counteraction of lower and upper jaws that results in sharpening of the cutting edge of infra- and supragnathals. Ptyctodonts possess crushing tooth plates. The cutting edges (i.e., "teeth") formed by semidentine and the supporting bone are structurally continuous. There is no indication of tooth replacement; instead, the elements grow by addition of tissue distal to the cutting edge (Ørvig 1980; Vézina 1986).

The gill arches are only partially ossified. There are probably five arches with ventral (ceratobranchials) and dorsal (epibranchials) elements. A groove on the inside of the submarginal may indicate a dorsal, ossified portion of the epihyal (Goujet 1984a; Forey and Gardiner 1986), and a postero-ventrally directed groove may indicate the continuation of the epihyal. The epihyal does not support the jaw articulation, thereby suggesting that a full gill slit may have existed between the mandibula and hyoid arch. A different arrangement of the jaw articulation was proposed by Forey and Gardiner (1986), who hypothesized that the ptyctodont jaw articulation was autostylic and supported by the anterior end of the ceratohyal, a unique situation within gnathostomes. In contrast, Young (1986) restored an epihyal close to the palatoquadrate and interpreted the bone on the inside of the submarginal as opercular cartilage.

Development

Although the structure of placoderm skulls is well known, there is little information about cranial development because few ontogenetic series are available. Developmental descriptions are restricted to size changes from juveniles to adults (Werdelin and Long 1986; Vézina 1986).

CHONDRICHTHYES

Monophyly and Relationship to Other Groups

Recent Chondrichthyes, or cartilaginous fishes, are represented by elasmobranchs and holocephalans (table 5.2) which share one unique, derived character—presence of prismatically calcified cartilage in the endocranium, the visceral skeleton, and the skeleton of the fins. There are several other features that typify, but are not exclusive to, the group (Maisey 1986). Presence of a neck canal is typical of placoid scales, but it appears only sporadically in early chondrichthyan scales (Vieth 1980), and migrates from the base to the neck during ontogeny (Karatajuté-Talimaa 1973). Typical placoid scales have been described from Lower Silurian deposits (430 mya) of Mongolia (Karatajuté-Talimaa et al. 1990). The presence of specialized nutritive foramina in the basal plate of the teeth

TABLE 5.2   Classification of fossil and extant Chondrichthyes

Subclass Subterbranchialia	Order Symmoriida
Cohort Iniopterygia	Order Eugeneodontida
Cohort Holocephali	Order Orodontida
Order Chondrenchelyidea	Order Petalodontida
Order Cochliodontida	Order Squatinactida
Order Psammodontida	Order Desmiodontida
Order Copodontida	Cohort Euselachii
Order Helodontida	Order Ctenacanthiformes
Order Menaspoidea	Order Hybodontiformes
Order Chimaerida	Order Hexanchiformes
Suborder Chimaerina	Subcohort Neoselachii
Subclass Elasmobranchii	Superorder Heterodontimorphii
Cohort unnamed	Superorder Galeomorphii
Order Xenacanthida	Superorder Squalomorphii
Order Cladoselachida	Superorder Squatinomorphii
Order Coronodontida	Superorder Batomorphii

may be related to the former character, because teeth are derived from scales. Revolving tooth replacement occurs in elasmobranchs as well as in some acanthodians (Miles 1973a: *Ptomacanthus;* replacement of symphysial tooth whorls after Zangerl 1981). The length of the septum between the gill filaments is a function of the existence of an opercle or opercular flap. In holocephalans and dipnoans, nearly the entire length of the gill filaments is separated by the septum; the septum is longer than the gill filaments in primitive actinopterygians and shortened in more advanced actinopterygians. Extremely long septa are typical for elasmobranchs that lack a common opercular chamber; the lateral extension of each septum beyond the attachment of the gills closes the gill slit to form a row of small "opercular" chambers (Woskoboinikoff 1932). There are additional unique, shared derived postcranial features that support the monophyly of chondrichthyans (Maisey 1986).

Earlier authors considered chondrichthyans to be primitive because cartilage is the ontogenetic precursor of replacement bone. However, Romer (1942, 1969) demonstrated that cartilage is an embryonic adaptation, and we now know that bone tissue occurs within chondrichthyans (Zangerl 1968; Peignoux-Deville et al. 1982). Chondrichthyans have been proposed to be the sister group of (1) placoderms (Stensiö 1959, 1963b; Moy-Thomas and Miles 1971; Jarvik 1980; Goujet 1982), (2) acanthodians (Nelson 1968; Jarvik 1977, 1980), (3) teleostomes (Zangerl 1981; Young 1986), and (4) placoderms + teleostomes (Forey 1980; Gardiner 1984a). Young (1986) hypothesized (see above) that placoderms are the sister group of all other gnathostomes and that the chondrichthyans are related to teleostomes. The relationship between acanthodians and chondrichthyans is a subset of the teleostome-chondrichthyan relationship. Nelson (1968) favored such a relationship based on two features of gill arches—viz., their posterior position and posteriorly directed pharyngo-branchials. Jarvik (1977, 1980) postulated a close relationship of acanthodians to modern euselachians (Squalomorphii) based on many features, most of which are primitive or ambiguous (Maisey 1984, 1986). The most reasonable hypothesis at present postulates chondrichthyans to be the sister group of teleostomes as a whole. This is based on possession of the following characters in both teleostomes and chondrichthyans: (1) fusion of ethmoid region to endocranium, (2) postorbital connection between palatoquadrate and endocranium, (3) dental lamina and true dentine, and (4) similar positions of internal rectus and superior oblique eye muscles.

Exocranium

Chondrichthyans lack an actual exocranium. Their heads may be covered by scales, which may be enlarged somewhat, and are less antero-posteriorly directed than the body scales. With the exception of menaspoid holocephalans, the head scales generally are not fused to form plates even in early elasmobranchs; however, the circumorbital plates in cladoselachians (in which the skin of the body is nearly naked) are an exception (Dean 1909; Zangerl 1981). Circumorbital plates are represented by many small plates in a double row surrounding the orbit. Zangerl distinguished these from a sclerotic ring which occurs in the form of "weakly calcified connective tissue (perhaps cartilage)" (Zangerl 1981, 4) in symmoriids. In *Menaspis*, a menaspoid holocephalan, an unknown number of separate plates form the head shield. However, the head shield is composed of a single plate in *Deltoptychius*, another menaspoid holocephalan.

Endocranium

It is generally accepted that the chondrichthyan endocranium is a single unit, and that the occurrence of an otico-occipital fissure (fig. 5.4B) is a synapomorphy for xenacanth elasmobranchs (Schaeffer 1981) and convergent to the structure of the same name in teleostomes. Based on sister-group relationships between holocephalans and elasmobranchs, it is assumed that possession of a moderately long otico-occipital region is primitive for chondrichthyans and still existing in euselachians. Therefore, possession of a shortened (Eugeneodontida, Neoselachii) or elongated (Xenacanthida and "*Cladodus*") otico-occipital region is a synapomorphic condition of these groups. If the dichotomy between elasmobranchs and holocephalans occurred within chondrichthyans and not at their base (Maisey 1986) and

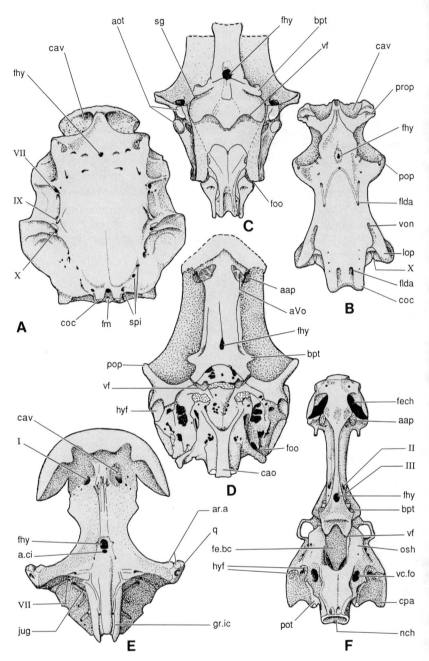

Fig. 5.7. Endocranium of gnathostomes in ventral view. A. Arthrodiran placoderm *Dicksonosteus arcticus* Goujet (after Goujet 1984b, fig. 6). B. Xenacanth elasmobranch *Xenacanthus* sp. (after Schaffer 1981, fig. 6). C. Acanthodian *Acanthodes bronni* Kner (after Miles 1973b, fig. 5). D. Palaeonisciform actinopterygian *Mimia toombsi* Gardiner and Bartram (after Gardiner 1984b, fig. 50). E. Dipnoan *Chirodipterus wildungensis* Gross (after Säve-Söderbergh 1952, fig. 1). F. Osteolepiform crossopterygian *Eusthenopteron foordi* Whitewaves (after Jarvik 1980, figs. 88B and 93A).

the xenacanths are the most primitive chondrichthyans (Mader 1986), then the following may be true. The presence of an otico-occipital fissure may be primitive among chondrichthyans and, therefore, a symplesiomorphy of chondrichthyans and teleostomes. Similarly, the presence of the postorbital articulation with the otic process of the palatoquadrate may be a symplesiomorphy of the two groups. Neither feature is present in placoderms. Given the former phylogenetic arrangement, an elongated otico-occipital region (figs. 5.1C, 5.5B, 5.7B) is primitive (Romer 1964), whereas the shortened otico-occipital region is derived.

The lack of chondrification of the anterior wall of the cranial cavity in front of the pineal foramen (fig. 5.4C: precerebral fontanelle) is a unique feature of the chondrichthyan endocranium. Chondrichthyans also lack a nasal capsule floor. The orbital is surrounded by a thickened ring which forms preorbital and prominent postorbital processes where the palatoquadrate attaches with the ethmoidal and postorbital articulations. An eyestalk is present in neoselachians, and assumed to have been present in Paleozoic elasmobranchs (Gross 1937; Schaeffer 1981). An open endolymphatic fossa occurs in the dorsal midline (fig. 5.4C) of the endocranium of elasmobranchs, but is absent in holocephalans.

Lateral otic processes (figs. 5.4C, 5.5B, 5.7B) occur in elasmobranchs but not in holocephalans. Far posterior in the region of the lateral otic processes (Maisey 1980), the epihyal articulates with the endocranium in elasmobranchs (fig. 5.5B: hyf) in contrast to the articulation behind the orbit in placoderms and teleostomes (fig. 5.5A,D-F: hyf). The occipital arch forms paired occipital condyles (in contrast to the exoccipital condyles of tetrapods) for the articulation with the first centrum.

The chondrichthyan endocranium (Compagno 1973, 1977, 1988) is limited in its diversity, being a single unit. The otico-occipital region can change in length in relation to the length of the whole endocranium from long (over 50%) to short (to much less than 50%); it is short in neoselachians except in Heterodontimorphii (50%). The nasal capsules and the orbits are always quite large, although relative size differences can be observed.

Variations occur in the formation of processes, rostral (rostrum, in many sources), pre- and postorbital processes, and the size of the precerebral fontanelle. Pre- and postorbital processes are small in most elasmobranchs; they can extend laterally, and even far, as in the hammerhead sharks, the Sphyrinidae (family within the Galeomorphii), and mobulid rays (family within the Batomorphii). In Sphyrinidae, the pre- and postorbital processes form narrow stripes which connect distally; the preorbital process is joint with the distally extended nasal capsule. The nasal capsule is ventrally closed (Compagno 1988). In mobulid rays, the lateral extension is formed by a compact structure. In most batomorphs the distal part of the preorbital process is separated from the nasal capsule; it forms a separate cartilage. In Torpedinoidea, the preorbital process is enlarged and branched into many separate processes which bridge the area between the reduced rostral process and the preorbital process.

The rostral process is a structure of the Neoselachii excluding the Heterodontimorphii. It is formed either by a median ventral process, by two lateral processes combined with a median ventral one (all three are fused anteriorly), or by a troughlike structure. Elongation of the rostral process occurs within different neoselachian groups, in Mitsukurinidae within Galeomorphii, in Pristiophoriformes within Squalimorphii, and in Batomorphii, and also in the Paleozoic shark *Bandringa* (Zangerl 1969). The sawsharks, the Pristiophoriformes, have a solid, heavily calcified rostral process with lateral teeth; the rostral process is much longer than the neurocranium proper. In rhinobatid and rajid batomorphs, the length of the rostral process exceeds also the length of the neurocranium; here the precerebral fontanelle is elongated as it is in other batomorphs. A special case is the Paleozoic shark *Ornithoprion* with a long mandibular rostrum separated from the Meckelian cartilage (Zangerl 1981).

Visceral Skeleton

The mandibular arch of elasmobranchs is formed by two free cartilaginous elements (fig. 5.6B), the palatoquadrate and Meckel's cartilage. The palatoquadrate is fused to the endocranium in holocephalans (holostylic), and is either free or fused in iniopterygians. Teeth or tooth plates are not attached to these elements, but instead move in connective tissue above them. For this reason, teeth can be replaced continuously. The articulation of the palatoquadrate with the endocranium is variable; Maisey (1980) noted rostral, ethmoidal, orbital, palatobasal, and postorbital articulations, not all of which occur in a single specimen. Because the epihyal articulates with the palatoquadrate in all elasmobranchs to some degree, all are hyostylic. Amphistyly is a special case of hyostyly in which the palatoquadrate is more firmly attached to the braincase; in advanced sharks, the epihyal supports the more freely movable palatoquadrate ("typical" hyostyly).

The palatoquadrate and Meckel's cartilage form a double joint with an articular knob at the posterior end and a joint pan on the posterior medial side of the palatoquadrate. Meckel's cartilage forms the cotyle to accept the quadrate head, and the dorsal process to articulate with the joint pan on the medial side of the palatoquadrate. Lateral to the palatoquadrate and Meckel's cartilage, there are a number of labial cartilages (five in *Hybodus*, but three or fewer in Recent sharks) to which some superficial jaw muscles attach. The jaw articulation may be placed below or behind the otico-occipital region (Compagno 1988). The position is not related to the length of the otico-occipital region; so of course it is below a long otico-occipital region. In sharks with a short otico-occipital region, it can lie below (e.g., Scyliorhinidae and Carcharhinidae within Galeomorphii) or far behind the region (e.g., Sphyrhinidae, Pseudocarchariidae, and Mitsukurinidae within Galeomorphii).

The hyoid arch consists of epi-, cerato- and median basihyal in elasmobranchs; a hypohyal is absent in chondrichthyans (fig. 5.8B). Holocephalans are the only gnathostomes with a pharyngohyal. According to Maisey (1984), even though the pharyngohyal is a serial homologue of the pharyngobranchials, its presence in holocephalans is a specialization and not a primitive feature. Maisey (1986) even suggested that the pharyngohyal of holocephalans is homologous with the epihyal of elasmobranchs, and that the epihyal of holocephalans is homologous with the interhyal of elasmobranch, but later he interpreted it as part of the ceratohyal (Maisey 1989). There is a half gill slit, a spiracle, between epihyal and palatoquadrate in chondrichthyans (closed in adult holocephalans); a complete first gill slit as postulated by Zangerl and Williams (1975) and Zangerl and Case (1976) for some Paleozoic sharks, is generally not accepted (Maisey 1986). The gill arches posterior to the spiracle have a complete set of posteriorly directed pharyngo-, epi-, cerato-, and hypobranchials, and a median basibranchial (fig. 5.8B). Except for holocephalans and some Paleozoic sharks (cladoselachians and symmoriids), there is a gap between the basihyal and basibranchials corresponding to the anteriorly directed ceratohyal and posteriorly directed hypobranchials. The posterior gill arches are modified in some extant sharks; thus, the pharyngo- and epibranchial or the cerato- and hypobranchial may fuse within one arch or between the two last arches. Extrabranchials are present outside the gill arches, but they are rarely illustrated.

The gill arches are narrowly spaced below the posterior endocranium in Subterbranchialia (Zangerl 1981), but widely spaced in elasmobranchs so that the shoulder girdle (scapulocoracoid) is widely separated from the skull. Subterbranchialia have an opercular flap supported by hyoidean rays, but hyoidean rays occur in different Paleozoic elasmobranchs (Maisey 1986).

Development

The ontogenetic development of the endocranium and visceral skeleton has been described for several elasmobranchs (cf. compilations in de Beer 1937 and Holmgren 1940). Because the total length of the embryos and the number of days posthatching are unreliable indications of developmental stage (Jollie 1971), developmental descriptions are sometimes contra-

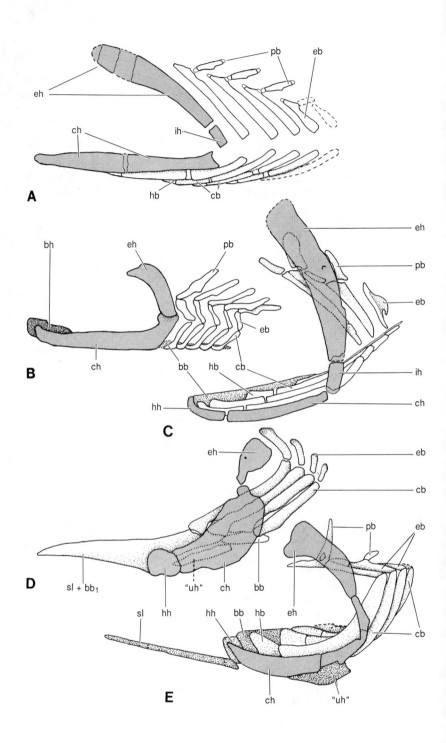

dictory. Nonetheless, some generalizations can be made about sequential development of elements.

The paired parachordals chondrify first on either side of the anterior notochord (de Beer 1931; El-Toubi 1949; fig. 5.9A: chordal skull). Subsequently, each parachordal cartilage develops two or three dorsal extensions (fig. 5.9B) that form the anterior and posterior parts of the auditory capsule and the occipital arch. An isolated orbital cartilage appears in the prechordal skull. Ventral to the orbital and parachordal cartilages, the paired trabeculae cranii, polar cartilages, and elements of the visceral skeleton (palatoquadrate, Meckel's cartilage, epihyal, and ceratohyal) form. The trabeculae cranii are considered to be pharyngeal elements of the mandibular arch by many authors (e.g., Jollie 1971); later they are incorporated into the endocranium. If this interpretation is correct, then possession of trabeculae cranii is, in fact, the same as the diagnostic feature of gnathostomes—viz., possession of biting jaws.

Subsequent development (fig. 5.9C) involves fusions of the orbital and parachordal cartilages via the acrochordal cartilages, and fusion of the trabeculae via the polar cartilages (Holmgren 1940; El-Toubi 1949). The lateral and dorsal endocranial walls are formed through expansion of the orbital cartilages, the auditory capsules, and occipital cartilages. Ultimately, these structures fuse with one another, leaving only small foramina for nerves and blood vessels. The trabeculae cranii grow forward into the rostral region to form the laminae orbitonasales, which surround the nasal sacs on each side, and the rostral cartilages (Jollie 1971; fig. 5.9D). The paired trabeculae fuse with one another ventral to the brain to form a plate; subsequently, fusion between the lateral margin of the plate and the orbital cartilage forms the inner part of the orbit. A supraorbital cartilage forms lateral to the orbital cartilage and the anterior part of the auditory capsule; subsequently, it fuses with the endocranium to form the dorsal and anterior wall of the orbit.

Two cartilages appear lateral to the auditory capsule—the lateral commissure proximally, and the spiracular cartilage distally (fig. 5.9C-E). Eventually the lateral commissure and then the spiracular cartilage are incorporated into the lateral wall of the endocranium. In order of occurrence,

---

Fig. 5.8. (*opposite*). Gill basket of gnathostomes in lateral view. A. Acanthodian *Acanthodes bronni* Kner (combination of Miles 1973b, figs. 15, 17; and Jarvik 1977, fig. 8). B. Hybodont elasmobranch *Hybodus* sp. (after Maisey 1982, fig. 9D; and 1983, figs. 16B, C, E). C. Palaeonisciform actinopterygian *Mimia toombsi* Gardiner and Bartram (combination of Gardiner 1984b, figs. 108, 119, with figs. 104 and 55). D. Dipnoan *Griphognathus whitei* Miles (combination of Miles 1977, figs. 138b, a with fig. 134a). E. Osteolepiform rhipidistian *Eusthenopteron foordi* Whiteaves (combination of Jarvik 1954, fig. 23, and Jarvik 1980, figs. 109, 110).

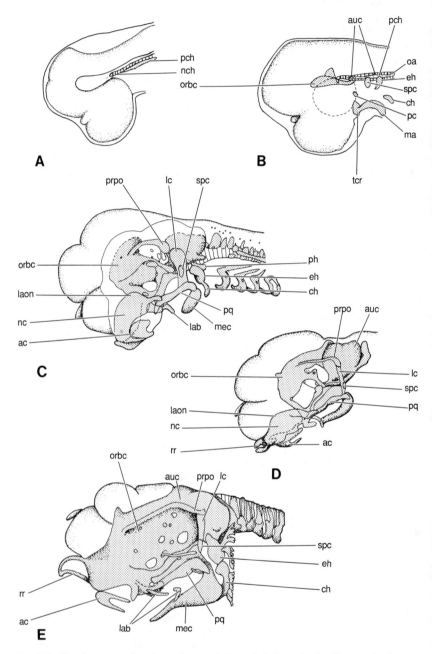

Fig. 5.9. Development of endocranium and visceral skeleton in *Scyllium canicula* (Linné) in lateral view (simplified after Holmgren 1940). Length: A, 18 mm; B, 23.5 mm; C, 27.5 mm; D, 31.0 mm; E, 40.0 mm.

the endocranium closes dorsally via the tectum synoticum that unites the anterior parts of the auditory capsules, in the occipital region via the tectum occipitale, and finally, in the orbital region via the tectum orbitale.

The above description demonstrates that the separately appearing units sequentially lose their individuality by fusion with each other into the cartilaginous endocranium. Space between the units disappears with fusion before the neurocranium surrounds the brain dorsally. In embryonic stages (fig. 5.9E), all separately formed units are already fused so that no fissures appear in the definitive cartilaginous neurocranium.

Chondrification of the visceral skeleton proceeds in an anterior-to-posterior direction. Thus, the elements to appear first are the palatoquadrate, Meckel's cartilage, and the epi- and ceratohyal (fig. 5.9B). These are succeeded by the pharyngo-, epi-, and ceratobranchials (fig. 5.9C), and finally by the hypo- and basibranchials. The more lateral elements, labial cartilages (fig. 5.9D-E), extrahyal, and extrabranchial cartilages appear contemporaneously with the hypo- and basibranchials.

TELEOSTOMI

Monophyly and Relationship to Other Groups

The Teleostomi (table 5.3) comprise the Acanthodii and the Osteichthyes (including tetrapods). Herein, I follow Miles's (1973b) placement of acanthodians within teleostomes (contra Nelson 1968 and Jarvik 1977), based on the presence of the following characters: (1) cranial otico-occipital fissure, (2) anterior position of lateral commissure, (3) anterior (pineal

TABLE 5.3   Classification of Teleostomi

Class Acanthodii	Subclass Sarcopterygii
Order Climatiida	Infraclass Dipnoi
Order Ischnacanthida	Infraclass Crossopterygii
Order Acanthodida	Actinistia
Class Osteichthyes	Onychodontiformes
Subclass Actinopterygii	Porolepiformes
Cladistia	Osteolepiformes
Palaeonisciformes	Panderichthyiformes
Acipenseriformes	Tetrapoda
Neopterygii	
Ginglymodi	
Halecostomi	
Halecomorphi	
Teleostei	
(Classification and phylogeny of lower Actinopterygii not settled)	

organ) and posterior (cranial fissure) dorsal fontanelles, (4) paired paroc-cipital (craniospinal) process, (5) spiracular groove in basisphenoid region, (6) articulation of hyomandibula above jugular vein, (7) basal articulation of palatoquadrate, and (8) a series of dermal branchiostegal rays in hyoid gill cover. Miles (1973b) cited the presence of an interhyal as an additional feature, but Maisey (1986) considered the feature primitive for gnathos-tomes because questionably it occurs in one fossil cladoselachian. Maisey (1989) reinterpreted the so-called interhyal in cladoselachians to be the separated posterior end of the ceratohyal.

The sister group of the Teleostomi are the Chondrichthyes (see above). Because the sister-group relationship between placoderms and teleostomes proposed by Gardiner (1984a) is based on general features (Young 1986), it is not accepted.

Exocranium

The primitive pattern of the teleostome exocranium is a mosaic. The head of acanthodians is covered by scales or tesserae; the group did not acquire a stabilized bone pattern during their 180-million-year history (Early Silurian–Middle Permian). The anterior part of the skull roof of primitive sarcopterygians is a bone mosaic, as is the anterior part of the lower jaw of primitive dipnoans. Stabilization of the skull-roof pattern proceeds an-teriorly. Actinopterygians are the only teleostome group that lacks a bone mosaic in its most primitive representatives. The cheek region reflects a similar situation—i.e., scales or tesserae in acanthodians (except *Dipla-canthus* and *Culmacanthus*), many small bones in dipnoans, and fewer bones in crossopterygians and actinopterygians. The exocranial pattern must have evolved independently in all three groups of osteichthyans.

Endocranium

Teleostomes are distinguished from other gnathostomes primarily on the basis of endocranial features. The endocranium is partially divided by fis-sures (fig. 5.5C-F), and thus is not solid as in chondrichthyans or solid with a small anterior portion as in placoderms. The otico-occipital fissure (from which the vagus nerve, cranial nerve X, exits) separates the occipital and otic regions. Another fissure (ventral part = ventral fissure, and lateral part = oticosphenoid fissure) marks the division between the otic and orbitotemporal regions. The anterior dorsal fontanelle (fig. 5.4B, D, F) is the opening for the pineal and parietal organ; the posterior dorsal fonta-nelle corresponds to the dorsal part of the otico-occipital fissure.

Visceral Skeleton

The endoskeletal mandibular arch is formed by the palatoquadrate and Meckel's cartilage. The palatoquadrate ossifies from three centers—viz., the autopalatine, metapterygoid, and quadrate; only the latter is known in dipnoans, because the palatoquadrate is fused to the endocranium. The palatoquadrate articulates with the endocranium via the otic process (paratemporal articulation), the ascending process (postorbital articulation), the basal (palatobasal articulation), and the apical process (ethmoidal articulation). The latter is absent in acanthodians; the palatoquadrate is unossified anteriorly in *Acanthodes*. Meckel's cartilage ossifies in two centers to form the mentomeckelian anteriorly and the articular posteriorly; in adults, the entire cartilage may be ossified. The hyoid and posterior branchial arches are composed of a ventral series (unpaired median basibranchials, paired hypohyal/hypobranchials and ceratohyal/ceratobranchials) and a dorsal series (epihyal/epibranchial and pharyngobranchials except in dipnoans). The presence of an interhyal between the cerato- and epihyals commonly is considered to be a typical teleostome feature.

ACANTHODII

Monophyly Relationship to Other Groups

Acanthodians (table 5.3), which appeared in the Early Silurian (430 mya), are among the earliest known gnathostomes. They are a small group of typical teleostomes with fin spines anterior to every fin except the caudal fin and with additional, paired fin spines between the pectoral and pelvic fins. The monophyly of the group is based on its possession of two features: (1) fin spines in front of pectoral and pelvic fin, and (2) box-in-box scales (i.e., scales in which new layers of bone and dentine or mesodentine are deposited concentrically around each previous scale).

The acanthodians have been thought to be related to chondrichthyans or osteichthyans. The relationship to chondrichthyans is based mainly on primitive characters, and the proposed relationship to osteichthyans is not as convincing as the many supporting data of Miles (1973b) might suggest. Miles listed the following synapomorphies for acanthodians and osteichthyans: (1) paired paroccipital processes (process on dorsal side of lateral occipital ossification in acanthodians), (2) anterior position of lateral commissure, (3) articulation of epihyal above jugular vein, (4) basisphenoid with spiracular groove and internal carotids, (5) basal articulation of palatoquadrate, and (6) series of dermal branchiostegal rays extending onto the hyoid gill cover. An otico-occipital fissure also occurs in xenacanth chondrichthyans (Schaeffer 1981), but it appears on the dorsal side of the neurocranium only and is missing on the ventral surface. This morphological dissimilarity indicates convergent formation which is supported phylogenetically, too, by appearance in one chondrichthyan group only.

Maisey (1986) adds three other features to the foregoing list of six synapomorphies: anterior and posterior hemibranchs incompletely separated by gill septum, absence of branchial skeleton external to gills, and pore canals in lateral-line canals. Three otoliths occur in acanthodians and osteichthyans (Schultze 1990); their presence could be used as a synapomorphy if the condition were known for primitive acanthodians, but that is the problem for most of the characters which are known only from *Acanthodes*, the most advanced last survivor of the group.

Exocranium

Acanthodians lack a stabilized cranial bone pattern. Scales extend onto the head, and are enlarged to tesserae in some forms (fig. 5.2B). Tesserae and scales are reduced in advanced acanthodians, so that the head lacks a dermal cover except around the orbit. Here, four to six large circumorbital bones are formed, or in some cases, numerous small bones are interspersed among a few large bones. In some taxa, the infraorbital canal passes through the circumorbital bones. The branchiostegal rays pass continuously from the gular region to the hyoidean opercular region, which is covered by long, narrow, branchiostegal-like plates. In primitive acanthodians, additional gill covers lie posterior or postero-dorsal to the hyoidean opercular cover (fig. 5.2B).

Endocranium

The endocranium is known only in the youngest, most advanced genus—*Acanthodes* from the Early Permian. The middle and posterior parts are ossified perichondrally. The endocranium is divided into orbito-otic and occipital regions by the otico-occipital fissure (fig. 5.5C). The orbito-otic region is composed of a dorsal ossification (with a postorbital process and two articular knobs for the postorbital articulation of the palatoquadrate on its lateral side) and a small ventral ossification. There is a keyhole-shaped opening for the pineal organ in the dorsal surface of the dorsal ossification (fig. 5.4B). In adults, the dorsal ossification extends laterally around the otic capsule; in this area, the jugular vein runs in a groove and the epihyal articulates. A ventral ossification may occur between the otico-occipital and ventral fissures. Anterior to the ventral fissure, the basisphenoid is ossified (fig. 5.7C). It is pierced by the buccohypophysial foramen. The basal process of the antero-ventral part of the metapterygoid articulates laterally with the basipterygoid process on the basisphenoid; the spiracular groove extends dorsally posterior to the basipterygoid process. There are one ventral and two lateral ossifications in the occipital region. The ventral ossification underlies the notochord and forms the groove for the dorsal aorta on its ventral side.

Visceral Skeleton

The palatoquadrate and Meckel's cartilage are known from many forms, but the branchial skeleton is known only in *Acanthodes*. In most acanthodians, the palatoquadrate is single. In *Acanthodes,* an autopalatine, metapterygoid, and quadrate were identified by Miles (1973b). Using the processes as landmarks, it seems likely that the autopalatine is unossified, and that the deep anterior ossification represents only the metapterygoid (fig. 5.6C). Meckel's cartilage also bears an anterior mentomeckelian and a posterior articular ossification in this taxon. In all acanthodians except ischnacanthids, a complicated double articulation with anterior and posterior process connects the palatoquadrate and lower jaw. The palatoquadrate articulates with the endocranium via a basal process of the antero-ventral part of the metapterygoid and an otic cotylus of the dorsal part of the metapterygoid (two cotyli in *Acanthodes*). There is a mandibular split ventral to Meckel's cartilage in some acanthodians. Dermal toothed jaw bones and tooth spirals at the symphysis are restricted to ischnacanthid acanthodians. The dentigerous jaw bone grows anteriorly, adding new toothlike serrations at its anterior end. Acanthodid acanthodians do not possess teeth.

The hyoid arch and four or five branchial arches articulate with one elongate basibranchial. The ceratohyal and epihyal (= hyomandibula of tetrapods) ossify as two elements each. An interhyal is developed, but a hypohyal is unknown (fig. 5.8A). Each posterior arch develops a hypobranchial. Each ceratobranchial is represented by two elements. A posteriorly directed pharyngobranchial articulates with the epibranchial.

Development

Size series of some acanthodid acanthodians (*Acanthodes bridgei, A. bronni, A. lundi,* and *Howittacanthus kentoni*) are known. The scale cover develops from the tail region toward the head from small to large specimens (Zidek 1976, 1985). Three otoliths occur in small specimens of *Acanthodes.* In larger specimens, the otoliths are covered progressively (i.e., as a function of overall size) by ossification of the otic region (Heidtke 1990); thus, one to three otoliths are described in different species. Hence, the disagreement over the number of otoliths in acanthodians has its origin (Schultze 1990).

OSTEICHTHYES

Monophyly and Relationship to Other Groups

The Osteichthyes comprise two groups, the Actinopterygii and the Sarcopterygii (table 5.3). The sarcopterygians are composed of the Dipnoi and the Crossopterygii. Although it is widely accepted that actinopterygians are the sister group of sarcopterygians, the relationship between dipnoans and crossopterygians is controversial. Thus, Schultze (1987) accepts the more traditional view that dipnoans are the sister group of crossopterygians, whereas Maisey (1986) and Chang (1991) place dipnoans within crossopterygians as the sister group of porolepiforms. Osteichthyans are united by an array of characters that distinguish them from other gnathostome fishes (Lauder and Liem 1983; Maisey 1986; Schultze 1987), as follows: (1) prearticular dentate, (2) margins of upper and lower jaws bearing teeth (outer dental arcade) on dermal bones lateral to palatoquadrate and Meckel's cartilage, (3) canal-bearing premaxilla and/or antorbital, (4) anteriorly directed infrapharyngobranchials, (5) suprapharyngobranchials on first two gill arches, (6) presence of hypohyal, (7) gular plates, (8) subopercular and opercular plates, and (9) many branchial and postcranial features.

Osteichthyans and chondrichthyans are the two major groups of extant gnathostomes (Goodrich 1909). Schaeffer (1975) considered possession of a cleaver-shaped palatoquadrate and postorbital attachment of the palatoquadrate with the endocranium to be synapomorphies uniting osteichthyans and chondrichthyans and distinguishing them from placoderms. Young (1986) listed six features for such a sister-group relationship (see above), even though he favored a placoderm-chondrichthyan sister-group arrangement. Alternatively, Jarvik (1980) considered dipnoans to be the sister group of holocephalans with his Plagiostomi together with placoderms, elasmobranchs, and acanthodians (Schultze and Trueb 1981), and Lagios (1979) and Wiley (1979) considered actinistians and chondrichthyans to be sister groups. Because dipnoans and actinistians have features characteristic of osteichthyans, these hypotheses do not seem well founded. Generally, it is conceded that of the two fossil groups, the acanthodians and placoderms, osteichthyans are the sister group of the former (Miles 1973b; Lauder and Liem 1983; see above). The alternate hypothesis, in which osteichthyans are the sister group to placoderms (Forey 1980; Gardiner 1984a), is based on generalized features, some of which occur in agnathans (Young 1986).

Exocranium

Each osteichthyan group has distinct exocranial and endocranial patterns. The pattern of osteolepiform crossopterygians, especially that of panderichthyiforms, most closely resembles the tetrapod pattern (Westoll 1943; Schultze and Arsenault 1985). Panderichthyiforms have three pairs of median bones on the skull roof—postparietals, parietals, and frontals—in positions corresponding to those of primitive tetrapods. Other crossopterygians lack a discrete pair of frontals; instead, the front part of the skull is covered by a mosaic of bones. In these taxa, the postparietals cover the otic region (fig. 5.1E) and the parietals surround the pineal-parietal organ (fig. 5.3D). Because the pattern in dipnoans is so different from that of crossopterygians and tetrapods, Forster-Cooper (1937) identified skull roof and cheek bones by letters and numbers, respectively. The skull-roof pattern of actinopterygians is similar to that of crossopterygians; therefore, Romer (1945) and Jollie (1962) assigned corresponding names to the bones. The nomenclature currently applied to actinopterygian skull bones derives from an incorrect application of that used in mammals, and is misleading (Schultze and Arsenault 1985). If one bases homology on positional relationships of bones to one another and to the neurocranium, one most postulate that the common ancestor of osteichthyans possessed a postparietal and parietal. If dipnoans are placed as a sister group of crossopterygians or within crossopterygians, then one would have to postulate that the mosaic skull-roof pattern of this group was derived from the basic, simpler pattern of the osteichthyan ancestor. Alternatively, one could postulate that the actinopterygian pattern and the tetrapod pattern of crossopterygians were derived independently, in which case independent systems of nomenclature should be employed. I choose to follow the first approach.

A mosaic pattern of bones on the snout seems to be primitive for all osteichthyans, even though it is unknown among primitive actinopterygians. Consolidation of paired bones along the midline starts posteriorly with two bones in front of the extrascapulars. This is true of primitive dipnoans too; however, in most dipnoans, an unpaired median bone, the B-bone, lies in the midline. Extrascapulars with the occipital commissure of the lateral-line system lie behind the endocranium and are not solidly enclosed in the skull roof. Although the presence of a tooth-bearing outer dental arcade (premaxilla, maxilla, dentary) is cited as a common character of Osteichthyes, dipnoans lack all three bones and actinistians lack a maxilla. On the other hand, all osteichthyans possess a tooth-bearing prearticular.

In all three groups there has been a general tendency to reduce the number of cranial bones throughout their evolutionary history. In Devonian actinopterygians, dipnoans, and coelacanths, there are more exocranial bones and greater ossification of the neurocranium than in extant forms. The coelacanth *Latimeria* represents an extreme case of reduction; in this taxon, the cheek bones are without direct contact with each other.

Endocranium

The endocranium of osteichthyans ossifies perichondrally and endochondrally. Ossification proceeds in a posterior-to-anterior direction, and perichondral ossification precedes endochondral ossification. Thus, in actinopterygians, the anterior ethmoidal region is unossified or bears only weak perichondral ossification. The endocranium is partly divided into regions by fissures (see Teleostomi, Endocranium). The otico-occipital fissure is lined perichondrally in contrast to acanthodians (Gardiner 1984b). The ventral fissure in actinopterygians and dipnoans is homologous with the ventral part of the intracranial joint of crossopterygians, and separates the otic and orbitotemporal regions. In advanced actinopterygians and dipnoans, the ventral fissure is posterior in position. The location of the fissure is correlated with the development of the posterior myodome in actinopterygians, and questionably associated with a feeding adaptation in dipnoans (Gardiner 1984b). The otico-occipital region may be single as one unit or be divided into many ossification centers. Primitive actinopterygians and dipnoans lack separate ossification centers (except one, *Dipnorhynchus,* in which Campbell and Barwick (1982) described three ossification centers in the otic region), whereas advanced actinopterygians and crossopterygians have many ossification centers. It is disputed whether in the course of evolution, the number of ossification centers has tended to increase (e.g., the ethmoid region) or decrease (e.g., the otic and occipital regions). In the occipital region, a supraoccipital is known only in teleostean actinopterygians, some crossopterygians, and tetrapods. The occipital region is variable in its segmental structure. Primitively, there seem to be three segments in osteichthyans, but there may be more or fewer among extant actinopterygians. In extant dipnoans, there are three segments in *Neoceratodus* and one in *Lepidosiren,* and there is only one in the extant actinistian *Latimeria.*

Primitively in osteichthyans, a massive lateral commissure penetrated by the jugular canal forms the lateral wall of the trigeminofacialis chamber in the otic region. The facet for the epihyal lies dorsal to the jugular canal in actinopterygians and straddles it in sarcopterygians. A spiracular groove is developed in primitive actinopterygians together with an open spiracle on the skull roof, but a spiracular groove is rudimentary or missing in sarcopterygians. Except for dipnoans, the endolymphatic ducts are closed in osteichthyans. Paired fossae bridgei are not a common feature of osteichthyans, occurring only in actinopterygians. Crossopterygians have paired posttemporal fossae for axial musculature, and dipnoans lack both fossa bridgei and posttemporal fossa. Although a posterior myodome is absent in the otic region of primitive osteichthyans, it occurs in actinopterygians. Two pairs of anterior myodomes are found in some primitive actinopterygians, actinistians, and few rhipidistians. Primitively, these structures may be absent; based on their variable positions in different osteichthyans, they seem to have developed independently in various taxa. Endochondral ossification invades the nasal capsule of crossopterygians, but not that of actinopterygians.

Visceral Skeleton

The mandibular and hyoid arches are covered laterally by dermal bones. The dermal covers of the mandibular arches of actinopterygians, dipnoans, and crossopterygians are each distinctive (fig. 5.2C-E), but the endoskeletal bauplan is similar in each group. The dermal hyoid cover (operculogular series) extends posteriorly to cover posterior gill arches laterally. An opercle and subopercle occur in all osteichthyans, but there are differences in the bones that lie between the subopercle and gulars. The prearticular on the medial surface of Meckel's cartilage and the pterygoid (= endopterygoid) on the medial side of the palatoquadrate (upper jaw) are present in all osteichthyans, whereas the occurrence of ossifications (i.e., dermal plates with teeth) on the gill arches varies within groups. An unpaired median parasphenoid covers the roof of the mouth.

ACTINOPTERYGII

Monophyly and Relationship to Other Groups

Among the many features that distinguish actinopterygians (table 5.3) from sarcopterygians are the following: (1) Composition of the external side of the lower jaw in which the dentalosplenial occupies the position of the dentary, splenial, and postsplenial, and carries the anterior portion of the mandibular canal; (2) absence of squamosal; (3) dermohyal on dorsal portion of hyomandibula; (4) preopercular sensory canal not connected to infraorbital canal by jugal canal; (5) even number of extrascapulars (always in pairs, no median); (6) ganoine, an epidermal derivative, present as an outer layer on scales and bones; and (7) acrodin tips on teeth (with the possible exception of *Cheirolepis*). On the basis of these features, the cladistians *Polypterus* and *Erpetoichthys* are actinopterygians (Lauder and Liem 1983; Gardiner 1984b; Maisey 1986); allocation of the cladistians to a separate osteichthyan group, the Brachiopterygii (Jarvik 1980), is unjustified (Schultze and Trueb 1981).

Although actinopterygians are easily recognizable within osteichthyans on the basis of the foregoing characters, it is difficult to determine whether the features are synapomorphies, because the acanthodian outgroup possesses few, if any, of the characters. In distinction to acanthodians, the scales and bones of actinopterygians and sarcopterygians have a derived, outer epidermal covering; this is a thin layer of "true" enamel in sarcopterygians and a multilayered covering of ganoine in actinopterygians. The surface of "true" enamel shows hexagonal impressions of the boundaries between the basal epidermal cells, whereas the surface of ganoine has tubercles corresponding to the center of the basal epidermal cells (see below). There is a connection (= jugal canal) between the preopercular and infraorbital canal in acanthodians and sarcopterygians; its loss in actinopterygians is a derived feature. Because acanthodians have no acrodin on teeth, this character is clearly a derived feature of actinopterygians.

Exocranium

The largest part of the skull-roof of actinopterygians is occupied by two pairs of bones, which are usually called "parietal" and "frontal." Because the topographic relationship of these bones to endocranial structures (fig. 5.1B) is similar to that of the postparietal and parietal in tetrapods and rhipidistians, I apply herein the nomenclature proposed by Romer (1945) and Jollie (1962) (see Schultze and Arsenault 1985; and Jollie 1986). The postparietal carries posterior and middle pit lines. The supra-orbital sensory canal ends in the postparietal of primitive actinopterygians (fig. 5.3B), whereas it connects to the occipital portion of the main lateral line in the intertemporal in advanced actinopterygians. Anteriorly, the su-praorbital sensory canal passes through the parietal, which surrounds a pineal foramen, and continues into the nasal, where it passes between the anterior and posterior nasal openings to join the ethmoidal commissure in the premaxilla (in the rostrodermethmoid in advanced actinopterygians). An unpaired median bone, the rostral, lies in front of the parietals and between the anterior nasal openings in primitive actinopterygians. *Chei-rolepis* has additional small bones in the snout region, a bone mosaic typical of primitive sarcopterygians which is unknown in other primitive actinopterygians; the pineal foramen pierces a separate bone, which lies between the parietals, in *Cheirolepis*. The posterior margin of the skull is formed by an even number of extrascapulars (two in primitive and four in advanced actinopterygians) which carry the occipital commissure. The main lateral line passes lateral to the postparietal and parietal through the supratemporal and intertemporal. The preopercular canal connects in the supratemporal to the main lateral line, and the infraorbital canal branches off in the intertemporal to pass through the circumorbital bones, the dermosphenotic (postorbital of rhipidistians and tetrapods), jugal, and lacrimal (fig. 5.2C). The jugal and lacrimal are divided into smaller bones known as infraorbitals (usually 1–5) in advanced actinopterygians. In advanced actinopterygians, a small bone, the antorbital, occupies the area between the posterior nasal opening and orbit; it carries an additional branch of the infraorbital canal. Dorsal to the orbit are additional bones, the supraorbitals. The orbit is large, and the eyeball is surrounded by four sclerotic plates (two or none in advanced actinopterygians). The cheek region is occupied by a dorsal extension of the posterior maxilla, the preopercle, and the dermal dermohyal, which is attached to the epihyal. In some advanced actinopterygians, the preopercle is separated from the posterior infraorbitals by additional suborbital bones. The preopercle carries the preopercular canal, which is connected to the main lateral canal, rather than the infraorbital canal as in sarcopterygians. The preopercular canal continues as the mandibular canal in the lower jaw. The cheek region is rigid in primitive actinopterygians. In advanced actinopterygians, the cheek bones are separated from each other, the maxilla and premaxilla become movable (protrusible mouth), and additional bones, supramaxilla(e) (two are characteristic for teleostean actinopterygians), appear above the maxilla.

Variation of the exocranium is extreme within actinopterygians (see Gregory 1933 for a broad presentation of actinopterygian skulls). The exocranium varies in proportions, in relation of bones to each other, in number of bones, and shape and thickness of bones. In *Polypterus*, the most primitive extant actinopterygian (Cladistia in table 5.3), accessory bones occur lateral to the medial pairs of extrascapulars, supratemporotabulars, and parietals, which are numerous and variable in number (Jollie 1984b); the postparietals appear as blastema, but are obliterated during growth of *Polypterus* (Pehrson 1947). There is a very long cheek region with a broad preopercle and two bones below it and posterior to the maxilla, of which the posterior one can be homologized with the quadratojugal, whereas the anterior one is an additional bone. The Acipenseriformes have numerous additional bones in the snout region which vary intraspecifically in shape and number (Jollie 1980); the snout is elongated to a long rostrum formed by many independent ossifications in Polyodontidae (Grande and Bemis 1991). The Ginglymodi (*Lepisosteus*) develop a bone mosaic in the cheek region, which occupies the place of the large preopercle of *Polypterus*. The anteriorly elongated upper jaw of *Lepisosteus* is bordered by many toothed small bones, lacrimals or infraorbitals, which carry the infraorbital canal and fuse with the maxilla (Jollie 1984a). Within teleosts, the number of bones is reduced, with the exception of some Scorpaeniformes, but even in this group and others like the Dactylopteriformes and Siluriformes the bony cover is formed by enlarged bones only. Change in size and proportions of these bones results in the great variability of the teleostean skull. Commonly, the cheek region between orbit and opercle is short; nevertheless it can be very elongated as in some osteoglossomorphs, such as *Arapaima, Notopterus,* and *Mormyrops* or in synbranchid eels. In *Arapaima*, the elongated cheek region is covered by elongated infraorbitals, whereas the lateral side of the palatal bones is merely covered by skin in the other genera.

In different teleostean groups, the snout is elongated as in Ginglymodi or other lower actinopterygians (e.g., saurichthyids, aspidorhynchids). The elongation can be formed by premaxilla and dentalosplenial (e.g., in the Belonidae, needlefishes). In teleosts with small premaxillae, maxillae, and dentalosplenial, the parietal with the mesethmoid in the upper side of the snout and articular (Mormyridae, elephantfishes), or preopercle (Acanthuridae, surgeonfishes; Balistidae, leatherjackets, and others) or preopercle and quadrate (Syngnathiformes, trumpetfishes, cornetfishes, snipefishes, pipefishes, and seashores; and Aulorhynchidae, tubesnouts) in the lower side of the snout are elongated.

At the other extreme, the skull can be very deep, as in Zeiformes and in some Perciformes; here the median supraoccipital reaches between the postparietals to form a deep crest. In flatfishes, the Pleuronectiformes, ventral and dorsal margins of the head become the lateral margins. The skull is asymmetrical by ontogenetic movement of one eye to the upper side; the skull roof lies on one side, but the other bones keep their positions. Deep sea fishes reduce the skull bones to narrow stripes with the extreme in some Lophiiformes, the anglerfishes. As a whole the teleosts have greater freedom in the variability of the skull bones than lower actinopterygians. The skull bones are tightly sutured to a boxlike skull in lower actinopterygians, whereas many bones in the heads of teleosts are not in close contact with their neighbors. That gives great possibility for differential growth and thus for great diversity in skull shapes of teleosts.

Endocranium

Typically, the main body of the actinopterygian endocranium is formed by the otic and orbitotemporal regions, with the occipital and ethmoidal regions being short additions to the posterior and anterior ends, respectively. The occipital region is limited anteriorly by the occipital fissure (fig. 5.5D), which is completely uninterrupted in primitive actinopterygians. The fissure is confluent dorsally with the posterior dorsal fontanelle, and extends latero-ventrally into the vestibular fontanelle and the ventral otic fissure. Thus, the dorsal extent of the occipital region is abbreviated (fig. 5.4D), but its ventral component is long (fig. 5.7D). The ventral surface is concave to house the dorsal aorta. The vagus nerve (cranial nerve X) exits from the occipital fissure.

The otico-orbitotemporal region is formed by a single ossification in primitive actinopterygians (Gardiner 1984b), but by many separate ossifications in advanced actinopterygians, especially teleosts (Patterson 1975). The epihyal (hyomandibular) articulates in an oblique facet anterior and dorsal to the jugular groove in primitive actinopterygians, whereas its position is horizontal in advanced actinopterygians. The spiracle runs in a groove from the oticosphenoid fissure to the cranial roof in front of the lateral commissure and opens on the surface in primitive actinopterygians, whereas it is enclosed in a canal and ends blind in advanced actinopterygians; it is bounded anteriorly by the postorbital process. The lateral commissure forms the lateral wall of the trigemino-facialis chamber and is penetrated by the jugular canal. The jugular canal and the canals for the branches of the facial (cranial nerve VII) and trigeminal (cranial nerve $V_{2,3}$) nerves open in the posterior orbital wall. Except in primitive actinopterygians, the posterior myodome enters the posterior orbital wall. The openings for the optic, oculomotor, and trochlear nerves (cranial nerves II–IV, respectively) open adjacent to, and near the back of, the medial wall of the orbit. The left and right orbits are separated by a narrow median wall.

Dorsally, an anterior dorsal fontanelle may be present as an extension of the pineal foramen (fig. 5.4D). The endolymphatic duct has a blind end in the otic region, but Gardiner (1984b) described an opening for the endolymphatic duct in the posterior dorsal fontanelle in one Devonian actinopterygian. Fossae bridgei—characteristic for advanced actinopterygians—are absent in primitive actinopterygians (fig. 5.4D). They can connect with the lateral cranial cavities which house a hemopoietic organ. In advanced actinopterygians there is a posttemporal fossa that is separated from, or confluent with, the fossa bridgei.

The basisphenoid surrounds the pituitary fossa laterally and ventrally. The pituitary fossa opens via a large foramen in the parasphenoid in primitive actinopterygians (fig. 5.7D). A basipterygoid process that articulates with the palatoquadrate is present. The oticosphenoid fissure separates the ventro-dorsal portion of the basisphenoid from the lateral commissure in Devonian actinopterygians (Gardiner 1984b).

The ethmoid region is perichondrally ossified in primitive actinopterygians, and bears many canals for nerves and blood vessels. On its posterior wall, the ethmoid bears two pairs of anterior myodomes, one dorsal and one ventral to the olfactory nerve canal (fig. 5.5D). The nasal capsule is surrounded by a thin perichondral ossification in actinopterygians, whereas additional endoskeletal ossifications occur in teleosts.

Visceral Skeleton

The endoskeletal mandibular arch is formed primitively by two elements (fig. 5.6D), the palatoquadrate (= upper jaw) and Meckel's cartilage (= lower jaw). The palatoquadrate bears two articulations with the neurocranium: (1) an ethmoidal articulation (between autopalatine and lateral ethmoid), which becomes double in higher actinopterygians, and (2) a palatobasal articulation (between the basal process of metapterygoid and basipterygoid process), which is lost in advanced actinopterygians. The palatoquadrate of advanced actinopterygians ossifies from three centers— the halecostomian autopalatine, metapterygoid, and quadrate. It is invested medially by two series of dermal bones; the outer series is composed of the vomer, dermopalatines, and ectopterygoid, and the inner series is constituted by the endopterygoid (= pterygoid) and tooth plates fused to the metapterygoid, the so-called dermometapterygoid. The lateral dermal cover is composed of the premaxilla, maxilla, infraorbitals, preopercular, dermohyal, and quadratojugal (fig. 5.2C). In advanced actinopterygians, the bones of the cheek region are reduced such that only soft tissue covers the space between the infraorbitals and preopercle, which is associated with the opercular series. The premaxilla and maxilla are mobile.

The condyle of the quadrate articulates in the glenoid fossa of the posterior end (articular) of Meckel's cartilage. In addition to the two Meckelian ossifications, there is a third ossification (the retroarticular) in advanced actinopterygians; in the latter, the retroarticular and angular can take part in the formation of the glenoid fossa. The tooth-bearing bone of actinopterygians, the dentalosplenial, carries the mandibular canal, and therefore represents the dentary + splenial + postsplenial of crossopterygians. The angular and surangular (lost in advanced actinopterygians) lie posterior to the dentalosplenial. The surangular is not a canal-bearing bone as in crossopterygians. The number of coronoids dorsal to Meckel's cartilage varies from many in primitive actinopterygians to none in advanced taxa.

The jaw articulation is primitively placed below the posterior part of the skull. Palaeonisciforms possess an oblique suspensorium; it means that the postero-dorsal margin of the palatoquadrate reaches from the postero-ventrally placed jaw articulation antero-dorsally to the region behind the orbit. The oblique preopercle (fig. 5.2C) follows the postero-dorsal margin of the palatoquadrate. The postero-ventral position of the jaw articulation results in a wide gape of the mouth. The jaws are shortened and placed behind the orbit in Acipenseriformes, resulting in a ventral mouth as in sharks. In Ginglymodi, the jaw articulation lies in front of the orbit, and the dentalosplenial is differently elongated depending on the species. Elongation of premaxilla, sometimes together with elongation of maxilla, and of dentalosplenial can be found in some lower actinopterygians (e.g., *Saurichthys,* aspidorhynchids) and in different teleosts (e.g., Belonidae, needle-fishes). In some cases the upper jaw is more elongated than the lower jaw (e.g., Xiphidae, swordfishes; Istiophoridae, billfishes), whereas in others only the lower jaw is elongated (Hemiramphidae, halfbeaks). In very few forms is the jaw articulation placed far behind the head so that the mouth becomes very large (Saccopharyngidae, swallowers) or enormous (Eurypharyngidae, gulpers); in the latter case the jaws are six to eight times the length of the neurocranium. In contrast, the jaws can be small in many teleosts, as in Syngnathidae where small premaxillae, maxillae, and dentalosplenials lie far anteriorly at the end of an elongated snout. The maxillae are free from the cheek bones in halecostomes so that the jaws could differentiate widely, especially in teleosts. This is one reason, if not the main one, for the explosive radiation of teleosts. In many ostariophysans and neoteleosts, the premaxillae become movable and protrusible, giving these teleosts further feeding advantages (Alexander 1967).

The hyoid arch and four branchial arches articulate with a long, unpaired basibranchial (fig. 5.8C). The fifth branchial arch is reduced (merely a ceratobranchial in Devonian actinopterygians) in primitive actinopterygians; in advanced actinopterygians, the branchial arches are reduced further in posterior-to-anterior direction. The epihyal (= hyomandibula) and interhyal form the dorsal portion of the hyoid arch; the symplectic connects the epihyal with the quadrate in advanced actinopterygians. The epihyal articulates with the endocranium. Of the posterior branchial arches, the first infrapharyngobranchial articulates with the neurocranium, whereas the other pharyngobranchials (supra- and infrapharyngobranchials) are connected to the neurocranium via connective tissue only. Tooth plates on the branchial arches are often more important for mastication than the teeth on the jaws in advanced actinopterygians. The urohyal, a tendon bone, is known only in advanced actinopterygians (Arratia and Schultze 1990).

The operculogular series forms a continuous series from the dorso-lateral opercle to the subopercle, branchiostegals, and the medio-ventral gular (figs. 5.2C, 5.10A). Gulars are lost in advanced actinopterygians.

Development

The development of the skull and visceral skeleton of many actinopterygian taxa has been described (cf. de Beer 1937, for a review). There are many similarities in the development of the endocranium and cartilaginous visceral skeleton of actinopterygians and elasmobranchs. The appearance of the paired parachordals is followed by that of the trabeculae cranii and polar cartilages (fig. 5.11A). The trabeculae extend anteriorly as laminae orbitonasales and fuse to form a median plate. Unlike elasmobranchs, in actinopterygians the occipital arch chondrifies separately (fig. 5.11B) dorsal to the notochord and posterior to the parachordals; the arch grows antero-dorsally to fuse dorsally with the auditory capsules. The separate chondrification of the occipital arch and its late inclusion into the cartilaginous neurocranium may explain the presence of an otico-occipital fissure in actinopterygians. Each auditory capsule appears as a separate cartilage above the parachordal (fig. 5.11A), and subsequently fuses with the parachordal (fig. 5.11B). The orbital cartilage appears later in actinopterygians than in elasmobranchs, and is represented either by an isolated element or by an outgrowth of the antero-dorsal corner of the auditory capsule (fig. 5.11C). Ossification of the endocranium proceeds in a posterior-to-anterior direction (i.e., from the occipital region forward).

Chondrification of the visceral skeleton proceeds in an anterior-to-

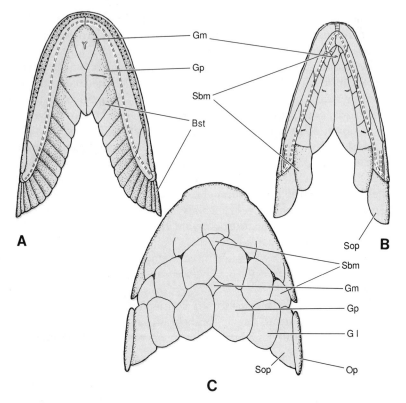

Fig. 5.10. Gular region of osteichthyans. A. Palaeonisciform actinopterygian *Moythomasia nitida* Gross (after Jessen 1968, fig. 1C). B. Osteolepiform crossopterygian *Eusthenopteron foordi* Whiteaves (after Jarvik 1980, fig. 121C). C. Dipnoan *Speonesydrion iani* Campbell and Barwick (after Campbell and Barwick 1984b, fig. 26).

posterior direction (from the mandibular arch to the posterior branchial arches) and from distal to proximal; thus the lateral elements appear before the medial elements (hypohyals, basihyal, basibranchials). The symplectic forms as an antero-ventral extension of the epihyal, and later separates from this element. Ossification of the cartilage starts later than the formation of dermal bones (compare fig. 5.11B with 5.11C, D).

The first dermal bones to appear are those associated with feeding. Teeth appear prior to the formation of their bony base. The appearance of the dentalosplenial is followed by that of the maxilla, and the premaxilla, parasphenoid, dermopalatine, and vomer shortly thereafter (fig. 5.11G). The ectopterygoid appears later (fig. 5.11H). Early in ontogeny, many other dermal bones form in association with the sensory-line system (fig. 5.11E, F). Single sensory-line bones originate from a few distinct nu-

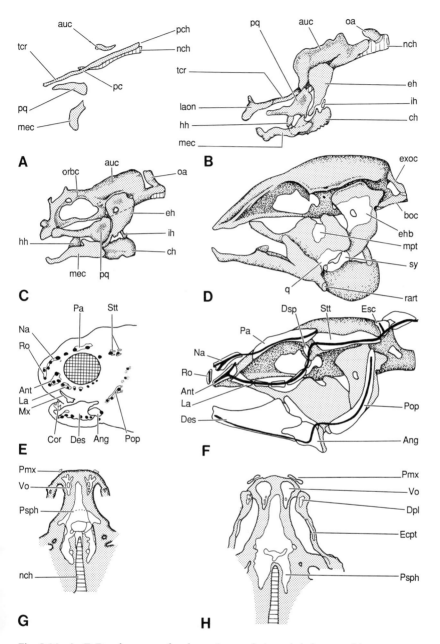

Fig. 5.11. A–F. Development of endocranium and visceral skeleton and its ossifications in *Amia calva* Linné in lateral view (simplified after Pehrson 1922, 1940). A. 8–8.8 mm length. B. 10–11 mm length. C. 13.6–14.0 mm length. D. 13.8 mm length, beginning ossification of cartilage. E. 31.5–34.5 mm length, appearance of dermal bones. F. 31.5–34.5 mm length, formation of sensory-line bones. G–H. Formation of palatal bones in *Amia calva* Linné in ventral view (simplified after Pehrson 1940); G, 10.4 mm length; H, 12.0 mm length.

clei associated with blastema related to neuromasts. These nuclei fuse together into a single bone without leaving a trace of the fusion; this process
has been described in different actinopterygians by Pehrson (1940, 1944,
1958).

SARCOPTERYGII

Monophyly and Relationship to Other Groups

Primitive dipnoans and crossopterygians (i.e., actinistians, rhipidistians,
and tetrapods; table 5.3) possess the following advanced features in common (Maisey 1986; Schultze 1987): (1) true enamel as their superficial
layer on scales and bones; (2) cosmine, a combination of enamel and
dentine with pore-canal system; (3) sclerotic ring with more than five
plates; (4) single broad basibranchial; (5) series of submandibular plates;
(6) articulation of epihyal straddling jugular canal; (7) epi- and interhyal
decoupled from hyoid bar; and (8) postcranial features. "True" enamel
and cosmine occur in the most primitive actinistian (Cloutier 1991a),
whereas cosmine is lost in all other actinistians, many lineages of rhipidistians, and tetrapods, and within dipnoans. The pore-canal system, a
specialized sensory (but not electroreceptive [Borgen 1989 contra Thomson
1975]) system within cosmine, occurs in only one group besides sarcopterygians. In this group, the cephalaspid agnathans, the pore-canal system is morphologically distinct and found in mesodentine and bone (Gross
1956; Schultze 1969) rather than in dentine and enamel. Another feature
is the "urohyal" that is preformed in cartilage; within actinopterygians, a
dermal urohyal is restricted to teleosts (Arratia and Schultze 1990 contra
Gardiner 1984b).

Both actinopterygians and sarcopterygians possess a superficial layer
of hard tissue derived from the epidermis on their scales and bones, and a
macromeric bone pattern. The "ectodermal enamel" of osteichthyans has
a surface pattern distinct (Schultze 1977) from that of actinopterygians
(ganoine with tubercles derived from the center of basal epidermal cells)
and sarcopterygians ("true" or "tetrapod-like" enamel with hexagonal impressions of the prismatic boundaries of basal epidermal cells). "Ectodermal enamel" as formation of the basal epidermal layer is a primitive
feature of osteichthyans, but the difference between the surface of ganoine
and "true" enamel is phylogenetically significant for both groups (contra
Smith 1989) and should indicate a difference in deposition of the crystallites in both tissues. Even though the hard tissue and the bone pattern are
different in both groups, it cannot be decided which formation of both
features in both groups is primitive and which advanced, because the out-
group does not possess either one. The dermal bone pattern on the head

differs among groups of sarcopterygians. On the cheek, the sarcopterygians possess the primitive connection (jugal canal) between the preopercle and infraorbital canal as in acanthodians, but they lack the connection between the preopercle and main lateral-line canal that is present in actinopterygians and acanthodians. Both actinopterygians and sarcopterygians are advanced in comparison to acanthodians, and their sister-group relationship generally is accepted.

Exocranium

Dipnoans and crossopterygians have distinct exocranial patterns. From the bone mosaic of primitive dipnoans (*Diabolepis, Uranolophus, Dipnorhynchus*) and crossopterygians (*Miguashaia, Powichthys*), the typical exocranial pattern of each group was developed in derived representatives. In dipnoans (fig. 5.3C), paired I-bones were established first, anterior to the five extrascapulars (two Z-, two H-, and one A-bone); these were followed by paired J-bones and a median, unpaired B-bone. In more derived taxa, the B-bone was enlarged and came to separate the I-bones, and large anterior bones appeared. In crossopterygians (fig. 5.3D), paired postparietals anterior to three extrascapulars were established first (fig. 5.1E); the postparietals extended to the intracranial joint, in front of which the parietals developed. In both dipnoans and crossopterygians, the number of lateral skull-roof bones carrying the lateral line is greater in primitive taxa than in advanced taxa. The main lateral line is forked into infraorbital and the supraorbital lines in early forms of both groups. Dipnoans have more (10 or more) bones in a short cheek region than do crossopterygians (8 or fewer). The maxilla and premaxilla are absent in dipnoans; among crossopterygians, the maxilla is absent in actinistians. The pattern of the skull-roof, cheek, and jaw bones evolved independently in dipnoans and crossopterygians from a mosaic of bones so that comparison between the pattern of advanced forms in both groups is not possible (compare fig. 5.3C with 5.3D).

Endocranium

There are more differences than similarities in the endocrania of dipnoans and crossopterygians. The dipnoan endocranium (fig. 5.5E) is a single unit to which the palatoquadrate is fused; in crossopterygians (fig. 5.5F), the ventral fissure extends dorsally to form an intracranial joint, thereby separating the endocranium into two separate units. The otico-occipital fissure is closed perichondrally in dipnoans, partially closed in rhipidistians, and is represented as a suture in actinistians. The openings of the endolymphatic ducts in the dorsal endocranium of primitive dipnoans may be homologous to the posterior fontanelle present in crossopterygians. The ventro-lateral part (vestibular fontanelle) of the otico-occipital fissure is open in rhipidistians, but closed in dipnoans. There is no aortic canal on the ventral side of the occipital region as in actinopterygians because the dorsal aorta bifurcates behind the occiput in sarcopterygians. A supraoccipital is present in crossopterygians, but not in dipnoans.

On the postero-dorsal surface of the otic region there are paired posttemporal fossae with axial musculature in crossopterygians (fig. 5.4F); structures in the same region in dipnoans (fig. 5.4E) carry adductor muscles and are not homologous to the fossae in crossopterygians. In crossopterygians and advanced dipnoans, the hyomandibular facet is double and straddles the jugular canal on the lateral side of the otic region; the facet is single in primitive dipnoans. The lateral commissure is not clearly visible in dipnoans because the palatoquadrate is fused to the lateral side of the endocranium. The ventral fissure has a posterior portion in dipnoans and advanced actinopterygians. However, in crossopterygians the fissure gives rise to an intracranial joint (fig. 5.5F).

Endochondral ossification extends into the ethmoidal region in sarcopterygians, and a rich canal system is found in the snout of primitive members of the group. Two pairs of anterior myodomes occur below the olfactory nerve canal in some crossopterygians, but not in dipnoans.

Visceral Skeleton

The upper part of the mandibular arch, the palatoquadrate, is fused to the endocranium in dipnoans (fig. 5.6E), but free in crossopterygians (fig. 5.6F). Thus, only the quadrate can be identified in dipnoans. In contrast, three palatoquadrate ossification centers are identifiable in some crossopterygians (actinistians), but primitively, there is only one large ossification. In crossopterygians, the palatoquadrate bears four endocranial articulations (figs. 5.5F, 5.6F): (1) an ethmoidal articulation between the autopalatine and ethmoid (may become divided into two articulations); (2) the palatobasal articulation between the basal and basipterygoid processes; (3) the postorbital articulation between the ascending and suprapterygoid processes; and (4) the paratemporal articulation behind the intracranial joint. Additional articulations occur in some crossopterygians.

The lingual and buccal dermal covers of the palatoquadrate differ in dipnoans and crossopterygians; the only palatal similarity shared is the presence of a parasphenoid and pterygoids in both groups. Except in the most primitive dipnoans (*Diabolepis, Uranolophus*), the parasphenoid lies posterior below the otico-occipital region of the endocranium, whereas in crossopterygians, it lies anterior below the ethmosphenoid.

Meckel's cartilage ossifies as a single unit in dipnoans, whereas it arises from two ossification centers that give rise to the anterior mentomeckelian bone and posterior articular bone in crossopterygians. Both groups possess a prearticular on the medial surface of Meckel's cartilage, but other mandibular bones are difficult to compare. Coronoids and dentary occur in crossopterygians (fig. 5.2E), but not in dipnoans (fig. 5.2D). The infradentaries (splenial to surangular of crossopterygians, or "splenial" to "surangular" of dipnoans) have different relations to sensory lines in both groups; whereas dipnoans have a fully developed oral canal, crossopterygians do not. The mandibular canal passes through the angular to the splenial in crossopterygians, whereas both the mandibular and oral canals pass through the "angular" to the "splenial" in dipnoans.

The branchial skeleton is reduced in extant sarcopterygians, but in those fossil forms in which a branchial skeleton is known, it is well developed. The hyoid arch is formed by the hypohyal, ceratohyal, and epihyal in dipnoans (fig. 5.8D), whereas crossopterygians (fig. 5.8E) possess an additional interhyal. The epihyal (hyomandibular) articulates with the endocranium via one head in primitive dipnoans, but via two heads (as in crossopterygians) in advanced dipnoans. In the following arches, hypo- and pharyngobranchials occur only in crossopterygians. The median ventral series is composed of only a few elements: one basibranchial in porolepiforms and dipnoans, and two basibranchials in osteolepiforms. An elongated, antero-median element is interpreted as a sublingual in osteolepiforms, but it is thought to represent a sublingual and first basibranchial in dipnoans (Miles 1977). Presence of a "urohyal" preformed in cartilage is common to both groups (Arratia and Schultze 1990).

The operculogular series varies in size but not composition. The submandibulars are broad in dipnoans (fig. 5.10C), but narrow in osteolepiforms (fig. 5.10B); submandibulars are unknown in actinistians.

DIPNOI

Monophyly and Relationship to Other Groups

The dipnoans are a distinct group of osteichthyans having many unique features (Schultze and Campbell 1987). The bone patterns of the skull-roof (fig. 5.3C), cheek (fig. 5.2D), and lower jaw (fig. 5.2D) are so different that a separate system of nomenclature developed by Forster-Cooper (1937) and Jarvik (1967) is applied here. The palate is uniquely characterized by broad pterygoids that occasionally are flanked by small bones and incurrent and excurrent nasal openings. These, along with many other features, distinguish dipnoans from all other gnathostomes.

Within sarcopterygians, the dipnoans are considered to be either the sister group of crossopterygians (e.g., Schultze 1987) or porolepiform rhipidistians (Maisey 1986; Chang 1991). In support of the former hypothesis, all crossopterygians possess (1) an intracranial joint, (2) three extrascapulars, and (3) a double-headed hyomandibula, whereas dipnoans possess their own suite of synapomorphies. Proponents of a sister-group relationship between dipnoans and porolepiforms argue that *Diabolepis* (an Early Devonian osteichthyan from China with premaxillae and external nasal openings; Chang and Yu 1984) and *Youngolepis* (a primitive rhipidistian or primitive porolepiform from the early Devonian) possess three uniquely shared derived characters: (1) rostral tubuli, (2) an immobilized intracranial joint, and (3) cosmine pore-canal structure (Maisey 1986) and Westoll lines. It should be pointed out that the presence of rostral tubuli is not known in all taxa, immobilization of the intracranial joint occurs independently in tetrapods, and cosmine is a primitive feature for all sarcopterygians.

Exocranium

In contrast to Devonian dipnoans, the three extant dipnoan genera have reduced exocrania and cartilaginous endocrania. Possession of median, unpaired bones that are flanked by two series of paired bones is a characteristic feature of dipnoans.

The skull-roof of primitive dipnoans is covered with numerous bones in addition to the bone mosaic of the snout. All dipnoans possess an unpaired, median B-bone that is surrounded by paired I-, J-, and C-bones (figs. 5.1D, 5.3C). The lateral-line bones lie laterally adjacent to these bones, and the occipital commissure passes through (the H-bones in *Uranolophus, Speonesydrion,* and *Dipnorhynchus*) the I-bones and bone A behind bone B. In advanced dipnoans, the number of bones is reduced and the occipital commissure passes from I- to I-bone through bone B, or posterior to the skull-roof bones, as in the extant Australian lungfish, *Neoceratodus.* The relation between skull-roof bones and lateral-line canals is lost completely in the extant African, *Protopterus,* and South American lungfish, *Lepidosiren.* In *Neoceratodus,* the skull-roof is covered by two median bones taking the spaces of bones B + C and E + F respectively, flanked by a bone occupying the area of bones I + J + K, and a lateral bone representing bones X + Y. The skull-roof bones of *Protopterus* and *Lepidosiren* cannot be homologized with those of *Neoceratodus* except for bones E + F; bones appear in two levels, a pair of superficial bones and two paired bones on the neurocranium which Holmgren and Stensiö (1936) interpreted as cartilaginous bones, not dermal skull-roof bones. The lateral one occupies the position of a quadrate. As in primitive actinopterygians, the supraorbital sensory canal does not connect to the main lateral line in the most primitive dipnoans; it ends in J, whereas it meets the main lateral line in bone X in all other dipnoans in which the infraorbital branches off in bone X. The infraorbital canal passes through a series (4, 5, 6, 7, 1) of circumorbital bones before it reaches the snout (fig. 5.2D). The infraorbital bones, 4, 5, 6 + 7, and 1, are developed in *Neoceratodus;* they do not suture with each other. They are missing in *Protopterus* and *Lepidosiren*. A maxilla and a separate premaxilla are not developed. In bone 5, the jugal canal branches off and continues as the preopercular canal through a series of small bones to reach the lower jaw as the mandibular canal. The series of small bones is present in *Neoceratodus,* but the bones are separated from each other, whereas they are lacking in *Protopterus* and *Lepidosiren*. The mandibular canals of both sides meet below the symphysis of the lower jaw between their connections with the oral canal in the dorsal portion of the lower jaw. The lateral aspect of the skull (cheek, fig. 5.2D), like the skull roof, poses nomenclatural problems; therefore, a numbered system of bone identification was introduced by Forster-Cooper (1937). The snout is ossified as a block (Devonian taxa) or formed in soft tissue (Late Devonian and Post-Devonian taxa).

Endocranium

The endocranium and the palatoquadrate form a single unit. If one accepts *Diabolepis* as a dipnoan or the sister taxon of all other dipnoans, the fusion of the palatoquadrate and endocranium is a synapomorphy of all dipnoans above *Diabolepis,* and the following characterization refers to the latter taxa. The exocranium sits on crests of the otic region, and is fused to the endocranium in the snout region (fig. 5.4E). The snout region is drained by an extensively developed vascular system (Campbell and Barwick 1987) and ossified in Devonian forms; it is unossified in some Late Devonian and all post-Devonian dipnoans. The nasal capsule is not enclosed in the ethmoidal region; the ethmoid forms the roof of the nasal capsule only. The sphenoid region is continuous with the otic region, there being no indication of a fissure between the two. Campbell and Barwick (1982) identified separate ossifications for the ventral, posterior, and lateral otic, and for the quadrate in an Early Devonian dipnoan. The hyomandibula has a single attachment to the lateral otic in Early Devonian dipnoans (Campbell and Barwick 1982, 1987), and a double attachment in Late Devonian forms (Miles 1977). The opening of the ductus endolymphaticus on the roof of the otic region (fig. 5.4E) is a primitive feature of Devonian dipnoans that also occurs in placoderms and chondrichthyans, but not in extant dipnoans. Similarly, the buccohypophysial canal opens on the ventral side of the sphenoid region (fig. 5.7E) in Devonian dipnoans, but not in extant dipnoans. The strong adductor musculature originates from spaces between the crests on the roof of the otic region (Luther 1913; Miles 1977; Campbell and Barwick 1987, fig. 19). A trace of the otico-occipital fissure marks the division between the occipital and otic regions (fig. 5.5E). The occipital region is short in Devonian dipnoans, but posteriorly lengthened along with the parasphenoid in extant forms.

Visceral Skeleton

Because the palatoquadrate is fused to the neurocranium, only the quadrate can be identified with certainty. The medial and lateral dermal covers of the palatoquadrate differ from those of other osteichthyans except for the pterygoid and parasphenoid, which are the same as in other osteichthyans. The parasphenoid is an elongate element that lies between the pterygoids in the Early Devonian genus *Uranolophus* (Denison 1968; Schultze 1992), whereas in most other dipnoan genera it is a short, plow-shaped bone that lies posterior to the pterygoids. The elements lateral to the anterior part of the pterygoids cannot be homologized directly with bones in other osteichthyans (Campbell and Barwick 1984a; contra Rosen et al. 1981); both nasal openings, incurrent and excurrent, lie between these bones.

Meckel's cartilage ossifies as a single piece in primitive dipnoans. The medial side of the cartilage is covered only by the prearticular. Coronoids and marginal dentary teeth are absent. The external side (fig. 5.2D) is formed by lateral-line-bearing bones which may or may not be comparable with those of other osteichthyans (Jarvik 1967; Campbell and Barwick 1984a).

A median, unpaired element of the branchial skeleton extends far forward between the lower jaws. This element is thought to represent the sublingual and basibranchial (fig. 5.8D) by Miles (1977) based on comparison with the osteolepiform *Eusthenopteron* (fig. 5.8E); a second median element lies posteriorly adjacent to the anterior bone. The hypohyal, a broad ceratohyal, and short epihyal form the hyoid arch in the dipnoan *Griphognathus*. The posteriorly adjacent four branchial arches lack hypobranchials, and their dorsal portions consist only of epibranchials. A "urohyal" that is preformed in cartilage articulates with the anterior median element.

The operculogular series is formed by large plates, as is the submandibular series (fig. 5.10C).

Development

The development of the endocranium and visceral skeleton of *Neoceratodus* and lepidosirenids has been described in detail (Fox 1965; Bertmar 1966). Endocranial chondrification is marked by the appearance of trabeculae cranii, and the mandibular, hyoid, and first two branchial arches. From its initial appearance, the parachordal cartilage is connected with the anterior and posterior portions of the auditory capsule and orbital cartilage via the acrochordal cartilage. The trabeculae are free initially, and only later become connected with the orbital and acrochordal plates, at which stage they are fused to form the trabecular plate. The orbital cartilage and auditory capsule fuse early in ontogeny. The palatoquadrate forms an additional bridge between the two parts of the endocranium. Via fusions of the basal, ascending, and otic processes of the palatoquadrate with the endocranium, a single endocranial unit is established early in ontogeny. The nasal capsule is surrounded dorsally by processes of the trabeculae cranii—viz., the lateral (trabecular horn), dorsal (taenia lateroethmoidalis), and postero-lateral (processes ectethmoideus) processes. Posterior to the palatoquadrate, the lateral commissure appears as a discrete cartilage, as does the epihyal subsequently; both fuse with the endocranium eventually. Concomitant with the fusion of the orbital cartilage and auditory capsule, branchial arches 3–5 chondrify. Subsequent developments results, first, in separation of the epi- and ceratobranchials, followed by appearance of the basihyal, hypohyals, and a precardial cartilage.

As in actinopterygians, the early appearance of dermal bones is associated with feeding. A premaxilla and maxilla do not occur in dipnoans; thus, the first dermal elements that appear are the vomerine teeth, pterygoids, and parasphenoid, followed by the prearticular and "dentary." The first paired and unpaired skull-roof bones appear when the endocranial roof already is partially closed. The opercle and subopercle appear contemporaneously with the latter.

CROSSOPTERYGII

Monophyly and Relationship to Other Groups

The monophyly of the crossopterygians (including tetrapods) is controversial; Schultze (1987) favored this hypothesis, whereas Rosen et al. (1981) and Maisey (1986) opposed it. Schultze (1987) cited three synapomorphies for crossopterygians (table 5.3): (1) intracranial joint, (2) three extrascapulars, and (3) double-headed hyomandibula. The presence of an intracranial joint between the sphenoid and otic regions is a derived feature of actinistians, onychodontiforms, porolepiforms, and osteolepiforms. Roček (1986) reported that some embryonic lissamphibians develop a precursor to it, but adult tetrapods do not possess an intracranial joint. Among youngolepid, primitive porolepiforms, an intracranial joint is absent in *Youngolepis,* but present in *Powichthys.* Dipnoans show no embryonic indication of an intracranial joint, and it also is missing in *Diabolepis.* Three extrascapulars occur in primitive actinistians, onychodontiforms, porolepiforms, and osteolepiforms; tetrapods lack extrascapulars, and primitively, dipnoans possess five. The presence of a double-headed hyomandibula is a homoplastic character of advanced dipnoans (Campbell and Barwick 1987).

Accepting crossopterygians as a monophyletic group (table 5.3), the tetrapods are included as the sister group of osteolepiform or panderich-thyiform crossopterygians (Schultze 1987; Panchen and Smithson 1987, but they exclude actinistians from crossopterygians). One external nasal opening combined with an internal opening (choana) on the palate is known only in these three groups, whereas both incurrent and excurrent nasal openings occur on the palate of dipnoans. The latter situation differs from that of tetrapods, and is derived independently from the choana in osteolepiforms and tetrapods, because *Diabolepis,* the closest sister group of dipnoans, still possesses two external nasal openings (Chang and Yu 1984). Maisey (1986) and Chang (1991) considered dipnoans to be the sister group of porolepiforms within crossopterygians based on similarities between *Diabolepis* and *Youngolepis,* the most primitive porolepiform. Only a few features support such an arrangement (e.g., immobilization of intracranial joint, which is only partly correct, because an intracranial joint is present in *Powichthys* [sister taxon of *Youngolepis*], whereas such a joint occurs in parallel in tetrapods), and the arrangement requires many reversals.

Exocranium

The skull-roof of crossopterygians most closely resembles that of tetrapods, having paired postparietals carrying the middle and posterior pit lines, and paired parietals surrounding the pineal foramen and carrying the supraorbital canal (fig. 5.3D). Paired frontals are formed only in pan-derichthyid crossopterygians, which are related most closely to tetrapods (Schultze and Arsenault 1985). In early crossopterygians, as in dipnoans, the snout is covered by many large plates. The posterior margin of the skull is formed by an uneven number of large extrascapulars (three, secondarily increased in advanced actinistians). The tabular and supratemporal flank the postparietals, and the intertemporal and supraorbitals (= postfrontal and prefrontal of primitive tetrapods) flank the parietals. Some crossoptery-gians possess an extratemporal suturing the tabular postero-laterally. The main lateral-line canal passes through the tabular, supratemporal, and in-tertemporal; in the latter, the canal divides into the supraorbital and infra-orbital canals. Posterior passage of the supraorbital canal into the parietal and postparietal as occurs in early actinopterygians and early dipnoans is unknown in crossopterygians. The postorbital jugal and squamosal sur-round the orbit posteriorly and ventrally, whereas the supraorbitals (post- and prefrontals of tetrapods) surround it dorsally and anteriorly. The orbita is small in adults, and the eyeball is covered with a ring built of many sclerotic bones so that the eye appears small. Most crossopterygians (i.e., actinistians, onychodontiforms, porolepiforms) possess two external nasal openings; osteolepiforms and panderichthyiforms have only one. In the latter, the functional second opening, like the choana of tetrapods, lies inside the mouth on the palate surrounded by the premaxilla, maxilla, vomer, and dermopalatine. The supraorbital line passes medially to the external nasal openings rather than between them as in actinopterygians. A series of bones (tectals) that do not bear canals lies lateral to the nasals and dorsal to the nostril(s).

The cheek region is movably connected to the skull roof. The spiracular slit opens between the tabular and squamosal. The squamosal with its jugular pitline is a typical crossopterygian bone (fig. 5.2E); porolepiforms and onychodontiforms possess two or more squamosals. The preopercular canal that originates from the infraorbital canal in the jugal passes through the squamosal to the preoperculum into the lower jaw. The quadratojugal separates the maxilla from the preoperculum. Only in some panderichthyiforms does the quadratojugal contact the jugal, thereby separating the squamosal from the maxilla, as in tetrapods. Coelacanths, the only crossopterygians surviving until today, are conservative during their evolutionary history. The rate of morphological changes decreases markedly in late Paleozoic time, and stays nearly constant afterward until today (Schaeffer 1952; Cloutier 1991b). The cheek region of the extant coelacanth *Latimeria* shows main differences to Paleozoic forms in the reduction of the size of the cheek bones. The bones do not articulate with each other anymore, but are separated by skin from each other.

The outside of the lower jaw is formed by a tooth-bearing dentary and four infradentaries (surangular, angular, postsplenial, and splenial) which carry the mandibular canal. A short oral canal may branch off in the surangular. The inside of the lower jaw is invested by the prearticular, which is separated dorsally from the dentary by three coronoids. The coronoids bear teeth that are larger than those on the dentary and prearticular. The teeth are covered by enamel.

Endocranium

The endocranium of crossopterygians is divided into two units by the intracranial joint, a dorsal extension of the ventral fissure (fig. 5.5F). A pair of subcephalic muscles joins the endocranial units. The palatoquadrate bridges the intracranial joint to articulate with the ethmosphenoid and otic regions. An intracranial joint occurs in actinistians, onychodontiforms, porolepiforms, and osteolepiforms. In the primitive porolepiform *Youngolepis,* an intracranial joint is absent (Chang 1982), but it is present in the sister genus *Powichthys* (Jessen 1980). The joint is thought to fuse during development in tetrapods (Roček 1986).

The nasal capsule in actinistians and onychodontiforms has two external openings that are lateral or dorso-lateral in position. The posterior opening is part of a larger ventro-lateral or ventral endocranial fenestra in porolepiforms, osteolepiforms (fig. 5.7F), panderichthyiforms, and tetrapods. In porolepiforms, the posterior external nasal opening corresponds to the dorsal portion of the ventro-lateral endocranial fenestra, whereas the choana in the three latter groups is an opening of the ventral portion of the ventro-lateral endocranial fenestra. This implies origin of the choana independent from the posterior external nasal opening (Jarvik 1942, 1981 versus Schmalhausen 1968 and Rosen et al. 1981). In actinistians, a cavity with three external openings (rostral organ, possibly an electrosensory organ) lies above the nasal capsule. In all crossopterygians, including primitive tetrapods, there is a buccohypophyseal opening on the ventral side (fig. 5.7F), and a pineal/parietal foramen on the dorsal side (fig. 5.4F) of the sphenoid region.

The optic, oculomotor, and trochlear nerves (cranial nerves II–IV, respectively) exit the neurocranium from the posterior part of the sphenoid region anterior to the ascending process of the palatoquadrate. The palatoquadrate articulates with the ethmosphenoid via three processes—viz., the autopalatinal attachment, and the basal and ascending processes (fig. 5.5F). The trigeminal nerve (cranial nerve $V_{2,3}$) opens either in the posterior sphenoid region (e.g., the primitive porolepiform *Powichthys;* Jessen 1980), in the intracranial fissure (e.g., the primitive porolepiform *Youngolepis;* Chang 1982) or joint (e.g., actinistians; Jarvik 1980), or in the anterior otic region (fig. 5.5F, osteolepiforms; Jarvik 1980).

The notochord extends anteriorly beneath the posterior endocranial unit (the otico-occipital) in the notochordal pit of the postero-ventral end of the ethmosphenoid. The ventral part of the otic region extends anteriorly, lateral to the sphenoid region, and articulates with the processus connectens. The palatoquadrate articulates with the anterior otic region at the paratemporal process. The hyomandibula has two dorsal heads which articulate with two grooves on the lateral commissure of the otic region above and below the groove for the jugular vein. The epaxial musculature extends dorsally anterior into the posttemporal fossa, which is bounded laterally by the crista parotica (fig. 5.4F). The posttemporal fossa seems to have evolved independently in different groups because it is missing in primitive actinistians and primitive porolepiforms such as *Youngolepis* (Chang 1982), but present in advanced actinistians, porolepiforms, and osteolepiforms. The dorsal surface of the otico-occipital is variable within crossopterygians. Thus, it is smooth in primitive actinistians and the porolepiform *Youngolepis,* but bears grooves and ridges in advanced porolepiforms (Jarvik 1980) and a network of grooves for the occipital artery in osteolepiforms (fig. 5.4F). The otico-occipital encloses the mid- and hindbrains, and the otic capsule. In actinistians, the endolymphatic duct opens on the dorsal surface of the otic region; the existence of such a connection in porolepiform or osteolepiforms is disputed. The medial, crescent-shaped fenestra in the osteolepiform *Eusthenopteron* (fig. 5.4F) and the similar fenestra in the primitive porolepiform *Youngolepis* (Chang 1982) are interpreted to be a dorsal opening of a supraotic cavity. The occipital fissure separates the otic and occipital regions in porolepiforms (Chang 1982) and osteolepiforms (fig. 5.5F); the fissure is filled by cartilage in osteolepiforms and obliterated in actinistians. The vagus nerve (cranial nerve X) lies in the occipital fissure.

Visceral Skeleton

Although the palatoquadrate (fig. 5.6F) is formed by one ossification in rhipidistians, it forms from three ossification centers in actinistians except in the most primitive actinistian, *Miguashaia*, as it does in advanced actinopterygians. The metapterygoid and quadrate are connected by cartilage in the Recent actinistian *Latimeria*, and the entopterygoid bridges the gap between the autopalatine and the posterior margin formed by the quadrate and metapterygoid. On the lingual side of the palatoquadrate, the same series of dermal bones (except for the dermometapterygoid that supposedly is present) is formed in crossopterygians as in actinopterygians. In the buccal cover of the palatoquadrate of rhipidistians, the infraorbitals of actinopterygians are termed the lacrimal, jugal, and postorbital; the maxilla is separated from the preopercle by one or more squamosals and the quadratojugal (fig. 5.2E). The jugal separates the maxilla from the squamosal in advanced rhipidistians, panderichthyiforms, and tetrapods (Vorobyeva and Schultze 1991). Actinistians possess a reduced lateral palatoquadrate cover. The jugal and postorbital form the ventral and posterior margin of the orbit; the squamosal, quadratojugal, and preopercle form the cheek region. A maxilla is absent.

Meckel's cartilage ossifies in two portions—the anterior mentomeckelian and posterior articular bones—but forms one unit in adult rhipidistians. Laterally, the rhipidistian jaw is covered by a tooth-bearing dentary and a ventral series of four bones, the surangular, angular, postsplenial, and splenial; the latter carry the mandibular canal, and a short oral canal occurs in the surangular (fig. 5.2E). In actinistians, the series is reduced to two bones, the angular and splenial. Actinistians possess many coronoids (with the posterior one greatly enlarged), whereas rhipidistians, including tetrapods, possess only three.

In the branchial skeleton, the median series varies from one basibranchial (porolepiforms, actinistians) to two (osteolepiforms); there is an additional anterior median sublingual in osteolepiforms (fig. 5.8E). The ceratohyal is ossified in two parts in osteolepiforms, as it is in advanced actinopterygians; it is a bladelike element in porolepiforms. The epihyal (hyomandibula) articulates by two heads with the endocranium in rhipidistians and actinistians. A bone, the so-called symplectic, forms a tandem articulation behind the quadrate with the lower jaw in actinistians. The following branchial arches carry infra- and suprapharyngobranchials on the two first epibranchials in osteolepiforms, as they do in actinopterygians; there is only one epibranchial in actinistians. A median unpaired "urohyal" of cartilaginous origin articulates with the ventral side of the basibranchial.

A series of submandibulars is intercalated between the lower jaw and the operculogular series (fig. 5.10B). In porolepiforms, a few branchiostegals are formed between the subopercle and gular, whereas a larger bone, the submandibulobranchiostegal, lies between the submandibulars and gulars in osteolepiforms. With the exception of the most primitive actinistian, which has a subopercle, actinistians possess only an opercle and a pair of gulars.

Development

Little is known of developmental series in fossil or extant crossopterygians. Juvenile *Latimeria,* the living actinistian, develop intraoviductally from 9 cm eggs to newborns about 42.5 cm long that lack a yolk sac (Millot and Anthony 1974; Smith et al. 1975; Balon et al. 1988). Fossil actinistians are recorded to be ovoviviparous or viviparous (Watson 1927) or oviparous (Schultze 1985; sequence from egg to juveniles with yolk sac to fully developed juveniles of *Rhabdoderma*). Juvenile *Latimeria* have large orbits; orbit size decreases with growth, whereas head length grows isometrically relative to standard length (McAllister and Smith 1978). Similar observations have been published on fossil crossopterygians, in which the size differences of orbit and head length between small juveniles and adults are even more pronounced (Schultze 1984). Juvenile specimens of the osteolepiform *Eusthenopteron* possess large orbits and a short cheek region; bones surrounding the orbit grow in a positively allometric pattern—i.e., they become larger in adult forms, while the orbit is reduced in size. Juvenile *Eusthenopteron* look like primitive actinopterygians (Palaeonisciformes). The same is the case for juvenile onychodontiforms (Jessen 1967: *Strunius*) and porolepiforms (compare Schultze 1973 with Schultze and Arsenault 1987: *Quebecius*).

EVOLUTIONARY TRENDS

Extensive mineralization (calcification or ossification) of endo- and exoskeleton characterizes the basal, Devonian jawed fishes. Though we may miss some unmineralized early forms, there is a trend toward reduced or lack of mineralization in the endo- and exoskeleton in younger forms of each group. This explains why the endoskeleton of Devonian or Late Paleozoic forms can be studied in detail, whereas the endoskeleton is often unknown in younger, extinct forms. Studies of the endoskeleton of more derived fishes must be confined, for the most part, to extant forms because the endoskeleton is made of unmineralized cartilage. As in the phylogenetic history of tetrapods, the number of exoskeletal bones is reduced from Devonian to extant jawed fishes.

Within placoderms, arthrodires exhibit this trend toward a reduced number of exoskeletal bones during the Devonian (Miles 1969: development from actinolepid to pachyosteomorph level). Miles (1969) interpreted this development as contributing to an increasingly efficient feeding mechanism. In other placoderms, this trend is not seen; either they remain unchanged, like the heavily armored antiarchs, or they are too incompletely known (Ptyctodontida, Rhenanida, Petalichthyida), or their known occurrence is very brief within the Devonian (Stensioellida, Pseudopetalichthyida, Acanthothoraci, Phyllolepida).

In chondrichthyans, the neurocranium and visceral skeleton were well calcified with prismatic cartilage in Paleozoic forms and primitive euselachians (Hybodontoidea). There are some Paleozoic forms with exoskeletal ossification on the head, large denticles (Iniopterygia), circumorbital plates (Cladoselachida), or even plates (Menaspoidea). Calcification, except for vertebral centra, is much reduced in Mesozoic and more modern chondrichthyans. The fossil record of these forms is almost limited to teeth and denticles.

The Acanthodii change from forms with heavily tessellated heads (Climatiida) to forms that lack a scale covering on the head (Acanthodida). In the endoskeleton, an opposite trend toward increased mineralization may be indicated; the only preserved neurocranium and visceral skeleton is found in the youngest form, *Acanthodes,* from the Permian (270 mya).

The trend toward reduced mineralization is most evident within the osteichthyans. The old grade division of actinopterygians into Chondrostei, Holostei, and Teleostei represents a continuum from primitive forms with strongly ossified exoskeleton and neurocranium to more lightly built skulls with fewer bones and a cartilaginous neurocranium. The result is increased mobility of individual skull bones, and the feeding mechanism is improved and differentiated, especially within teleosts (Lauder 1982). Postcranial ossification of the heavy exoskeletal scale armor shifts inward to ossifications around the notochord, the vertebrae. Similar evolutionary changes can be observed in sarcopterygians. The neurocranium is not ossified in post-Devonian dipnoans and the number of bones is reduced. The snout, which is a single heavily ossified element early in the Devonian, is unossified in Late and post-Devonian dipnoans. Actinistians show a similar trend. Many bones of the cheek of the extant *Latimeria* have no direct contact with each other and are mobile within the soft tissue. Other crossopterygian groups (Porolepiformes, Osteolepiformes) show reduction in the thickness of skeletal elements (loss of enamel and dentine) within the Devonian and Late Paleozoic. Further trends to reduce the number of ossifications in the neurocranium and exocranium are continued in their offspring, the tetrapods.

ACKNOWLEDGMENTS

The author is indebted to the review and criticisms of D. Goujet, Paris, to the improvement of his English by L. Trueb, Lawrence, Kansas, and to the preparation of the figures by G. Arratia, Lawrence, Kansas.

LIST OF ABBREVIATIONS

A, B, C	bones A, B, C, etc. of dipnoans	ch	ceratohyal
aap	attachment for autopalatine process of palatoquadrate	c.l	lateral crista
		c.m	median crista
ac	annular cartilage	Co	circumorbital
a.ci	arteria carotis interna	coc	occipital condyle
Ang	angular	Cor	coronoid
"Ang"	"angular" of dipnoans	cna	rhinocapsular bone
Ant	antorbital	cpa	crista parotica
aot	otic attachment for palatoquadrate	De	dentary
		dend	ductus endolymphaticus
ar.a	articular articulation for lower jaw	Des	dentalosplenial
		Dhy	dermohyal
ar.e	ethmoidal articulation	dor	dorsal otic ridge
ar.pa	paratemporal articulation	Dpl	dermopalatine
ar.po	postorbital articulation	Dsp	dermosphenotic
art	articular	eb	epibranchial
auc	auditory capsule	Ecpt	ectopterygoid
aVo	attachment for vomer	eh	epihyal (hyomandibula)
bb	basibranchial	ehb	ossification of epihyal
bh	basihyal	Esc	extrascapular
boc	basioccipital	exoc	exoccipital
bpt	basipterygoid process	fe.bc	fenestra basicranialis
bsp	basisphenoid ossification	fech	fenestra endochoanalis
Bst	branchiostegal ray	fe.na	fenestra nasalis
cao	aortic canal	fend	endolymphatic fossa
cav	cavity for nasal capsule	fhy	hypophyseal foramen
cb	ceratobranchial	fhym	foramen of hyomandibular branch of cranial nerve VII
cc	central sensory canal	flda	foramen for lateral dorsal aorta
c.dl	dorso-lateral crista		
CE	central	fm	foramen magnum

fmm	fossa for masseter muscle	NU	nuchal
fmt	fossa for temporalis muscle	oa	occipital arch
foo	fissure otico-occipitalis	oc	oral (sensory) canal
fo.pi	pineal fontanelle	occ	occipital commissure
fo.po	posterior dorsal fontanelle	ocr	occipital crest
f.pi	pineal foramen	Op	opercle
f.po	posttemporal fossa	op	orbital pedicel
fso	foramen superficial ophthalmic nerve	orbc	orbital cartilage
		osh	otical shelf
Gl	lateral gular	otic	otic region
Gm	median gular	Pa	parietal
Gp	principal gular	par	paratemporal articulation facet
gr.ic	groove for internal carotids		
hb	hypobranchial	pb	pharyngobranchial
Hgc	hyoid gill cover	pc	polar cartilage
hh	hypohyal	pch	parachondral cartilage
hyf	facet for epihyal (hyomandibula)	pf	precerebral fontanelle
		ph	pharyngohyal
ih	interhyal	PI	pineal plate
ij	intracranial joint	pmc	postmarginal (sensory) canal
Io	infraorbital	PMG	postmarginal
ioc	infraorbital (sensory) canal	Pmx	premaxilla
It	intertemporal	PN	postnasal
jc	jugular canal	PNU	paranuchal
Ju	jugal	Po	postorbital
jug	groove for jugular vein	poc	preopercular (sensory) canal
La	lacrimal	Pop	preopercle
lab	labial cartilage	pop	postorbital process
laon	lamina orbitonasalis	popa	anterior postorbital process in placoderms
lc	lateral commissure		
ll	main lateral line	popp	posterior postorbital process in placoderms
loc	lateral occipital ossification		
lop	lateral otic process	Por	postrostral
ma	mandibular arch	pot	postotical process
mc	mandibular (sensory) canal	Pp	postparietal
mec	Meckel's cartilage	pp	posterior "pit-line"
me	mentomeckelian	pq	palatoquadrate
MG	marginal	pre	ectethmoid process
mpt	metapterygoid	PRO	preorbital
Mx	maxilla	prop	preorbital process
Na	nasal	prpo	postorbital process
na	anterior endocranial nasal opening	"Psp"	"postsplenial" of dipnoans
		Psph	parasphenoid
nac	fenestra endonarina communis	PSU	postsuborbital
		psup	suprapterygoid process
nc	nasal capsule	psv	supravagal process
nch	notochord/notochordal canal	PTO	"postorbital" of placoderms

q	quadrate	SU	suborbital
Qj	quadratojugal	sy	symplectic
rart	retroarticular	T	tabular
Ro	rostral	tcr	trabeculae cranii
RO	rostral plate of placoderms	"uh"	chondral "urohyal" of
rr	rostral cartilages		sarcopterygians
Sang	surangular	vc.fo	vestibular fontanelle
"Sang"	"surangular"	vf	ventral fissure
	of dipnoans	Vo	vomer
Sbm	submandibulars	voc	ventral occipital ossification
sg	spiracular groove	von	ventral otic notch
Sgc	subsidiary gill covers	I	olfactory nerve
sic	spiracular canal	II	optic nerve
sl	sublingual	III	oculomotor nerve
SM	submarginal	IV	trochlear nerve
soc	supraorbital (sensory) canal	$V_{2,3}$	trigeminal nerve
Sop	subopercle	VII	facial nerve
spc	spiracular cartilage	IX	glossopharyngeal nerve
spi	foramina for spinal nerves	X	vagus nerve
Sq	squamosal	1, 2, 3,	
St	supratemporal	4 etc.	bones surrounding orbit and
Stt	supratemporotabular		covering cheek in dipnoans

REFERENCES

Alexander, R. McN. 1967. The functions and mechanisms of the protrusible upper jaws of some acanthopterygian fish. Journal of Zoology, London 151: 43–64.

Arratia, G., and H.-P. Schultze. 1990. The urohyal: Development and homology within osteichthyans. Journal of Morphology 203: 247–282.

———. 1991. The palatoquadrate and its ossifications: Development and homology within osteichthyans. Journal of Morphology 208: 1–81.

Balon, E. K., M. N. Bruton, and H. Fricke. 1988. A fiftieth anniversary reflection on the living coelacanth, *Latimeria chalumnae:* Some new interpretations of its natural history and conservation status. Environmental Biology of Fishes 23 (4): 241–280.

Bertmar, G. 1966. The development of skeleton, blood-vessels, and nerves in the dipnoan snout, with a discussion on the homology of the dipnoan posterior nostrils. Acta Zoologica, Stockholm 47: 81–150.

Borgen, U. J. 1989. Cosmine resorption structures on three osteolepid jaws and their biological significance. Lethaia 22: 413–424.

Campbell, K. S. W., and R. E. Barwick. 1982. The neurocranium of the primitive dipnoan *Dipnorhynchus sussmilchi* (Etheridge). Journal of Vertebrate Paleontology 2: 286–327.

———. 1984a. The choana, maxillae, premaxillae, and anterior palatal bones of early dipnoans. Proceedings of the Linnean Society of New South Wales 107: 147–170.

————. 1984b. *Speonesydrion*, an Early Devonian dipnoan with primitive tooth-plates. Paleo Ichthyologica 2: 1–48.

————. 1987. Paleozoic Lungfishes: A review. Journal of Morphology suppl. 1: 93–113.

Chang M.-M. 1982. *The Braincase of* Youngolepis, *a Lower Devonian Crosso-pterygian from Yunnan, South-Western China.* Stockholm: Department of Geology, University of Stockholm.

————. 1991. "Rhipidistians," dipnoans, and tetrapods. In *Origins of the Major Groups of Tetrapods: Controversies and Consensus,* H.-P. Schultze and L. Trueb, eds. Ithaca, N.Y.: Cornell University Press, pp. 3–28.

Chang M.-M., and Yu X. 1984. Structure and phylogenetic significance of *Diabolichthys speratus* gen. et sp. nov., a new dipnoan-like form from the Lower Devonian of eastern Yunnan, China. Proceedings of the Linnean Society of New South Wales 107: 171–184.

Cloutier, R. 1991a. Interrelationships of Palaeozoic actinistians: Patterns and trends. In *Early Vertebrate Studies and Related Problems in Evolutionary Biology,*Chang M.-M., Zhang G., and Liu Y., eds. Beijing: Science Press, pp. 379–426.

————. 1991b. Patterns, trends, and rates of evolution within the Actinistia. Environmental Biology of Fishes 32: 23–58.

Compagno, L. J. V. 1973. Interrelationships of living elasmobranchs. In *Interrelationships of Fishes,* P. H. Greenwood, R. S. Miles, and C. Patterson, eds. Zoological Journal of the Linnean Society, 53 (suppl. 1): 15–61.

————. 1977. Phyletic relationships of living sharks and rays. American Zoologist 17: 303–322.

————. 1988. *Sharks of the Order Carcharhiniformes.* Princeton: Princeton University Press.

Dean, B. 1909. Studies on fossil fishes (sharks, chimaeroids, and arthrodires). Memoirs of the American Museum of Natural History 9: 211–287.

de Beer, G. R. 1931. The development of the skull of *Scyllium canicula.* Quarterly Journal of Microscopical Science 74: 591–646.

————. 1937. *The Development of the Vertebrate Skull.* Oxford: Oxford University Press.

Denison, R. H. 1968. The evolutionary significance of the earliest known lungfish *Uranolophus.* In *Current Problems of Lower Vertebrate Phylogeny,* T. Ørvig, ed. Nobel Symposium 4. Stockholm: Almquist and Wiksell, pp. 247–257.

————. 1975. Evolution and classification of placoderm fishes. Breviora 432: 1–24.

————. 1978. Placodermi. In *Handbook of Paleoichthyology,* H.-P. Schultze, ed., vol. 2. Stuttgart: Gustav Fischer Verlag, pp. vi, 1–128.

————. 1983. Further consideration of placoderm evolution. Journal of Vertebrate Paleontology 3: 69–83.

El-Toubi, M. R. 1949. The development of the chondrocranium of the spiny dog-fish, *Acanthias vulgaris (Squalus acanthias).* Part I. Neurocranium, mandibula, and hyoid arches. Journal of Morphology 84: 227–279.

Forey, P. 1980. *Latimeria:* A paradoxical fish. Proceedings of the Royal Society of London B 208: 369–384.

Forey, P. L., and B. G. Gardiner. 1986. Observations on *Ctenurella* (Ptyctodontida) and the classification of placoderm fishes. Zoological Journal of the Linnean Society 86: 43–74.

Forster-Cooper, C. 1937. The Middle Devonian fish fauna of Achanarras. Transactions of the Royal Society of Edinburgh 59: 223–239.

Fox, H. 1965. Early development of the head and pharynx of *Neoceratodus* with a consideration of its phylogeny. Journal of Zoology 146: 470–554.

Gardiner, B. G. 1984a. The relationships of placoderms. Journal of Vertebrate Paleontology 4: 379–395.

———. 1984b. The relationships of the palaeoniscid fishes, a review based on new specimens of *Mimia* and *Moythomasia* from the Upper Devonian of Western Australia. Bulletin of the British Museum (Natural History), Geology 37: 173–427.

Goodrich, E. S. 1909. Cyclostomes and fishes. In *A Treatise on Zoology*, E. R. Lancester, ed., vol. 9. Edinburgh: R. & R. Clark.

Goujet, D. 1975. *Dicksonosteus*, un nouvel arthrodire du Dévonien du Spitsberg: Remarques sur le squelette viscéral des Dolichothoraci. Colloques internationaux de Centre national de la recherche scientifique, 218, Problèmes actuels de paléontologie (Évolution des Vertébrés): 81–100.

———. 1982. Les affinités des placoderms, une revue des hypothèses actuelles. Géobios, Mémoire spécial 6: 27–38.

———. 1984a. Placoderm interrelationships: a new interpretation, with a short review of placoderm classifications. Proceedings of the Linnean Society of New South Wales 107: 211–243.

———. 1984b. *Les poissons placoderms du Spitsberg: Arthrodires Dolichothoraci de la formation de Wood Bay (Dévonien Inférieur)*. Cahiers de paléontologie, sec. Vertébrés. Paris: Éditions du CNRS.

Graham-Smith, W. 1978. On the lateral lines and dermal bones in the parietal region of some crossopterygians and dipnoan fishes. Philosophical Transactions of the Royal Society of London B 282: 41–105.

Grande, L., and W. E. Bemis. 1991. Osteology and phylogenetic relationships of fossil and Recent paddlefish (Polyodontidae) with comments on the interrelationships of Acipenseriformes. Journal of Vertebrate Paleontology 11 (1) (suppl.), Memoir 1.

Gregory, W. K. 1933. Fish skulls: A study of the evolution of natural mechanisms. Transactions of the American Philosophical Society 23 (2): 75–481.

Gross, W. 1937. Das Kopfskelett von *Cladodus wildungensis* Jaekel. 1. Teil. Endocranium und Palatoquadratum. Senckenbergiana 19: 80–107.

———. 1956. Über Crossopterygier und Dipnoer aus dem baltischen Oberdevon im Zusammenhang einer vergleichenden Untersuchung des Porenkanalsystems paläozoischer Agnathen und Fische. Kungliga Svenska VetenskapsAkademiens Handlingar (4) 5: 1–140.

———. 1962. Peut-on homologuer les os des arthrodires et des téléostomes? Colloques internationaux de Centre national de la recherche scientifique 104, Problèmes actuels de paléontologie (Évolution des Vertébrés): 69–74.

Heidtke, U. 1990. *Studien über Acanthodes (Pisces: Acanthodii) aus dem saar-*

pfälzischen Rotliegend (?Ober-Karbon—Unter-Perm, SW-Deutschland). Pollichia-Buch 19. Bad Dürkheim, Germany: Pfalzmuseum für Naturkunde.

Holmgren, N. 1940. Studies on the head in fishes: Embryological, morphological, and phylogenetical researches. Part I. Development of the skull in sharks and rays. Acta zoologica, Stockholm 21: 51–267.

Holmgren, N., and E. Stensiö. 1936. Kranium and Visceralskelett der Acranier, Cyclostomen und Fische. In *Handbuch der vergleichenden Anatomie der Wirbeltiere,* L. Bolk, E. Göppert, E. Kallius, and W. Lubosch, eds., vol. 4. Berlin: Urban and Schwarzenberg, pp. 233–250.

Janvier, P. 1981. The phylogeny of the Craniata, with particular reference to the significance of fossil "Agnathans." Journal of Vertebrate Paleontology 1: 121–159.

Jarvik, E. 1942. On the structure of the snout of crossopterygians and lower gnathostomes in general. Zoologiska Bidrag från Uppsala 21: 235–675.

———. 1954. On the visceral skeleton in *Eusthenopteron* with a discussion of the parasphenoid and palatoquadrate in fishes. Kungliga Svenska Vetenskaps-Akademiens Handlingar (4) 5: 1–104.

———. 1967. On the structure of the lower jaw in dipnoans: With a description of an early Devonian dipnoan from Canada, *Melanognathus canadensis* gen. et sp. nov. Journal of the Linnean Society of London, Zoology 47: 155–183.

———. 1977. The systematic position of the acanthodian fishes. In *Problems in Vertebrate Evolution,* S. M. Andrews, R. S. Miles, and A. D. Walker, eds. London: Academic Press, pp. 199–225.

———. 1980. *Basic Structure and Evolution of Vertebrates.* Vol. 1. London: Academic Press.

———. 1981. *Basic Structure and Evolution of Vertebrates.* Vol. 2. London: Academic Press.

Jessen, H. 1967. Die Crossopterygier des Oberen Plattenkalkes (Devon) der Bergisch-Gladbach—Paffrather Mulde (Rheinisches Schiefergebirge) unter Berücksichtigung von amerikanischem und europäischem *Onychodus*-Material. Arkiv för Zoologi 18: 305–389.

———. 1968. *Moythomasia nitida* Gross and *M.* cf. *striata* Gross, devonische Palaeonisciden aus dem Oberen Plattenkalk der Bergisch-Gladbach—Paffrather Mulde (Rheinisches Schiefergebirge). Palaeontographica A 128: 87–114.

———. 1980. Lower Devonian porolepiforms from the Canadian Arctic with special reference to *Powichthys thorsteinssoni* Jessen. Palaeontographica A 167: 180–214.

Jollie, M. 1962. *Chordate Morphology.* New York: Reinhold Books.

———. 1971. Some developmental aspects of the head skeleton of the 35–37 mm *Squalus acanthias* foetus. Journal of Morphology 133: 17–40.

———. 1980. Development of Head and Pectoral Girdle Skeleton and Scales in *Acipenser.* Copeia 1980 (2): 266–249.

———. 1984a. Development of Cranial and Girdle Bones of *Lepisosteus* with a Note on Scales. Copeia 1984 (2): 476–502.

———. 1984b. Development of the head and pectoral skeleton of *Polypterus* with a note on scales (Pisces, Actinopterygii). Journal of Zoology, London 204: 469–507.

———. 1986. A primer of bone names for the understanding of the actinopterygian head and pectoral girdle skeletons. Canadian Journal of Zoology 64: 365–379.

Karatajuté-Talimaa, V. N. 1973. *Elegestolepis grossi* gen. et sp. nov., ein neuer Typ der Placoidschuppe aus dem Oberen Silur der Tuwa. Palaeontographica A 143: 35–50.

Karatajuté-Talimaa, V. N., L. I. Novitskaya, K. S. Rozman, and Z. Sodov. 1990. [*Mongolepis*—A new Lower Silurian genus of elasmobranchs from Mongolia]. Paleontologicheskiy zhurnal 1990 (1): 76–86. [In Russian. English translation: Paleontological Journal 24 (1), 1991]

Lagios, M. D. 1979. The coelacanth and the Chondrichthyes as sister groups: A review of shared apomorph characters and a cladistic analysis and reinterpretation. In *The Biology and Physiology of the Living Coelacanth*, J. E. McCosker and M. D. Lagios, eds., Occasional Papers of the California Academy of Sciences 13: 425–444. San Francisco: California Academy of Sciences.

Lauder, G. V. 1982. Patterns of evolution in the feeding mechanism of actinopterygian fishes. American Zoologist 22: 275–285.

Lauder, G. V., and K. F. Liem. 1983. The evolution and interrelationships of the actinopterygian fishes. Bulletin of the Museum of Comparative Zoology 150: 95–197.

Luther, A. 1913. Über die vom N. trigeminus versorgte Muskulatur der Ganoiden und Dipneusten. Acta Societatis scientiarum fennicae 41: 1–72.

Mader, H. 1986. Schuppen und Zähne von Acanthodiern und Elasmobranchiern aus dem Unter-Devon Spaniens (Pisces). Göttinger Arbeiten zur Geologie und Paläontologie 28: 1–59.

Maisey, J. G. 1980. An evaluation of jaw suspension in sharks. American Museum Novitates 2706: 1–17.

———. 1982. The anatomy and interrelationships of Mesozoic hybodont sharks. American Museum Novitates 2724: 1–48.

———. 1984. Chondrichthyan phylogeny: A look at the evidence. Journal of Vertebrate Paleontology 4: 359–371.

———. 1986. Heads and tails: A chordate phylogeny. Cladistics 2: 201–256.

———. 1989. Visceral skeleton and musculature of a Late Devonian shark. Journal of Vertebrate Paleontology 9: 174–190.

McAllister, D. E., and C. L. Smith. 1978. Mensurations morphologiques, dénombrements méristiques et taxonomie du coelacanthe, *Latimeria chalumnae*. Naturaliste canadien 105: 63–76.

Miles, R. S. 1969. Features of placoderm diversification and the evolution of the arthrodire feeding mechanism. Transactions of the Royal Society of Edinburgh 68: 123–170.

———. 1971. The Holonematidae (placoderm fishes): A review based on new specimens of *Holomena* from the Upper Devonian of Western Australia. Philosophical Transactions of the Royal Society of London 263: 101–234.

———. 1973a. Articulated acanthodian fishes from the Old Red Sandstone of England, with a review of the structure and evolution of the acanthodian shoulder-girdle. Bulletin of the British Museum (Natural History), Geology 24: 115–213.

———. 1973b. Relationships of acanthodians. In *Interrelationships of Fishes,* P. H. Greenwood, R. S. Miles, and C. Patterson, eds. London: Academic Press, pp. 63–103.

———. 1977. Dipnoan (lungfish) skulls and the relationships of the group: A study based on new species from the Devonian of Australia. Zoological Journal of the Linnean Society 61: 1–328.

Miles, R. S., and G. C. Young. 1977. Placoderm interrelationships reconsidered in the light of new ptyctodontids from Gogo, Western Australia. In *Problems in Vertebrate Evolution,* S. M. Andrews, R. S. Miles, and A. D. Walker, eds. London: Academic Press, pp. 123–198.

Millot, J., and J. Anthony. 1974. Les oeufs du Coelacanthe. Science et nature 121: 3–4 (+ color cover photograph).

Moy-Thomas, J. A., and R. S. Miles. 1971. *Palaeozoic Fishes.* 2d ed. London: Chapman and Hall.

Nelson, G. 1968. Gill-arch structure in *Acanthodes.* In *Current Problems of Lower Vertebrate Phylogeny,* T. Ørvig, ed., Nobel Symposium 4. Stockholm: Almquist and Wiksell, pp. 129–143.

Nelson, J. S. 1984. *Fishes of the World.* 2d ed. New York: John Wiley and Sons.

Ørvig, T. 1980. Histologic studies of ostracoderms, placoderms, and fossil elasmobranchs. 3. Structure and growth of the gnathalia of certain arthrodires. Zoologica scripta 9: 141–159.

Panchen, A. L., and T. R. Smithson. 1987. Character diagnosis, fossils, and the origin of tetrapods. Biological Review 62: 341–438.

Patterson, C. 1975. The braincase of pholidophorid and leptolepid fishes, with a review of the actinopterygian braincase. Philosophical Transactions of the Royal Society of London B 269: 275–579.

Pehrson, T. 1922. Some points in the cranial development of teleostomian fishes. Acta zoologica, Stockholm 3: 1–63.

———. 1940. The development of dermal bones in the skull of *Amia calva.* Acta Zoologica, Stockholm 21: 1–50.

———. 1944. Some observations on the development and morphology of the dermal bones in the skull of *Acipenser* and *Polyodon.* Acta zoologica, Stockholm 25: 27–48.

———. 1947. Some new interpretations of the skull in *Polypterus.* Acta zoologica, Stockholm 28: 399–455.

———. 1958. The early ontogeny of the sensory lines and the dermal skull in *Polypterus.* Acta zoologica, Stockholm 39: 241–258.

Peignoux-Deville, J., F. Lallier, and B. Vidal. 1982. Evidence for the presence of osseous tissue in dogfish vertebrae. Cell Tissue Research 222: 605–614.

Poplin, C. 1974. *Étude de quelques paléoniscidés pennsylvaniens du Kansas.* Cahiers de paléontologie. Paris: Éditions du CNRS.

Roček, Z. 1986. An "intracranial" joint in frogs. In *Studies in Herpetology,* Z. Roček, ed. Prague: Charles University, pp. 49–52.

Romer, A. S. 1942. Cartilage: An embryonic adaptation. American Naturalist 76: 394–404.

———. 1945. *Vertebrate Paleontology.* 2d ed. Chicago: University of Chicago Press.

———. 1964. The braincase of the Paleozoic elasmobranch *Tamiobatis.* Bulletin of the Museum of Comparative Zoology, Harvard University 131: 89–105.

———. 1969. *Notes and Comments on Vertebrate Paleontology.* Chicago: University of Chicago Press.

Rosen, D. E., P. L. Forey, B. G. Gardiner, and C. Patterson. 1981. Lungfishes, tetrapods, paleontology, and plesiomorphy. Bulletin of the American Museum of Natural History 167: 159–276.

Säve-Söderbergh, G. 1952. On the skull of *Chirodipterus wildungensis* Gross, an Upper Devonian Dipnoan from Wildungen. Kungliga Svenska Vetenskaps-Akademiens Handlingar 4 (3): 1–29.

Schaeffer, B. 1952. Rates of evolution in the coelacanth and dipnoan fishes. Evolution 6: 101–111.

———. 1975. Comments on the origin and basic radiation of the gnathostome fishes with particular reference to the feeding mechanism. Colloques internationaux de Centre national de la recherche scientifique 218, Problèmes actuels de paléontologie (Évolution des Vertébrés): 101–109.

———. 1981. The xenacanth shark neurocranium, with comments on elasmobranch monophyly. Bulletin of the American Museum of Natural History 169: 1–66.

Schaeffer, B., and K. S. Thomson. 1980. Reflections on agnathan-gnathostome relationships. In *Aspects of Vertebrate History: Essays in Honor of Edwin Harris Colbert,* L. L. Jacobs, ed. Flagstaff: Museum of Northern Arizona Press, pp. 19–33.

Schmalhausen, I. I. 1968. *The Origin of Terrestrial Vertebrates.* New York: Academic Press.

Schultze, H.-P. 1969. *Griphognathus* Gross, ein langschnauziger Dipnoer aus dem Oberdevon von Bergisch-Gladbach (Rheinisches Schiefergebirge) und von Lettland. Geologica et palaeontologica 3: 21–79.

———. 1973. Crossopterygier mit heterozerker Schwanzflosse aus dem Oberdevon Kanadas, nebst einer Beschreibung von Onychodontida-Resten aus dem Mitteldevon Spaniens und aus dem Karbon der U.S.A. Palaeontographica A 143: 188–208.

———. 1977. Ausgangsform und Entwicklung der rhombischen Schuppen der Osteichthyes (Pisces). Paläontologische Zeitschrift 51: 152–168.

———. 1984. Juvenile specimens of *Eusthenopteron foordi* Whiteaves, 1881 (osteolepiform rhipidistian, Pisces) from the Upper Devonian of Miguasha, Quebec, Canada. Journal of Vertebrate Paleontology 4: 1–16.

———. 1985. Reproduction and spawning sites of *Rhabdoderma* (Pisces, Osteichthyes, Actinistia) in Pennsylvanian deposits of Illinois, USA. Neuvième Congrès international de stratigraphie et de géologie du Carbonifère, Washington, and Champaign-Urbana, Compte Rendu 5: 326–330.

———. 1987. Dipnoans as sarcopterygians. Journal of Morphology suppl. 1: 39–74.

————. 1990. A new acanthodian from the Pennsylvanian of Utah, U.S.A., and the distribution of otoliths in gnathostomes. Journal of Vertebrate Paleontology 10: 49–58.

————. 1992. A new long-headed dipnoan (Osteichthyes, Pisces) from the Late Devonian of Iowa, U.S.A. Journal of Vertebrate Paleontology 12: 42–58.

Schultze, H.-P., and M. Arsenault. 1985. The panderichthyid fish *Elpistostege:* A close relative of tetrapods? Palaeontology 28: 293–309.

————. 1987. *Quebecius quebecensis* (Whiteaves), a porolepiform crossopterygian (Pisces) from the Late Devonian of Quebec, Canada. Canadian Journal of Earth Sciences 24: 2351–2361.

Schultze, H.-P., and K. S. W. Campbell. 1987. Characterization of the Dipnoi, a monophyletic group. Journal of Morphology Suppl. 1: 25–37.

Schultze, H.-P., and L. Trueb. 1981. Review of *Basic Structure and Evolution of Vertebrates* by Erik Jarvik. Journal of Vertebrate Paleontology 1: 389–397.

Shishkin, M. S. 1973. *The Morphology of the Early Amphibia and Some Problems of the Lower Tetrapod Evolution.* Moscow: Nauka.

Smith, C. L., C. S. Rand, B. Schaeffer, and J. W. Atz. 1975. *Latimeria,* the living coelacanth, is ovoviviparous. Science 190: 1105–1106.

Smith, M. M. 1989. Distribution and variation in enamel structure in the oral teeth of sarcopterygians: Its significance for the evolution of a protoprismatic enamel. Historical Biology 3: 97–126.

Stensiö, E. A. 1945. On the heads of certain arthrodires. II. On the cranium and cervical joint of the Dolichothoraci (Acanthaspida). Kungliga Svenska VetenskapsAkademiens Handlingar (3) 22 (1): 3–10.

————. 1959. On the pectoral fin and shoulder girdle of the arthrodires. Kungliga Svenska VetenskapsAkademiens Handlingar (4) 8 (1): 1–229.

————. 1963a. Anatomical studies on the arthrodiran head. Part 1. Preface, geological and geographical distribution, the organization of the head in the Dolichothoraci, Coccosteomorphi, and Pachyosteomorphi. Taxonomic appendix. Kungliga Svenska VetenskapsAkademiens Handlingar (4) 9: 1–419.

————. 1963b. The brain and cranial nerves in fossil, lower craniate vertebrates. Skrifter utgitt av Det Norske Videnskaps-Akademi i Oslo, I. Matematisk-Naturvidenskapelig Klasse, Ny Serie 13: 1–120.

————. 1969. Elasmobranchiomorphi. Placodermata. Arthrodires. In *Traité de Paléontologie,* J. Piveteau, ed., vol. 4 (2). Paris: Masson, pp. 71–692.

Thomson, K. S. 1975. On the biology of cosmine. Bulletin of the Peabody Museum of Natural History 40: 1–59.

Vézina, D. 1986. Les plaques gnathales de *Plourdosteus canadensis* (Placodermi, Arthrodira) du Dévonian supérieur du Québec (Canada): Remarques sur la croissance dentaire de la mécanique masticatrice. Bulletin de Muséum national d'histoire naturelle, Paris (4) 8, sec. C (3): 367–391.

Vieth, J. 1980. Thelodontier, Acanthodier, und Elasmobranchier-Schuppen aus dem Unter-Devon der Kanadischen Arktis (Agnatha, Pisces). Göttinger Arbeiten zur Geologie und Paläontologie 23: 1–69.

Vorobyeva, E. I., and H.-P. Schultze. 1991. Description and systematics of panderichthyid fishes with comments on their relationship to tetrapods. In *Origins of the Major Groups of Tetrapods: Controversies and Consensus,* H.-P. Schultze and L. Trueb, eds. Ithaca, N.Y.: Cornell University Press, pp. 68–109.

Watson, D. M. S. 1927. The reproduction of the coelacanth fish, *Undina.* Proceedings of the Zoological Society of London 1927: 453–457.

———. 1937. The acanthodian fishes. Philosophical Transactions of the Royal Society of London B 228: 49–146.

Werdelin, L., and J. A. Long. 1986. Allometry in the placoderm *Bothriolepis canadensis* and its significance to antiarch evolution. Lethaia 9: 161–169.

Westoll, T. S. 1938. Ancestry of the tetrapods. Nature 141: 127–128.

———. 1943. The origin of the tetrapods. Biological Review 18: 78–98.

Whiting, H. P. 1972. Cranial anatomy of the ostracoderms in relation to the organization of larval lampreys. In *Studies in Vertebrate Evolution,* K. A. Joysey and T. S. Kemp, eds. Edinburgh: Oliver and Boyd, pp. 1–20.

Wiley, E. O. 1979. Ventral gill arch muscles and the interrelationships of gnathostomes, with a new classification of the Vertebrata. Zoological Journal of the Linnean Society 67: 149–179.

Woskoboinikoff, M. M. 1932. Der Apparat der Kiemenatmung bei den Fischen: Ein Versuch der Synthese in der Morphologie. Zoologische Jahrbücher, Abteilung Anatomie und Ontogenie der Tiere 55: 315–488.

Young, G. 1986. The relationships of placoderm fishes. Zoological Journal of the Linnean Society of London 88: 1–57.

Zangerl, R. 1968. The morphology and the developmental history of the scales of the Paleozoic sharks *Holmesella?* sp. and *Orodus.* In *Current Problems of Lower Vertebrate Phylogeny,* T. Ørvig, ed., Nobel Symposium, 4. Stockholm: Almquist and Wiksell, pp. 399–412.

———. 1969. *Bandringa rayi,* a new ctenacanthoid shark from the Pennsylvanian Essex fauna of Illinois. Fieldiana: Geology 12 (10): 157–169.

———. 1981. Chondrichthyes I. Paleozoic Elasmobranchii. In *Handbook of Paleoichthyology,* H.-P. Schultze, ed., vol. 3A. Stuttgart: Fischer.

Zangerl, R., and G. R. Case. 1976. *Cobelodus aculeatus* (COPE), an anacanthous shark from the Pennsylvanian black shales of North America. Palaeontographica A 154: 107–157.

Zangerl, R., and M. Williams. 1975. New evidence on the nature of the jaw suspension in Paleozoic anacanthous sharks. Palaeontology 18: 333–341.

Zidek, J. 1976. Kansas Hamilton quarry (Upper Pennsylvanian) *Acanthodes,* with remarks on the previously reported North American occurrences of the genus. University of Kansas, Paleontological Contributions 83: 1–41.

———. 1985. Growth in *Acanthodes* (Acanthodii: Pisces)—data and implications. Paläontologische Zeitschrift 59: 147–166.

6

Patterns of Cranial Diversity among the Lissamphibia

LINDA TRUEB

INTRODUCTION

AS ORIGINALLY CONCEIVED by the editors of these volumes, a chapter was to be written describing the patterns of cranial diversity in amphibians. Herein, the Amphibia is considered to comprise the Loxommatidae and the Temnospondyli, and to exclude the Nectridea, Aïstopoda, and Microsauria, the relationships of which are uncertain (Gauthier et al. 1989). The Loxommatids and temnospondyls represent a vast taxonomic and morphological array of lower tetrapods. The former group is extinct and represented by such taxa as *Baphetes, Loxomma,* and *Megacephalus.* The Temnospondyli comprises an immense assemblage of fossil taxa (e.g., trimerorachoids, dendrerpetontids, eryopids, rhinesuchoids, capitosauroids, trematosauroids, plagiosauroids, etc.) in addition to the fossil and living lissamphibians (i.e., Gymnophiona + Batrachia, sensu Trueb and Cloutier 1991a). Although some progress has been made in inferring the phylogenetic relationships among the surviving temnospondyls and a few of their fossil relatives, overall, relationships within this extensive group of lower tetrapods are obscure. To attempt a summary of patterns of cranial diversity in such an extensive and systematically enigmatic group of animals is premature and far beyond the scope of a single-authored contribution and a single chapter in a volume of this sort. A more reasonable, but nonetheless challenging assignment, was to attempt an assessment of the diversity of the smaller and more coherent (i.e., monophyletic) group, the extant members of the Lissamphibia.

As defined by Trueb and Cloutier (1991a), the Recent Lissamphibia is composed of the Apoda (caecilians), the Caudata (salamanders), and the Anura (frogs and toads). Trueb and Cloutier's phylogenetic analyses of the inter- and intrarelationships of the Lissamphibia revealed that among the fossil temnospondyl amphibian taxa, lissamphibians are related most

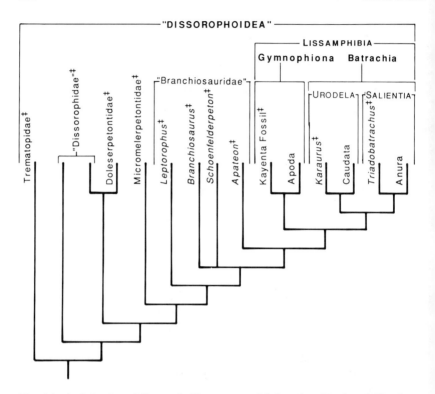

Fig. 6.1. A phylogeny of dissorophoid temnospondyls based on Trueb and Cloutier (1991a). Double dagger indicates fossil taxa.

closely to dissorophoid taxa (fig. 6.1); they share possession of a medio-lateral tooth-replacement pattern and possession of a large orbit (although this feature is reversed in apodans). One group of dissorophoids, the "Branchiosauridae," is paraphyletic with respect to the Lissamphibia (Trueb and Cloutier 1991b); thus, dissorophids are not the lissamphibian sister group as has been postulated previously. "Branchiosaurids" (repre-sented by *Leptorophus, Schoenfelderpeton, Branchiosaurus,* and *Apateon* in the analysis of Trueb and Cloutier 1991a) share several cranial features in common with lissamphibians. If present, the palatine is not exposed in lateral view of the skull and articulates with the maxilla only by means of an antero-lateral process of the palatine, and the narial opening is large (except in apodans, in which the character is reversed). Among "branchiosaurids," *Apateon* (fig. 6.2) is postulated to the sister taxon of the Lissamphibia; this relationship is corroborated by the possession of pedicellate teeth in both groups; however, this is a homoplastic feature that also diagnoses doleserpetontids (*Tersomius, Doleserpeton,* and *Amphibamus*) and one that is reversed in the fossil urodele *Albanerpeton.*

Fossil and Recent lissamphibians are diagnosed by several cranial characters in addition to some postcranial features. Lissamphibians lack five skull bones (postparietal, postorbital, jugal, tabular, and supratemporal) and none has a discrete palatine as an adult. Moreover, if an ectopterygoid is present, it articulates with the maxilla. Primitively, pre- and postfrontal bones articulate with one another. Plesiomorphically, lissamphibians lack a parietal foramen, and the parietal organ is either covered by bone or lies within a fenestra between the dermal bones (frontals, parietals, frontoparietals) roofing the frontoparietal fontanelle of the endocranium. A discrete articular bone is absent in the mandible of all adult lissamphibians except urodeles and a squamosal embayment absent in all except the salientians; the presence of these characters in urodeles and salientians may represent reversals.

Within the Lissamphibia (fig. 6.1), the Urodela [*Karaurus* + Caudata] is the sister group of the Salientia [*Triadobatrachus* + Anura]. The Batrachia [Urodela + Salientia] differs from the Gymnophiona in the absence of the postfrontal in the skull roof, the ectopterygoid in the palate, and the surangular and splenial in the lower jaw.

Having listed these similarities, I have exhausted the list of cranial commonalities of living amphibians; the three groups are remarkably different from one another. Caecilians are reclusive amphibian "snakes" which, as the analogy suggests, lack limbs, and have long, narrow skulls characterized by a well-developed exocranium (unlike snakes), a reduced orbit, and primitively, a profusion of teeth (fig. 6.2). Salamanders usually are visualized as attenuate, four-limbed amphibians that are generalized relative to their sister groups. Although, as a group, they lack the spectacular and obvious specializations of caecilians and anurans, salamanders are by no means homogeneous (and by implication, uninteresting). Only among salamanders do we find obligate neotenes, as well as tetrapods that have lost their lungs (the majority of salamander species). The morphological consequences of these phenomena on the cranial morphology of salamanders is shown herein to be substantial.

As one herpetological pundit put it, "a frog is a frog, is a frog" (Inger 1967, 369). Despite the familiar morphological modifications of anurans for saltatorial locomotion—i.e., "the tremendous morphological gap [that] separates them from all other amphibians"—I must disagree with Inger's comment (1967, 369) that "the Salientia [Anura] constitute an un-

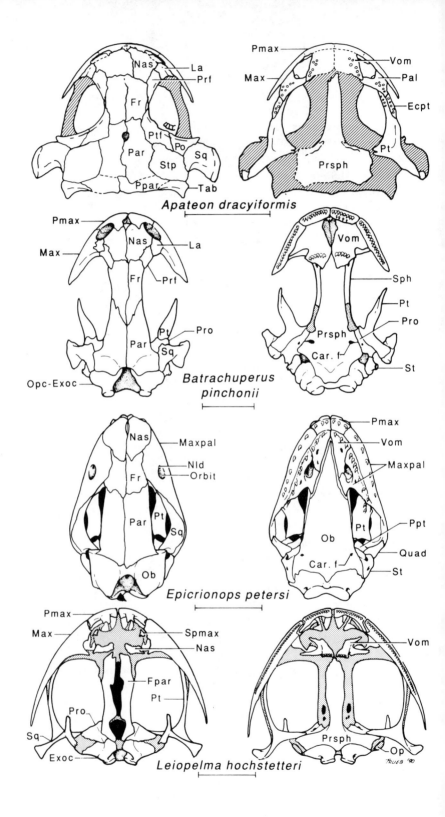

Apateon dracyiformis

Batrachuperus pinchonii

Epicrionops petersi

Leiopelma hochstetteri

TRUEB '90

usually invariable, narrow, isolated group morphologically." The diversity of modifications of anuran crania is as numerous as the species, and the variation so widespread that it produces a plethora of patterns.

In order to identify and describe trends or patterns of morphological change within a group, we first must be assured that the group is monophyletic—i.e., that all of its members share a common ancestor. This implies that we have a working hypothesis of the phylogenetic history of the organisms, and can identify the historical constraints (i.e., synapomorphies or shared-derived characters) that diagnose them. Simply put, we must have identified a phylogenetic pattern before we can infer morphological trends and evolutionary processes. There is a substantial body of evidence supporting the monophyly of the Lissamphibia (Trueb and Cloutier 1991a, b, and references therein). However, the quality of our understanding of the phylogenetic histories of the extant lissamphibian groups varies; caecilians are the best known, anurans the least. Nonetheless, I have selected the best available documented phylogeny for each order, and based my discussion of evolutionary trends in the cranium on that hypothesis. The reader doubtless will note that the cohesiveness of these discussions bears a direct relationship to the quality of the phylogenetic scheme on which it is based.

The chapter is divided into five major sections. The first describes the fundamental structure of the lissamphibian cranium as a preface to the following three sections that deal with the crania of each of the orders. Each of the latter is organized in the same way. Introductory comments include a statement of the size and composition of the order, along with references to pertinent literature. For the most part, citations are limited to primary literature, which in turn will provide more extensive lists of useful references. Descriptions of architectural diversity are followed by discussion of observed patterns of diversity. Each of the descriptions of diversity begins with a discussion of general features of the order, and is followed by descriptions of the endocranium, exocranium, composite endo- and exocranial units, dentition, and hyobranchial apparatus. Tables

---

Fig. 6.2. (*opposite*) Representative amphibian skulls. Left column, dorsal views. Right column, ventral views. *Apateon dracyiformis* is a fossil branchiosaurid; as proposed by Trueb and Cloutier (1991a), the genus is the sister group of the Lissamphibia. Drawing adapted from Boy (1986); cross-hatching represents ventral (left) and dorsal (right) surfaces, respectively. *Batrachuperus pinchonii* is a primitive hynobiid salamander. Drawing adapted from Carroll and Holmes (1980). *Epicrionops petersi* is a primitive rhinatrematid caecilian; redrawn from Nussbaum (1977). Black areas internal to skull are open. *Leiopelma hochstetteri* is a primitive leiopelmatid anuran; drawing modified from Stephenson (1951). Stipple-patterned areas represent cartilage; black areas represent cranial foramina or fenestrae. Bars equal 5 mm. See Appendix for abbreviations.

summarize differences in cranial features within each of the orders. The concluding section is a brief discussion comparing patterns of diversification among the three orders.

THE BASIC CRANIAL PLAN OF LISSAMPHIBIANS AND ITS COMPONENTS

Endocranium

Technically, the endocranium includes all parts of the skull that are cartilaginous and/or performed in cartilage. This includes the neurocranium (including the auditory capsules), middle-ear structures, palatoquadrate, and parts of the olfactory capsule, and mandible, as well as structures that stabilize the upper jaw against the neurocranium and olfactory capsule. Certain architectural units of the cranium, such as the suspensorium and mandible, are sufficiently complex integrations of endo- and exocranial elements that they are described separately below.

Neurocranium and Auditory Capsules. In a simplistic analogy, the neurocranium and auditory capsules of all living amphibians can be envisioned as a T-shaped, cubical container. The shaft of the "T" represents the neurocranium; the auditory capsules, which flank the neurocranium posterolaterally, form the head of the "T." Both the tubular neurocranium and bulbous auditory capsules are preformed in cartilage. Subsequently, the cartilage is replaced by bone that arises from a variable number of ossification centers. The extent of ossification of the neurocranium and auditory capsules is highly variable.

The neurocranium can be divided conveniently into anterior and posterior portions, with the optic foramen (or anterior margin of the basicranial fenestra, if present in the adult) marking the boundary between the two parts, as well as the area of fusion of the posterior parachordals with the anterior trabeculae (= prechordal cartilages) early in development. The trabeculae fuse below the brain to form the anterior neurocranial floor or ethmoid plate and produce a dorsal extension (preoptic root) that forms the sides of the anterior braincase. Fusion of the preoptic root with the dorsal orbital cartilage forms the antero-lateral–antero-medial margin of the frontoparietal fontanelle. The antero-medial braincase roof is variably termed the ethmoid plate (anurans) or tectum internasale (salamanders). The frontoparietal fontanelle is emarginate anteriorly in primitive caecilians (e.g., *Ichthyophis glutinosus*); thus, the brain lacks a cartilaginous roof. In the cartilaginous housing for the anterior part of the brain, two to six centers of ossification arise to produce, in the adult, the sphenethmoids.

In adult amphibians, these bones partially or totally encircle the brain anterior to the optic foramen. They form the margins of the anterior half or third of the frontoparietal fontanelle dorsally and the basicranial fenestra ventrally, and in anurans and caecilians bear paired olfactory foramina anteriorly for the forward passage of the olfactory nerves from the brain.

The floor of the neurocranium posterior to the optic foramen forms in cartilage by fusion of the posterior portions of the parachordal rods, and is termed the hypochordal commissure (caecilians and some anurans) or basal plate (salamanders and most anurans). The medial margins of the unfused parachordals along with the leading margin of their midventral fusion delineate the posterior half of the basicranial fenestra. The anterior portion of each parachordal produces two dorsal extensions—the pila metoptica behind the optic foramen and the pila antotica between the oculomotor foramen anteriorly and prootic foramen posteriorly—that form the lateral braincase anterior to the auditory capsules. The pilae are united dorsally to one another and the preoptic root anteriorly by the orbital cartilage. The auditory capsules form as subspherical cartilaginous structures that lie postero-laterally adjacent to the parachordals to which they fuse. The capsule is separated from the pila antotica by the prootic foramen. The medial wall of each auditory capsule forms the postero-lateral wall of the braincase, which bears one to three auditory foramina. The jugular foramen lies postero-medial to the auditory capsule between the capsule and the floor of the neurocranium. The dorso-medial margin of the auditory capsule (taenia tecta marginalis) is continuous with the orbital cartilage; together these cartilages form the lateral margins of the frontoparietal fontanelle. The posterior margin of the fontanelle is formed by a dorsal bridge between the posterior portions of each otic capsule—the tectum synoticum; this structure is absent in primitive caecilians (e.g., *Ichthyophis glutinosus*). The foramen magnum is formed by the tectum synoticum (if present) dorsally and the basal plate or hypochordal commissure ventrally.

Several centers of ossification appear in this cartilaginous framework to form the auditory capsule and posterior neurocranium. The principal bones common to lissamphibians are paired prootics and exoccipitals. The prootics form all but the postero-medial osseous walls of the auditory capsules; the exoccipitals form around the foramen magnum, complete the auditory capsules posteriorly, and produce paired occipital condyles at the ventro-lateral "corners" of the foramen magnum. In most lissamphibians, the exoccipitals are fused indistinguishably with prootics in the adult. Two other centers of ossification—the opisthotic and pleurosphenoid—have been identified as contributing to the posterior neurocranium of some amphibians; however, if these elements are present, they usually are indistinguishable in adults owing to fusion with one another and the remaining posterior neurocranial elements.

Ear. The inner ear is housed in the auditory capsule. The middle ear is defined as the cavity located lateral to the capsule and posterior to the palatoquadrate body; it is derived from Visceral Pouches I and/or II, and houses the ear ossicles or plectral apparatus. The presence and nature of the plectral apparatus is variable in lissamphibians, and much remains to be learned about the development and homologies of the ossicles among the extant orders. In its simplest anatomical state, the plectrum consists of an expanded footplate that lies in the fenestra ovalis (= oval window) of the auditory capsule and a distal stylus that is directed antero-laterally; traditionally, this structure is called the stapes or columella. The base of the stylus may bear a stapedial foramen for the passage of the stapedial artery and/or the hyomandibular trunk of the facial nerve (C.N. VII). Two structures may be associated with the base of the stapes in the fenestra ovalis—the pars interna plectri and the operculum. The pars interna plectri is a cartilaginous base of the stylus that is elaborated around and within the anterior margin of the fenestra ovalis. If present as a discrete element, the operculum lies in the fenestra ovalis posterior to the stapes. Usually the operculum is cartilaginous; however, if the stapes is absent, the operculum may be partially ossified and fill the fenestra ovalis. The distal end of the stylus either is associated with the posterior aspect of the suspensorium (caecilians and salamanders) or lies within the squamosal embayment and bears an elaboration of cartilaginous processes that may connect it to the tympanic annulus (anurans). The details of these relationships are described below.

Olfactory Capsule. The olfactory capsule actually is a composite endo- and exocranial structure, being composed of a complicated and extremely variable configuration of cartilages that are associated with the upper jaw, external naris, and nasal sacs, as well as the dermal elements that surround the capsule. Occasionally, a single dermal bone, the septomaxilla, is incorporated into the capsule. The nasal cartilages arise as anterior and dorsal outgrowths of the cranial trabeculae that give rise to the anterior neurocranium, as described above.

Amphibians possess an anterior, cup-shaped cartilage (alary or cupular) associated with the external naris. The dorsal rim of the cup supports the external naris anteriorly, whereas its base forms the anterior wall of the olfactory capsule. The configuration of the alary cartilage and its orientation are highly variable depending upon the position of the external naris and the shape of the snout.

Most of the remaining olfactory cartilages are involved with encapsulating the olfactory organs, and consist of the following: (1) a vertical plate(s)—the septum nasi—separating the olfactory organs medially; (2–3) dorsal and ventral plates—the tectum nasi and solum nasi—that form part of the roof and floor of the capsule, respectively; (4) a transverse plate—the planum antorbitale or lamina orbitonasalis—that separates the olfactory capsule from the orbit; and (5) a dorsal, diagonally oriented bar of cartilage—the oblique cartilage—that joins the alary cartilage to the tectum nasi posteriorly.

Stabilization of the Anterior Part of the Upper Jaw. In adult lissamphibians, support of the upper jaw primarily is a function of the suspensorium (see description below); however, the planum antorbitale provides an anterior brace. It is a robust extension of the ethmoidal cartilage that extends laterally or antero-laterally from the neurocranium to the maxilla, thereby bracing the jaw against the braincase and forming the posterior wall of the nasal capsule. The planum also may be buttressed against the upper jaw by the presence of cartilaginous processes that extend anteriorly (anterior maxillary process) and posteriorly (posterior maxillary process) from it along the lingual margin of the maxilla. Although additional supporting structures are variable among amphibians, most have one or two rodlike prenasal cartilages that extend anteriorly from the solum nasi to the premaxillae of the upper jaw.

Exocranium

The exocranium consists of those cranial elements that are membranous (or dermal) in origin and that nearly always overlie endocranial structures. Dermal bones comprise the skull table, the snout and cheek regions, the upper jaw, and part of the palate. Dermal, or exocranial, elements also are integral components of composite structures such as the suspensorium and lower jaw. As a group, lissamphibians are characterized by a marked reduction in the numbers of exocranial elements relative to early tetrapods and lungfish. Thus, they invariably lack temporal, intertemporal, supratemporal, tabular, postorbital, postparietal, and jugal bones, and the palatine is not represented as a discrete elements in adults.

Skull Table. The skull table of living amphibians is represented by a simple, medial series of dermal roofing bones that consists of nasals, frontals, and parietals in an anterior-to-posterior sequence (fig. 6.2). The nasals always are paired and overlie the olfactory capsules. The frontals overlie the anterior neurocranium between the orbits, thereby covering the anterior part of the frontoparietal fontanelle and forming the dorsal margin of the orbit in the absence of postfrontals. The parietals are located posterior to the frontals and the orbit, and cover the posterior portion of the frontoparietal fontanelle. Medial fusion of the frontals and the parietals occasionally produces azygous elements, and anurans are characterized by fusion of the frontal and the parietal to form a single bone, the frontoparietal. Additional elements that contribute to the skull table in some amphibians are the prefrontal, postfrontal, and dermal sphenethmoid. The prefrontal lies laterally adjacent to the posterior part of the nasal and anterior part of the frontal, and may form the dorso-medial margin of the orbit. When it is present, the postfrontal lies lateral to the frontal and forms the dorsal margin of the orbit. The dermal sphenethmoid is a neomorphic bone formed in some amphibians between the nasals and frontals (or frontoparietals) above the sphenethmoid.

Snout. Herein, the snout is defined as that part of the skull anterior to the orbits; as such, it incorporates the anterior part of the skull table—i.e., the nasals. Although the fundamental function of the nasal in amphibians is to roof the olfactory capsule, it usually contributes to the lateral aspect of the snout in conjunction with the maxilla, and prefrontal, lacrimal, and septomaxilla (depending on the presence and condition of the latter three elements). The nasal nearly always provides bony support for the external narial opening, and in the absence of a prefrontal, it forms the anterior margin of the orbit.

The maxilla and premaxilla generally are thought of with respect to their tooth-bearing function in the upper jaw. Nonetheless, both are involved intimately in support and protection of the olfactory capsule in amphibians. The maxilla covers the ventro-lateral aspect of the olfactory capsule, whereas the premaxilla usually forms the rostrum anteriorly. Both bones are triradiate in cross section, bearing a pars dorsalis (facial flange of maxilla; alary process of premaxilla), pars dentalis (ventral dental ridge), and pars palatina (lingual palatal shelf). The peripheral margin of the olfactory capsule lies between the facial flanges and palatal shelves of both bones.

The palatal aspect of the snout is composed of the marginal contributions of the maxillae and premaxillae (as described above) and the paired vomers ventrally. The vomer usually bears teeth, forms a bony floor of the olfactory capsule, provides internal support for the olfactory eminence, and usually forms part or all of the bony margin of the choana.

Three bones are variably present and involved in the snout in amphibians—the prefrontal, lacrimal, and septomaxilla. Strictly speaking, the prefrontal is considered part of the dorsal skull table, but like the lacrimal, its primary contribution to the cranium in amphibians is in the provision of lateral coverage of the olfactory capsule. When present, the lacrimal lies between the nasal and premaxilla and forms the posterior margin of the external narial opening. The septomaxilla is a particularly problematic component of the amphibian snout. It is sporadic in its occurrence, and when present, it may be a superficial or an internal element. If superficial, the septomaxilla covers the antero-lateral aspect of the olfactory capsule and forms the posterior border of the external narial opening. Usually, however, the septomaxilla is a tiny element that lies within the olfactory capsule; here, it is associated intimately with a labyrinth of cartilages involved with support of the various olfactory cava and the nasolacrimal duct.

Neurocranial Region of the Palate. The dermal palate exclusive of the snout region and bones involved in the suspensorium consists solely of the parasphenoid. The bone invariably is present, although it may be fused with endocranial elements (e.g., prootic, sphenethmoid). The anterior end of the parasphenoid lies near, or anterior, to the level of the planum antorbitale; posteriorly, the bone terminates anterior to the exoccipitals. It may bear postero-lateral, winglike plates that underlie the auditory capsules. The anterior shaft of the parasphenoid is termed the cultriform process, whereas the postero-lateral parts are the alae.

Upper Jaw. The upper jaw, or maxillary arcade, is highly variable in its configuration and composition among amphibians. Three pairs of bones usually comprise the upper jaw—the premaxillae (antero-medially), maxillae (laterally), and quadratojugals (posteriorly). Only one pair is present in all amphibians—the premaxillae. Owing to loss of the quadratojugals, the maxillary arcade may be incomplete posteriorly. When present, teeth are borne on both the premaxilla and maxilla.

Composite Endo- and Exocranial Units

Mandible. The chondrocranial precursor of the lower jaw is Meckel's cartilage, parts of which persist in nearly all adult amphibians. Ossification of the anterior tip of Meckel's cartilage produces the mentomeckelian (= mentomandibular) bones on either side of the mandibular symphysis. In some amphibians, the postero-dorsal surface of Meckel's cartilage ossifies in the area of its articulation with the palatoquadrate. The remainder of the mandible is composed of dermal bones that invest Meckel's cartilage. Although as many as seven centers of dermal ossification have been identified in the formation of the lower jaw of some amphibians (angular, complementale, coronoid, dentary, prearticular, splenial, and supra-angular in caecilians; Wake and Hanken 1982), in metamorphosed adults, the mandible consists of only two dermal elements—a lateral, tooth-bearing bone (pseudodentary of caecilians and dentary of salamanders and anurans;

Duellman and Trueb 1986), and a medial bone (pseudoangular of caecilians, prearticular [= goniale or coronoideium] of salamanders, and angulosplenial of anurans; Duellman and Trueb 1986) that sheathes the medial, ventral, and posterior surfaces of Meckel's cartilage.

Suspensorium. The suspensorium consists of the complex of exo- and endocranial elements that are involved in the suspension of the jaws from the neurocranium and, in particular, the stabilization of the upper jaw against the neurocranium. The suspensorium has been studied fairly extensively in salamanders and anurans (see Pyles 1987, for review), but little is known for caecilians. The nomenclature of the suspensorium is especially confusing; in this discussion, the terminology of Pyles (1987) is followed.

The endocranial core of the suspensorium is the body of the palatoquadrate (= quadrate in some sources) cartilage and its various processes. The palatoquadrate cartilage appears early in development as a vertical procartilaginous bar located anterior to the first visceral pouch and lateral to the union of the pila antotica and auditory capsule. A medial outgrowth of the palatoquadrate, the ascending process, connects with the dorsomedial part of the pila antotica of the neurocranium; although the ascending process persists in adult salamanders, it is lost in adult anurans and never forms in caecilians. In adult lissamphibians, the palatoquadrate is a column of cartilage that is located lateral or antero-lateral to the auditory capsule. Dorsally, the palatoquadrate body usually is connected to the auditory capsule via an otic process. Ventro-medially, the palatoquadrate bears a basal (salamanders and caecilians) or pseudobasal (anurans) process that articulates directly or via the basitrabecular process of the neurocranium with the antero-ventral area of the basal plate or otic capsule. The ventral or postero-ventral surface of the palatoquadrate is termed the articular process (= quadrate process in some sources); the articular process may be partially ossified as the quadrate bone. The final process is the pterygoid process, which extends anterior–antero-laterally from the ventro-medial aspect of the palatoquadrate body and may join the posterior maxillary process (see above) along the lingual surface of the maxilla in the region of the orbit.

Nearly all lissamphibians bear at least two exocranial bones associated with the palatoquadrate and its processes. These are the squamosal and pterygoid, although the latter is absent in some salamanders. The squamosal invests the lateral, and usually the dorsal aspect of the palatoquadrate, and also may form part or all of the posterior orbital margin. The pterygoid is associated with the medial aspect of the palatoquadrate, the pterygoid process, and the basal or pseudobasal process. One other dermal bone occurs in some salamanders—a metapterygoid (= epipterygoid in some sources) that invests the distal ascending process.

Dentition

Teeth commonly are present on the maxillae, premaxillae, vomers, and dentaries. Less frequently, they may be borne on the neopalatines (anurans) and coronoid bone, if it is present in the mandible. The ectopterygoid, pterygoid, and parasphenoid lack true dentition, although the latter two elements may bear toothlike, bony odontoids in some taxa.

Hyobranchial Apparatus

The structure of the hyobranchial apparatus is so diverse among adults of the extant orders of amphibians that it eludes generalization, other than to point out that it is invariably present. The hyoid lies in musculature of the floor of the mouth, and is connected via the ceratohyal to the suspensory region or ventral auditory area of the cranium by muscles and ligaments in caecilians and salamanders, and by a synchondrotic fusion in most anurans. Examination of the cartilaginous hyobranchial apparatus of developing or larval amphibians reveals certain structural commonalities not apparent in adults. There are two midventral elements—Basibranchial I (anterior) and II (posterior). Associated with the latter is a series of paired, postero-laterally oriented elements. The most anterior and most robust are the ceratohyals. Posterior to the ceratohyals there are hypobranchials in salamanders and anurans; salamanders usually have two pairs of hypobranchials, whereas in anurans, the hypobranchials are fused to form a plate. Hypobranchials are not apparent in caecilians. Four pairs of ceratobranchials are present in most larval amphibians. These elements are associated with the distal ends of the hypobranchials, if the latter are present. In the absence of epibranchials, ceratobranchials are the terminal elements of the hyobranchial series.

CRANIAL OSTEOLOGY OF THE APODA

Living representatives of the order Apoda (caecilians) comprise six families containing 34 genera and 162 species (Frost 1985). There is a surprising amount of literature available on the cranial morphology of these generally poorly known, burrowing amphibians. Reviews of, and citations to, early literature may be found in Nussbaum (1977) and Wake and Hanken (1982). A general description of caecilian skull structure is presented by Duellman and Trueb (1986), and a photographic atlas of 48 species is available in Taylor (1969b).

Several classifications have been proposed recently for apodans. Those of M. Wake (1985, 1986) and Duellman and Trueb (1986) agree at the familial level with that of Taylor (1968, 1969a) as amended by Nussbaum (1977, 1979) and Nussbaum and Wilkinson (1988). The following discus-

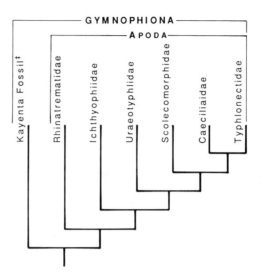

Fig. 6.3. A phylogeny of the Gymnophiona from Duellman and Trueb (1986) and Trueb and Cloutier (1991a). Double dagger indicates fossil taxa.

sion is based on the phylogenetic arrangement of these authors (fig. 6.3), rather than those proposed by Laurent (1986) and Lescure et al. (1986).

Caecilians: Diversification of a Fossorial Morphotype

Much has been made of the fact that, except for a few aquatic typhylonec-tids, caecilians are fossorial. (See Nussbaum 1977, and Wake and Hanken 1982, for commentaries and reviews.) This generalization has provided a ready explanation for the peculiarities of cranial structure characteristic of the group. However, to characterize all caecilians simply as "fossorial" is facile and uninformative, given their obvious diversification in cranial structure. Owing to their secretive nature, information on the habits of caecilians is scarce and anecdotal. Nonetheless, a brief survey of the litera-ture has revealed that the most primitive (i.e., least apomorphic) families are "surface cryptic" (sensu Ramaswami 1941). Thus, *Epicrionops petersi* (Rhinatrematidae) was found in gravel layers of a water seepage located between layers of rock at the base of a cliff adjacent to a rocky stream (W. E. Duellman, field notes, 1968). Another rhinatrematid, *Rhinatrema bivittatum*, was found under a stone that was immersed partially in water at the edge of a clear-water creek (Nussbaum and Hoogmoed 1979). Simi-larly, Ramaswami (1941) pointed out that the ichthyophiid *Ichthyophis* is not a typical burrower that digs by its head; instead, it lives under rotten vegetation where there is sufficient moisture. Ramaswami (1947) reported finding adults of *I. monochrous* in a small pool of water and under a dead log beside a mountain stream, whereas larvae were found in loose soil under grass. The more advanced caeciliaids seem to be more specialized burrowers. Thus, *Gegeneophis carnosus* was found 23–25 cm below the surface in wet earth (Ramaswami 1942), and various species of *Microcaecilia* were reported to have been found in rotting logs, in the upper soil layer in rainforest, and as deep as 50 cm in the soil (Nussbaum and Hoogmoed 1979).

Architectural Diversity

General Features. Caecilian skulls are distinguished by their robust, highly ossified structure and fusiform shape. The exocranium is extensive and may include a postfrontal bone, in contrast to other lissamphibians (fig. 6.4). Caecilians have a well-developed "cheek" region between the palatoquadrate and orbit, which is composed of the squamosal and occasionally, the maxillopalatine (fig. 6.5). When evident superficially, the orbit in caecilians is extremely small in contrast to those of salamanders and anurans (fig. 6.2). The order also is characterized by having an opening for the tentacle; the tentacular foramen or groove either is associated with the antero-ventral margin of the orbit or lies between the orbit and the external narial opening (figs. 6.6–6.7). The jaw articulation lies anterior to the auditory capsule, and the mandible bears a retroarticular process; muscles that insert on the retroarticular process provide for a dual jaw-closing mechanism that is unique among amphibians (Nussbaum 1983; Bemis et al. 1983).

Endocranium. *Neurocranium and Auditory Capsules.* The anterior braincase is formed by the sphenethmoid (= orbitosphenoid in some sources). The bone is formed from as many as six centers of ossification and the names of these centers frequently are used to designate parts of the sphenethmoid in the adult. Thus, "orbitosphenoid" refers to the lateral sphenethmoid on each side, "mesethmoid" to the antero-medial portion, "basisphenoid" to the ventro-medial area arising from paired ossifications, and "supraethmoid" to the dorso-medial part. The entire posterior neurocranium, including the auditory capsules, is a single element in the adult—the os basale (fig. 6.4). Ontogenetically, the os basale arises by fusion of several centers of ossification, including the exoccipitals, prootics, parasphenoid, and possibly, the opisthotics and pleurosphenoids (see de Beer 1937). The auditory capsule of caecilians is relatively narrow compared to those of salamanders and anurans. As a consequence, the neurocranium (including the auditory capsules) is more tubular than T-shaped.

Ear. The relatively little that is known about caecilian ears is summarized by Wever (1985). Caecilians lack a fenestra rotunda. All but one family (Scolecomorphidae; fig. 6.6) possess a stapes and oval window. The plec-

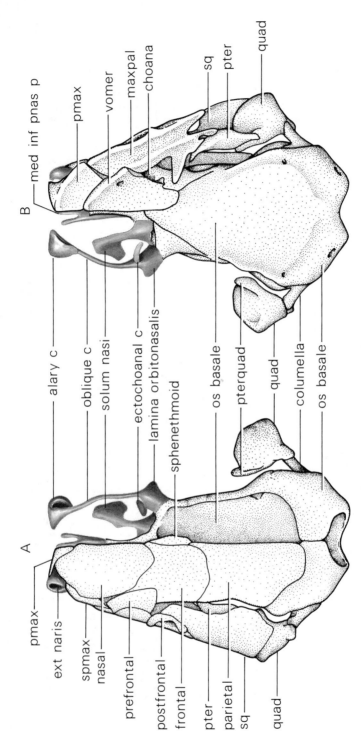

Fig. 6.4. Skull of the apodan *Ichthyophis glutinosus* (Ichthyophiidae) with dermal bones removed from the right side to reveal underlying chondrocranial elements; bones are stippled and cartilaginous elements shown in gray. A. Dorsal. B. Ventral. Redrawn from a graphic reconstruction by Visser (1963), and reproduced from Duellman and Trueb (1986) with permission of McGraw-Hill Book Company. See Appendix for abbreviations.

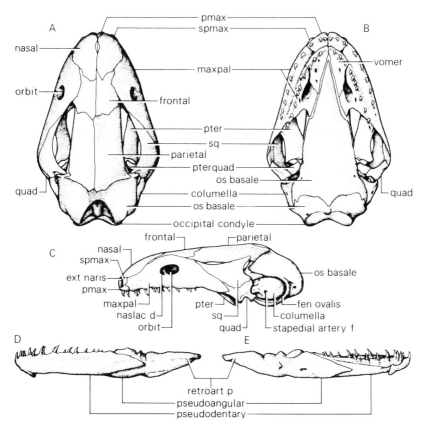

Fig. 6.5. Skull of the apodan *Epicrionops petersi* (Rhinatrematidae) in dorsal (A), ventral (B), and lateral (C) views. Mandible in lateral (D) and medial (E) views. Redrawn from Nussbaum (1977) and reproduced from Duellman and Trueb (1986) with permission of McGraw-Hill Book Company. See Appendix for abbreviations.

tral apparatus is simple, consisting of a short, but robust, stapes and broad footplate that lies in the fenestra ovalis. Presence of a stapedial foramen is variable. The stapes is oriented antero-laterally; distally, it either articulates with, or is fused to, the palatoquadrate. In adults, there is no evidence of a separate operculum, although Marcus (1935) proposed that it was incorporated into the footplate developmentally, and Barry (1954) suggested that the footplate was homologous to the operculum of other amphibians—a proposal that has not been accepted widely.

Olfactory Capsule. The nasal regions of six species of caecilians were examined by Jurgens (1971). Relative to the capsules of salamanders and anurans, those of caecilians are attenuate and characterized by a minimal

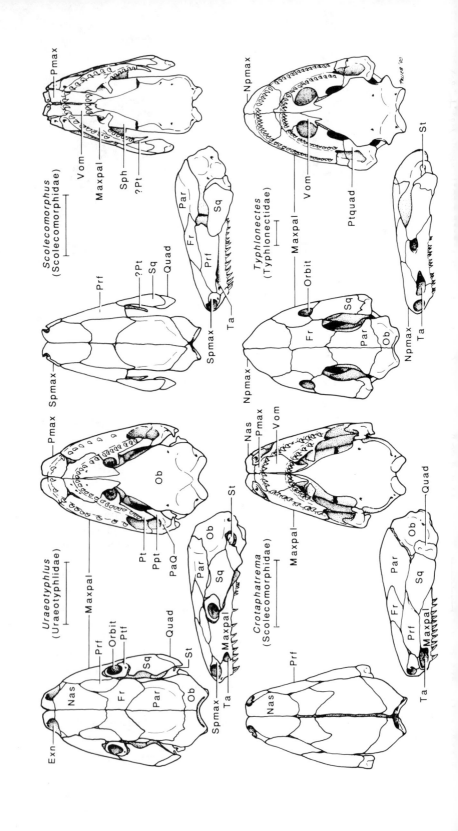

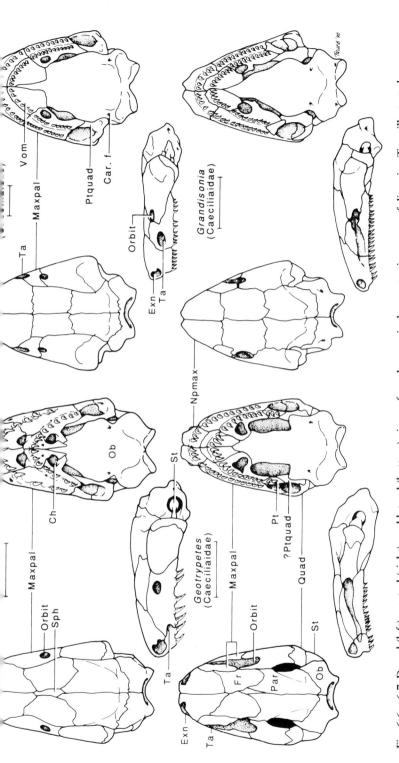

Fig. 6.6.–6.7 Dorsal (left), ventral (right), and lateral (bottom) views of apodan crania demonstrating range of diversity. Taxa illustrated: Uraeotyphlidae (*Uraeotyphlus narayani* adapted from Nussbaum 1979); Scolecomorphidae (*Scolecomorphus vittatus* and *Crotaphatrema bornmuelleri* adapted from Nussbaum 1985); Typhlonectidae (*Typhlonectes natans* adapted from Carroll and Currie 1975); and Caeciliaidae (*Caecilia albiventris* adapted from Carroll and Currie 1975, *Dermophis mexicanus* adapted from Wake and Hanken 1982, and *Geotrypetes seraphini* and *Grandisonia alternans* adapted from Carroll and Currie 1975).

amount of internal cartilaginous support (fig. 6.4); the latter probably is a structural correlate of the nearly complete exocranial covering of the snout (cf. description below). The capsules are narrowly separated medially by a partially ossified septum nasi. The posterior wall is formed by the sphenethmoid (medially) and the planum antorbitale laterally (= lamina orbitonasalis). Although the alary (= cupular) cartilage is well developed, the tectum nasi, solum nasi, and oblique cartilage are minimal. There is little elaboration of cartilaginous processes from the solum to support the nasal sacs; instead support is provided by medial processes of the septomaxilla (and presumably the nasopremaxilla or maxillopalatine if the septomaxilla is not discrete).

Stabilization of the Anterior Part of the Upper Jaw. In caecilians, support of the upper jaw is limited to the antero-lateral extension of the planum antorbitale from the sphenethmoid and a short, antero-medial extension of the septum nasi—the medial inferior prenasal cartilage—that abuts the premaxillae anteriorly (fig. 6.4).

Exocranium. *Skull Table.* The skull is roofed completely in caecilians by paired nasals (or nasopremaxillae), frontals, and parietals (figs. 6.4–6.7). A parietal foramen is absent. Three families (Ichthyophiidae, Uraeotyphlidae, and Scolecomorphidae; table 6.1) also possess prefrontals, and two families (Ichthyophiidae and Uraeotyphlidae) have postfrontals (= oculars of Taylor 1969a, and postorbitals elsewhere). In those caecilians with completely roofed temporal regions—i.e., stegokrotaphic representatives of the Scolecomorphidae and Caeciliaidae—the squamosal is expanded dorsomedially to articulate with the frontals and the parietals. A final component is the dorsal surface of the sphenethmoid, which is exposed between the frontals and/or nasopremaxillae in some caeciliaids.

Snout and Neurocranial Region of Palate. The snout in caecilians is distinctive among living amphibians owing to its length, the frequent presence of a tentacular foramen, and nearly complete coverage by dermal bones (fig. 6.2). The number of dermal bones present in the snout is variable among adult caecilians (table 6.1). There may be as few as three (nasopremaxilla, maxillopalatine, and vomer) or as many as seven—premaxilla, nasal, septomaxilla, maxillopalatine, prefrontal, postfrontal, and vomer (figs. 6.6–6.7). Although a separate lacrimal is absent in adults, it has been reported to exist as a separate center of ossification that fuses with the maxillopalatine in at least one taxon (Marcus et al. 1935).

The lateral aspect of the snout is especially variable with respect to the position and nature of the tentacular opening, the bone(s) participating in the anterior margin of the orbit and the posterior margin of the narial opening, and the shape of the rostrum. If the mouth is terminal, the rostrum is blunt and does not project beyond the tooth-bearing part of the upper jaw. In caecilians having slightly subterminal mouths, the rostrum tends to be rounded anteriorly, whereas in those with markedly subterminal mouths, the rostrum is distinctly pointed. If the septomaxilla is discrete, it forms the posterior margin of the naris; otherwise, the narial opening lies within the compound nasopremaxilla. If an orbital opening is present, it usually lies between the squamosal and maxillopalatine, or enclosed in the maxillopalatine (rhinatrematids); occasionally, however, part or all of its margin may be formed by the postfrontal (ichthyophiids and uraeotyphlids). The tentacle lies in a groove or foramen. Tentacular grooves are associated with the orbit and lie in the maxillopalatine, whereas a tentacular foramen may lie in the maxillopalatine or between the nasopremaxilla and the maxillopalatine.

The ventral snout region of caecilians characteristically differs from those of salamanders and anurans in being completely floored by robust lingual shelves of the premaxillae, maxillopalatines, and large, triangular vomers (= prevomers in some sources) (fig. 6.2). Furthermore, the palate is provided with a row of teeth medial to, and paralleling, the marginal dentition; these teeth lie on the vomer and maxillopalatine. The major sources of variation in the anterior caecilian palate involve the number and disposition (i.e., whether a diastema exists between the vomerine and maxillopalatine teeth) of the inner row of teeth, the bones that participate in the formation of the choana, and the relationship between the vomers and parasphenoid (figs. 6.6–6.7). Generally, the choana is bordered by the vomer antero-medially and the maxillopalatine laterally. The maxillopalatine bears a postchoanal flange that forms the posterior margin of the choana; in some taxa, the flange encircles the entire choana, thereby excluding the vomer from the choana. The vomers always articulate with one another antero-medially, but there is considerable variation in the extent of the medial articulation between the bones (table 6.1). The medial articulation may be complete, or nearly complete, so that the paired vomers overlie the anterior part of the cultriform process of the parasphenoid. Alternately, the medial margins of the vomers may diverge posteriorly from one another to expose part of the parasphenoid or actually flank its antero-lateral margins.

Upper Jaw. Unlike salamanders and many anurans, the maxillary arcade of adult caecilians always is complete. Toothed premaxillae (or nasopremaxillae) and maxillopalatines invariably are present. The posterior elements of the upper jaw are variable. The squamosal is a broad element that forms the "cheek" of caecilians behind the eye; in many taxa, the squamosal participates in the upper jaw because it lies between the maxil-

TABLE 6.1 Survey of cranial characters of caecilian families based on Nussbaum (1977, 1979) and Taylor (1969a)

Character	Rhinatrematidae	Ichthyophiidae	Uraeotyphlidae	Scolecomorphidae	Caeciliaidae	Typhlonectidae
1. Premaxilla	Discrete	Discrete	Discrete	Fused with nasals	Fused with nasals	Fused with nasals
2. Septomaxillae	Discrete	Discrete	Discrete	Discrete	Fused with adjacent bones	Fused with adjacent bones
3. Prefrontals	Absent	Present; usually articulating with septomaxilla	Present; not articulating with septomaxilla	Present; articulating with septomaxilla	Absent or fused	Absent or fused
4. "Postfrontals"	Absent/fused	Present or absent/fused	Present	Absent/fused	Absent/fused	Absent/fused
5. Temporal fossa	Large	Small	Small	Large or closed	Small or closed	Large
6. Squamosal-frontal contact	Absent	Present	Present	Absent	Present	Present
7. Squamosal notch for os basale process	Present	Absent	Absent	Absent	Absent	Absent
8. Palatoquadrate articulating with maxillopalatine	Yes	No	No	No	No	No
9. Mouth position	Terminal	Recessed	Subterminal	Subterminal	Subterminal	Subterminal
10. Vomer: posterior separation of	Wide	In contact	In contact	In contact	Wide or in contact	Wide
11. Vomer length	Midchoana	Beyond midchoana	Beyond midchoana	Midchoana	Midchoana or beyond	Beyond midchoana
12. Maxillopalatine: postchoanal flange	Present	Present	Present	Present	Present or absent	Present
13. Postchoanal flange: partial or complete	Partial	Partial	Partial	Partial	Partial or complete	Partial

foramen ovalis						
15. Stapedial foramen	Present	Present	Absent	Absent	Absent	Absent
16. Pterygoid	Present	Present	Present	Absent/fused	Present, but tends to fuse	Present, but tends to fuse
17. Pterygoid: size	Large	Moderate	Moderate	—	Moderate to small	Small
18. Basitrabecular process	Absent	Present	Present	Present	Present	Present
19. Basitrabecular process: size	—	Small	Small	Small	Large	Large
20. Retroarticular process: size	Short	Long	Long	Long	Long	Long
21. Retroarticular process: shape	Straight	Curved	Curved	Curved	Curved	Curved
22. Pseudoangular bones: internal process	Present	Present	Present	Absent	Present	Present
23. Splenial teeth	Present	Present or absent	Present	Absent	Present or absent	Present
24. External exposure of eye socket	Present	Present	Present	Absent	Present or absent	Present
25. Vomeropalatine tooth diastema	Absent	Absent	Absent	Present or absent	Present or absent	Absent
26. Ceratobranchial elements	2/3 (I–III, or I–I)	3 (I–IV)	3 (I–IV)	3 (I–IV)	3 (I–IV)	3 (I–IV)
27. Ceratobranchials III and IV	III and/or IV absent	III and IV fused	III and IV fused	III and IV fused	III and IV fused	III and IV fused
28. Expansion of Ceratobranchials III and IV	—	Present, slight	Present, moderate	Absent	Present, broad	Present, broad
29. Ceratohyal, Basibranchial I and Ceratobranchial I	United	United	United	United	Separate	Separate

lopalatine anteriorly and the ossified palatoquadrate posteriorly. In other taxa, the squamosal is excluded from the margin of the upper jaw by a dermal bone that lies ventral to the squamosal, articulates with the maxillopalatine, and is united synostotically to the ossified palatoquadrate posteriorly. The identity of this posterior jaw element is questionable. According to Marcus et al. (1935) and de Villiers (1936), a separate center of ossification, which they identified as the quadratojugal, exists in this area in *Hypogeophis* (Caeciliaidae); thus, the compound bone of the adult was termed a quadrate-quadratojugal. Other authors have called the terminal element of the upper jaw a "quadrate" or "pterygoquadrate."

Composite Endo- and Exocranial Units. *Mandible.* The mandible of all adult caecilians is characterized by the presence of a retroarticular process, a dentate pseudodentary, and a robust pseudoangular (fig. 6.5D, E). The bones are firmly attached to each other, although a remnant of Meckel's cartilage may persist between the pseudodentary and pseudoangular in a few species. The pseudoangular bears a U-shaped facet that articulates with the articular process of the palatoquadrate. The retroarticular process of the pseudoangular provides for the insertion of the m. interhyoideus posterior; contraction of this muscle pulls the process postero-ventrally, thereby pivoting the anterior part of the mandible upward around the palatoquadrate. The dual jaw-closing mechanism of caecilians, described by Nussbaum (1983) and Bemis et al. (1983), is unique among lissamphibians.

The homologies between the pseudodentary and pseudoangular and the mandibular bones of other amphibians are difficult to assess. According to Marcus et al. (1935), the pseudodentary of *Hypogeophis* (Caeciliaidae) is composed of the fused dentary, splenial, coronoid, supra-angular, and mentomeckelian, whereas the pseudoangular is composed of the fused angular, prearticular, articular, and complementale. In their study of another caeciliaid (*Dermophis mexicanus*), Wake and Hanken (1982) failed to observe centers of ossification for either the prearticular or supra-angular, and questioned the existence of a center representing the complementale.

Suspensorium. The suspensoria of only a few caecilians have been described in detail (see review in Nussbaum 1977). Our understanding of the system is hampered not only by lack of information, but also by the specialized nature of the suspensorium and uncertainty regarding the number, identity, and homologies of its components in those taxa that have been investigated. The only ossified endochondral elements that all adult caecilians possess in common with other lissamphibians are the palatoquadrate and the articular and pterygoid processes of the palatoquadrate. An ascending process of the palatoquadrate is absent. The otic process apparently is lost in all adults, and the basal process of the palatoquadrate and basitrabecular process of the neurocranium are sporadic in their occurrence. Some caecilians possess a columellar process of the palatoquadrate that is associated with the stapes. This process is unique to this group among the Lissamphibia, as is the resulting association of the stapes with the suspensorium.

The ossification of the pterygoid process of the palatoquadrate and associated bones is highly variable (figs. 6.4–6.7) and has caused considerable confusion. Occasionally (e.g., caeciliaids; fig. 6.7), the pterygoid process is synostotically united with the body of the palatoquadrate, thereby leading to the term "pterygoquadrate" for the entire assemblage. If the ossified pterygoid process is discrete from the palatoquadrate such that two bones lie in series between the palatoquadrate and maxillopalatine, the posterior member has been interpreted as a pterygoid (= ossified pterygoid process of the palatoquadrate, herein) and the anterior member as an ectopterygoid (= pterygoid, herein) (e.g., Carroll and Currie 1975). If an ectopterygoid exists in caecilians, it is represented by a center of ossification incorporated into the maxillopalatine (Marcus et al. 1935), and is not a free element in adults (Nussbaum 1977). In some caecilians (e.g., some typhlonectids and caeciliaids), there is complete fusion between the palatoquadrate, pterygoid process, and pterygoid, such that the so-called pterygoquadrate articulates with the maxillopalatine. In others (e.g., scolecomorphids), a discrete pterygoid seems to have been lost; thus, a medial brace among the palatoquadrate, maxillopalatine, and neurocranium does not exist.

The squamosal is an integral part of the caecilian suspensorium and well developed in all species. The squamosal covers the lateral aspect of the palatoquadrate, as well as the temporal region, to create a "cheek." The bone always bears a robust articulation with the maxillopalatine anteriorly and the ossified palatoquadrate posteriorly. If the temporal region is roofed (i.e., a stegokrotaphic skull), the squamosal articulates with the lateral margins of the frontal and parietal. If the temporal region is open (i.e., a zygokrotaphic skull), the squamosal may bear an incomplete articulation(s) with the frontal and/or parietal (e.g., rhinatrematids, uraeotyphylids, typhlonectids, some scolecomorphids), or lack an articulation with the skull table entirely (e.g., *Scolecomorphus*).

The following generalizations can be made about the suspensorium of caecilians. Postero-dorsal stabilization of the palatoquadrate seems to be provided in all taxa except scolecomorphids (which lack stapes) by a syndesmotic, synchondrotic, or synostotic association of the palatoquadrate and stapes. Further dorsal stabilization is a function of the dorsal margin of the squamosal, which is articulated variably with the frontal and/or parietal. Anterior support is provided by the articulation of the squamosal with the maxillopalatine. Medial abutment of the upper jaw against the neurocranium may be absent. If present, it is a function of two bones—the ossified pterygoid process of the palatoquadrate and the pterygoid—which may be syndesmotically or synostotically united to one another. Together these elements abut the palatoquadrate and maxillopalatine against the neurocranium in one of three ways. If a basitrabecular (= basipterygoid in some sources) process is absent, a syndesmotic union may exist between the neurocranium in the region of the otic capsule and the pterygoid process and pterygoid. If the neurocranium bears a basitrabecular process, it may be syndesmotically united to the pterygoid process of the palatoquadrate, or articulated with, or fused to, the basal process of the palatoquadrate.

Dentition. All caecilians bear teeth on the mandible (pseudodentary), upper jaw (premaxilla or nasopremaxilla, and maxillopalatine), and palate (vomer and maxillopalatine). The palatal teeth form an inner series that generally parallels the labial series of the upper jaw. Unlike the latter, however, the palatal series may bear a diastema between the vomerine and maxillopalatine dentition (scolecomorphids). Characteristically, caecilians bear numerous teeth that are homogeneous in size and form in the mature individual. However, in some caeciliaids and all scolecomorphids, the number of teeth is markedly diminished and the sizes of the individual teeth much enlarged. And in *Rhinatrema,* the teeth are heterogeneous in that the number of maxillopalatine teeth is reduced, and the individual teeth are enlarged and recurved (Nussbaum 1977).

Relatively little attention has been paid to mandibular teeth in caecilians. All have a labial series of teeth, and representatives of each family except the scolecomorphids have a lingual complement of so-called splenial teeth. Taylor (1977) noted that in the 23 species he examined the splenial teeth usually are small and number between 1 and 18 per side.

Hyobranchial Apparatus. The hyobranchial apparatus of caecilians differs from those of salamanders and anurans in that there is no evidence in the adult or young of separate hypohyals or hypobranchials (fig. 6.8). Thus, the hyobranchia of larvae consist of two basibranchial elements flanked laterally (in an anterior-to-posterior sequence) by paired ceratohyals and two to four ceratobranchials. The hyobranchium remains cartilaginous in the adult, but its configuration changes slightly. The second basibranchial either fuses with the first or is lost. The first basibranchial fuses with, and thereby unites, the ceratohyals. Each pair of ceratobranchials fuses midventrally. Further, the first pair of ceratobranchials may be united

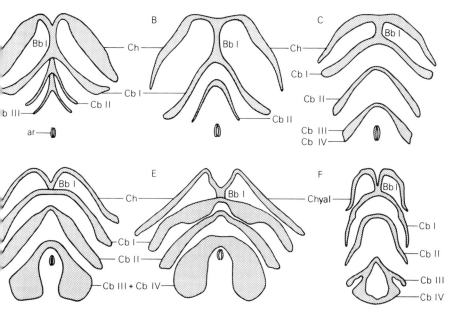

Fig. 6.8 Hyobranchial skeletons of apodans in ventral view redrawn from Nussbaum (1977), and reproduced from Duellman and Trueb (1986) with permission of McGraw-Hill Book Company. A. *Epicrionops* (Rhinatrematidae). B. *Rhinatrema* (Rhinatrematidae). C. *Ichthyophis* (Ichthyophiidae). D. *Gymnophis* (Caeciliaidae). E. *Typhlonectes* (Typhlonectidae). F. *Scolecomorphus* (Scolecomorphidae). See Appendix for abbreviations.

antero-medially with the basibranchial and ceratohyals (rhinatrematids, ichthyophiids, uraeotyphlids, scolecomorphids) or not (caeciliaids, typhlonectids). The posterior ceratobranchials (III and IV) are the most variable part of the hyobranchium. Ceratobranchials III and IV are reduced or lost in rhinatrematids, and fused in the remaining caecilians. The fused ceratobranchials may be slender (scolecomorphids), slightly expanded (ichthyophiids), moderately expanded (uraeotyphlids), or broadly expanded (caeciliaids and typhlonectids).

The Primitive Caecilian Cranium. It is especially significant that the two most primitive genera, the rhinatrematids *Epicrionops* and *Rhinatrema,* seem not to be accomplished burrowers. Based on Nussbaum's (1979) well-corroborated phylogeny of caecilians (fig. 6.3), it is evident that these taxa differ from the caecilian stem species or hypothetical ancestor only in the configuration of the posterior part of their hyobranchial apparatus (table 6.1). Thus, we can infer that, plesiomorphically, caecilians had a zygokrotaphic (i.e., with large temporal fossa), kinetic skull. The braincase was fully ossified, and fused to the parasphenoid. The mouth was terminal. Extensive temporal fossae probably allowed passage of paired m. adductor mandibulae from the mandible to the dorsal surface of the skull.

Although the hypothetical ancestor possessed discrete premaxillae, septomaxillae, prefrontals, postfrontals, and perforate stapes, the maxilla and palatine were fused to form the maxillopalatine. The suspensorium was robust, being composed of a well-developed palatoquadrate that articulated directly with the maxillopalatine laterally. Dorsal stabilization of the suspensorium involved articulation of the palatoquadrate with the stapes posteriorly and articulation of a postero-dorsal process of the squamosal with a notch in the os basale. In the absence of a basitrabecular process of the neurocranium, the palatoquadrate was connected to the neurocranium medially via a syndesmotic union of the pterygoid process of the palatoquadrate with the neurocranium. The maxillopalatine was braced against the braincase by the pterygoid.

The orbit was not covered by bone, and the tentacle exited the skull via a tentacular foramen or groove associated with the anterior margin of the orbit. The teeth were bicuspid and recurved. A full complement of labial and palatal teeth was present, and the mandible was characterized by marginal dentition, as well as a well-developed row of splenial teeth. The mandible bore a short, straight retroarticular process, onto which an interhyoideus posterior muscle presumably inserted to provide for a dual jaw-closing mechanism.

The hyobranchial apparatus was cartilaginous. This may be associated with the poorly developed tongue characteristic of caecilians, the elaboration of the dual jaw-closing mechanism, and the apparent relegation of the hyobranchium as an attachment for muscles involved in raising and lowering the floor of the mouth to facilitate force-pump respiration.

It seems reasonable to infer from these data that the hypothetical ancestral caecilian, like the basal rhinatrematid clade, was only partially fossorial—that like *Rhinatrema* and *Icthyophis,* it may have lived in loose soil, beneath surface litter, and in littoral habitats. The solidly fused braincase of the fusiform, but blunt-snouted, skull would have been sufficiently robust to move through friable substrates. The kineticism of the suspensorium, along with the poorly developed retroarticular process of the mandible, suggests that early caecilians may have been more efficient at grasping prey on the surface than in restricted subterranean situations.

Patterns of Derivation among Living Caecilians. The primary evolutionary trend among caecilians is one of increasing stegokrotaphy among ichthyophiids, uraeotyphlids, scolecomorphids, and caeciliaids. Secondary zygokrotaphy characterizes the typhlonectids. Table 6.1 summarizes characteristics of the six families.

Stegokrotaphy. Trends toward stegokrotaphy involve complexes of morphological specializations that are first evident in ichthyophiids and uraeotyphlids, and reach their zeniths in scolecomorphids and caeciliaids. The elaboration of the skull toward a stegokrotaphic, akinetic condition generally is associated with (1) reduction of the number of cranial elements through fusion of centers of ossification, (2) expansion of bones to cover or reduce the size of the orbit, roof the temporal fossa partially or totally, and separate the exit of the tentacle from the orbit, and (3) strengthening or modification of the suspensorium. Because the evolutionary expression of stegokrotaphy in the highly apomorphic African Scolecomorphidae differs in many significant regards from that of the caeciliaids, the two families are discussed separately below.

Primitive Stegokrotaphy (Icthyophiidae and Uraeotyphlidae). The skulls of ichthyophiid and uraeotyphlid caecilians are distinguished from the zygokrotaphic skull of rhinatrematids by lateral expansion of the frontal and parietal, and dorsal elaboration of the squamosal to roof the temporal fossa partially, or nearly completely (some ichthyophiids). The squamosal also expands ventrally to form a brace in the maxillary arcade between the maxillopalatine anteriorly and the quadrate posteriorly. The expansion of the squamosal with the increase in its articular surfaces presumably strengthens the suspensorium. Internally, the suspensorium is strengthened by the acquisition of a small basitrabecular process of the neurocranium that articulates syndesmotically with the pterygoid process of the palatoquadrate postero-laterally and the pterygoid antero-laterally, thereby bracing the upper jaw against the skull.

Stegokrotaphy in the Scolecomorphidae. The intrafamilial relationships of this peculiar family are unknown. Of the two genera included in the family, *Scolecomorphus* possesses a zygokrotaphic skull, whereas that of *Crotaphatrema* is obviously more robust (Nussbaum 1985). For the purposes of this discussion, I am assuming that the skull of *Scolecomorphus* is less derived than that of *Crotaphatrema*. The crania of both genera share derived features associated with stegokrotaphic trends—fusion of the premaxilla with the nasals, loss or incorporation of the postfrontals with other cranial bones, and marked expansion of the squamosal. Unlike any other caecilian, however, the prefrontal in scolecomorphids is vastly expanded in the dorso-lateral region of the skull. The bone covers the orbit in both genera, and together with the maxillopalatine forms a bony lateral canal that houses the tentacle, which exits the skull anteriorly. As in most other caecilians, the tentacle exits the skull via a foramen. Scolecomorphids, in contrast to other caecilians, seem to have an exceedingly weak suspensorium. The palatoquadrate is robust, but it lacks a pterygoid process in *Scolecomorphus vittatus,* and has only a small process in *Crotaphatrema lamottei;* the basitrabecular processes of both taxa are small, and pterygoids either are reduced or missing. Further, the stapes, which acts as a suspensory unit in other caecilians, is absent in this family. Thus, scolecomorphids seem to have achieved a degree of kineticism in the suspensory apparatus that is unique among caecilians; the significance of this peculiar condition is unknown.

Stegokrotaphy in the Caeciliaidae. Reduction in the number of cranial elements occurs by way of the fusion of the premaxilla with the nasal to produce a nasopremaxilla, and loss of the septomaxilla and prefrontal through fusion with either the maxillopalatine or nasopremaxilla (which bone is unknown). The fate of the postfrontal, which is associated with the orbit in ichthyophiids and uraeotyphlids, also is unknown; however, examination of the topology of caecilian skulls lacking this bone suggests that it may fuse either with the maxillopalatine or the squamosal, or with both.

Dorsal expansion of the squamosal combined with lateral elaboration of the frontal and/or parietal effects complete closure of the temporal fossa in caeciliaids. Reduction in the size of the orbit or covering of the orbit in caeciliaids is associated with absence (presumably through fusion with adjacent elements) of the pre- and postfrontals, and a more anterior position of the tentacular foramen.

Stegokrotaphy is characterized by development of a more robust suspensorium in caeciliaids. The squamosal increases in size and bears extensive articulations with the frontal, parietal, maxillopalatine, palatoquadrate, and stapes. The pterygoid process of the palatoquadrate is ossified and articulates with the neurocranium by means of a basitrabecular process. Although the pterygoid is only moderate or small in caeciliaids, it completes an arcade of support between the maxillopalatine and the basitrabecular process of the neurocranium.

Secondary Zygokrotaphy. One family of caecilians, the typhlonectids, is characterized by character reversals that are associated with the independent evolution of zygokrotaphic skulls from a presumably stegokrotaphic ancestor. The typhlonectids comprise four genera of South American caecilians. As perusal of table 6.1 suggests, the family is allied closely to its terrestrial sister group, the caeciliaids, by similarities of the skull and hyobranchium. The resemblances suggest that typhlonectids were derived from a fossorial, stegokrotaphic ancestor, and that the zygokrotaphic skull characteristic of the family is associated with its aquatic habits and may have evolved by reduced ossification of four dermal bones—the frontal, parietal, squamosal, and maxillopalatine.

Typhlonectids retain a robust suspensorium. However, to a greater or lesser degree, the lateral margins of the frontal and parietal and the dorsal margin of the squamosal are emarginated to produce a temporal fossa. In addition, the orbit is large, and the tentacular groove is open, or only partially shielded by the maxillopalatine.

CRANIAL OSTEOLOGY OF THE CAUDATA

The order Caudata (sensu Trueb and Cloutier 1991a) is composed of 12 families and 91 genera; of these, 3 families and 29 genera are represented only by fossils (Estes 1981); thus, living salamanders comprise a total of 9 families containing 62 genera and 352 species (Frost 1985). The closest approximation to a synthesis of the cranial osteology of salamanders is that contained in Duellman and Trueb (1986). Although these authors reviewed pertinent descriptive literature, the contributions of Carroll and Holmes (1980), Estes (1981), and Jurgens (1971) and the references cited therein should not be overlooked. Of the three orders of amphibians, relatively the least is known about the development, diversity, and evolutionary trends of the cranial skeleton in salamanders; the most complete and useful reviews available are those of Wake and Özeti (1969) on salamandrids, Tihen (1958) on ambystomatids (including *Rhyacotriton* and *Dicamptodon*), Wake (1966) on plethodontids, and Larsen (1963) on a variety of taxa of neotenic and transformed salamanders.

Useful reviews of proposed caudate phylogenies appear in Estes (1981) and Duellman and Trueb (1986). It is clear that an understanding of the evolutionary relationships of the extant families is obfuscated by the occurrence of paedomorphic taxa. All members of four of the nine families retain larval characters as adults—the Sirenidae, Amphiumidae, Proteidae, and Cryptobranchidae. At least some members of three other families or groups—the Plethodontidae, Ambystomatidae, and Dicamptodon (*D. copei*)—are considered to be paedomorphic. Only two groups seem to lack obvious paedomorphs—the "hynobiids," and the Salamandridae—although populations of some species of the latter families are facultatively neotenic. The phylogeny adopted here (Cloutier, n.d.; fig. 6.9) differs from that of Duellman and Trueb (1986) in several important respects. The Sirenidae is considered to be the most highly derived salamander family, and the Amphiumidae and Proteidae are sister groups of one another. The Dicamptodontidae is not recognized, and "hynobiids" are considered paraphyletic (indicated herein by enclosure of the familial name in quotation marks). In overall construction, this phylogeny agrees with others proposed during the past 15 years (e.g., Edwards 1976; Milner 1983; Duellman and Trueb 1986) in its placement of "hynobiids" and cryptobranchids

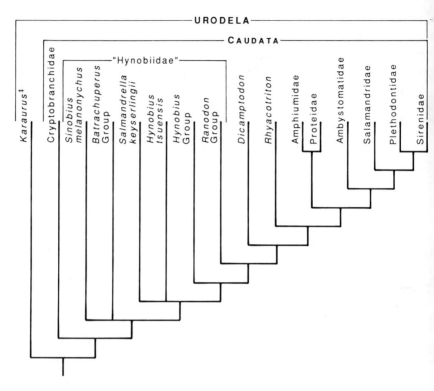

Fig. 6.9 A phylogeny of the Urodela from Cloutier (in preparation). Double dagger indicates fossil taxa.

at the base of the tree, Rhyacotriton and Dicamptodon at the midlevel of the tree, and ambystomatids, salamandrids, and plethodontids as more highly derived taxa.

Salamanders: Diversification of Semiterrestrial Generalists

Despite the fact that salamanders lack some of the plesiomorphic features that characterize caecilians, there is little doubt that as a group, caudates are the least specialized lissamphibians; in their basic design, caudates probably are the most similar to the hypothetical lissamphibian ancestor (Trueb and Cloutier 1991a). But it should not be inferred from this statement that salamanders are morphologically homogeneous. To the contrary, the diversity of caudate morphotypes far exceeds that found in either caecilians or anurans, both of which are constrained historically by suites of morphological features that are associated with their specialized modes of locomotion.

From a basic tailed, elongate, and four-limbed design that is moderately effective for movement on both land and in water (i.e., semiterrestrial habits), various major lineages of salamanders have evolved specializations for totally aquatic and terrestrial lifestyles. Other clades seem to cross, or lie between, adaptive zones. The aquatic zone is populated by cryptobranchids, proteids, amphiumids, and sirenids, all of which are large or long (ca. 250–1500 mm total length) and obligate neotenes in the sense of possessing gill slits (except in *Andrias* and *Megalobatrachus*). Sirenids and amphiumids have converged upon an eel-like morph in which the body is greatly elongated, the head long and narrow, and the limbs reduced (hind limbs absent in sirenids). Of the aquatic salamanders, the proteids probably are the least derived, although their heads tend to be narrow and their limbs small relative to the sizes of their bodies. The purely terrestrial zone is largely the province of plethodontids, many of which are arboreal specialists. Plethodontids are distinguished by their smaller size (ca. 27–350 mm total length), direct development of bolitoglossine and plethodontine plethodontids, and absence of lungs. The semiterrestrial zone is frequented by *Dicamptodon,* and some members of the "hynobiids," salamandrids, and ambystomatids—salamanders that are relatively generalized in structure and that return to the water to breed. However, each of the three latter groups contains some representatives that have different adaptive specializations. Thus, some ambystomatids (e.g., *Ambystoma mexicanum*) are neotenic denizens of the aquatic zone. Among the "hynobiids" are salamanders (e.g., *Batrachuperus pinchonii*) that are fully transformed, but exclusively stream inhabitants. In contrast to ambystomatids, most salamandrids that have moved out of the semiterrestrial zone have tended to become more terrestrial in some cases acquiring thick, verrucose skin (e.g., *Triturus*) and in others, live birth of young (e.g., *Salamandra atra*).

The question arises how, if at all, diversity of cranial structure is correlated with the general morphological and ecological diversity described above. Perusal of studies of salamander feeding and the structures associated with feeding (Regal 1966; Özeti and Wake 1969; Larsen and Guthrie 1975; Lombard and Wake 1976, 1977; Erdman and Cundall 1984; Lauder and Shaffer 1985; Cundall et al. 1987) reveals that salamanders inhabiting different adaptive zones have distinctive modes of feeding. The way in which the organism feeds is primarily dependent on the presence or absence of branchial apertures, the development and structure of the tongue, the structure of the hyobranchium, location of the jaw articulation, and the dentitional pattern. Much of the cranial variability in salamanders can be correlated with the adaptive zone inhabited by the organism and its mode of feeding and respiration.

Architectural Diversity

General Features. Unlike caecilians, salamanders tend to have broad, depressed gymnokrotaphic skulls characterized by an open temporal region, large orbit lacking a posterior margin, absence of a "cheek," and incomplete upper jaw (fig. 6.2). In many of these features they resemble some or all anurans; however, the skull roof of most salamanders is more complete than that of most anurans. Salamanders lack the fusion of cranial components that characterizes caecilians, and the stapes of transformed adults is connected to the squamosal rather than the quadrate. Moreover, discrete palatine and quadratojugal bones are absent in the adults (but see below). The jaw articulation usually lies well anterior to the posterior limits of the skull, and the mandible retains separate prearticular and articular elements in contrast to those of caecilians and anurans. Salamanders are unique among amphibians in possessing a four-faceted articulation of the exoccipital with the cervical vertebra; in addition to the occipital condyles, they possess a tuberculum interglenoideum, which is a well-developed anteroventral process of the atlas that projects into the foramen magnum to articulate with paired facets of the exoccipitals.

Endocranium. *Neurocranium and Auditory Capsules.* The anterior braincase is formed by the sphenethmoid (= orbitosphenoid or orbitotemporal in some sources) (fig. 6.10). Because the sphenethmoids apparently are formed from one center of ossification medial to the eye on each side of the skull (Bonebrake and Brandon 1971), it is probable that the sphenethmoid is homologous to the ossification center identified as the orbitosphenoid in caecilians. Nonetheless, in salamanders, the sphenethmoid is paired, with each bone forming the side of the neurocranium between the optic and/or oculomotor foramen posteriorly and the orbitonasal foramen at the anterior margin of the orbit; it forms bony margins to the anterolateral edges of the frontoparietal (dorsal) and basicranial (ventral) fontanelles, respectively.

The formation of the posterior neurocranium is relatively poorly understood. Three paired centers of ossification have been identified in *Ambystoma*—the prootic, opisthotic, and exoccipital (Bonebrake and Brandon 1971). If the braincase is ossified anterior to the auditory capsule, the ossification apparently represents the prootic. Like its anterior counterpart, the sphenethmoid, the prootic is paired and, if present, forms a bony margin to the postero-lateral margin of the frontoparietal and basicranial fontanelles. The prootic also is thought to form the anterior face of the auditory capsule. The opisthotic forms the dorsal, ventral, and lateral parts of the otic capsule, whereas the exoccipital forms the postero-medial walls around the foramen magnum and the occipital condyles. In adult salamanders, the two or three bones present are completely fused (table 6.2A, B).

Ear. The configuration of the ear in adult salamanders, as well as its development, are highly variable. The most useful recent summaries of the ear morphology of salamanders are those of Monath (1965), Lombard (1977), and Wever (1985). Salamanders possess a fenestra rotunda and fenestra ovalis. The plectral apparatus is variably composed of a bony stapes (lacking a stapedial foramen) and an operculum, which may be cartilaginous or bony, and independent or fused to adjacent elements (table 6.2A, B). Ontogenetically, the stapes (absent in salamandrids and sirenids) appears prior to the operculum and bears a stylus that projects antero-dorsally from the auditory capsule to unite with the squamosal via a synchondrotic or ligamentous attachment. During development, the attachment of the stapes may shift to the quadrate (e.g., the proteid *Necturus*). Additionally, in neotenic taxa such as *Cryptobranchus* (Cryptobranchidae) and *Amphiuma* (*Amphiumidae*), the stapes may bear ligamentous connections to the ceratohyal.

Plesiomorphically, the apparatus consists of a bony stapes that bears a distal stylus and an expanded footplate that lies in the anterior part of the fenestra ovalis; an operculum may be associated with the stapes in the posterior part of the fenestra. In more derived salamanders, the operculum tends to become reduced and/or fused with the lateral wall of the otic capsule. Salamandrids are characterized by the loss of the stapes and the retention of a bony or cartilaginous operculum that fills the fenestra ovalis. In plethodontids, the stapes is thought to be fused to the operculum (Monath 1965), which forms a plate in the fenestra ovalis; in some members of this family, the stylus of the stapes is well developed, whereas in others it is slender and short.

Olfactory Capsule. The nasal capsules of five species of salamanders (representing five families) were examined in detail by Jurgens (1971), who also summarized and discussed the results of previous studies. Salamanders differ from anurans and caecilians in usually having widely separated capsules that are considerably more robust than those of other lissamphibians. Like caecilians, they lack the intricate array of cartilages associated with the external naris of anurans; presumably, this is correlated with the presence of intrinsic narial muscles that control opening and closure of the naris in salamanders as contrasted to the mechanism in anurans, most of which lack direct muscular control (Gans and Pyles 1983; personal ob-

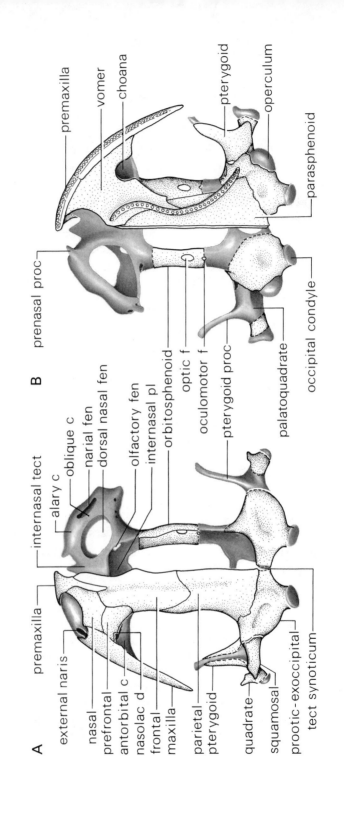

A

- premaxilla
- external naris
- nasal
- prefrontal
- antorbital c
- nasolac d
- frontal
- maxilla
- parietal
- pterygoid
- quadrate
- squamosal
- prootic-exoccipital
- tect synoticum

- internasal tect
- alary c
- oblique c
- narial fen
- dorsal nasal fen
- olfactory fen
- internasal pl
- orbitosphenoid
- optic f
- oculomotor f
- pterygoid proc
- palatoquadrate
- occipital condyle

B   prenasal proc

- premaxilla
- vomer
- choana
- pterygoid
- operculum
- parasphenoid

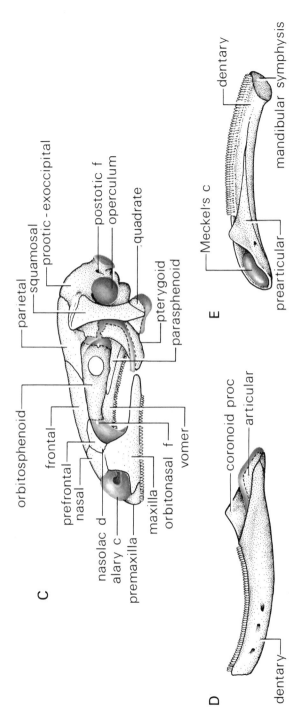

Fig. 6.10 Skull of the caudate *Salamandra salamandra* (Salamandridae) in dorsal (A), ventral (B), and lateral (C) views. Mandible in lateral (E) and medial (F) aspects. Dermal bones are removed from the right side to reveal underlying chondrocranial elements; bones are stippled and cartilaginous elements shown in gray. Redrawn from Francis (1934), and reproduced from Duellman and Trueb (1986) with permission of McGraw-Hill Book Company. See Appendix for abbreviations.

TABLE 6.2A Survey of cranial characters of adult salamanders

Character	Group				
	Cryptobranchidae	"Hynobiidae"	Dicamptodon	Rhyacotriton	Amphiumidae
1. Prootic/exoccipital/opisthotic	3 separate elements	3 separate elements	3 separate elements	3 separate elements	3 separate elements
2. Operculum	Absent/fused with stapes	Free with ossified stapes, or absent/fused	Free with ossified stapes	Free with ossified stapes	Absent/fused with stapes
3. Stapes	Present in adults; ligamentous attachment to squamosal or quadrate	Present in adults; free	Present in adults; free	Present in adults; free	Present in adults; ligamentous attachment to squamosal or quadrate
4. Lateral wall of nasal capsule	Complete	Complete	Incomplete	Incomplete	Incomplete
5. Lateral narial fenestra	Absent	Absent	Present	Present	Absent
6. Posterior wall of nasal capsule	Complete	Complete	Complete	Complete	Incomplete
7. Septomaxilla	Absent	Present	Present	Present	Absent
8. Naso-lacrimal duct	Absent	Present	Present	Present	Absent
9. Jacobson's organ	Present, poorly developed	Present	Present	Present	Present, poorly developed
10. Nasal	Present	Present	Present	Absent	Present
11. Medial articulation of nasals	Present	Present	Present	—	Absent
12. Prefrontal	Present	Present	Present	Present	Present
13. Lacrimal	Absent	Present	Present	Present	Absent
14. Premaxillae	Separate	Separate	Separate	Separate	Fused

15. Pars dorsalis of premaxilla: length	Short	Short	Short	Long	Long
16. Pars dorsalis of premaxilla: relation to skull roof	Overlaps nasals	Overlaps nasals	Separates prefrontals	Separates nasals	Separates nasals
17. Premaxillary dentition	Present	Present	Present	Present	Present
18. Maxilla	Present	Present	Present	Present	Present
19. Vomerine dentition placement	Marginal	Medial	Medial	Medial	Marginal
20. Quadratojugal	Absent	Present, but fused in adults, or absent	Absent	Absent	Absent
21. Angular	Present	Present or absent	Absent	Absent	Absent
22. Coronoid	Absent	Dentate bone present in larvae; absent in adults	Edentate bone present in adults	Absent	Absent
23. Articular	Absent	Present	Present	Present	Absent
24. Pterygoid	Present	Present	Present	Present	Present
25. "Palatopterygoid"	Absent	Absent	Present or absent	Absent	Absent
26. Metapterygoid	Absent	Present or absent	Absent	Absent	Absent
27. Basitrabecular process	?	Present	?	Present	?
28. Hypobranchial I and Ceratobranchial I	Fused into single rod	Fused into single rod	Separate	Separate	Fused into single rod
29. Ceratobranchial II	Present	Present	Absent	Absent	Present
30. Dentition	Pedicellate	Pedicellate	Pedicellate; compressed, bladelike	Pedicellate; conical	Pedicellate

TABLE 6.2B Survey of cranial characters of adult salamanders

Character	Group				
	Proteidae	Ambystomatidae	Salamandridae	Plethodontidae	Sirenidae
1. Prootic/exoccipital/prootic	Opisthotic separate	Fused	Fused	Fused	3 separate elements
2. Operculum	Free with ossified stapes	Free (bony or cartilaginous with ossified stapes, or absent/fused	Bony or cartilaginous, filling fenestra ovalis	Fused to stapes; united to otic capsule	Free with ossified stapes
3. Stapes	Present in adults; attached to quadrate	Present in adults; usually fused to skull, but may be free	Absent in adults	Present, reduced, or absent in adults	Present in adults; ?
4. Lateral wall of nasal capsule	Incomplete	Incomplete	Incomplete	Incomplete	Incomplete
5. Lateral narial fenestra	Absent	Present	Present	Present	Absent
6. Posterior wall of nasal capsule	Incomplete	Complete	Complete	Complete	Incomplete
7. Septomaxilla	Absent	Present	Absent	Present or absent	Absent
8. Naso-lacrimal duct	Absent	Present	Absent	Present	Absent
9. Jacobson's organ	Represented only by olfactory buds	Present	Present	Present	Large, well developed; ventral
10. Nasal	Absent	Present	Present	Present or absent	Present
11. Medial articulation of nasals	—	Absent	Absent	Absent	Absent

Character	1	2	3	4	5
12. Prefrontal	Absent	Present or absent	Present	Present	Absent
13. Lacrimal	Absent	Absent	Absent	Absent	Absent
14. Premaxillae	Separate	Separate or fused	Separate or fused	Separate	Separate
15. Pars dorsalis of premaxilla: length	Long	Long	Long	Long	Long
16. Pars dorsalis of premaxilla: relation to skull roof	Lateral to nasal, medial to frontal	Separates nasals	Separates nasals	Separates nasals	Overlaps frontal
17. Premaxillary dentition	Absent	Present	Present	Present	Present
18. Maxillae	Vestigial or absent	Present or absent	Present	Present	Absent
19. Vomerine dentition placement	Covering vomer	Medial or marginal	Medial or marginal	Medial or marginal	Marginal
20. Quadratojugal	Absent	Absent	Absent	Absent	Absent
21. Angular	Fused with prearticular	Fused with prearticular	Fused with prearticular	Fused with prearticular	Fused with prearticular
22. Coronoid	Present	Absent	Absent	Absent	Dentate bone present in adults
23. Articular	Absent	Absent	Present or absent	Present or absent	Absent
24. Pterygoid	Vestigial	Absent	Present	Present	Present
25. "Palatopterygoid"	?Present	?Present or absent	Absent	Absent	?Present
26. Metapterygoid	Absent	Absent	Absent	Absent	Absent
27. Basitrabecular process	?	Present	Absent	Present	?
28. Hypobranchial I and Ceratobranchial I	Separate	Separate	Separate or fused	Separate	Separate
29. Ceratobranchial II	?Present	Absent	Absent	Absent	Present or absent
30. Dentition	Nonpedicellate	Pedicellate	Pedicellate	Pedicellate	Pedicellate

servation). Salamanders also lack the ossification of the nasal cartilages (septum nasi) that frequently is found in anurans.

The medial walls of the nasal capsules arise from the trabecular plate (= planum internasale and planum basale in some sources) (fig. 6.10). Antero-ventrally, the trabecular plate of each side of the head terminates in a slender process, the inferior lateral prenasal process (= inferior prenasal cartilage), which rests against the lingual surface of the premaxilla. In most taxa (table 6.2A, B), a short dorso-medial bridge of cartilage (tectum internasale) unites the walls to form a septum nasi between the capsules; if present, the septum may be fenestrate (i.e., with a fenestra precerebralis) or not. The anterior margin of the septum nasi, together with the anterior portions of the medial nasal walls, define the cavum internasale within which the intermaxillary gland is located in terrestrial salamanders. The posterior border (lamina precerebralis) of the septum nasi, together with the posterior portions of the medial nasal walls, form the cavum cranii, which houses the anterior part of the brain that projects into the internasal region and the margins of the frontoparietal fontanelle anterior to the sphenethmoid.

Lateral and anterior extension of the medial wall of the nasal capsule forms a roof (tectum nasi), which is variably fenestrate, and therefore, incomplete in all salamanders. All taxa possess a dorsal narial fenestra, and all except the proteids, an anterior apical foramen for passage of the ramus medialis nasi through the anterior wall (alary or cupular cartilage) of the capsule. In the ventro-lateral region of the anterior part of the nasal capsule is the large fenestra endonarina communis that accommodates the external naris and nasal tube. In plethodontids, the fenestra is divided into anterior and posterior portions to accommodate the nasal tube anteriorly and the naso-lacrimal duct posteriorly.

The lateral wall of the nasal capsule is incomplete in proteids, sirenids, and amphiumids, and complete in "hynobiids" and cryptobranchids. In the remaining taxa there is a lateral narial fenestra that varies in size and position (table 6.2A, B).

The posterior wall of the capsule is composed dorsally of the planum antorbitale and ventrally of the lamina orbitonasalis, which is an antero-lateral extension of the trabecular plate at the anterior margin of the orbit. The way may be incomplete (proteids, amphiumids, and sirenids), or if complete, it bears a foramen (orbitonasal) for the passage of the ramus ophthalmicus profundus.

The floor of the nasal capsule is largely incomplete, bearing an immense endochoanal fenestra that is bordered anteriorly by the nariochoanal cartilage, medially by the medial wall of the capsule, posteriorly by the lamina orbitonasalis, and laterally by the ventro-lateral wall of the nasal capsule, the ectochoanal cartilage. The latter may be present, partly developed, or absent, depending upon the degree of development of the lateral wall of the nasal capsule.

The septomaxilla occurs sporadically in salamanders. It is absent in all taxa lacking naso-lacrimal ducts (table 6.2A, B) and in salamandrids. The bone is best developed in "hynobiids," and least well developed in ambystomatids and in those plethodontids in which it occurs.

Stabilization of the Anterior Part of the Upper Jaw. In all salamanders the lamina orbitonasalis and planum antorbitale brace the maxilla against the skull in the anterior orbital region. Anterior support of the snout is provided by abutment of the prenasal process and alary (= cupular) cartilage against the premaxilla. Lateral support depends upon the degree of development of the ventro-lateral margin (ectochoanal cartilage) of the olfactory capsule, which varies from absent to complete.

Exocranium. *Skull Table.* The composition of the skull table and the topological relationships of the component elements are variable among salamanders (figs. 6.11–6.12). As many as six pairs of bones may be involved—viz., premaxillae, nasals, prefrontals, frontals, parietals, and squamosals.

The partes dorsalis of the premaxillae are an integral component of the anterior skull table in all taxa except the cryptobranchids, most "hynobiids," and some salamandrids (e.g., *Notophthalmus*) in which the processes are not well developed. Among all remaining taxa except the sirenids, the partes dorsalis overlap the frontals and separate the nasals (or prefrontals in *Rhyacotriton*) medially. In sirenids, the partes laterally flank the long, slender nasals. In some taxa (e.g., *Dicamptodon* and *Rhyacotriton*), the partes are expanded broadly to roof most of the anterior snout, whereas in others, they are partly or wholly fused to one another (e.g., some plethodontids and *Amphiuma*) or bear an extensive medial articulation (e.g., *Ambystoma*, proteids).

Paired nasals occur in all salamanders except for adults of one species of *Rhyacotriton* (personal communication, D. C. Cannatella; Wake 1980; contra Duellman and Trueb 1986), and some plethodontids (Larsen 1963). The nasals usually lie anterior to the frontals and prefrontals (if present). Except for sirenids and *Rhyacotriton,* the nasals are relatively large. Plesiomorphically, they articulate with one another medially and are overlapped by the partes dorsalis of the premaxillae (table 6.2A, B). In more advanced taxa, the bones are separated broadly and lie laterally adjacent to the partes dorsalis of the premaxillae.

In the seven families in which it is present (table 6.2A, B), the prefrontal lies antero-laterally adjacent to the frontal and roofs the skull in the region of the planum antorbitale at the anterior margin of the orbit; in

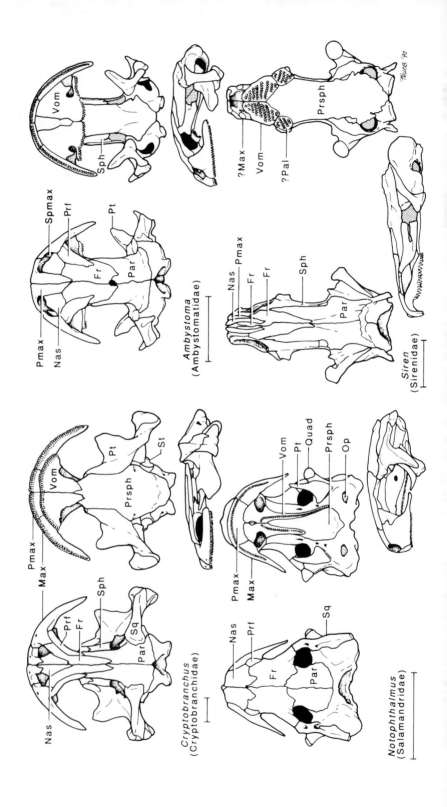

Cryptobranchus
(Cryptobranchidae)

Ambystoma (Ambystomatidae)

Notophthalmus (Salamandridae)

Siren (Sirenidae)

Pmax
Max
Vom
Pt
Prsph
St
Nas
Prf
Fr
Sph
Par
Sq

Pmax
Max
Vom
Pt
Quad
Prsph
Op
Nas
Prf
Fr
Par
Sq

Pmax
Nas
Spmax
Prf
Fr
Par
Pt

Nas
Pmax
Fr
Fr
Sph
Par

?Max
Vom
?Pal
Prsph

Fuetz 90

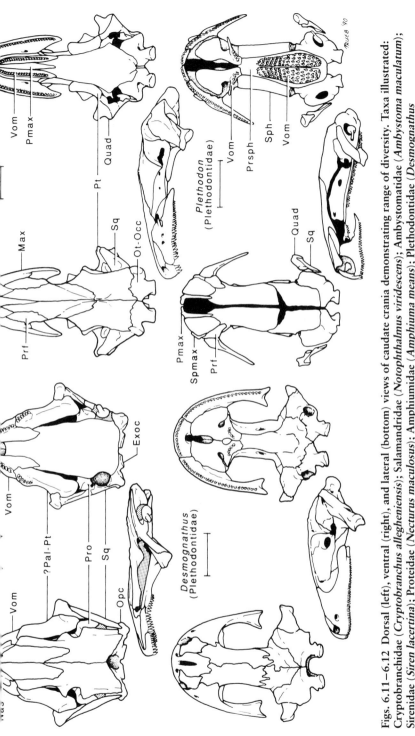

Figs. 6.11–6.12 Dorsal (left), ventral (right), and lateral (bottom) views of caudate crania demonstrating range of diversity. Taxa illustrated: Cryptobranchidae (*Cryptobranchus alleghaniensis*); Salamandridae (*Notophthalmus viridescens*); Ambystomatidae (*Ambystoma maculatum*); Sirenidae (*Siren lacertina*); Proteidae (*Necturus maculosus*); Amphiumidae (*Amphiuma means*); Plethodontidae (*Desmognathus quadramaculatus* and *Plethodon cinereus*). All drawings except plethodontids adapted from Carroll and Holmes (1980); *Plethodon* adapted from Larsen (1963), and *Desmognathus* drawn from UMMZ 182027. See Duellman and Trueb (1986) for illustrations of a diversity of plethodontid taxa. Stipple-patterned areas represent cartilage; black areas represent cranial foramina or fenestrae. Bars equal 5 mm. See Appendix for abbreviations.

some taxa, the bone participates in the anterior margin of the orbit, whereas in others, it is excluded from it.

All taxa possess separate, paired frontals, which usually lie postero-medial to the nasals and prefrontals if the latter are present. Exceptions to this arrangement are found in cryptobranchids, sirenids, and amphiumids in which the frontals extend antero-laterally to roof part of the nasal region (fig. 6.11). In *Cryptobranchus*, the frontal articulates with the maxilla and is flanked antero-medially by the nasal and postero-laterally by the prefrontal. In *Siren*, the anterior ends of the frontals are separated by paired nasals and partes dorsalis of the premaxillae, whereas in *Amphiuma*, the frontals are separated throughout their anterior half by the long slender pars dorsalis of the fused premaxillae. In the remaining salamanders, the frontals usually roof the anterior half of the braincase in the orbital region and overlap the parietals. Usually, the paired frontals have at least a partial articulation with one another; thus, the frontoparietal fontanelle is exposed partially by a fenestra in *Rhyacotriton*, and some "hynobiids," ambystomatids, and plethodontids. In most taxa in which the frontal region is roofed completely, a parietal foramen is absent. In one family, the salamandrids, the frontals of some taxa (e.g., *Notophthalmus*, *Tylototriton*) are elaborated to produce supraorbital flanges that extend postero-laterally to articulate with the squamosal, forming a squamosal-frontal arch that separates the adductor musculature and immobilizes the suspensorium (Carroll and Holmes 1980).

The final elements of the skull table are the paired parietals, which vary considerably in configuration and relative size among salamanders. In most, there is a complete medial articulation of the paired parietals that generally corresponds to the condition of the frontals (see discussion above). The parietals usually roof the posterior half of the braincase from the midorbital to the midotic region. Anterior elaboration of the parietal is evident in the cryptobranchids and proteids in which the element underlies most of the frontal and spans the orbital region of the braincase. Posterior elaboration is more subtle and involves lateral expansion across the otic capsule in the region of the posterior margin of the orbit (e.g., *Ambystoma*, some plethodontids) or across the otic capsule to establish an articulation with the squamosal (e.g., some "hynobiids," cryptobranchids, *Amphiuma*).

Snout and Neurocranial Region of Palate. The snout in most salamanders is short and broad (with the obvious exceptions of the amphiumids and sirenids), and relatively well covered by bone, although the external narial openings are large, and there usually is a midventral diastema anteriorly behind the premaxillae. The number of dermal bones present in the snout is variable among adult salamanders. There may be as few as four (vomer, nasal, parasphenoid, and premaxilla in proteiids) or as many as eight (vomer, nasal, parasphenoid, premaxilla, maxilla, septomaxilla, prefrontal, and lacrimal in "hynobiids"; see table 6.2A, B for distributions of elements).

The major source of diversity in the salamander snout involves the vomer, which is invariably present and dentate, but which seems to vary in its configuration and pattern of dentition, depending on the developmental status (larval versus adult), habits, and phylogenetic status of the salamander and the presence or absence of the maxilla (figs. 6.11–6.12). The marginal tooth pattern, typical of larvae and neotenes, is defined as one in which the teeth are located along the anterior edge of the vomer and either parallel or replace the dentition of the maxillary arcade. In the posterior tooth pattern, the vomerine teeth are situated in the postero-medial part of the vomer. The vomerine tooth patterns of "hynobiids" seem to share features of the anterior and posterior patterns in that in some taxa (e.g., *Liua shihi*), the tooth row is displaced postero-medially but nonetheless parallels the maxillary arcade, whereas in others (e.g., *Batrachuperus pinchonii*), the tooth row is located along the extreme postero-medial margin of the vomer and does not parallel the maxillary arcade. In all other salamanders except amphiumids and sirenids (see description below), the teeth are posterior in pattern, and in salamandrids and plethodontids they may be elaborated into a long, slender tooth row that extends posteriorly over nearly the entire length of the parasphenoid; the posterior tooth row of some plethodontids is separated from the anterior body of the vomer.

The second major source of variation in the vomer involves its shape, which in most salamanders tends to be broadly triangular, such that the anterior margin bears a broad articulation with the premaxilla and maxilla. The nature of the medial articulation between the vomers seems to be correlated with the anterior extent of the parasphenoid. A complete medial articulation between the paired elements occurs in cryptobranchids, whereas in most other taxa the vomers tend to articulate with one another postero-medially at the level of the planum antorbitale. Despite the fact that this arrangement usually results in an antero-medial fenestra between the premaxillae and vomers, the parasphenoid terminates at approximately the anterior level of the orbit in these taxa. Postero-lateral vomerine processes that support the posterior margin of the choana are absent in cryptobranchids and "hynobiids," poorly developed in ambystomatids, and well developed in salamandrids and most plethodontids.

In those salamanders either lacking a maxilla (e.g., the plethodontid *Eurycea*, sirenids, and proteids) or having an exceptionally long snout (amphiumids), the vomers are markedly different. In taxa lacking a maxilla, the vomers are displaced laterally, usually lack any medial articulation (short antero-medial articulation present in the proteid *Necturus*), and bear either a marginal row of teeth or a proliferation of teeth that covers a long, slender vomer (sirenids). Although amphiumids retain a maxilla, the vomer is a long, slender element that bears a row of teeth (paralleling the maxillary arcade) along its medial edge. In each of the aforementioned taxa, the parasphenoid extends anterior to the orbit beneath all or part of the vomer to form a bony floor to the olfactory region.

Aside from the vomer, the external snout region of salamanders varies depending on the presence or absence of the prefrontal, lacrimal, and maxilla, and the configuration of the premaxilla (table 6.2A, B; see discussion of skull table, above). In those taxa lacking a prefrontal and/or lacrimal, the pars facialis of the maxilla tends to be elaborated so that it articulates with the remaining bones of the anterior skull table to form a bony lateral covering for the olfactory capsule. The vomer is modified to act as the functional equivalent of the maxilla in salamanders lacking the latter element, although in sirenids, the olfactory capsule lacks a dermal lateral wall.

Upper Jaw. The upper jaw element that is always present in salamanders is the premaxilla (= intermaxilla in some sources); although usually paired, in some taxa the premaxillae are fused (table 6.2A, B). Most taxa retain a maxilla; in those lacking a maxilla, it is replaced functionally by a modified vomer. The maxillary arcade is incomplete in nearly all salamanders; two exceptions are the salamandrids *Echinotriton andersoni* and *Tylototriton verrucosus* (Nussbaum and Brodie 1982). If present, the maxilla bears ligamentous connections with the pterygoid (if present), quadrate, and quadratojugal (if present). All salamanders except some "hynobiids" lack the posterior element of the upper jaw, the quadratojugal. Quadratojugal ossifications have been reported to occur in *Batrachuperus mustersi* (Cloutier, in preparation) and *Onychodactylus japonicus* (Ryke 1950). However, in both of these taxa, the ossification is synostotically united to other bones in the adult; in the former, it is fused to the quadrate, and in the latter, with the squamosal.

Composite Endo- and Exocranial Units. *Mandible.* Even less is known about the structure of the lower jaw in salamanders than about the rest of the cranium. All taxa possess Meckel's cartilage, which ossifies anteriorly to produce the mentomeckelian bone at the mandibular symphysis; the mentomeckelian is synostotically united with the dentary bone (fig. 6.10D, E). In some taxa (table 6.2A, B), the posterior end of Meckel's cartilage ossifies as the articular bone, which articulates with the quadrate. The remainder of the mandible is composed of dermal elements—the tooth-bearing dentary lateral to Meckel's cartilage, and the prearticular medial to the cartilage. Additional elements that are present in some taxa are the angular and coronoid (table 6.2A, B).

Suspensorium. There is a limited amount of information available on the endocranial structure of the suspensoria of only a few taxa of salamanders (e.g., *Salamandra,* Francis 1934; *Rhyacotriton,* Cloete 1961; *Onychodactylus,* Ryke 1950). Based on these descriptions, however, it is evident that the suspensorial endoskeleton of caudates is more complex than that of either caecilians or anurans. The palatoquadrate consists of three regions. The dorsal pars quadrata is cartilaginous, whereas the ventral region ossifies as the quadrate bone. The ventral region bears an antero-medial process, the pterygoid process. Unlike its homologue in caecilians and anurans, the pterygoid process usually is not united synchondrotically with the posterior maxillary process anteriorly (except in some "hynobiids"). The dorsal pars quadrata bears two to four connections to the neurocranium. Dorsalmost is the otic process that is fused to the crista parotica except in *Cryptobranchus* and *Rhyacotriton.* The ascending process of the pars quadrata fuses to the pila antotica. A third process, the basal process, extends from the pars quadrata toward the base of the skull. In salamandrids and the plethodontid *Pseudotriton,* this process is fused to the neurocranium, whereas in other taxa for which there is information (table 6.2A, B), the process bears a diarthrotic joint with the basitrabecular process of the neurocranium. In addition, the stapes may be united to the palatoquadrate, thereby establishing a fourth connection between this element and the neurocranium.

The dermal elements associated with the suspensorium are variable (table 6.2A, B). The squamosal, which invests the palatoquadrate laterally and articulates with the skull roof, is always present. The pterygoid is present and well developed in all taxa except the plethodontids (fig. 6.12), in which it is absent, and the sirenids, in which it is vestigial. The pterygoid invests the basal and pterygoid processes of the palatoquadrate, and frequently articulates with the parasphenoid, but never articulates with the maxilla as it usually does in anurans. A third element, the metapterygoid, occurs in some "hynobiids" of the genera *Hynobius* and *Batrachuperus* (Cloutier, in preparation); this bone is unknown in all other salamanders, anurans, and caecilians. The metapterygoid is a small ossification that surrounds the distal portion of the ascending process of the palatoquadrate; it articulates with the dorsal margin of the pterygoid laterally and the lateral wall of the neurocranium and parietal medially to provide an additional abutment of the suspensorium against the braincase.

The occurrence and disposition of a fourth element, the palatine, is puzzling. According to Trueb and Cloutier (1991a), all lissamphibians lack a discrete palatine bone as adults. A so-called palatopterygoid bone has been identified in proteids and the plethodontid genus *Eurycea*, both of which lack a maxilla. In these taxa, the palatopterygoid bears marginal dentition, and functionally participates in the "maxillary arcade"; in the proteids, the bone articulates with the vomer anteriorly and the quadrate posteriorly to form a complete upper jaw and an integral part of the suspensorium. A so-called palatine has been identified in the sirenids (fig. 6.11); it is a small, round bone located posterior to the vomer and covered with teeth. Ephemeral centers of ossification have been identified as the palatine in some hynobiids and salamandrids (Cloutier, in preparation; Lebedkina 1979). Thus, it is possible that if ontogenetic information were available for those taxa possessing a palatopterygoid, we might confirm the dual origin of this element. In the case of the sirenids, it is possible that the presence of a palatine (if the element is identified correctly) is a reversal in this peculiar family.

In lateral aspect, the palatoquadrate and squamosal usually are oriented such that the ventral articular facet lies slightly anterior to the dorsal pars quadrata; thus, in most salamanders, the jaw articulation lies immediately antero-lateral to the otic capsule. In cryptobranchids and *Dicamptodon*, the articulation lies more posterior—i.e., lateral to the otic capsule; thus, the relative positions of the ends of the palatoquadrate are reversed, with the articular end posterior to the pars quadrata in lateral view. The jaw articulation is located well anterior to the otic capsule in sirenids, proteids, and some plethodontids (e.g., *Eurycea*).

Dentition. Although larval salamander teeth are nonpedicellate and undivided, the dentition of nearly all adults is predicellate and biscuspid; the exceptions are sirenids and some or all of the teeth of certain male plethodontid salamanders. Tooth-bearing elements include the bones of the upper jaw—premaxilla (except in sirenids), maxilla, and the palatopterygoid and vomer. Palatal dentition is limited to the vomer, but may extend over the parasphenoid in salamandrids and plethodontids, depending on the configuration of the vomer. In transformed adult salamanders, mandibular dentition is limited to the dentary; however, in some larvae and neotenes (e.g., the proteid *Necturus*), a dentate coronoid bone also is present. The distribution of teeth in salamanders is more variable than that of anurans or caecilians, but the morphology is more conservative than that of anurans, and in particular, caecilians.

Hyobranchial Apparatus. The basic hyobranchial pattern of salamanders (characterizing larvae, and with some modifications, neotenic taxa) consists of usually one but occasionally two medial rods, the basibranchials (= copulae), to which lateral elements are attached (fig. 6.13). In an anterior-to-posterior sequence, the proximal paramesial series is composed

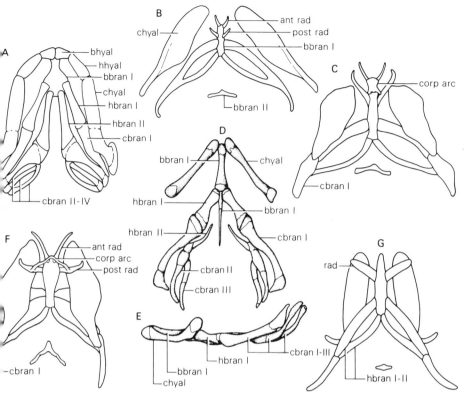

Fig. 6.13. Hyoid apparatus of some representative caudates. A. *Cryptobranchus alleganiensis* (Cryptobranchidae), ventral view. B. *Salamandra salamandra* (Salamandridae), ventral view. C. *Rhyacotriton olympicus* (familial allocation uncertain), dorsal aspect. D. *Proteus anguinus* (Proteidae), in ventral and lateral (E) views. F. *Ambystoma macrodactylum* (Ambystomatidae), dorsal view. G. *Aneides* sp. (Plethodontidae), ventral aspect. Drawings adapted from the following sources: (A) Jollie 1962; (B) Francis 1934; (C) Cloete 1960; (D–E) Marche and Durand 1983; (F) Papendieck 1954; (G) Hilton 1947. Illustration reproduced from Duellman and Trueb (1986) with permission of McGraw-Hill Book Company. See Appendix for abbreviations.

of a hypohyal and Hypobranchials I and II. The ceratohyal articulates with the distal end of the hypohyal, Ceratobranchial I with Hypobranchial I, and Ceratobranchial II with Hypobranchial II. Ceratobranchial III articulates medially with Ceratobranchial II, and similarly, Ceratobranchial IV with the medial end of Ceratobranchial III. The distal ends of the ceratohyal usually bear a ligamentous attachment to the suspensorium (not in plethodontids). Many authors have referred to ceratobranchials as epibranchials (see Duellman and Trueb 1986) in salamanders, thereby obscuring the homology of these elements with those of other lissamphibians and vertebrates in general. Reilly and Lauder (1988) presented convincing evidence that the putative epibranchials of salamanders in fact are cerato-branchials, and that epibranchials are known to occur only atavistically in one population of the salamandrid *Notophthalmus viridescens*.

Diversity in hyobranchial morphology primarily involves loss and fusion of elements, resulting in less complex hyobranchia. Thus, in most metamorphosed salamanders, hypohyal elements are missing, and the cer-atohyals usually are dissociated from the basibranchium (e.g., *Salamandra salamandra*), or occasionally articulate directly with the element (e.g., the proteid, *Proteus*). In metamorphosed salamanders that use their tongue to food (e.g., ambystomatids, salamandrids, plethodontids, *Rhyacotriton*, and *Dicamptodon*), the anterior basibranchial usually bears one or two pairs of slender lateral elements known as radials that are associated with tongue musculature. Although most transformed salamanders apparently retain two pairs of hypobranchials, the anterior pair is fused with their distal partners, the ceratobranchials in "hynobiids," and there is a ten-dency for simplification of the posterior hyobranchium by loss of Cerato-branchials II–IV, with III and IV being absent most frequently.

The Primitive Caudate Cranium of the Semiterrestrial Generalist. Al-though "hynobiids" represent an evolutionary grade, the precise inter-relationships of which we do not understand at present (Cloutier, in preparation), we can be reasonably certain that the cranial features of semiterrestrial generalists of these groups constitute an approximation of the primitive salamander morphotype. A detailed list of these features ap-pears in table 6.2A, B. Representatives of "hynobiids" are the only sala-manders that are known to possess a complete complement of cranial elements, along with a complete narial capsule, and unmodified premaxilla (i.e., absence of elaboration of partes dorsalis). Other characters of evolu-tionary significance are the presence in larvae of a quadratojugal and dentate coronoid, and in the adult, the lateral placement of the jaw articu-lation and presence of an articular, metapterygoid, basitrabecular process, and relatively unmodified hyobranchium, and simple pattern of palatal dentition.

"Hynobiids" are described by Regal (1966) as possessing a Type II tongue—i.e., one which is not well differentiated, but which possesses loose lateral and posterior margins and superficial ridges or papillae. Based on his observations of *Ambystoma tigrinum*, Regal hypothesized that the function of such a tongue basically is manipulative. Thus, through forces generated by the relatively unmodified hyoid, the tongue could be moved fore and aft, up and down, and sideways to hold and manipulate food against the palatal dentition; at the same time, the hyoid serves its other essential function—that of raising and lowering the floor of the mouth to create a buccopharyngeal pump for lung ventilation in the terrestrial amphibian. Although there are no detailed observations of feeding behavior in "hynobiids," the basic pattern described for *Ambystoma tigrinum* (Larsen and Guthrie 1975) is not dissimilar from the behavior reported for the "hynobiid" *Batrachuperus mustersi* (Reilly 1983).

Patterns of Cranial Architecture among Salamanders in the Aquatic Zone. The obligate inhabitants of the aquatic zone comprise a peculiar and diverse group derived from various clades of terrestrial or semiterrestrial ancestors. All are "gape-and-suck" feeders that possess a Type I tongue—a thickening of the buccal floor around the branchial elements typical of larvae (Regal 1966). Additionally, they have well-developed hyobranchia (lacking marked reduction of posterior components) that, together with the gill apparatus, provide for a controlled, unidirectional flow of water through the buccal cavity (Lauder and Shaffer 1985). Further, their dentition tends to be marginal, and in most, accessory palatal dentition is absent; if palatal dentition is present, it is marginal and parallels that of the maxillary arcade.

Two general types of skulls are found among these salamanders. Cryptobranchids have broad, flat crania with bluntly rounded and broad snouts, and the jaw articulation displaced far lateral and slightly posterior relative to that of all other salamanders except *Dicamptodon*. Recently, it was reported that unlike any other known amphibian, *Cryptobranchus* and *Andrias* (Cryptobranchidae) are capable of asymmetric movement of the hyoid apparatus that results in asymmetric depression of the lower jaw during prey capture (Cundall et al. 1987). Thus, despite the potentially extensive gape of these organisms, only part of the mouth is open at any given time during feeding, which may increase the efficiency of the gape-and-suck mechanism.

Sirenids, amphiumids, and proteids have depressed, elongate skulls with narrow snouts; the arrangement and composition of their snouts are dissimilar from one another and from those of all other known salamanders (see descriptions above and table 6.2A, B). The jaw articulation is located markedly anterior to the otic capsule in proteids, as it is in most larval salamanders, presumably resulting in a restricted gape. Owing to the attenuation of the skulls and location of the jaw articulation anterolateral to the otic capsule in sirenids and amphiumids, these taxa have much greater gapes than that of proteids. Presumably, this is associated with the presence of extraordinarily well developed dentition and the ability to strike moving or elusive prey rather than rely solely on stationary capture techniques as cryptobranchids, proteids, and larval salamanders do (Erdman and Cundall 1984).

Cranial Diversification Associated with the Terrestrial Zone. Representatives of two families of salamanders—the salamandrids and plethodontids—have made notable inroads into the terrestrial life zone. Members of both families possess modifications of the hyoid, tongue, and palate that are involved in feeding strategies, but of the two groups, the plethodontids (especially the bolitoglossines) are by far the most highly derived and terrestrial, as is discussed below.

Both families are characterized by elaboration of the vomerine dentition. In salamandrids, the postero-lateral portion of the vomerine dentigerous process is elongated into a slim projection that extends posteriorly to the otic region along the margin of the parsphenoid. In most plethodontids, the vomerine dentigerous process maintains an anterior transverse component, but the medial portion is elaborated into extensive series or patches of teeth that overlie the medial portions of the parasphenoid. In some taxa (e.g., *Plethodon jordani*, *Bolitoglossa subpalmata*), the posterior portions of the vomer presumably become separated from the anterior parts during development.

Modification of the hyoid involves simplification of the posterior hyobranchial skeleton by reduction with elaboration of the anterior components that, with their associated musculature, act to control the anterior tongue pad and propel it forward toward the mouth opening in terrestrial members of these families. In the cases of the most terrestrial salamandrids (*Salamandra*, *Chioglossa*, and *Salamandrina*), the ceratobranchials are absent, but the anterior parts of the hyobranchial apparatus and tongue are elaborated (Type III of Regal 1966). According to Özeti and Wake (1969), tongue protrusion involves little protraction of the hyobranchial apparatus, but instead depends more on flexibility of the posterior hyobranchium along with elaboration and the capability to rotate the anterior portions. Thus, the hyobranchium is still in place to drive the force-pump mechanism of lung ventilation in these forms that tend to have reduced lungs. Modification of the anterior hyobranchium allows the organisms to project the tongue (which is characterized by the presence of a free posterior flap) from the mouth to varying degrees.

As pointed out by Lombard and Wake (1976), loss of lungs has been the most significant factor in the development of the specialized feeding mechanism of plethodontid salamanders. Once the hyobranchium and its musculature were freed from their involvement in force-pump breathing to ventilate the lungs, these morphological components could be involved in the elaborate projectile tongue mechanism characteristic of most plethodontid salamanders. In these organisms, the hyobranchium is largely cartilaginous; the hyobranchium, together with its muscles and the elaborate tongue pad that is free of, or only loosely connected to, the lower jaw, form a projectile that allows these salamanders to capture prey.

CRANIAL OSTEOLOGY OF THE ANURA

The order Anura is composed of approximately 3,700 living species as-signed to 302 genera and 24 families (Duellman and Trueb 1986, as amended by Cannatella 1985). There is one extinct anuran family (the Palaeobatrachidae), and fossil representatives of 11 of the Recent families; in addition, there are six genera and six species of fossils that are not as-signed to families. Thus, there are totals of approximately 40 genera and 78 species of fossil anurans. There is a considerable body of literature in which anuran cranial features are described or figured. However, owing to the numbers and diversity of anuran taxa, there really are no satisfactory, comprehensive syntheses of variation across the order. The two broadest reviews appear in Trueb (1973) and Duellman and Trueb (1986); these publications also provide reasonably extensive citations to the literature. Earlier works that should be mentioned include Cope (1889), Boulenger (1897–98), Gaupp (1896), and W. K. Parker (1881).

Among the systematic accounts in which there are useful osteological descriptions and references to other literature are H. W. Parker (1934) on microhylids and Burton (1983) on asterophyinine microhylids. Informa-tion on leptodactyloids is available in Lynch (1971, 1978), and Davies (1987) for the leptodactylid *Uperoleia*. Tihen (1962) provided useful ob-servations on New World *Bufo,* McDiarmid (1969) on brachycephalids and some genera of bufonids, and Trueb (1971) on the bufonid *Rhampho-phryne.* Duellman (1970) illustrated the crania of many Middle American hylids; Trueb (1970) described the skulls of casque-headed hylids, Trueb and Tyler (1974) the Great Antillean hylids, and Trueb (1974) the hylid genus *Hemiphractus.* Pipoids have been described by Trueb and Canna-tella (1986) and Cannatella and Trueb (1988a, b).

In addition to these works, there exists a body of more purely de-scriptive anatomical literature on the internal and external features of anuran crania that postdates the anatomical studies of the Europeans at the turn of the century. Some of the best examples are found in the An-nals of the University of Stellenbosch and the South African Journal of Science by such authors as Du Toit, De Villiers, and many other workers (cf. references in Trueb 1973, and Jurgens 1971). The papers of Paterson (1939–1955), Pusey (1943), Stephenson (1951), Baldauf and coauthors (1955–1965), Trueb (1968), and Trueb and Cannatella (1982) follow in this tradition. Publications that deal with specific subsets of the anuran cranium that should be mentioned are Jurgens (1971) on the amphibian nasal capsule, Wever (1985) on the amphibian ear, and Trewavas (1933) on the hyoid and larynx of the Anura.

The phylogeny and classification of anurans is the least well under-stood of the three orders of Recent amphibians. The interrelationships of

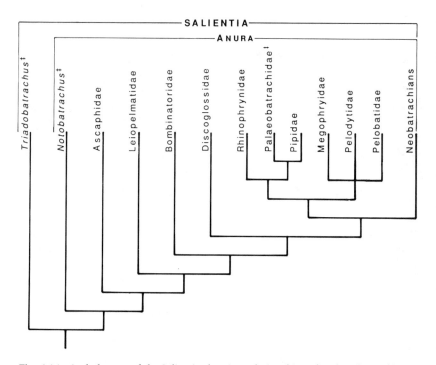

Fig. 6.14. A phylogeny of the Salientia showing relationships of archaeobatrachian anurans adapted from Cannatella (1985) and Trueb and Cloutier (1991a). Double dagger indicates fossil taxa.

the nine families of archaeobatrachians (fig. 6.14) have been addressed by Cannatella (1985), and his arrangement is accepted herein as a working hypothesis. This arrangement, however, accounts for only approximately 23 genera and 107 species (but 10 of the 24 families) of Recent anurans; the remaining 279 genera containing 3,600 species belong to the Neobatrachia. For the purposes of this discussion, the arrangement of the 15 families of neobatrachians proposed by Duellman and Trueb (1986) and amended by Ford (1989) is accepted (fig. 6.15). Neobatrachians can be divided into two broad groups—the ranoids and hyloids. The ranoids are comprised of the ranids, hyperoliids, rhacophorids, microhylids, and sooglossids; together, these taxa account for about 134 genera and 1,350 an-

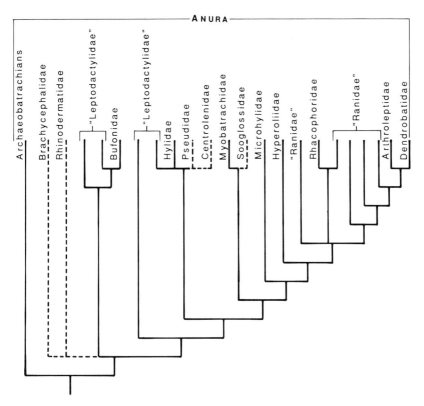

Fig. 6.15. A phylogeny of neobatrachian anurans adapted principally from Ford (1989). Dashed lines indicate provisional placement of families not considered by Ford based on the phylogenetic scheme of Duellman and Trueb (1986).

uran species. The remaining 10 families (ca. 145 genera and 1,970 species) are considered hyloids.

Anurans: Diversification of Saltatorial Specialists

Patterns of diversification are particularly difficult to identify and assay among anurans for two reasons. First, anurans share many derived traits associated with terrestrial existence, a saltatorial mode of locomotion, and specialized feeding mechanisms involving a protrusible tongue. Thus, anuran crania tend to be lightweight and depressed. The sensory organs have been elaborated relative to those of salamanders and caecilians, and the crania modified to accommodate these structures. The hyoid is associated more closely with feeding mechanisms than ventilation functions. Second, our clearest understanding of phylogenetic relationships currently is limited to discoglossoids and mesobatrachians, groups that, excluding the pipoids, have a limited amount of cranial diversity. Neobatrachians comprise the majority of anurans, and certainly the broadest spectrum of morphological diversification is to be found in this assemblage. Until we have a clearer concept of historical relationships within the Neobatrachia, it will be impossible to define evolutionary patterns of anatomical change, and comments necessarily are limited to broad generalizations.

Architectural Diversity

General Features. Like the skulls of salamanders, those of anurans tend to be broad, depressed, and gymnokrotaphic—i.e., characterized by an open temporal region, a large orbit that usually lacks a posterior margin, and lack of a "cheek" in most taxa (figs. 6.2, 6.16). The anuran cranium is much simpler than those of either salamanders or caecilians in that it consists of many fewer elements; thus, the frontal and parietal are represented by a single ossification, the frontoparietal, and the lacrimal, prefrontal, postfrontal, opisthotic, metapterygoid, coronoid, articular, prearticular, and mandibular dentition (except for one species) are absent. The skull table, palate, and snout of anurans tend to be incomplete. The maxillary arcade is variably complete or incomplete. The jaw articulation usually lies lateral or slightly postero-lateral to the otic capsule. The septomaxilla always is present as a discrete element of the nasal capsule. When present, the stapes is free, rather than attached to the squamosal or palatoquadrate. Most anurans possess a tympanic annulus in association with the stapes; this structure is unknown in all other vertebrates. The hyobranchium is a highly derived structure that bears little resemblance to the hyobranchia of either salamanders or caecilians; in adult anurans, it is modified into a plate in the floor of the mouth that, owing to the muscles attached to it, is involved in vocalization, ventilation, and feeding.

Not unexpectedly, given the much greater number of species of anurans relative to caecilians and salamanders, there is a great deal more diversity of cranial structure. Variation involves relative ossification of the crania, loss of discrete elements through fusion or failure to develop, reduction in the degree of development of other elements, and in some instances, appearance of novel dermal bones unknown in any other Recent amphibians. Among the latter are the neopalatine, interfrontal, internasal, dermal sphenethmoid, and prenasal.

Endocranium. *Neurocranium and Auditory Capsules.* The anterior braincase is formed by the sphenethmoid (fig. 6.17) which, developmentally, appears from a single center of ossification antero-medial to the eye on each side of the skull (Kemp and Hoyt 1969). Owing to its mode of de-

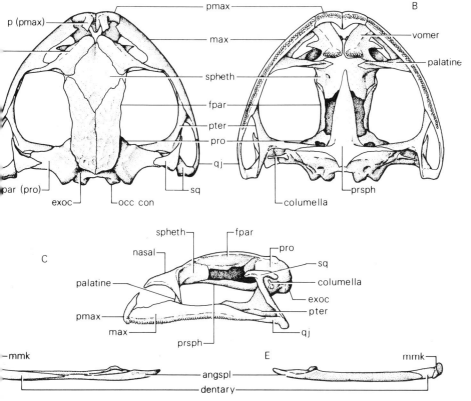

Fig. 6.16. Skull of the hylid frog *Gastrotheca walkeri* in dorsal (A), ventral (B), and lateral (C) views. Mandible in lateral (D) and medial (E) aspect. Reproduced from Duellman and Trueb (1986) with permission of McGraw-Hill Book Company. See Appendix for abbreviations.

velopment, the bone probably is homologous with the sphenethmoid of salamanders and the orbitosphenoid portion of the sphenethmoid of caecilians. In most adult anurans (table 6.3A, B), the two halves of the sphenethmoid are fused to form a single girdle bone; in those taxa noted as having a "divided" or "paired" sphenethmoid (e.g., *Ascaphus*, *Leiopelma*, most microhylids), the apparent division is the result of incomplete medial replacement of cartilage by bone. The sphenethmoid is synchondrotically or syostotically united to the septum nasi and planum antorbitale. Anterolaterally, it or the planum antorbitale is pierced by the orbitonasal canal. Dorsally, the sphenethmoid usually forms the bony and/or cartilaginous margins of the frontoparietal fenestra. Posteriorly, the bone may terminate at the anterior margin of the optic foramen or surround it. The length of the ossified portion of the sphenethmoid is highly variable.

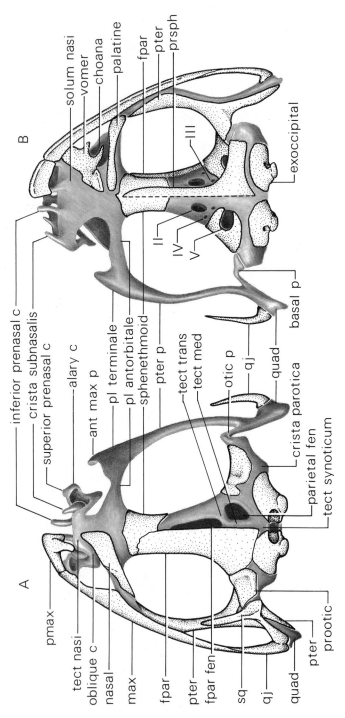

Fig. 6.17. Skull of the ranid frog *Rana esculenta* in dorsal (A) and ventral (B) aspects with dermal bones removed from right side to reveal underlying chondrocranial elements; bones are stippled and cartilaginous structures shown in gray. Redrawn from Gaupp (1896) and reproduced from Duellman and Trueb (1986) with permission of McGraw-Hill Book Company. See Appendix for abbreviations.

The posterior neurocranium is composed of two pairs of bones (fig. 6.17). The prootics lie behind the optic foramen and form the posterior braincase and all of the otic capsules except for the posterior walls. The latter, along with the occipital condyles and margin of the foramen magnum are formed by the exoccipitals. The postero-lateral and posterior margins of the frontoparietal fontanelle are formed dorsally by the prootic. Like the sphenethmoid, the prootic varies greatly in the degree of ossification in anurans. Thus, the ossified paired prootics frequently are separated by cartilage dorso- and ventro-medially, and there may be a cartilaginous hiatus between the prootics and exoccipitals in the dorsal region of the otic capsule. Similarly, the development and ossification of the crista parotica—the dorsal shelf extending from the otic capsule over the middle ear—is highly variable. In one anuran family, the pipids (table 6.3A, B), the prootic bears a ventral furrow through which the Eustachian tube extends. The exoccipitals always are present and the occipital condyles ossified, but ossification may be incomplete dorso-ventrally and dorsomedially around the foramen magnum.

Ear. Most anurans possess a more highly developed sense of hearing and derived auditory structure than either caecilians or salamanders; the ear is characterized by the presence of oval and round windows, an operculum that usually is separate from the stapes (= columella), and a tympanic annulus. The most primitive anurans (ascaphids and leiopelmatids) lack a stapes and tympanic annulus (table 6.3A, B), but it is unclear whether this is a primitive or derived feature; among the neobatrachians, the ear structure is variably present or absent, and if present, may be reduced.

The operculum is cartilaginous and lies in the posterior portion of the fenestra ovalis. It is thought to be present in all taxa, although it may be fused to the stapes in pipids (personal observation); in those taxa lacking a stapes (e.g., *Rhinophrynus*), the operculum usually is enlarged. The stapes consists of a proximal footplate located anterior to the operculum in the fenestra ovalis, and a distal bony stylus (pars media plectri) that bears a cartilaginous connection (pars externa plectri) to the tympanic annulus distally. The tympanic annulus is a cartilaginous, funnel-like structure that lies beneath the skin at the distal side of the middle ear and supports the tympanic membrane which is visible externally in some anurans.

Reduction of the auditory system in anurans seems to follow an obligate sequence involving loss of structures in a proximal–medial sequence. Thus, the tympanum may be absent, but the tympanic annulus and remainder of the plectral apparatus present (e.g., pipids). Usually, the absence of the tympanum is accompanied by absence of the tympanic annulus (table 6.3A, B), although the stapes may be present (e.g., the lep-

TABLE 6.3A Survey of cranial characters of anurans based primarily on Cannatella (1985), Trueb (1973), and Duellman and Trueb (1986)

Character	Family or group				
	Ascaphidae	Leiopelmatidae	Bombinatoridae	Discoglossidae	Megophryidae
1. Sphenethmoid	"Divided"	"Divided"	Single	Single	Single
2. Eustachian tube/bony prootic canal	Absent/Absent	Absent/Absent	Present/Absent	Present/Absent	Present/Absent
3. Stapes	Absent	Absent	Present or absent	Present	Present
4. Tympanic annulus	Absent	Absent	Present or absent	Present	Present
5. Septum nasi	Wide; cartilaginous	Wide; cartilaginous	Narrow; partly ossified	Narrow; partly ossified	Narrow; partly ossified
6. Neopalatine	Absent	Absent	Absent	Absent	Absent
7. Palatine process of pars facialis of maxilla	Absent	Absent	Present or absent	Present or absent	Present
8. Frontoparietal	Paired	Paired	Paired	Paired	Paired
9. Additional dermal cranial elements	Absent	Absent	Interfrontal or absent	Absent	Absent
10. Nasal	Sickle-shaped	Sickle-shaped	Sickle-shaped	Sickle-shaped	"Straight"
11. Vomer	Present; paired	Present; paired	Present; paired	Present; paired	Present; paired
12. Postchoanal ramus of vomer	Absent	Present	Present	Present	Absent
13. Quadratojugal	Absent	Absent	Present	Present	Present
14. Mentomeckelian	Present	Present	Present	Present	Present
15. Medial ramus of pterygoid	Present; slender	Present; slender	Present; slender	Present; slender	Present; slender
16. Dentition	Present; pedicellate, bicuspid	Present; pedicellate, bicuspid	Present; pedicellate, bicuspid	Present; pedicellate, bicuspid	Present; pedicellate, bicuspid

Character					
17. Parahyoid	Present; single	Present; single	Present; single	Present; paired	Absent
18. Endochondral ossification of hyoid plate	Absent	Absent	Present	Absent	Absent
19. Hyalia	Complete	Complete	Complete	Complete	Disjunct
20. Hyoglossal foramen	Absent	Absent	Absent	Absent	Absent
21. Antero-lateral process of hyoid	Absent	Present	Present	Present	Absent
22. Base of antero-lateral process of hyoid	—	Narrow	Wide	Wide	—
23. Fusion of antero-lateral process to hyale	—	Absent	Absent	Absent	—

TABLE 6.3B Survey of cranial characters of anurans based primarily on Cannatella (1985), Trueb (1973), and Duellman and Trueb (1986)

Character	Pelodytidae	Pelobatidae	Family or group Rhinophrynidae	Pipidae	Neobatrachians
1. Sphenethmoid	Single	Single	Single	Single	Single or "divided"
2. Eustachian tube/bony prootic canal	Present/absent	Present/absent	Absent/absent	Present/present	Present/absent
3. Stapes	Present	Present but may be reduced	Absent	Present	Absent or present; may be reduced
4. Tympanic annulus	Present	Present or absent	Absent	Present	Present or absent
5. Septum nasi	Narrow; partly ossified	Narrow; partly or wholly ossified	Narrow; bony; formed by nasals	Narrow; bony; formed by dermal bone in some	Narrow; partly ossified
6. Neopalatine	Absent	Absent	Absent	Absent	Present or absent
7. Palatine process of pars facialis of maxilla	Present	Present	Absent	Absent	Absent
8. Frontoparietal	Paired	Paired or azygous	Azygous	Azygous	Paired
9. Additional dermal cranial elements	Absent	Absent	Absent	Absent	Absent or prenasal, internasal, dermal sphenethmoid
10. Nasal	"Straight"	Sickle-shaped	Sickle-shaped	Large, subcircular	"Straight"

11. Vomer	Present; paired	Present; paired	Present; paired	Present or absent; azygous	Present or absent; paired
12. Postchoanal ramus of vomer	Present	Present	Present	Absent	Present or absent
13. Quadratojugal	Present	Present or absent	Present	Absent	Present (may be reduced) or absent
14. Mentomeckelian	Present	Present	Absent	Absent	Present
15. Medial ramus of pterygoid	Present; slender	Present; slender	Absent	Present; wide	Present; but may be reduced
16. Dentition	Present; pedicellate, bicuspid	Present; pedicellate, bicuspid	Absent	Present or absent; nonpedicellate, monocuspid	Present or absent; pedicellate, bicuspid
17. Parahyoid	Present; paired	Absent	Present; single	Absent	Absent
18. Endochondral ossification of hyoid plate	Absent	Absent	Absent	Absent	Absent
19. Hyalia	Disjunct	Disjunct	Disjunct	Present or absent; disjunct	Complete
20. Hyoglossal foramen	Absent	Absent	Absent	Present	Absent
21. Antero-lateral process of hyoid	Present	Present	Absent	Present or absent	Present
22. Base of antero-lateral process of hyoid	Wide	Wide	—	Wide or —	Wide
23. Fusion of antero-lateral process to hyale	Present	Present	—	Absent or —	Absent

todactylid *Telmatobius;* Trueb 1979), and if an annulus is present, the stapes always is present also. Plesiomorphically, the stapes is absent in living anurans, and among derived anurans it has been lost independently in many lineages (table 6.3A, B).

Olfactory Capsule. Explanation of the structure and variation of the anuran nasal capsule is available in Jurgens (1971) and Duellman and Trueb (1986) and references cited therein. Anurans differ from salamanders and caecilians in lacking intrinsic narial muscles (except for some pipids; Trueb, personal observation; Gans and Pyles 1983), and in the invariable presence of a discrete septomaxilla; closure of the nares is effected by action of intermandibular musculature on an array of narial cartilages (Gans and Pyles 1983), of which the most important probably are the alary and superior prenasal cartilages described below. The cartilaginous olfactory capsule of anurans is more extensive than that of caecilians but less complete than that of salamanders, and more complex than in either of the latter taxa. There is considerable variation in relative proportions and position of structures depending upon the position of the nares (dorsal, dorso-lateral, anterior) and the overall configuration of the snout; on the other hand, the basic plan and number of components of the anuran nasal capsule seem to be relatively constant.

The medial wall between the nasal capsules is the septum nasi, which is synchondrotically or synostotically united to the sphenethmoid posteriorly in nearly all anurans. Usually, the septum is narrow, although in some primitive and some derived taxa, it is wide (e.g., ascaphids, brachycephalids; table 6.3A, B); the septum always is solid (i.e., no medial cava), and highly variable with respect to its degree of ossification. A platelike dorso-lateral extension of the septum forms a roof (tectum nasi) that only anteriorly covers the entire nasal capsule between the external nares (fig. 6.17). The oblique cartilage diverges postero-laterally from the tectum postero-medial to the naris and supports its posterior margin; the oblique cartilage extends ventrally to join ventral narial cartilages in the region of the planum terminale. The posterior half of the cartilaginous nasal capsule between the planum terminale and planum antorbitale (posterior wall of the nasal capsule) is incomplete dorsally, laterally, and ventrally. The posterior wall of the nasal capsule and the posterior margin of the choana are composed of a transverse plate of cartilage, the planum antorbitale. The latter extends from the sphenethmoid to the maxilla laterally. Usually the planum is cartilaginous, although in a few taxa it may be mineralized, and in some pipids it is ossified. The postero-medial wall of the nasal capsule is formed by the sphenethmoid, which is pierced by the large olfactory foramen; at this level, the neurocranium nearly always is ossified.

At the level of the tectum nasi, the septum bears a ventral shelflike extension that represents the floor of the nasal capsule, which is most complete in the region of the oblique cartilage behind the naris. A number of small cartilaginous structures are associated with the anterior solum. The inferior prenasal cartilage (fig. 6.17) is a slender rod that extends antero-ventrally from the solum to the premaxilla. The crista subnasalis is an antero-lateral block of cartilage that forms an abutment between the maxilla and solum. At the level of the naris, the dorsal surface of the solum nasi produces an intricate pair of platelike cartilages that separate and support the nasal cava and that are associated with the septomaxilla. The dorsal is the lamina superior, and the ventral the lamina inferior. If the laminae are united medially to the septum, the connection is termed the crista intermedia. Despite its intimate association with the cartilaginous nasal capsule, the septomaxilla is believed to be a dermal element. It lies at, and slightly posterior to, the level of the naris and supports the anterior end of the naso-lacrimal duct as it diverges postero-laterally from the olfactory organ. In most anurans, the septomaxilla seems to be a U-shaped structure (medial and lateral rami of dorsal and ventral views) with the closed end lying anterior. The lateral ramus bears a dorsal crest that is variably developed, and a ventral spur that extends forward from the posterior end of the lateral ramus. In pipids, the septomaxilla is a long, relatively flat, arcuate element; perhaps coincidentally, pipids are the only known anurans in which the naso-lacrimal duct is absent in some taxa.

The antero-dorsal and antero-lateral walls of the nasal capsule are formed by the alary and superior prenasal cartilages. The former is a cup-shaped structure that protects the anterior end of the cavum principale and supports the anterior–antero-lateral margin of the naris. The superior prenasal cartilage is an irregularly shaped rod of cartilage that extends antero-medially from the alary cartilage to the premaxilla.

Stabilization of the Anterior Part of the Upper Jaw. The crista subnasalis, inferior prenasal cartilage, and planum antorbitale, along with the anterior and posterior maxillary processes of the planum, brace the maxillary arcade against the skull. Additional support is provided by the neopalatine (= anuran palatine in other sources) and palatine process of the maxilla (table 6.3A, B). In the absence of reduction of the two latter elements, the sphenethmoid ossification may invade the planum antorbitale, or in the case of some pipids, the planum antorbitale may be ossified.

Trueb and Cloutier (1991a) established that the Lissamphibia lack a discrete palatine as adults. But earlier, Cannatella (1985) noted that a free palatine was present only in neobatrachians (table 6.3A, B), and that *Barbourula* (Bombinatoridae), *Discoglossus* (Discoglossidae), the Megophryidae, Pelobatidae, and *Pelodytes* (Pelodytidae) possess a process that seems to arise from the lingual surface of the pars facialis of the maxilla and extends medially along the ventral surface of the planum antorbitale. Based on examination of larval *Pelobates fuscus,* Cannatella (1985) suggested that the process arises as part of the maxilla, and therefore, does not represent a fusion of a "palatine" bone with the maxilla as suggested by Rocek (1980). The presence of a slender bone underlying the planum antorbitale that usually articulates with the maxilla and sphenethmoid and that is edentate apparently is a morphological novelty of neobatrachians. Herein, I refer to this element as a *neopalatine* in distinction to the *palatine* of early tetrapods. Typically, the latter is a triangular or subtriangular bone that articulates with the maxilla, vomer, pterygoid, and ectopterygoid. The topographical relationship between the palatine and planum antorbitale in these extinct taxa is unknown; there is no evidence that the palatine bore an articulation with the sphenethmoid as the neopalatine does in most neobatrachians that possess the element. Although the neopalatine may bear a transverse ridge (serrated or smooth), the bone does not bear true teeth. In hypo-ossified anurans (e.g., the hylid *Pseudacris clarkii*), as well as hyperossified frogs such as *Brachycephalus* (Brachycephalidae), *Rhamphophryne* (Bufonidae), or *Corythomantis* (Hylidae), the neopalatine either is reduced or absent. Similarly, entire families such as the Dendrobatidae are characterized by reduction and loss of the neopalatine (Myers and Ford 1986).

Exocranium. *Skull Table.* Although the configuration of the skull table is extraordinarily variable in anurans, its composition is simple and relatively constant within the order (figs. 6.18–6.19). In most taxa, the skull table is composed of the dorsum of the sphenethmoid and a pair of frontoparietals; the frontoparietal is azygous in some pelobatids and in the pipoids (table 6.3A, B). Some bombinatorids (e.g., *Bombina orientalis;* Tschugunova 1981) possess an interfrontal bone between the anterior ends of the frontoparietals; the bone is small and lies posterior to the sphenethmoid over the anterior end of the frontoparietal fontanelle. Casque-headed hylids (e.g., *Triprion, Aparasphenodon*) possess a dermal sphenethmoid—a platelike bone that overlies the sphenethmoid and fuses to it during development (Trueb 1966, 1970). In most anurans, the nasals and squamosals would not be considered part of the skull table. However in some taxa with casqued heads (e.g., some bufonids, the leptodactylid *Ceratophrys,* casqued hylids such as *Hemiphractus*), the nasals are expanded to form the anterior margin of the orbit, cover the sphenethmoid, and in some cases, articulate with the frontoparietals and form part of the supraorbital flange. Similarly, the head of the squamosal may be expanded medially over the otic region.

Variation in the configuration of the skull table is primarily a function of the sizes and degree of ossification of the frontoparietals (and in some instances, the nasals). Plesiomorphically, the frontoparietals are slender, arcuate elements that overlie the dorso-lateral aspect of the braincase posterior to the sphenethmoid; although the paired elements may articulate with one another postero-medially, there usually is a frontoparietal fenestra between them exposing the underlying fontanelle. Expansion of the frontoparietal seems to occur in the following sequence: (1) medial growth in a posterior-to-anterior direction so that the frontoparietal fenestra is covered partially or totally; (2) postero-lateral expansion of the frontoparietal over the prootic in the region of the epiotic eminence; (3) elaboration of a supraorbital flange and growth of the frontoparietal over the sphenethmoid anteriorly; (4) growth of a postorbital process which, maximally developed, forms a shelf that may articulate with the squamosal over the otic region.

Unusual expansion of dermal roofing bones (occasionally including the squamosal and maxilla) is referred to as casquing. It is a relatively common phenomenon among anurans (e.g., many representatives of bufonids, pelobatids, leptodactylids, brachycephalids, and hylids). In all casque-headed anurans, there is some degree of sculpturing of the dermal bones; this is the result of exostosis, or proliferation of superficial bone. In its least well organized state, the bone is laid down in a loose, reticulate pattern, usually in the area of the initial center of ossification of the bone. With further elaboration (e.g., the casque-headed hylids; Trueb 1970), the surfaces of the bones may become organized into patterns of radiating ridges, prominent tubercles, etc. The developmental culmination of this pattern of hyperossification is co-ossification, a condition in which the dermis of the skin is largely replaced by bone so that the skin effectively is fused to the underlying cranial elements.

Snout and Neurocranial Region of the Palate. Relative to those of caecilians and salamanders, the snouts of anurans are short and broad (fig. 6.2), and in most taxa, only moderately protected by dermal elements (figs. 2.17– 2.19). Nasals, premaxillae, and maxillae are invariably present. Vomers may be reduced or absent. Neomorphic dermal bones occur in some casque-headed hylids; *Triprion* bears a rostral prenasal bone anterior to the premaxillae, and *Pternohyla fodiens* an internasal dorso-medial to the premaxillae.

The nasals are highly variable components of the snout, and have three basic configurations among anurans (table 6.3A, B). Plesiomorphically, the nasals are sickle-shaped—i.e., the anterior margins are concave, and the bones bear moderately long antero-medial processes (Cannatella 1985). In most meso- and neobatrachians, the nasals are straight—i.e., the bones lack a concave anterior margin and medial processes, but possess a maxillary process that extends ventro-laterally toward the maxilla along the

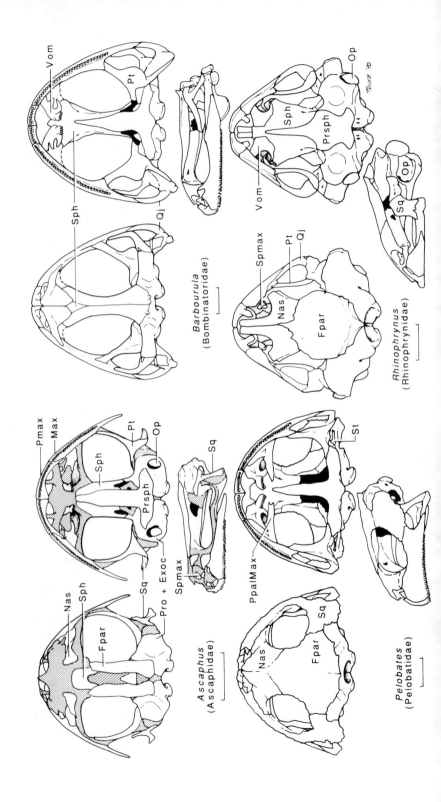

Barbourula
(Bombinatoridae)

Rhinophrynus
(Rhinophrynidae)

Ascaphus
(Ascaphidae)

Pelobates
(Pelobatidae)

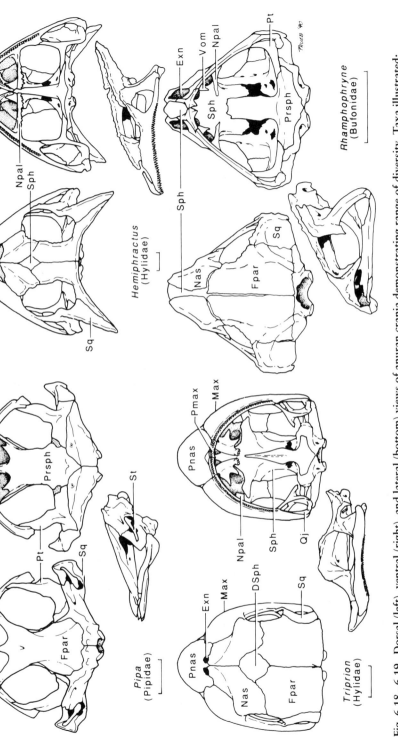

Fig. 6.18–6.19. Dorsal (left), ventral (right), and lateral (bottom) views of anuran crania demonstrating range of diversity. Taxa illustrated: Ascaphidae (*Ascaphus truei*, KU 215698); Bombinatoridae (*Barbourula busuagensis*, KU 79003); Pelobatidae (*Pelobates syriacus*, KU 146856); Rhinophrynidae (*Rhinophrynus dorsalis* adapted from Trueb and Cannatella 1982); Pipidae (*Pipa snethlageae* adapted from Trueb and Cannatella 1986; Hylidae (*Hemiphractus proboscideus* adapted from Trueb 1974, and *Triprion petasatus* adapted from Trueb 1970); and Bufonidae (*Rhamphophryne festae* adapted from Trueb 1971). Cross-hatched pattern indicates frontoparietal fenestra; stipple pattern indicates cartilage. Bars equal 5 mm. See Appendix for abbreviations.

anterior margin of the orbit. Some pipids (*Hymenochirus, Pseudhymeno-chirus*, and *Pipa*) are peculiar in possessing large subcircular nasals; also, *Xenopus* is the only known group of frogs in which the nasals are fused medially. Depending upon the extent of cranial ossification, there is considerable variation in the relative size of the nasals. Minimally (e.g., *Ascaphus*), the bone roofs the olfactory organ between the oblique cartilage and the planum antorbitale, thereby exposing most of the cartilaginous olfactory capsule dorsally and laterally. Maximally (e.g., casque-headed, co-ossified hylids), the nasals expand to articulate with one another medially, overlap the sphenethmoid, and articulate with the maxilla ventro-laterally. In some cases (e.g., the hylid *Corythomantis* and bufonid *Rhamphophryne*), the nasals grow antero-ventrally over or beside the premaxillae to form a bony rostrum.

The maxilla and premaxilla are important components of the snout that invariably are present. The paired premaxillae bear dorsal alary processes (or partes dorsalis) that basically are short vertical processes against which the superior prenasal process of the olfactory capsule rests. The processes vary in their relative length and in the angle of their orientation; thus, they may be inclined posteriorly or slightly anteriorly. The alary processes never are involved in the skull roof as they are in some salamanders. The maxilla bears a dorsal flange, the pars facialis, which is variably developed to protect the ventro-lateral aspect of the olfactory capsule. At the anterior margin of the orbit, the maxilla may bear a preorbital process that articulates with the maxillary process of the nasal. Both the maxilla and premaxilla bear horizontal, palatal shelves—the partes palatinae—that form the peripheral bony palate. There is considerable variation in the sizes of these palatal shelves, but typically, they are not well developed. The pars palatina of the premaxilla usually bears a medial palatine process that floors the olfactory capsule between the vomers.

If present, the vomers usually are paired elements that floor the olfactory capsule between the levels of the naris and choana. Among anurans, pipids are peculiar (table 6.3A, B) in lacking vomers except in the genus *Xenopus,* in which the vomer is a small, azygous element located posterior to the choanae. Maximally developed, the vomer is triradiate (anterior ramus and pre- and postchoanal rami) and bears a toothed dentigerous process postero-medially. There is considerable variation (particularly among neobatrachians) in the size of the vomer, the development of its rami, and the presence and pattern of the vomerine dentition. Vomerine reduction (except in pipids) usually involves (1) loss of the dentigerous process, (2) reduction or loss of the postchoanal ramus, (3) reduction or loss of the prechoanal ramus, and (4) loss of the anterior ramus, in this order. Elaboration, in contrast, usually involves medial expansion of the main body (i.e., anterior ramus) of the vomer, thereby decreasing the intervomerine gap. In the pelobatid *Spea* and apparently in some microhylids, the post-choanal ramus is expanded laterally across the planum antorbitale toward the maxilla (Cannatella 1985; Parker 1934). The pattern of vomerine dentition is especially variable. The dentigerous process may be narrow and medial or expanded in width to the postchoanal region of the planum antorbitale; the series of teeth may be curved or straight. The pair of dentigerous processes may lie in a transverse plane, or lie at an angle to one another, forming a shallow V-shape or its inverse. In the hylid genus *Hemiphractus*, the vomers bear odontoids, and if teeth are present they are represented by one to three fangs located anterior on the vomer (Trueb 1974).

Unlike salamanders and caecilians, the parasphenoid of anurans rarely is involved in the palate of the snout. Instead, the bone invests the ventral surface of the neurocranium posterior to the level of the planum antorbitale, bridging the cartilage usually present between the sphenethmoid and prootic. In all anurans except the pipoids, the parasphenoid bears postero-lateral wings or alae that underlie the anterior part of the otic capsule; thus, the parasphenoid of most anurans is T-shaped in distinction to its homologue in salamanders and caecilians. The bone is edentate, although it may bear medial serrations in some hyperossified neobatrachians (e.g., the hylids *Osteocephalus, Trachycephalus*).

Upper Jaw. All anurans retain premaxillae and maxillae in the maxillary arcade. The quadratojugal occurs sporadically (table 6.3A, B), and frequently is reduced in neobatrachians. In the case of some casque-headed hylids (e.g., *Hemiphractus*), the quadratojugal may be expanded to form part of the "cheek" characteristic of these anurans. Similarly in casque-headed anurans, the pars facialis of the maxilla may be greatly elaborated to cover the ventro-lateral aspect of the skull. The premaxilla never is involved in casquing, and may be covered by other bones (e.g., the prenasal in *Triprion*, fig. 6.19; the maxilla in some symphygnathine microhylids). Teeth may be present or absent; if present, they occur on both the maxilla and premaxilla.

Composite Endo- and Exocranial Units. *Mandible.* The lower jaw of anurans is relatively simplistic and composed of four elements (fig. 6.16D, E). The dentary is slender and edentate in all anurans except the hylid *Gastrotheca guentheri*, in which it bears true teeth; in some casqued taxa such as *Ceratobatrachus* (Ranidae) and *Hemiphractus* (Hylidae), the dentary is serrated to produce a series of toothlike odontoids. The larger bony component is the angulosplenial, which forms the articular surface of the mandible and extends forward along the lingual surface of the mandible; the homology of this element with mandibular elements of salamanders and caecilians is uncertain. Meckel's cartilage lies between the dentary and angulosplenial. Anteriorly, in all anurans except the pipoids (table 6.3A, B), the medial part of the infrarostrals of the larval chondrocranium ossify as the mentomeckelian bones (which, therefore, may not be homologous with the bones of the same name that form in Meckel's cartilage in sala-manders); occasionally, these are synostotically united with the adjacent dentaries.

Suspensorium. The suspensorium of anurans is less complex and robust than that of caecilians and salamanders. The palatoquadrate is cartilagi-nous, although the ventral articular portion may be ossified incompletely as the pars articularis or quadrate. The superior end of the palatoquadrate usually is attached to the otic capsule via the cartilaginous otic process. Ventrally, the element bears two other processes—the pseudobasal or basal and pterygoid processes. The pseudobasal process extends postero-medially to the otic capsule, with which it may articulate or be fused. The pterygoid process extends forward from the palatoquadrate to the maxilla, where it is in synchondrotic union with the posterior maxillary process.

Two dermal elements are invariably present and associated with the palatoquadrate—the squamosal and the pterygoid. The squamosal typi-cally is a triradiate bone, the ventral arm of which invests the palatoquad-rate laterally and always is present. The antero-dorsal zygomatic ramus is extraordinarily variable in its development. It is absent in only a few taxa (e.g., *Rhinophrynus*). Usually, it extends antero-ventrally toward the max-illa, forming an incomplete posterior margin to the orbit. In hyperossified taxa (e.g., the leptodactylids *Ceratophrys* and *Lepidobatrachus* among many others), the zygomatic ramus commonly is greatly expanded and has a robust articulation with the maxilla, thereby forming a "cheek." The condition of the zygomatic ramus in pipids is unique; the bone forms a funnel-shaped element fused to the ossified portion of the tympanic annu-lus that embraces the distal end of the stapes (Trueb and Cannatella 1986). The postero-dorsal squamosal arm, the otic ramus, is present in all but the most poorly ossified anurans (e.g., the leptodactylid *Notaden*). The otic ramus invests the lateral margin of the crista parotica, and usually bears a shelflike medial otic plate that overlies the dorso-lateral surface of the otic capsule. Not uncommonly, the head of the squamosal (i.e., dorsum of zy-gomatic and otic rami) are exostosed and casqued, and may contribute to the skull table (see description above).

The pterygoid is a triradiate palatal element that invests the pterygoid, articular, and pseudobasal or basal processes of the palatoquadrate. In so doing, it forms a three-cornered brace between the suborbital portion of the maxilla anteriorly and the otic capsule and palatoquadrate posteriorly. Variation in the pterygoid principally involves the presence and extent of development of the anterior and medial rami of the pterygoid. The medial ramus investing the pseudobasal process frequently is reduced so that it does not articulate with the otic capsule (table 6.3A, B); in one taxon, *Rhinophrynus*, it is absent. The anterior ramus is present in all anurans except the pipid genera, *Hymenochirus* and *Pseudhymenochirus*. The relationship of the anterior ramus to the maxilla is highly variable with respect to the level at which the two bones articulate with one another, and the length of the articulation in the orbital region. In one genus of bombinatorids (*Bombina*) as well as a few neobatrachians, the anterior ramus extends anteriorly along the maxilla and curves medially to invest the posterior margin of the planum antorbitale (Cannatella 1985). Pipids (table 6.3A, B) are unique among anurans in having the medial and posterior pterygoid rami greatly expanded to form an otic plate that partially or wholly floors the otic capsule and provides a bony floor to the eustachian canal. In some pipid taxa the otic plate is fused partially to the prootic bone.

Dentition. In anurans, teeth may be present on the maxilla, premaxilla, and vomer, but frequently are absent (e.g., bufonids; table 6.3A, B); only one taxon (*Gastrotheca guentheri*, a hylid) possesses teeth on the dentary. Plesiomorphically, the teeth are pedicellate and bicuspid. However, they may be modified into fanglike structures in some anurans such as the bombinatorids, the leptodactylid genus *Telmatobius*, and the hylid genus *Hemiphractus*. Pipid frogs possess the most derived dentition; the teeth (if present) are fanglike, monocuspid, and lack the joint between the crown and pedicel. In at least one pipid, *Pipa arrabali*, the teeth are fused to the maxilla and premaxilla (Cannatella 1985).

Hyobranchial Apparatus. In its basic design, the anuran hyobranchium consists of a cartilaginous hyoid plate that is attached to the ventral surface of the otic capsule via a pair of slender, recurved processes, the hyale, that originate from the antero-lateral corners of the plate (fig. 6.20). The anterior margin of the plate is concave; the area delimited by the anterior edge of the plate and the hyalia is the hyoglossal sinus, which accommodates the passage of the hyoglossus muscle from the ventral surface of the hyoid to the tongue dorsally. Typically, the hyoid plate bears three pairs of lateral processes. The cartilaginous antero-lateral processes may be absent (e.g., *Leiopelma;* table 6.3A, B), but usually are present and vary considerably in their configuration. Cartilaginous postero-lateral processes differ in their shapes, but always seem to be present. Similarly, the postero-medial processes (= thyrohyals) are invariably present and ossified, although their shape may vary slightly. The most thorough survey of anuran hyobranchial structure was published by Trewavas (1933).

    The major kinds of variation in anuran hyobranchial structure are

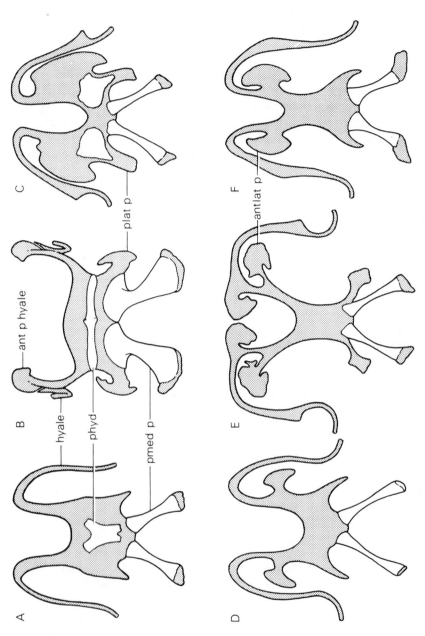

Fig. 6.20. Hyobranchial skeletons of anurans in ventral view. Bone is white and cartilage is stippled. A. *Leiopelma hochstetteri* (Leiopelmatidae). B. *Rhinophrynus dorsalis* (Rhinophrynidae). C. *Bombina variegata* (Bombinatoridae). D. *Leptodactylus ocellatus* (Leptodactylidae). E. *Heleioporus albopunctatus* (Myobatrachidae). F. *Bufo himalayanus*

summarized by Cannatella (1985; table 6.3A, B). Most archaeobatrachians possess a membranous bone on the ventro-medial surface of the hyoid plate; the bone either is single or paired. Whereas the hyalia are complete in most anurans, they are either absent or disjunct in several groups of mesobatrachians (table 6.3A, B). The tongueless pipids have the most highly derived and peculiar hyobranchia of anurans (see Cannatella and Trueb 1988; Cannatella 1985; and references therein for descriptions). In these frogs, the hyalia may be entirely absent or so reduced as to be unrecognizable. Medial fusion of the antero-basal parts of the hyalia results in the formation of a small hyoglossal foramen from the hyoglossal sinus. The posterior part of the hyobranchium (postero-medial processes with or without postero-lateral processes) may be separated from the anterior components. The antero-lateral processes may become greatly expanded (*Pipa*) and incorporate the postero-lateral processes (*Xenopus*), and become heavily mineralized (*Hymenochirus*).

Pipid Frogs. It is a common misconception and generalization that anurans are aquatic; in fact, most are only semiaquatic (primarily returning to the water to breed or escape predators; e.g., ranids, many bufonids) and many are terrestrial (having reproductive specializations that obviate the need of returning to water for breeding). The only truly aquatic frogs known are the pipids, which, although capable of movement across land between bodies of water, nearly always are found in the water. Members of the family possess many morphological features associated with an aquatic life-style (see Trueb and Cannatella 1986; Cannatella and Trueb 1988a, b; Trueb, in press), and these include cranial characters. The heads are depressed and wedge-shaped in lateral profile. The neurocranium tends to be complete ossified, and the dermal neurocranial bones modified; thus, the frontoparietal is azygous and expanded to cover the entire dorsum of the braincase, and the parasphenoid synostotically integrated into the ventral braincase. The structure of the occipital condyles and the articulation of the skull with the cervical vertebra are such that there is little possibility of dorso-ventral flexure of the skull on the axial column. The eustachian tube lies in a bony canal formed in the prootic and floored to varying degrees by an otic plate that originates from elaboration of the posterior and medial rami of the pterygoid. This plate occupies a position covered in part by the parasphenoid alae in other anurans. For reasons not yet understood, the septomaxillae of these frogs are long, flat, and sickle-shaped. Other peculiar features of the cranium seem to be related to feeding (the mechanism of which is unknown). The modifications of the hyobranchium (see description above) must be correlated with the absence of a tongue in pipids. The mandible lacks mentomeckelian bones, and the dentaries and angulosplenials tend to be narrowly separated at the symphysis. If present, the teeth are monocuspid fangs that lack a joint between the crown and pedicel; in some taxa, the teeth are fused to, rather than socketed within, the maxillae and premaxillae.

Nonpipid Anurans. The following generalizations concerning cranial diversity of nonpipid anurans are a combination of conclusions of Trueb and Alberch (1985) and Trueb (personal observations).

1. The degree of cranial ossification is unrelated to the size of the anurans. Thus, extraordinarily small frogs (e.g., *Brachycephalus*) may be as hyperossified as large taxa (e.g., the leptodactylid *Ceratophrys*). Conversely, relatively large anurans such as members of the leptodactylid genus *Telmatobius* frequently are hypo-ossified in comparison to others of a similar size.
2. There are certain correlates between feeding and life habits and degree of ossification. Carnivorous anurans (e.g., the hylid *Hemiphractus*, the leptodactylid *Caudiverbera*, the ranid *Pyxicephalus*) tend to be large, hyperossified frogs. Anurans such as *Scaphiopus* and some *Bufo* that live in arid or seasonally arid environments and/or microhabitats tend to have hyperossified skulls. In contract, stream inhabitants (e.g., *Ascaphus*, the leptodactylids *Telmatobius* and *Rheobatrachus*) tend to have hypo-ossified crania regardless of their body size.
3. Changes in the shapes of cranial components may be unrelated to the size of the organism, and to a certain extent, the degree of ossification. For example, in the hyperossified hylid *Triprion petasatus*, the pterygoid and neopalatine are reduced by comparison with those bones of most other hylid frogs.
4. Ossification of dermal and endochondral elements seems to be independent; thus, increases or decreases in ossification may affect both kinds of bone or either one, independent of the other. This results in anurans, such as many microhylids, in which dermal ossification is well developed around a poorly ossified braincase, or in centrolenids that generally have well-ossified braincases with a minimal development of surrounding dermal bones.
5. There seems to be an upper (but virtually no lower) limit to the amount of bone that is invested in the cranium; this results in some observable morphological patterns. For example, in casque-headed anurans, the structural support of the skull is provided by the exocranium, whereas the usual supporting bones, the neopalatine and pterygoid, frequently are reduced.
6. Loss of elements does not occur in large anurans (greater than 100 mm snout-vent length, e.g., the leptodactylid *Caudiverbera*). Skulls of small or miniature species often are characterized by paedomorphic traits;

thus, cranial elements that appear latest in the ontogenetic sequence may be reduced or missing. This includes elements such as the vomer, quadratojugal, neopalatine, and stapes.

7. Shape changes in cranial components related to reduction generally reflect the ontogenetic trajectory of the development of the element. Thus, reduction of the squamosal, for example, can be predicted to involve (a) loss of the zygomatic ramus, (b) loss of the otic plate, and (c) loss of the otic ramus—the reverse sequence of the developmental pattern.

8. Neomorphic dermal elements are not present in small or miniature species (less than 25 mm snout-vent length, e.g., brachycephalids) regardless of their degree of ossification. The presence of novel dermal elements always is associated with hyperossification in the forms of exostosis and casquing.

The generalizations listed above are dissatisfying in terms of their definition of evolutionary patterns. To greater and lesser degrees, they may prove to have predictive value as we unravel the historical patterns that have resulted in the tremendous diversity of anurans that exists today.

SUMMARY

As contrasted with their fossil dissorophoid relatives, living lissamphibians—represented by apodans, caudates, and anurans—are characterized by reduced crania, reorganization of the suspensorium, and a unique pattern of tooth replacement. The primary losses of bones involve the skull table with the absence of the postparietal, supratemporal, and tabular bones; the cheek also is reduced by the loss of the jugal. Anurans and caecilians also lack a separate articular bone in the lower jaw. Lissamphibians differ from their fossil relatives in having a premaxilla that bears a lingual shelf, the pars palatina. Pedicellate, bicuspid teeth occur in lissamphibians as well as doleserpetontids and the "branchiosaurid" sister group of the Lissamphibia, *Apateon;* however, only lissamphibians are known to replace teeth in a medial-to-lateral direction. Changes in the organization of the suspensory apparatus of modern amphibians are reflected by the pterygoid bone, which unlike those of other dissorophoids, bears a quadrate ramus that is oriented postero-laterally. Moreover, the anterior rami of the paired pterygoids articulate neither with one another nor with the vomers.

In contrast to caecilians, salamanders and anurans possess large orbits and moderate-sized external nares. They lack postorbital, postfrontal, and lacrimal bones in the skull roof, surangular and splenial bones in the mandible, and an ectopterygoid in the palate. The absence of these elements seems to be associated with (1) simplification of the mandible, and (2) a trend toward increased zygokrotaphy of the skull. Furthermore, the crania of the Batrachia tend to be shorter and broader, rather than long and narrow as in caecilians. Both salamanders and anurans possess complex hyobranchial apparatuses involved with manipulation of the tongues in feeding.

Salamanders lack some of the plesiomorphic features that characterize caecilians; nonetheless, on the whole they are less specialized than either caecilians or anurans. As a group, they are uniquely characterized by having an incomplete maxillary arcade and a pterygoid bone with a free anterior ramus; they differ from apodans and anurans in their possession of an independent articular bone in the lower jaw of adults of some taxa. Herein, salamanders are interpreted as the semiterrestrial generalists among modern amphibians. The diversification of their cranial structure seems to be correlated with different adaptive zones and modes of feeding and respiration. Thus, it is hypothesized that from a semiterrestrial generalist, cranial diversification proceeded along two adaptive (but several phyletic) lines. One is geared to aquatic life in which all organisms are gape-and-suck feeders, and either have broad, flat skulls or depressed, elongate skulls with narrow snouts. The other is associated with terrestriality; these organisms possess modifications of the hyoid, tongue, and palate unknown in other salamanders.

Anurans are without a doubt the most derived of the lissamphibians. They are characterized by reduction and loss of cranial elements, and broad, depressed, and lightweight skulls that seem to be associated with saltatorial locomotion and specialized feeding mechanisms involving a protrusible tongue. They lack separate frontal and parietal bones, a lacrimal, palatine, prefrontal, prearticular, and splenial. Unlike caecilians and salamanders, they have a distinct squamosal embayment, and the anterior ramus of the pterygoid articulates with the maxilla. Usually, the jaw articulation is located near, or posterior to, the posterior limits of the endocranium, rather than anterior to it as in salamanders and caecilians. The numbers and diversity of anuran species combined with our fundamental lack of understanding of the phylogeny and classification of the most numerous and derived families preclude broad statements about, or descriptions of, evolutionary trends in the cranial pattern(s) in this group.

ACKNOWLEDGMENTS

A number of my colleagues have contributed significantly to the completion of this review. I am particularly grateful to David Cannatella, Richard Cloutier, and Rebecca A. Pyles, who shared results of manuscripts in preparation or in press so that the present contribution would be as current as possible. Although the accuracy and completeness of the data presented here are solely the responsibility of the author, many of the ideas are outgrowths of discussions with Richard Cloutier, David Cannatella, Darrel R. Frost, William E. Duellman, Rebecca A. Pyles, and Linda S. Ford. To each of these individuals I extend my thanks for their interest and forbearance. Ronald Nussbaum of the University of Michigan Museum of Zoology provided specimens for examination and illustration. Completion of this work was supported by NSF grants BSR-85-08470 and 89-18161.

LIST OF ABBREVIATIONS

alary p	alary process
anglspl	angulosplenial
ant	anterior
ant p hyale *or* antlat p	anterior process of hyale
ant rad	anterior radius
antlat p	antero-lateral process of hyoid plate
ar	arytenoid cartilages
BbI	Basibranchial I
bbran I–II	Basibranchials I–IV
bhyal	basihyal
c	cartilage
Car. f	carotid foramen
Cb I–IV	Ceratobranchials I–IV
cbran I–IV	Ceratobranchials I–IV
Ch	choana
Chyal	ceratohyal
corp arc	corpus arcuata
cr par	crista parotica
DSph	dermal sphenethmoid
Ecpt	ectopterygoid
Exoc *or* exoc	exoccipital
Exn *or* ext nar	external naris
ext	external
f	foramen
fen	fenestra
Fpar *or* fpar	frontoparietal
Fr	frontal
hbran I–II	hypobranchials I–II
hhyal	hypohyal
KU	University of Kansas Museum of Natural History
La	lacrimal
Max *or* max	maxilla
Maxpal *or* maxpal	maxillopalatine
med inf pnas c	medial inferior prenasal cartilage

mmk	mentomeckelian bone
Nas	nasal
naslac d *or* Nld	naso-lacrimal duct
Npmax	naso-premaxilla
Npal	neopalatine
Ob	os basale
occ con	occipital condyle
Op	operculum
Opc-Exoc	Opisthotic-Exoccipital
Orbit	orbit
Ot-Occ	otic-occipital, representing fusion of prootic, opisthotic, and exoccipital
Pal	palatine
Pal-pt	palatopterygoid
PaQ	ascending process of quadrate
Par	parietal
phyd	parahyoid bone
pl	planum
plat p	postero-lateral process of hyoid plate
Pmax *or* pmax	premaxilla
pmed p	postero-medial process of hyoid plate
Pnas	prenasal
Po	postorbital
PoQ	processus oticus of quadrate
post rad	posterior radius
Ppar	postparietal
Ppt	pterygoid process of the quadrate
Prf	prefrontal
Pro *or* pro	prootic
Pro + Exoc	fused prootic and exoccipital
proc	process
Prsph *or* prsph	parasphenoid
Pt *or* pter	pterygoid
pterquad *or* Ptquad	pterygoquadrate
Ptf	postfrontal
Qj *or* qj	quadratojugal
Quad *or* quad	quadrate
rad	radius
retroart p	retroarticular process
Sph *or* spheth	sphenethmoid
Spmax	septomaxilla
Sq *or* sq	squamosal
St	stapes
Stp	supratemporal
Ta	tentacular aperture
Tab	tabular

tect   tectum
tect med   tectum medialis
tect trans   tectum transversalis
UMMZ   University of Michigan Museum of Zoology
Vom   vomer

REFERENCES

Bauldauf, R. J. 1955. Contribution to the cranial morphology of *Bufo w. woodhousei* Girard. Texas Journal of Science 7 (3): 275–311.

———. 1957. Additional studies on the cranial morphology of *Bufo w. woodhousei* Girard. Texas Journal of Science 9 (1): 84–88.

———. 1958. Contribution to the cranial morphology of *Bufo valliceps* Wiegmann. Texas Journal of Science 10 (2): 172–186.

Bauldauf, R. J., and E. C. Tanzer. 1965. Contributions to the cranial morphology of the leptodactylid frog, *Syrrhophus marnocki* Cope. Texas Journal of Science 17 (1): 71–100.

Barry, T. H. 1954. The ontogenesis of the sound-conducting apparatus of *Bufo angusticeps* Smith. Morphologisches Jahrbucher 97 (4): 478–544.

Bemis, W. E., K. Schwenk, and M. H. Wake. 1983. Morphology and function of the feeding apparatus in *Dermophis mexicanus* (Amphibia: Gymnophiona). Zoological Journal of the Linnean Society 77: 75–96.

Bonebrake, J. E., and R. A. Brandon. 1971. Ontogeny of cranial ossification in the small-mouthed salamander, *Ambystoma texanum* (Matthes). Journal of Morphology 133: 189–204.

Boulenger, G. A. 1897–98. *The Tailless Batrachians of Europe.* London: Ray Society.

Boy, J. A. 1986. Studien über die Branchiosauridae (Amphibia: Temnospondyli). 1. Neue und wenig bekannte Arten aus dem mitteleuropäischen Rotliegenden (?oberstes Karbon bis unteres Perm). Palaeontologische Zeitschrift 60 (1/2): 131–166.

Burton, T. C. 1983. The phylogeny of the Papuan subfamily Asterophryinae (Anura: Microhylidae). Ph.D. diss., University of Adelaide.

Cannatella, D. C. 1985. A phylogeny of primitive frogs (Archaeobatrachians). Ph.D. diss., University of Kansas.

Cannatella, D. C., and L. Trueb. 1988a. Evolution of pipoid frogs: Intergeneric relationships of the aquatic frog family Pipidae (Anura). Journal of the Linnean Society, Zoology 94: 1–38.

———. 1988b. Evolution of pipoid frogs: Morphology and phylogenetic relationships of *Pseudhymenochirus.* Journal of Herpetology 22 (4): 439–456.

Carroll, R. L., and P. J. Currie. 1975. Microsaurs as possible apodan ancestors. Zoological Journal of the Linnean Society 57 (3): 229–247.

Carroll, R. L., and R. Holmes. 1980. The skull and jaw musculature as guides to the ancestry of salamanders. Zoological Journal of the Linnean Society 68 (1): 1–40.

Cloete, S. E. 1961. The cranial morphology of Rhyacotriton olympicus (Gaige). Annals of the University of Stellenbosch 36: 114–145.

Cloutier, R. n.d. Changes in the osteology of Batrachuperus mustersi (Hynobiidae: Caudata) during ontogeny. Manuscript.

Cope, E. D. 1889. The Batrachia of North America. Bulletin of the United States National Museum 34: 1–525.

Cundall, D., J. Lorenz-Elwood, and J. D. Groves. 1987. Asymmetric suction feeding in primitive salamanders. Experientia 43: 1229–1231.

Davies, M. 1987. Taxonomy and systematics of the genus Uperoleia Gray (Anura: Leptodactylidae). Ph.D. diss., University of Adelaide.

de Beer, G. R. 1937. The Development of the Vertebrate Skull. London: Oxford Press.

de Villiers, C. G. S. 1936. Some aspects of the amphibian suspensorium with special reference to the paraquadrate and quadratomaxillary. Anatomischer Anzeiger 81: 225–247.

Duellman, W. E. 1970. The hylid frogs of Middle America. Monographs of the Museum of Natural History of the University of Kansas 1: 1–753.

Duellman, W. E., and L. Trueb. 1986. Biology of Amphibians. New York: McGraw-Hill Book Co.

Edwards, J. L. 1976. Spinal nerves and their bearing on salamander phylogeny. Journal of Morphology 148: 305–328.

Erdman, S., and D. Cundall. 1984. The feeding apparatus of the salamander Amphiuma tridactylum: Morphology and behavior. Journal of Morphology 181: 175–204.

Estes, R. 1981. Handbuch der Paläoherpetologie, pt. 2, Gymnophiona, Caudata. New York: Gustav Fischer Verlag.

Ford, L. S. 1989. The phylogenetic position of poison-dart frogs (Dendrobatidae): Reassessment of the neobatrachian phylogeny with commentary on complex character systems. Ph.D. diss., University of Kansas.

Francis, E. T. B. 1934. The Anatomy of the Salamander. London: Oxford University Press.

Frost, D. R. (ed.). 1985. Amphibian Species of the World: A Taxonomic and Geographic Reference. Lawrence, Kansas: Allen Press and the Association of Systematics Collections.

Gans, C., and R. Pyles. 1983. Narial closure in toads: Which muscles? Respiration Physiology 53: 215–223.

Gaupp, E. 1896. A. Ecker's und R. Wiedersheim's Anatomie des Frosches. 2 vols. Braunschweig: Friedrich Vieweg und Sohn.

Gauthier, J., D. Cannatella, K. de Queiroz, A. G. Kluge, and T. Rowe. 1989. Tetrapod phylogeny. In The Hierarchy of Life, B. Fernholm, K. Bremer, and Jörnvall, eds. Elsevier Science Publishers B.V. (Biomedical Division), pp. 337–353.

Hecht, M. K., and J. L. Edwards. 1976. The methodology of phylogenetic inference above the species level. In Patterns in Vertebrate Evolution, M. K. Hecht, P. C. Goody, and B. M. Hecht, eds. New York: Plenum Press, pp. 3–51.

Hilton, W. A. 1947. The hyobranchial skeleton of Plethodontidae. Herpetologica 3: 191–194.

Inger, R. F. 1967. The development of a phylogeny of frogs. Evolution 21: 369–384.

Jollie, M. 1962. *Chordate Morphology*. New York: Reinhold Publishing Co.

Jurgens, J. D. 1971. The morphology of the nasal region of Amphibia and its bearing on the phylogeny of the group. Annals of the University of Stellenbosch 46 (ser. A, no. 2): 1–146.

Kemp, N. E., and J. A. Hoyt. 1969. Sequence of ossification in the skeleton of growing and metamorphosing tadpoles of *Rana pipiens*. Journal of Morphology 129 (4): 415–444.

Larsen, J. H., Jr. 1963. The cranial osteology of neotenic and transformed salamanders and its bearing on interfamilial relationships. Ph.D. diss., University of Washington.

Larson, J. H., Jr., and D. J. Guthrie. 1975. The feeding system of terrestrial tiger salamanders (*Ambystoma tigrinum melanostictum* Baird). Journal of Morphology 147: 137–154.

Lauder, G. V., and H. B. Shaffer. 1985. Functional morphology of the feeding mechanism in aquatic ambystomatid salamanders. Journal of Morphology 185: 297–326.

Laurent, R. F. 1986. Ordre des Gymnophiones. In *Traité de zoologie*, P.-P. Grassé and M. Delsol, eds. Paris: Masson, pp. 595–608.

Lebedkina, N. S. 1979. *Evolution of the Amphibian Skull*. Moscow: Nauka. [In Russian]

Lescure, J., S. Renous, and J.-P. Gasc. 1986. Proposition d'une nouvelle classification des amphibiens gymnophiones. Memoires de la Société zoologique de France 43: 145–177.

Lombard, R. E. 1977. Comparative morphology of the inner ear in salamanders (Caudata: Amphibia). Contributions to Vertebrate Evolution 2: 1–140.

Lombard, R. E., and D. B. Wake. 1976. Tongue evolution in the lungless salamanders, family Plethodontidae. I. Introduction, theory, and a general model of dynamics. Journal of Morphology 148: 265–286.

———. 1977. Tongue evolution in the lungless salamanders, family Plethodontidae. II. Function and evolutionary diversity. Journal of Morphology 153: 39–90.

Lynch, J. D. 1971. Evolutionary relationships, osteology, and zoogeography of leptodactyloid frogs. Miscellaneous Publication of the University of Kansas Museum of Natural History 53: 1–238.

———. 1978. A re-assessment of the telmatobiine leptodactylid frogs of Patagónia. Occasional Paper of the Museum of Natural History of the University of Kansas 72: 1–57.

Marche, C., and J. P. Durand. 1983. Recherches comparatives sur l'ontogenèse et l'évolution de l'appareil hyobranchial de *Proteus anguinus* L., proteidae aveugle des eaux souterraines. Amphibia-Reptilia 4: 1–16.

Marcus, H. 1935. Zur Entstehung der Stapesplatte bei *Hypogeophis*. Anatomischer Anzeiger 80: 142–146.

Marcus, H., E. Stimmelmayr, and G. Porsch. 1935. Beiträge zur Kenntnis der Gymnophionen. XXV. Die Ossifikation des *Hypogeophis* schädels. Morphologisches Jahrbucher 76: 375–420.

McDiarmid, R. W. 1969. Comparative morphology and evolution of the neotropical frog genera *Atelopus, Dendrophryniscus, Melanophryniscus, Oreophrynella,* and *Brachycephalus.* Ph.D. diss., University of Southern California.

Milner, A. R. 1983. The biogeography of salamanders in the Mesozoic and early Caenozoic: A cladistic-vicariance model. In *Evolution, Time, and Space: The Emergency of the Biosphere,* R. W. Simms, J. H. Price, and P. E. S. Whalley, eds. London: Academic Press, pp. 431–468.

Monath, T. 1965. The opercular apparatus of salamanders. Journal of Morphology 116: 149–170.

Myers, C. W., and L. S. Ford. 1986. On *Atopophrynus,* a recently described frog wrongly assigned to the Dendrobatidae. American Museum of Natural History Novitates (2843): 1–15.

Nussbaum, R. A. 1977. Rhinatrematidae: A new family of caecilians (Amphibia: Gymnophiona). Occasional Paper of the Museum of Zoology, University of Michigan 682: 1–30.

―――. 1979. The taxonomic status of the caecilian genus *Uraeotyphlus* Peters. Occasional Paper of the Museum of Zoology, University of Michigan 687: 1–20.

―――. 1983. The evolution of a unique dual jaw-closing mechanism in caecilians (Amphibia: Gymnophiona) and its bearing on caecilian ancestry. Journal of Zoology, London 199: 545–554.

―――. 1985. Systematics of caecilians (Amphibia: Gymnophiona) of the family Scolecomorphidae. Occasional Paper of the Museum of Zoology, University of Michigan 713: 1–49.

Nussbaum, R. A., and E. D. Brodie, Jr. 1982. Partitioning of the salamandrid genus *Tylototriton* Anderson (Amphibia: Caudata) with a description of a new genus. Herpetologica 38: 320–332.

Nussbaum, R. A., and M. S. Hoogmoed. 1979. Surinam caecilians, with notes on *Rhinatrema bivittatum* and the description of a new species of *Microcaecilia* (Amphibia, Gymnophiona). Zoologische Mededelingen, Leiden 54: 217–235.

Nussbaum, R. A., and M. Wilkinson. 1988. On the classification and phylogeny of caecilians (Amphibia: Gymnophiona): A critical review. Herpetological Monographs 2: 1–42.

Özeti, N., and D. B. Wake. 1969. The morphology and evolution of the tongue and associated structures in salamanders and newts (family Salamandridae). Copeia (1): 91–123.

Papendieck, H. I. C. M. 1954. Contributions to the cranial morphology of Ambystoma macrodactylum Baird. Annals of the University of Stellenbosch 30: 151–178.

Parker, H. W. 1934. *A Monograph of the Frogs of the Family Microhylidae.* London: British Museum (Natural History).

Parker, W. K. 1881. On the structure and development of the skull in the Batrachia. Part III. Philosophical Transactions of the Royal Society, London 1: 1–266.

Paterson, N. F. 1939. The head of *Xenopus laevis.* Quarterly Journal of Microscopical Science 81: 161–234.

―――. 1945. The skull of *Hymenochirus curtipes.* Proceedings of the Zoological Society of London 15 (3–4): 327–354.

————. 1955. The skull of the toad, *Hemipipa carvalhoi* Mir.-Rib. with remarks on other Pipidae. Proceedings of the Zoological Society of London 125 (1): 223–252.

Pusey, H. K. 1943. On the head of the leiopelmid frog, *Ascaphus truei*. Quarterly Journal of Microscopical Science 84: 106–185.

Pyles, R. A. 1987. Morphology and mechanics of the jaws of anuran amphibians. Ph.D. diss., University of Kansas.

Ramaswami, L. S. 1941. Some aspects of the cranial morphology of *Uraeotyphlus narayani* Seshachar (Apoda). Record of the Indian Museum 43 (II): 143–207.

————. 1942. An account of the head morphology of *Gegenophis carnosus* (Beddome), Apoda. Journal, Mysore University, sect. B, Contribution 9, Zoology 3 (24): 205–220.

————. 1947. Apodous Amphibia of the Eastern Ghats, South India. Current Science 16: 8–10.

Regal, P. J. 1966. Feeding specializations and the classification of terrestrial salamanders. Evolution 20: 392–407.

Reilly, S. M. 1983. The biology of the high altitude salamander *Batrachuperus mustersi* from Afghanistan. Journal of Herpetology 17 (1): 1–9.

Reilly, S. M., and G. V. Lauder. 1988. Atavisms and the homology of hyobranchial elements in lower vertebrates. Journal of Morphology 195: 237–245.

Roček, Z. 1981 [1980]. Cranial anatomy of frogs of the family Pelobatidae Stannius, 1856, with outlines of their phylogeny and systematics. Acta Universitatis Carolinae 1980: 1–164.

Ryke, P. A. J. 1950. Contribution to the cranial morphology of the Asiatic urodele Onychodactylus japonicus (Houttuijn). Annals of the University of Stellenbosch 26: 2–21.

Stephenson, E. M. T. 1951. The anatomy of the head of the New Zealand frog, *Leiopelma*. Transactions of the Zoological Society of London 27 (2): 255–305.

Taylor, E. H. 1968. *The Caecilians of the World*. Lawrence: University of Kansas Press.

————. 1969a. A new family of African Gymnophiona. University of Kansas Science Bulletin 48: 297–305.

————. 1969b. Skulls of Gymnophiona and their significance in the taxonomy of the group. University of Kansas Science Bulletin 48 (15): 585–687.

————. 1977. The comparative anatomy of caecilian mandibles and their teeth. University of Kansas Science Bulletin 51 (8): 261–282.

Tihen, J. A. 1958. Comments on the osteology and phylogeny of ambystomatid salamanders. Bulletin of the Florida State Museum, Biological Science 3 (1): 1–50.

————. 1962. Osteological observation on New World *Bufo*. American Midland Naturalist 67 (1): 157–183.

Trewavas, E. 1933. The hyoid and larynx of the Anura. Philosophical Transactions of the Royal Society of London B 222 (10): 401–527.

Trueb, L. 1966. Morphology and development of the skull in the frog *Hyla septentrionalis*. Copeia (3): 562–573.

————. 1968. Cranial osteology of the hylid frog, Smilisca baudini. University of Kansas Publications of the Museum of Natural History 18 (2): 11–35.

————. 1970. Evolutionary relationships of casque-headed tree frogs with co-ossified skulls (family Hylidae). University of Kansas Publications of the Museum of Natural History 18 (7): 547–716.

————. 1971. Phylogenetic relationships of certain neotropical toads with description of a new genus (Anura, Bufonidae). Los Angeles County Museum Contributions in Science 216: 1–40.

————. 1973. Bones, frogs, and evolution. In *Evolutionary Biology of the Anurans: Contemporary Research on Major Problems,* J. L. Vial, ed. Columbia: University of Missouri Press, pp. 65–132.

————. 1974. Systematic relationships of Neotropical horned frogs, genus *Hemiphractus* (Anura: Hylidae). Occasional Paper of the Museum of Natural History of the University of Kansas 29: 1–60.

————. 1979. Leptodactylid frogs of the genus *Telmatobius* in Ecuador with the description of a new species. Copeia (4): 714–733.

Trueb, L. In press. Historical constraints and morphological novelties in the evolution of the skeletal system of aquatic anurans of the family Pipidae. Journal of Zoology London. Submitted for symposium volume.

Trueb, L., and P. Alberch. 1985. Miniaturization and the anuran skull: A case study of heterochrony. In *Vertebrate Morphology,* H.-R. Duncker and G. Fleischer, eds. New York: Gustav Fischer Verlag, pp. 113–121.

Trueb, L., and D. C. Cannatella. 1982. The cranial osteology and hyolaryngeal apparatus of *Rhinophrynus dorsalis* (Anura: Rhinophrynidae) with comparisons to Recent pipid frogs. Journal of Morphology 171: 11–40.

————. 1986. Systematics, morphology, and phylogeny of genus *Pipa* (Anura: Pipidae). Herpetologica 42 (4): 412–449.

Trueb, L., and R. Cloutier. 1991a. A phylogenetic investigation of the inter- and intrarelationships of the Lissamphibia (Amphibia: Temnospondyli). In *Origins of the Higher Groups of Tetrapods: Controversy and Consensus,* H.-P. Schultze and L. Trueb, eds. Ithaca: Cornell University Press, pp. 175–188.

————. 1991b. Toward an understanding of the amphibians: Two centuries of systematic history. In *Origins of the Higher Groups of Tetrapods: Controversy and Consensus,* H.-P. Schultze and L. Trueb, eds. Ithaca: Cornell University Press, pp. 223–313.

Trueb, L., and M. J. Tyler. 1974. Systematics and evolution of the Greater Antillean hylid frogs. Occasional Paper of the Museum of Natural History of the University of Kansas 24: 1–60.

Tschugunova, T. J. 1981. Interfrontalia in *Bombina orientalis* (Blgr.) and *Bombina bombina* (L.). In *Herpetological Investigations in Siberia and the Far East,* L. J. Borkin, ed. Moscow: Academy of Science, USSR, Zoological Institute, pp. 117–121.

Visser, M. H. C. 1963. The cranial morphology of Ichthyophis glutinosus (Linné) and Ichthyophis monochrous (Bleeker). Annals of the University of Stellenbosch 38 (3, ser. A): 67–102.

Wake, D. B. 1966. Comparative osteology and evolution of the lungless salamanders, family Plethodontidae. Memoirs of the Southern California Academy of Science 4: 1–111.

———. 1980. Evidence of heterochronic evolution: A nasal bone in the Olympic salamander, *Rhyacotriton olympicus*. Journal of Herpetology 14 (3): 292–295.

Wake, D. B., and N. Özeti. 1969. Evolutionary relationships in the family Salamandridae. Copeia: 124–137.

Wake, M. H. 1985. Order Gymnophiona. In *Amphibian Species of the World*, D. Frost, ed. Lawrence: Allen Press and the Association of Systematics Collections, pp. 619–641.

———. 1986. A perspective on the systematics and morphology of the Gymnophiona (Amphibia). Memoires de la Société zoologique de France 43: 21–38.

Wake, M. H., and J. Hanken. 1982. Development of the skull of *Dermophis mexicanus* (Amphibia: Gymnophiona), with comments on skull kinesis and amphibian relationships. Journal of Morphology 173: 203–223.

Wake, M. H., and G. Z. Wurst. 1979. Tooth crown morphology in caecilians (Amphibia. Gymnophiona). Journal of Morphology 159: 331–342.

Wever, E. G. 1985. *The Amphibian Ear*. Princeton: Princeton University Press.

7

Patterns of Diversity in the Reptilian Skull

OLIVIER RIEPPEL

INTRODUCTION

THE REPTILIA HAS LONG BEEN CONSIDERED a paraphyletic assemblage, comprising all amniotes that are neither birds nor mammals. This situation has changed with Gauthier, Kluge, and Rowe's (1988a, b) definition of a monophyletic Reptilia, including birds but excluding mammal-like reptiles and mammals (fig. 7.1). Their analysis basically corroborates Reisz's (1980; see also Heaton and Reisz 1986) views, which treated the Synapsida (including all mammal-like reptiles and their descendants) as a sister group of the Eureptilia, the latter comprising the Anapsida (Captorhinomorpha and turtles) plus the Diapsida (see also Gaffney 1980). The classification of a few Paleozoic reptiles such as mesosaurs, millerettids, pareiasaurs, and procolophonians remains problematic; they have been grouped as "Parareptilia" by Gauthier, Kluge, and Rowe (1988b).

"Reptiles" were subdivided by Olson (1947) into two major "lineages," his Parareptilia (including the Diadectomorpha, Procolophonia, Pareiasauria, and Chelonia), and his Eureptilia (comprising all other groups, including synapsids). The Diadectomorpha have now been classified with amphibians (Heaton 1980; Panchen and Smithson 1988), i.e., outside amniotes (Gauthier, Kluge et al. 1988b). But the status of the Parareptilia and the relationships of turtles remain a subject of debate. Recently, Reisz and Laurin (1991) have argued that the Testudines are the sister group of procolophonians rather than of captorhinomorphs (Gaffney and Meeker 1983; see also Gaffney and Meylan 1988).

The Diapsida have recently come under considerable scrutiny (Gauthier 1984, 1986; Gauthier, Estes et al. 1988; Benton 1985; Evans 1988): a number of diapsid fossils, most prominently the earliest diapsid, *Petrolacosaurus,* from the Upper Pennsylvanian of Kansas (Reisz 1981) are classified outside the Neodiapsida, the latter including a series of fossils plus the Sauria (Gauthier, Kluge et al. 1988a), which subdivide into two major clades (fig. 7.1). The Archosauromorpha include the Rhynchosauria, the Prolacertiformes, and the Archosauria, the latter comprising pterosaurs, dinosaurs, crocodiles, and birds. The Lepidosauromorpha include the Lepidosauria, the latter comprising the Sphenodontida and the Squamata. The Younginiformes have been classified within the Lepidosauromorpha, but recently evidence has accumulated indicating their status as a sister group of the Sauria (Archosauromorpha plus Lepidosauromorpha) (Zanon 1990; Laurin 1991).

The Squamata are currently subdivided into the Lacertilia (paraphyletic, fig. 7.2), Amphisbaenia, and Serpentes (fig. 7.3), three groups of controversial interrelationships. The cladistic analysis of diapsid interrelationships has also thrown a number of marine Mesozoic reptiles such as ichthyosaurs, nothosaurs, plesiosaurs, and placodonts, formerly classified as Euryapsida and/or Parapsida, into focus. A more detailed account of diapsid interrelationships will be given below in the discussion of dermatocranial structure.

COMPARATIVE MORPHOLOGY OF THE REPTILE SKULL

Types of Bone in the Reptile Skull

Three types of ossifications, viz., dermal, cartilage, and membrane bone, can be distinguished in the reptile skull (Patterson 1977). Dermal bone (exoskeletal) is ontogenetically and/or phylogenetically related to the basement membrane of the epidermis: it forms the dermatocranium. Cartilage bone (endoskeletal) ossifies in preformed cartilaginous elements and is represented by ossifications of the neurocranium. "Membrane bone" refers to endoskeletal ossifications which are not preformed in cartilage, but which are homologous to structures preformed in cartilage at a more inclusive level of the taxonomic hierarchy (in contrast to dermal bone, which in reptiles shows a similar histogenesis). An example is the floor of the neurocranium of reptiles, which displays a large basicranial fenestra, within which the central part of the basisphenoid ossifies as membrane bone. Starck (1979) distinguished a fourth type of ossification, i.e., *Zuwachsknochen*, representing (endoskeletal) membrane ossifications added to cartilage bone or to their membrane bone representatives respectively; the alary process of the prootic (discussed below) is an example.

The Neurocranium: General Characteristics

The development of the neurocranium is primarily related to the development of sense organs and the brain (fig. 7.4). For descriptive purposes it is convenient to distinguish the basicranium from the primary lateral braincase walls. The basicranium is formed by the trabeculae cranii anteriorly,

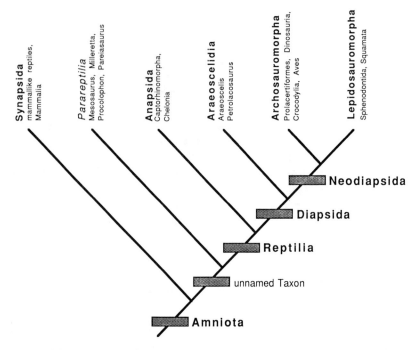

Fig. 7.1. The interrelationships of Amniota. (Based on Gauthier, Kluge et al. 1988 a, b)

the parachordal cartilages (basal plate) posteriorly and the acrochordal cartilage in between (Rieppel 1978c; but see Bellairs and Kamal 1981).

Anteriorly, the trabeculae cranii merge into the internasal septum separating the two nasal capsules from one another. The structure and systematic implications of the nasal capsule in lepidosaurs was discussed by Pratt (1948). More posteriorly, the trabeculae cranii form the base of the interorbital septum and associated orbitosphenoid cartilages. The otic capsules chondrify around the developing labyrinth and establish a contact with the parachordal cartilage (basal plate) by means of the basicapsular commissure. The medial wall of the otic capsule is last to chondrify, and it remains unossified or incompletely ossified in the adult skull of many taxa such as captorhinomorphs (Price 1935; Heaton 1979), turtles (Gaffney 1972, 1979), and early diapsids (Evans 1986). Posteriorly, the braincase incorporates occipital vertebrae (de Beer 1937). Chondrifications roofing the occipital and otic region of the braincase (tectum posterior and tectum synoticum) develop between the occipital arches and otic capsules. The tectal roof may carry an anterior ascending process thought to be related to metakinesis: it is generally present in lizards, but lacking in snakes,

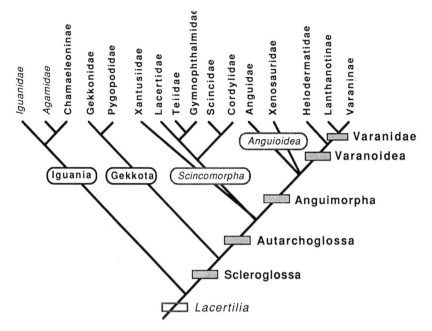

Fig. 7.2. A conservative approach to lizard interrelationships, based mainly on Estes et al. 1988. The Iguania have recently been reviewed by Frost and Etheridge (1989); for gekkotan interrelationships see Kluge (1987)

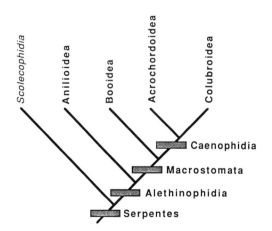

Fig. 7.3. The interrelationships of snakes. (Based on Rieppel 1988)

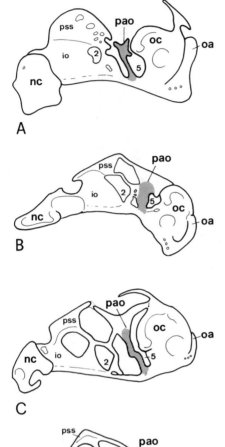

Fig. 7.4. The neurocranium in reptiles; the pila antotica is shaded. A. *Emys orbicularis*. B. *Crocodylus porosus*. C. *Sphenodon punctatus*. D. *Acanthodactylus boskianus*. E. *Natrix natrix*. Abbreviations: ci, carotis internus foramen; io, interorbital septum; nc, nasal capsule; oa, occipital arch; oc, otic capsule; pao, pila antotica; pss, planum supraseptale; x, fenestra X; 2, nervus opticus; 5, nervus trigeminus. (A redrawn after B. W. Kunkel in Bellairs and Kamal 1981, fig. 73; B after K. Shiino in Bellairs and Kamal 1981, fig. 82; C, after G. Werner in Bellairs and Kamal 1981, fig. 44; D, after A. M. Kamal and A. M. Abdeen in Bellairs and Kamal 1981, fig. 19; E, after Bäckström 1931, fig. 8)

which have obliterated metakinesis. However, the processus ascendens is lacking in geckos (Bellairs and Kamal 1981) with a highly kinetic skull.

The Basicranium. The trabeculae cranii are laid down as paired structures, fused at their anterior tip as they merge into the internasal septum. During subsequent development, they fuse from front to back to form an unpaired cartilaginous rod, the trabecula communis. In chelonians and crocodiles, a mesenchyme condensation is observed between the developing trabeculae, known as intertrabecula (Shaner 1926; Pehrson 1945; Bellairs 1958), which eventually is incorporated into the trabecula communis.

The posterior ends of the trabeculae remain separate and diverge to meet the lateral edges of the acrochordal cartilage, which develops behind the hypophysis, within the plica ventralis of the embryonic brain and at the anterior tip of the notochord. From the posterior end of the trabeculae project the basitrabecular (basipterygoid) processes, which will take part in the palatobasal articulation. The acrochordal cartilage separates the anterior hypophyseal fenestra from the posterior basicranial fenestra lying between the anterior portions of the parachordals (basal plate). The acrochordal cartilage eventually ossifies as dorsum sellae, while the hypophyseal as well as the basicranial fenestrae become closed by membrane ossification (part of the basisphenoid) and by the underlying parasphenoid. The anterior surface of the dorsum sellae bears pits where the retractor eye muscles take their origin (Säve-Söderbergh 1946). The dorsum sellae is low and the sella turcica shallow in reptiles with reduced eyes and eye muscles such as burrowing lizards and amphisbaenians (Gans 1978; Rieppel 1978a). A similar condition obtains in snakes (Rieppel 1979b), which have lost their retractor bulbi muscle (Underwood 1970, 49).

The internal carotid runs along the latero-ventral aspect of the basicranium; at the level behind the basipterygoid process the internal carotid gives off the cerebral carotid, which pierces the sella turcica, and itself continues anteriorly as palatine artery, which is joined by the Vidian nerve (ramus palatinus of the facial nerve). As the parasphenoid comes to underlie the basicranium, its lateral wings enclose the internal carotid together with the palatine nerve within the Vidian canal (Shishkin 1968). The closure of the Vidian canal remains incomplete in early reptiles (captorhinomorphs: Heaton 1979), in a variety of early diapsids, including archosauromorph taxa (Evans 1986), and in *Sphenodon*. Complete closure of the Vidian canal is a squamate synapomorphy, although the situation in the primitive snake genus *Typhlops* remains debatable (Rieppel 1979a, 1988; Bellairs and Kamal 1981). Part of the controversy results from the difficulty in identifying the parasphenoid in squamate embryos (Kesteven 1940), a problem which deserves further study: lateral wings of the parasphenoid have been claimed to be absent in snakes (de Beer 1937; Bellairs and Kamal 1981) which, if true, would raise problems of homology of the Vidian canal in lizards and alethinophidian snakes (see Rieppel 1988, 43; and fig. 1).

In reptiles that show extensive fusion of the dermal palate to the basicranium, the internal carotid together with the Vidian nerve are also trapped in an intracranial course. In crocodilians, the palatine ramus of the facial nerve passes through a canal in the basisphenoid, termed "parabasal" canal by Romer (1956, 143).

This canal is already observed in the Late Triassic protosuchid crocodile *Eopneumatosuchus,* where it shares the same topographical relations as does the Vidian canal in squamates (Crompton and Smith 1980, 208). The internal carotid enters the basicranium in the occiput through a foramen caroticum posterius within the basioccipital (*Eopneumatosuchus*) or the opisthotic-exoccipital (in modern crocodiles). More anteriorly, the carotid joins the palatine nerve within the parabasal canal before it enters the pituary fossa (Romer 1956, 142; Bellairs and Kamal 1981, 236).

In turtles, the internal carotid is trapped in the canalis caroticus internus contained within the pterygoid or lying between the pterygoid and basisphenoid (Gaffney 1979, 101), depending on the pattern of ossification of the pterygoid bone (Nick 1912); the extent of the canal varies with the different posterior extension of the pterygoid in pleurodires and cryptodires (Gaffney 1975). Fossil evidence suggests that during phylogeny the pterygoid extended backward prior to the posterior elongation of the internal carotid canal (Rieppel 1980c, and references therein). Ontogenetically this must again be related to different ossification patterns of the pterygoid bone.

Sauropterygians are yet another group of reptiles with a closed dermal palate, trapping the internal carotid and the Vidian nerve in an intracranial course. In *Simosaurus* (personal observation), the pterygoid is fused to the basicranium over its entire length; the point of entry of the internal carotid into the pterygoid-basicranial suture is unclear, but anteriorly the carotid canal bifurcates and opens within the basisphenoid (foramen for the cerebral carotid in the sella turcica) and lateral to it in the pterygoid (foramen for the palatine artery). A third anterior foramen in the pterygoid may have served the exit of the Vidian nerve, which may have joined the internal carotid along its intracranial course. Similar conditions may be expected in other sauropterygians such as plesiosaurs and perhaps placodonts, but no detailed information is available.

Orbitotemporal Ossifications. The cartilage in the orbitotemporal region of the reptile neurocranium is fenestrated and/or reduced to a variable degree. Among extant taxa, turtles develop the most extensive cartilaginous sidewall of the braincase at least during some ontogenetic stage (fig. 7.4A); later it is partially reduced and replaced by a secondary lateral braincase wall formed by parietal down-growths (Rieppel 1976a). At the other end of the spectrum, snakes show the complete reduction of the lateral braincase wall in the orbitotemporal region (fig. 7.4E): vestigial and transient orbital cartilages have only rarely been reported in snake embryos (Bellairs 1949b). Orbitotemporal cartilages may give rise to various ossifications in the lateral braincase wall of adult lizards (the orbitosphenoid of Oelrich 1956; "trifid ossification" of Romer 1956).

The base of the antotic pila (shaded in fig. 7.4) ossifies as clinoid process in most reptiles. In captorhinids, the clinoid process forms part of the basisphenoid ossification (Price 1935; Heaton 1979), the generalized condition at the level of the Reptilia, also found in turtles (Gaffney 1972). In the Late Jurassic turtle genus *Plesiochelys* and in *Emydura*, the clinoid process is tall and appears to incorporate most of the embryonic antotic pila (Gaffney 1976; 1979, 137). As far as is known, the Euryapsida (sauropterygians and placodonts) retain the generalized condition (Rieppel 1989b). In lepidosauromorph reptiles, the clinoid process remains largely confined to the basisphenoid ossification with some possible contribution of the prootic. In early archosauromorphs, the clinoid process becomes associated with the prootic ossification (Evans 1986), while in later archosaurs the pila antotica ossifies as pleurosphenoid, completing the osseous lateral wall of the braincase as in extant crocodiles (and birds).

A separate pleurosphenoid ossification (fig. 7.5B) has been described in the lateral wall of the amphisbaenian braincase (Zangerl 1944), but it probably represents the anterior alar process of the prootic (Rieppel 1981b, 523–524; see also fig. 7.5A), an anterior expansion of the prootic (*Zuwachsknochen*) otherwise characterizing autarchoglossan (fig. 7.2) lizards (Gauthier 1982). On the other hand, the Amphisbaenia are diagnosed as a monophyletic group by the contribution of a membrane bone, the orbitosphenoid, to the formation of the closed braincase wall (Bellairs and Gans 1983).

The lateral wall of the alethinophidian (fig. 7.3) braincase incorporates an element lying within the prootic incisure, lateral to the Gasserian ganglion and between the maxillary and mandibular divisions of the trigeminal nerve (fig. 7.5C–E). The bone, which is of membrane origin but which may incorporate cartilage associated with the lateral edge of the basal plate (de Beer 1926; Bäckström 1931; Bellairs and Kamal 1981; Haluska and Alberch 1983), has sometimes been compared to the lacertilian epipterygoid, although the latter shows different topographical relationships with respect to the branches of the trigeminal nerve (fig. 7.5E–F; see comments on the epipterygoid of the amphisbaenian *Trogonophis* below, and Rieppel 1976b).

Ventrally, the laterosphenoid bone articulates with the lateral wing of

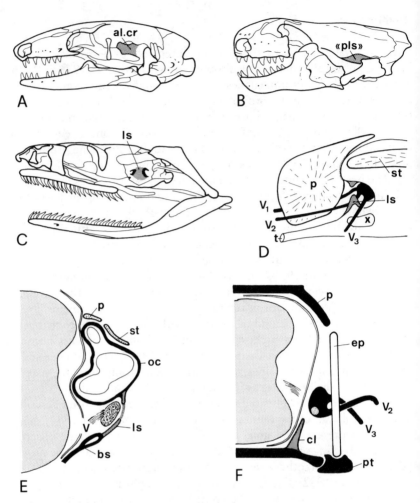

Fig. 7.5. The closure of the lateral braincase wall in squamate reptiles.
A. *Typhlosaurus cregoi,* a skinkid lizard showing an enlarged alary crista on the prootic. B. *Amphisbaena alba* with the "pleurosphenoid," an anterior extension of the prootic. C. *Nerodia rhombifera,* showing the laterosphenoid bone. D. The development of the alethinophidian laterosphenoid bone and its relations to the branches of the trigeminal nerve. E. A transverse section through the orbitotemporal region of the skull of *Natrix natrix* on day 21 of incubation. F. A diagrammatic representation of the cavum epiptericum in lizards. Abbreviations: al.cr, alary crista of the prootic; bs, basisphenoid; cl, clinoid process (ossified base of the pila antotica) on the basisphenoid; ep, epipterygoid; ls, laterosphenoid; oc, otic capsule; p, parietal; pls, pleurosphenoid; pt, pterygoid; st, supratemporal; t, trabecula cranii; x, fenestra X in the parachordal plate; V_1, opthalmic branch of the trigeminal nerve; V_2, maxillary branch of the trigeminal nerve; V_3, mandibular branch of the trigeminal nerve. (A, redrawn after Rieppel 1981a, fig. 8; B, after Rieppel 1979e, fig. 1; C, after Cundall 1987, fig. 4-10; D, after Bellairs and Kamal 1981, fig. 69; E, original; F, original)

the basal plate, i.e., of the basisphenoid-parasphenoid complex. The lateral wing of the basicranium (missing in scolecophidians which also lack the laterosphenoid: McDowell 1967) has been been interpreted as a dorsally deflected basitrabecular process (in order to support the equation of the laterosphenoid with the lacertilian epipterygoid: Brock 1929; Brock retracted that position in 1941; see also McDowell 1967, 1975). However, this conjecture of homology is refuted by the occurrence of basitrabecular cartilages in conjunction with the lateral wings of the basal plate in *Eryx* (Kamal and Hammouda 1965a; but see comments by Bellairs and Kamal 1981) and *Sanzinia* (Genest-Villard 1966). Dorsally, the laterosphenoid of snakes develops in continuity with a ventral membranous extension (*Zuwachsknochen*) of the prootic. The latter may be compared to the anterior extension (alar process) of the prootic in autarchoglossan lizards and amphisbaenians mentioned above.

There is still considerable disagreement as to the interpretation of the laterosphenoid bone. Its homology with the lacertilian epipterygoid cannot be supported on topographical grounds. Bellairs and Kamal (1981) consider it a neomorph derivative of the splanchnocranium, and the space medial to it, housing the Gasserian ganglion, as the cavum epiptericum. Rieppel (1989a) treated the element as a taxic homology (synapomorphy) diagnostic for alethinophidian snakes, with no (or unknown) transformational relations to cranial structures in other squamates; the Gasserian ganglion is claimed to lie in an intramural but extradural space (de Beer 1926). On the basis of its dorsal continuity with a membranous "prootic extension" of the otic capsule, and of its ventral continuity with the lateral edge of the parachordal (basal) plate, the laterosphenoid is interpreted to lie level with the primary lateral braincase wall, from which the dura would have shrunken away owing to the complete reduction of orbitotemporal cartilages (Rieppel 1976b; compare figs. 7.4E and 7.5E).

The Otico-Occipital Region. The occipital arch rises up from the basal plate behind the otic capsule, enclosing the roots of the hypoglossal nerve within a variable number of foramina. It eventually ossifies as exoccipital, establishing a dorsal contact with the posterior part of the otic capsule, which eventually ossifies as opisthotic. The space between the otic capsule, basal plate, and occipital arch is the fissura metotica: it forms the metotic foramen (Rieppel 1985) in the adult skull of generalized reptiles (captorhinids: Price 1935; Heaton 1979; early diapsids: Evans 1980, 1986; turtles: Rieppel 1980c, 1985; and *Sphenodon*), transmitting the glossopharyngeal and vagus nerves along with the jugular vein. The metotic fissure has become subdivided in a number of reptile clades to separate an anterior recessus scalae tympani (transmitting the glossopharyngeal nerve in most lizards) from the posterior jugular or vagus foramen. In crocodiles, the fissura metotica becomes subdivided by the development of a subcapsular process extending anteriorly from the occipital arch (from the lateral edge of the basal plate, according to Shiino 1914). Birds have been claimed to share a similar development, a conjecture of homology which was used to support the disputed sister-group relationship of crocodiles and birds (Whetstone and Martin 1979; see also Rieppel 1985).

The fissura metotica is again subdivided in squamate reptiles. The separation of an anterior recessus scalae tympani (occipital recess, sensu Oelrich 1956) from the posterior vagus foramen is effected differently in lizards and snakes. In lizards, the posterior part of the otic capsule is applied to the lateral margin of the basal plate; in snakes, a strut of cartilage grows down the medial wall of the otic capsule to meet the basal plate (Kamal 1971; Rieppel 1988). The difference of developmental pathways might indicate the independent subdivision of the metotic fissure in lizards and snakes. The metotic fissure is also subdivided in the Amphisbaenia, but no developmental data are available.

The Splanchnocranium

The Palatoquadrate. The palatoquadrate in *Lacerta*, described by Gaupp (1900), can be considered to represent the paradigmatic condition with which to compare the fate of the element in all other reptiles.

In an early embryo of *Lacerta*, the palatoquadrate arch consists of an anterior pterygoid process, extending anteriorly dorsal to the anlage of the pterygoid bone and atrophying during later stages of development. Lateral to the basitrabecular process, the palatoquadrate forms the ascending process, which eventually ossifies as epipterygoid or columella cranii. Ventrally, the ascending process of the palatoquadrate articulates with the distal tip of the basitrabecular process by the intermediate of the basal process. The basal process becomes detached from the palatoquadrate during early developmental stages and is accommodated within the pterygoid notch as meniscal cartilage. It forms a synovial joint with the basitrabecular (basipterygoid) process, completing the palatobasal articulation which in turn forms the floor of the cavum epiptericum (fig. 7.5F). The latter represents an extracranial space, bounded laterally by the ascending process (i.e., epipterygoid) and medially by the primary lateral wall of the braincase (i.e., pila antotica). It is traversed by the ophthalmic branch of the trigeminal nerve and by the head vein. The maxillary and mandibular branches of the trigeminal nerve pass out behind the epipterygoid and continue their course lateral to it (fig. 7.5F). During early developmental stages, the epipterygoid is in a transient cartilaginous connection with the quadrate process of the palatoquadrate, which eventually ossifies as quadrate bone.

In the turtle embryo *Chelydra serpentina* (stage 19 of Yntema 1968), there is a well-developed pila antotica, forming the primary lateral wall of the braincase. It atrophies during later stages of development, and a secondary lateral wall of the braincase is formed by the ascending process of the palatoquadrate, which articulates with the crista basipterygoidea ventrally, and which meets a lateral down-growth of the parietal dorsally (Rieppel 1976a). The ascending process of turtles remains relatively broad and low, and thus resembles an early stage of differentiation of the epipterygoid in *Lacerta*. Owing to the lack of developmental studies, the occurrence of an epipterygoid in pleurodire turtles is not known.

The palatoquadrate of crocodiles consists of a large quadrate process and a slender anterior pterygoid process. The latter bears a vestigial ascending process. No epipterygoid ossifies in the adult skull. The space which corresponds to the cavum epiptericum is not bounded laterally (Bellairs and Kamal 1981).

Within amphisbaenians a small epipterygoid bone has been described for *Trogonophis* only (Bellairs 1949a), articulating with the dorsal surface of the pterygoid some distance in front of the palatobasal articulation. The position of the epipterygoid bone with respect to the maxillary branch of the trigeminal nerve is unusual in *Trogonophis,* as the nerve passes medial to the bone rather than lateral to it as in lizards (Bellairs and Kamal 1981).

In snake embryos, the palatoquadrate is atrophied, with the exception of the quadrate cartilage. However, there is some controversy concerning the homology of the laterosphenoid bone (see above).

The Sound-Transmitting Apparatus. In modern reptiles, the sound-transmitting apparatus is formed by a medial bony stapes (columella auris) and a distal cartilaginous extrastapes (extracolumella), developing from two separate rudiments, the otostapes medially and the hyostapes laterally. Some lizards show a synovial joint between these two components. The extracolumella is related to the tympanic membrane by means of an insertion plate, typically consisting of four processes arranged in a cruciform pattern (Werner and Wever 1972; Wever 1978). Two further processes characterize the lacertilian columella, at least in its embryonic condition: these are the dorsal process, from the tip of which derive the intercalary cartilage participating in the movable quadrate suspension, and the internal process, which projects antero-ventrally toward the quadrate bone. The latter two processes develop in continuity with the medial rudiment, the otostapes. However, the joint between stapes and extracolumella develops just medial to these two processes, so that in later stages the dorsal process (the base of which fails to chondrify in lizards but not in *Sphenodon*) and the internal process appear to belong to the extracolumella (hyostapes).

The bony stapes is composed of a footplate, accommodated within the fenestra ovalis, and a lateral shaft, which may be pierced by a foramen transmitting the stapedial artery. Because the occurrence of a stapedial foramen is plesiomorphous at the level of the Amniota (Goodrich 1930), the foramen must have secondarily reappeared in a number of squamates (Greer 1976), most probably as a result of paedomorphosis (Estes 1983; Rieppel 1984a).

Snakes lack the tympanic membrane and the extracolumella. The stapes of snakes typically contacts an articular process on the quadrate which develops from a separate cartilaginous nodule, the stylohyal of Parker (1879): it represents the intercalary cartilage (the tip of the dorsal process of the otostapes: Brock 1929; de Beer 1937; Rieppel 1980d) fused to the quadrate. The cartilaginous distal end of the ophidian stapes is not homologous to the lacertilian extracolumella. It has been compared to the base of the dorsal process of the otostapes (Brock 1929; Kamal and Hammouda 1965b), but if the course of the chorda tympani is constant, it must represent the internal process of the lacertilian otostapes (Rieppel 1980d).

In early tetrapods, the stapes is a massive structure bracing the braincase against the cheek in a primitively metakinetic skull (Carroll 1980; Reisz 1981). In *Eocaptorhinus*, the stapes is a strong element, carrying a relatively large footplate accommodated within a stapedial recess along the posterior margin of the fenestra ovalis (fenestra ovalis externa of Heaton 1979, 56–57), and lightly sutured to the prootic and basisphenoid anteriorly. This is not a construction suitable for the transmission of high-frequency airborne sound. In other captorhinomorph genera such as *Hylonomus* (Carroll 1964) and *Paleothyris* (Carroll 1969a), the stapes is somewhat lighter, but a middle ear with an efficient transducer mechanism for airborne sound developed only later, and apparently two times independently within reptiles: in turtles and diapsids (Reisz 1981). A light stapes consisting of a small footplate and an elongated shaft, connected to a relatively large tympanum suspended within a posterior concavity of the quadrate bone, is currently recognized as a synapomorphy of the Neodiapsida (Benton 1985, 112). The large ratio of tympanum surface to stapedial footplate area provides an efficient impedance-matching mechanism permitting the reception of high-frequency airborne sound (Wever 1978).

There are, however, a number of squamates which have lost the impedance-matching mechanism and modified the middle ear. In acontine scincs (genera *Acontias, Acontophiops,* and *Typhlosaurus*), in *Dibamus,* in the anguid genus *Anniella,* and in amphisbaenians, the stapedial footplate is large and accommodated in a ventro-laterally placed fenestra ovalis, while the occipital recess (lateral aperture of the recessus scalae tympani) is reduced to a small foramen transmitting the glossopharyngeal nerve (see Wever 1978, for pressure compensation mechanisms). These changes may result from size constraints rather than represent particular adaptations: all the lizards mentioned are miniaturized, perhaps in adaptation to fossorial or burrowing habits (Rieppel 1984b), but small representatives of the terrestrial or arboreal chamaeleonine genera *Brookesia*, *Rhampholeon*, and *Chamaeleo* show similar modifications of the ear capsule (personal observation).

In acontine scincs the shaft of the stapes extends laterally posterior to the quadrate (fig. 7.13A-C) to contact an extracolumella which is related to a fibrous plate expanding below the skin of the cheek region. In *Anniella*, the stapes abuts the quadrate (Toerien 1950). In the Dibamidae, the stapes (lacking an extracolumella: Rieppel 1980d) abuts a posterior articular process of the quadrate (fig. 7.13D), an arrangement recalling the ophidian condition (Gasc 1968). In amphisbaenians the stapes is connected to an elongated extracolumella passing behind and lateral to the quadrate and extending anteriorly into a dermal thickening lateral to the lower jaw; only in *Bipes* does the short stapedial shaft terminate in a fibrous terminal disk lying behind the quadrate (Wever and Gans 1972). The elongated extracolumella of *Amphisbaena* is thought to be homologous to the epihyal (Wever and Gans 1973).

It has been suggested that the modifications in the impedance-matching middle ear of snakes indicate a burrowing ancestry of the group, but Berman and Regal (1967) have argued that these modifications are correlated with the development of a high degree of cranial kinesis, involving extensive quadrate movement. Snakes differ from all other squamates by the development of a crista circumfenestralis (Estes et al. 1970; Baird 1970), a bony rim surrounding the relatively large fenestra ovalis as well as the lateral aperture of the recessus scalae tympani (Rieppel 1979b), thus defining a pericapsular recess housing the stapedial footplate.

The Neodiapsida are diagnosed by a posteriorly excavated (concave) quadrate and by the presence of a retroarticular process on the lower jaw. Both structures serve the suspension of a tympanic membrane. Generalized Sauropterygia retain the same morphology, but more advanced members of the group either reduce the size of the tympanum or lose it altogether, probably in relation to their capacity for rapid dives to greater depths (Rieppel 1989b). Turtles show a peculiar suspension of the tympanum on a funnel-shaped cavity formed by the quadrate and the adjoining squamosal (fig. 7.6), which separates a lateral tympanic cavity from the medial pericapsular recess (Wever and Vernon 1956).

In the sea turtle *Chelonia mydas,* there is no tympanic membrane, and most of the tympanic cavity is filled by a fatty tissue (Ridgeway et al. 1969), presumably compensating for the relative vacuum that builds up in the middle ear during diving. A tympanum suspension somewhat similar to

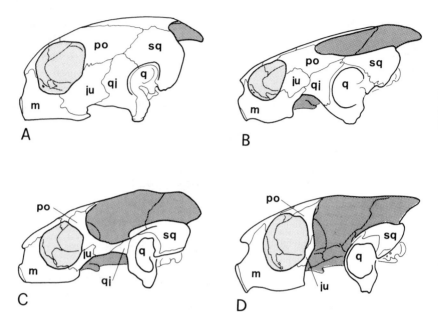

Fig. 7.6. The emargination of the temporal region in the dermatocranium of the Chelonia. A. *Chelonia mydas.* B. *Chrysemys (Pseudemys) concinna.* C. *Geomyda mouhotii.* D. *Terrapene ornata.* Abbreviations: ju, jugal; m, maxilla; po, postorbital; q, quadrate; qj, quadratojugal; sq, squamosal. (A, redrawn after Gaffney 1979, fig. 214; B, after Gaffney 1979, fig. 229; C, after Gaffney 1979, fig. 236; D, after Gaffney 1979, fig. 252)

that of turtles, i.e., on a funnel-shaped quadrate, is observed in some groups of mosasaurs, marine varanoid reptiles from the Upper Cretaceous (Russell 1967). It is unknown whether this structure is related to diving. In mosasaurs, the tympanic membrane may be calcified to prevent rupture during rapid diving excursions (Russell 1967).

The Dermatocranium: General Characteristics

The skull roof, bony covering of the cheek region, dermal palate, and tooth-bearing bones lining the primary jaws are all components of the dermatocranium. Throughout reptiles, a general trend toward a reduction and fenestration of the dermatocranium can be observed in correlation with an expansion of the jaw adductor musculature. Captorhinomorphs are characterized by a complete roofing of the temporal region (anapsid) condition: (fig. 7.7A), an essentially closed occiput with small post-temporal fenestra (Reisz 1981, 63), and the palate is essentially closed with no suborbital fenestrae and relatively narrow interpterygoid vacuities (fig. 7.11A). In turtles and diapsid reptiles, both the temporal region and the occiput become opened through fenestration or emargination (see below), whereas in early synapsids (characterized by a single lower temporal fossa: fig. 7.7D), the occiput is even more closed than in captorhinomorphs, owing to the platelike configuration of the constituent elements, which is a diagnostic feature of the clade (Heaton 1980; Reisz 1980, 1981).

The palate, articulating with the base of the braincase at the palato-basal articulation, is opened by the formation of suborbital fenestrae (diagnostic of diapsids) and by a widening of the interpterygoid vacuities

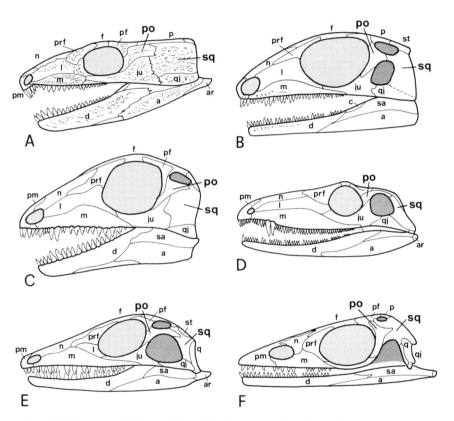

Fig. 7.7. The temporal fenestration of the dermatocranium in reptiles.
A. *Eocaptorhinus platyceps,* anapsid. B. *Petrolacosaurus kansensis,* the earliest diapsid. C. *Araeoscelis gracilis,* modified diapsid. D. *Varanosaurus acutirostris,* synapsid. E. *Youngina capensis,* diapsid. F. *Pachypleurosaurus edwardsi,* modified diapsid. Abbreviations: a, angular; ar, articular; c, coronoid; d, dentary; f, frontal; ju, jugal; l, lacrimal; m, maxilla; n, nasal; p, parietal; pf, postfrontal; pm, premaxilla; po, postorbital; prf, prefrontal; q, quadrate; qj, quadratojugal; sa, surangular; sq, squamosal; st, supratemporal. (A, redrawn after Heaton 1979, fig. 2; B, after Reisz 1981, fig. 2; C, after Reisz et al. 1984, fig. 3; D, after Romer and Price 1940, fig. 3; E, after Carroll 1981, fig. 9; F, after Carroll and Gaskill 1985, fig. 14)

(fig. 7.11). Reduction of the dermal palate is usually correlated with increasing cranial kinetism. An opposite trend is observed in the formation of a closed secondary palate, usually correlated with immobilization or fusion of the palatobasal articulation.

The most prominent bone in the primitive reptile palate is the pterygoid. A transverse and dentigerous flange developed by the middle portion of the pterygoid has been identified as the hallmark of the "reptilian" grade of evolution (Carroll 1969b, c). Although the palatal dentition was reduced or lost in many reptile groups, the transverse pterygoid flange continues to serve as site of origin of the pterygoideus superficialis muscle; its formation is related to the development of the static pressure system of jaw mechanics, distinguishing most fossil and extant reptiles from amphibians (Olson 1961; Carroll 1969c).

As it lies superficial to both neurocranium and splanchnocranium, it is the dermatocranium which in most reptiles determines the shape of the head, sometimes modified to form often bizarre structures (spines, horns, etc.) which function as defensory devices or as signals in the context of social behavior. Particular mention may be made of the formation of a frill in the ceratopsian dinosaurs and in chameleons. The superficial similarity of frill formation has been used to reconstruct the jaw adductor musculature in ceratopsians (Lull 1908; Haas 1955; see also Ostrom 1966). These considerations neglected some fundamental differences in the structural plan of the temporal region in these two reptile groups (Rieppel 1981a). While the frill of chameleons does allow an expansion of the area of origin of the jaw adductor musculature, that of ceratopsians apparently served a dual function: the strong epaxial neck musculature inserted into its posterior surface, whereas the anterior surface may have served thermoregulation.

PATTERNS OF SKULL STRUCTURE AND THEIR TAXONOMIC IMPLICATIONS

The Reduction of the Dermatocranium

The dermatocranium is the component of the skull which historically has been most widely used in reptile systematics and classification. Major reptilian lineages have been recognized on the basis of the configuration of the temporal region of the skull, while at a lower taxonomic level, the presence or absence of individual bones, as well as their shape, is of importance in systematics.

Captorhinomorph reptiles, representing the most generalized condition at the level of the Reptilia, show a completely closed temporal region of the dermatocranium. This is known as the anapsid condition (fig. 7.7A).

The whole bulk of the jaw adductor musculature must have been accommodated between the lateral wall of the neurocranium and the superficial dermatocranium. This space opens posteriorly through post-temporal fossae, bordered dorsally and laterally by the dermatocranium, medially and ventrally by the neurocranium (paroccipital process). In early "stem-reptiles," these fossae remain small (Carroll 1969a; Heaton 1979). From their area of origin, the fibers of the jaw adductor musculature pass to the lower jaw through the subtemporal fossa, bounded by the dermal palate (pterygoid bone) medially and the lower margin of the dermal cheek region (jugal and quadratojugal bones) laterally.

Within the Reptilia the dermatocranium has repeatedly been opened up in various clades following different patterns. Two basic mechanisms of reduction have been identified, and both are correlated with an expansion of the origins of jaw adductor muscles beyond the original confines of the dermatocranium. This permits an increase of muscle mass, i.e., of the numbers of fibers involved in a complex pinnate system, or an increase in length of individual fibers, or both. The physiological cross section of a muscle determines the force it can generate, while fiber length determines the excursion range and the rate of relative shortening (Gans and de Vree 1987).

Temporal Emargination. The first mechanism of reduction is emargination, as exemplified by turtles (Romer 1956; Kilias 1957; Gaffney 1979). Emargination of the originally closed temporal region proceeds from the lower margin of the cheek in a dorsal direction and/or from the upper margin of the post-temporal fossa in an anterior direction (fig. 7.6). Emargination may reduce the dermal covering to a slender temporal arcade (fig. 7.6C), or even completely open the temporal region (fig. 7.6D).

Some controversy surrounds the question whether turtles are, indeed, anapsids (as suggested by the oldest known turtle, *Proganochelys*: Gaffney 1990), or whether they might represent modified diapsids, in which case the complete dermal covering of the cheek region would be secondary where it occurs in the group. Lakjer (1926) used the presence of a quadrato-maxillary ligament in turtles to homologize the ventral embayment of the cheek with a lower temporal fossa. Diapsids, however, are diagnosed by the presence of an upper temporal fossa (see below); and that turtles emarginated the posterior temporal fossa, rather than opened an upper temporal fenestra, is indicated by the relation of the posteriorly expanding external jaw adductor muscle to the (overlying) superficial epaxial neck musculature (Rieppel 1990).

Emargination of the post-temporal fossa permits the expansion of the jaw adductor muscles in a postero-dorsal direction along a posteriorly expanded supraoccipital spine; lateral emargination of the cheek region permits the expansion of a bulging superficial muscle portion onto the lateral surface of the lower jaw (Schumacher 1973). As the external adductor extends from its postero-dorsal origin with a more or less horizontal orientation of the central tendon toward the lower jaw with a more vertical orientation of the insertional tendon, the muscle turns around a pulley system which was used by Gaffney (1975) to diagnose the Cryptodira as opposed to the Pleurodira. In cryptodire turtles, the prootic carries a trochlear process on the antero-dorsal aspect of the paroccipital process, which forms a synovial joint with the transilient cartilage of the adductor tendon system (Schumacher 1973; Gaffney 1979, 15; this joint is not developed in juvenile *Chelydra:* Rieppel 1990). In pleurodires, the transilient cartilage of the insertional tendon is supported by the processus trochlearis pterygoidei, a lateral expansion of the pterygoid bone reaching into the subtemporal fossa (Schumacher 1973; Gaffney 1979, 104–105).

Temporal Fenestration. Temporal fenestrae initially form at three bone junctions (Reisz 1981): the upper temporal opening develops between the parietal, postorbital, and squamosal, the lower temporal opening lies between the squamosal, jugal, and quadratojugal. Carroll (1982, 97) found no reason to relate the formation of temporal fossae to a change in the configuration of jaw adductor muscles or of jaw mechanics; rather, they would have lightened the skull and "concentrated the areas of ossification for maximum resistance to the forces resulting from feeding and manipulating prey." These areas are indicated by thickened internal cranial ridges in the early diapsid genus *Petrolacosaurus* (Reisz 1981, fig. 25). Temporal fenestration might also be related to the provision of a mechanically advantageous angle for muscle fiber insertion into the periosteum of the dermatocranium (Frazzetta 1968; Tarsitano and Oelofson 1985; Tarsitano et al. 1989).

The generalized condition is represented by anapsid reptiles, lacking temporal fenestration. The Synapsida, or mammal-like reptiles and mammals, are characterized by the presence of a single, lower temporal opening (fig. 7.7D). The Diapsida were initially diagnosed by the presence of both upper and lower temporal openings; a basal dichotomy within the Diapsida splits the group into the Archosauromorpha and Lepidosauromorpha (Gauthier 1984; Benton 1985; see fig. 7.1). The archosaurs include the extant crocodiles, while lepidosaurs comprise *Sphenodon* as well as lizards, amphisbaenians, and snakes. In contrast to *Sphenodon* (fig. 7.8C), lizards retain an upper temporal arcade only (fig. 7.8D), which separates the upper temporal opening from the wide open cheek: Williston (1914, 1917) believed the latter to be the result of emargination from below and therefore grouped the lizards and their squamate relatives within his "Parapsida" (amphisbaenians and snakes have further modified the structure of the skull by the loss of the upper temporal arcade). Williston's (1914,

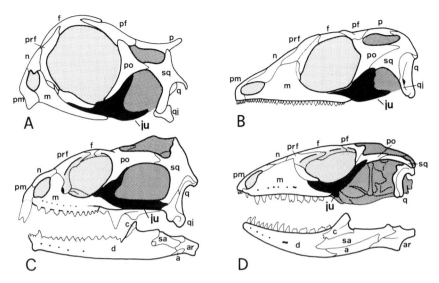

Fig. 7.8. The reduction of the lower temporal arcade in diapsid reptiles.
A. *Sphenodon punctatus,* embryo. B. *Gephyrosaurus bridensis,* Lower Jurassic.
C. *Sphenodon punctatus,* adult. D. *Tupinambis nigropuncatus.* Abbreviations: a,
angular; ar, articular; c, coronoid; d, dentary; f, frontal; ju, jugal; m, maxilla;
n, nasal; p, parietal; pf, postfrontal; pm, premaxilla; po, postorbital; prf, prefrontal;
q, quadrate; qj, quadratojugal; sa, surangular; sq, squamosal. (A, redrawn after
Howes and Swinnterton 1901, p. 3, fig. 10; B, after Evans 1980, fig. 1; C, after
M. Jollie in Robb 1977, fig. 2; D, after Rieppel 1980e, fig. 1)

1917) assumptions about the history of the lizard skull appeared to be
refuted by the discovery of *Prolacerta* from the Lower Triassic of South
Africa (Parrington 1935). This reptile shows a diapsid skull with an incomplete lower temporal arcade—the posterior process of the jugal no longer
meets the quadratojugal below the lower temporal fossa. This was taken
as evidence of a diapsid origin of lizards. The reduction of the lower temporal arcade and its replacement by a quadrato-maxillary ligament permits the expansion of a superficial portion of the external jaw adductor
onto the lateral surface of the surangular (Rieppel and Gronowski 1981).

Since the time of the description of *Prolacerta,* a great variety of early
diapsids from the Upper Permian and Triassic have come to light, some difficult to classify (Evans 1984, 1988; Benton 1985). One salient feature
emerging from the study of these fossils is that many early diapsids are characterized by an incomplete lower temporal arcade. The taxa in question
include the prolacertimorph (Archosauromorpha) genera *Protorosaurus*
(Seeley 1887), *Prolacerta* (Parrington 1935), *Kadimakara* (Bartholomai
1979), *Macrocnemus* (Kuhn-Schnyder 1962), *Malerisaurus* (Chatterjee
1986), *Tanystropheus* (Wild 1973), and *Tanytrachelos* (Olsen 1979); the

pleurosaur genera *Palaeopleurosaurus* and *Pleurosaurus* (Carroll 1985); the sphenodontid genera *Gephyrosaurus* (Evans 1980; see also fig. 7.8B), some (juvenile?) *Clevosaurus* (Robinson 1973; Fraser 1988), some *Planocephalosaurus* (Fraser 1982), and some *Diphydontosaurus* (Whiteside 1986); the "flying reptiles" *Coelurosauravus* (Evans and Haubold 1987), *Kuehneosaurus* (Robinson 1962), and *Icarosaurus* (Colbert 1966, 1970); and the thalattosaur genera (Neodiapsida incertae sedis) *Askeptosaurus* (Kuhn-Schnyder 1952), *Clarazia, Hescheleria* (Rieppel 1987a), and *Thalattosaurus* (Merriam 1905). Carroll (1985, 26) classified the Pleurosauridae with the Sphenodontidae within the Sphenodontia, concluding that the incomplete lower temporal arcade may well represent the plesiomorph condition within the group. This view is corroborated by the application of cladistic techniques (Whiteside 1986; Fraser 1988), which have shown *Gephyrosaurus* (with an incomplete lower temporal bar) to be the sister group of all other Sphenodontida. This arrangement implies that the complete lower temporal arcade and the resulting monimostyly of the quadrate is secondary in those sphenodontids where it occurs. That a secondary lower temporal arch should develop in *Sphenodon* may be explained by reference to specializations of the dentition (Robinson 1976) and jaw mechanics (Gorniak et al. 1982), allowing for a powerful shearing bite in the absence of a streptostylic quadrate (Whiteside 1986; Fraser 1988).

The Diapsida are classically diagnosed by the presence of two temporal fossae, as shown by the earliest representative of the group, *Petrolacosaurus* from the Upper Pennsylvanian of Kansas (fig. 7.7B). As early synapsids share a lower temporal fossa with diapsids, the diagnosis of the latter group was modified to refer to the presence of an upper temporal fossa only (Reisz 1981). A reinvestigation of the Lower Permian reptile *Araeoscelis* (Reisz et al. 1984) showed this genus to combine the presence of a single upper temporal fenestra and a fully closed lower cheek region (fig. 7.7C) with a number of postcranial characteristics relating it to *Petrolacosaurus*. The two genera were therefore grouped as Araeoscelidia, included within the Diapsida as a sister group of the Neodiapsida (sensu Benton 1985). By implication *Araeoscelis* becomes a diapsid, in contrast to the view of Williston (1917), who included the genus within his Parapsida along with a number of marine Mesozoic reptiles (see below). Within the Diapsida, either *Araeoscelis* is of generalized structure, or it has secondarily closed the lower temporal fossa in adaptation to durophagous habits (Carroll 1981, 371; Reisz et al. 1984).

If the Diapsida are diagnosed by the presence of a single upper temporal fossa (Benton 1985, 107), the problem of the Parapsida and Euryapsida is in some sense defined away. The Sauropterygia (pachypleurosaurs, "nothosaurs," plesiosaurs, and pliosaurs) and the Placodontia combine the presence of an upper temporal opening with a ventrally emarginated cheek. Romer (1968b) held the sauropterygians to be derived from a form like *Araeoscelis* by ventral emargination of the cheek. An alternative hypothesis views the sauropterygian skull to be derived from a fully diapsid condition by the reduction of the lower temporal arcade (Jaekel 1910; Kuhn-Schnyder 1967, 1980; Carroll 1981). Placodonts, on the other hand, were believed to never have had a lower temporal arch, and hence were denied any close relationship to sauropterygians (Kuhn-Schnyder, 1967, 1980; Carroll 1981; Sues 1987b; but see Romer 1971). Modern cladistic analysis supports a sister-group relation of sauropterygians and Placodonts (the two forming the monophyletic Euryapsida), but hypotheses of fenestration versus emargination of the lower cheek region in either clade remain inconclusive on grounds of parsimony (Rieppel 1989b; Zanon, n.d.). As documented by the recent description of the ichthyosaur-like reptile *Hupehsuchus* from the Triassic of China (Carroll and Dong Zhi-Ming 1991), temporal fenestration and emargination can occur in conjunction in diapsid skulls. The inclusion of the Euryapsida within the Diapsida (Neodiapsida) is furthermore substantiated by the congruence of other, cranial and postcranial, characteristics (Sues 1987a, b; Rieppel, 1989b).

The ichthyosaurs likewise combine the presence of a single upper temporal opening with a ventral emargination of the cheek. Their temporal opening was believed to be of a different type than that of the "euryapsids," bordered laterally by the supratemporal rather than by the squamosal: they were therefore referred to a separate group, the Parapsida, by Colbert (1955). Romer (1968a) demonstrated that the upper temporal opening of ichthyosaurs lies in its usual position, bounded laterally by squamosal and postorbital. Again it must be concluded that ichthyosaurs are diapsids (Mazin 1982; Massare and Callaway 1990), irrespective of any hypothesis about process (Tarsitano 1982, 1983; see also McGregor 1902) accounting for the ventral opening of the cheek, and irrespective of the problem of their relationships to the sauropterygians.

The Formation of a Secondary Palate

In the primitive tetrapod skull, the internal nares lie anteriorly in the palate, below the neurocranial nasal capsules; in *Eocaptorhinus* (Heaton 1979) and other captorhinomorphs (Clark and Carroll 1973) it is bordered by the maxilla laterally, by the vomer medially, and by the palatine posteriorly (fig. 7.11A). A variety of reptile groups have developed a secondary palate, among which are turtles, crocodiles, advanced mammal-like reptiles, and some lizards.

The vaulted palate of turtles is characterized by deep choanal grooves, running from the anteriorly placed internal nares toward the glottis lying behind the tongue. Bramble and Wake (1985, 235) believe that these struc-

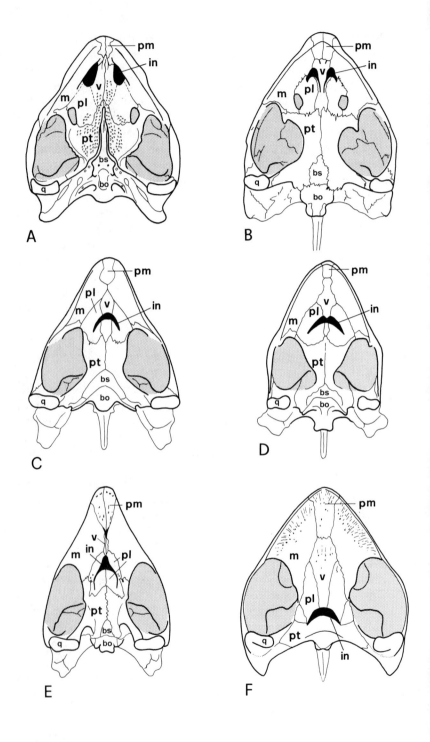

tural relations facilitate ventilation by the formation of air passages which are separated from the oral cavity accommodating the fleshy tongue. The system becomes optimized by a bony ventral closure of the choanal grooves. In turtles, a secondary palate (fig. 7.9) is developed in various subgroups, to a variable degree, and in a variable pattern (Romer 1956; Gaffney 1979); the systematic implications, if any, remain to be investigated.

Since the work of Huxley (1875), the position of the internal nares has played a major role in the classification of crocodiles. In the Triassic genus *Protosuchus*, type of the family Protosuchidae, suborder Protosuchia, the secondary palate is still very rudimentary (fig. 7.10A): the internal naris lies adjacent to the anterior maxillary teeth, bordered medially by vomer and palatine (Crompton and Smith 1980, 196). The Mesosuchia, a paraphyletic assemblage including marine crocodiles from the Jurassic and Cretaceous, are characterized by a more posterior position of the internal nares (fig. 7.10B): they come to lie between the posterior portions of the palatine bones, or on the posterior margins of the latter. In the Eusuchia, first appearing in the Cretaceous, the secondary palate has been further expanded, the internal nares now being fully enclosed by the pterygoid bones (fig. 7.10C). In 1868, Eudes-Deslongchamps discovered that the internal nares of an embryonic alligator lie at a position comparable to that of the Mesosuchia, and are shifted posteriorly during subsequent developmental stages (Buffetaut 1977): a classic case of "Haeckelian recapitulation" by terminal addition (confirmed by personal observation). A functional interpretation of the secondary palate is possible at least for modern crocodiles, where the internal nares lie behind a skin fold supported by the pterygoids and separating the mouth cavity from the pharynx. This permits breathing with submerged jaws, the typical lurking position of crocodiles.

Within lizards, Lakjer (1927) distinguished the palaeochoanate from the neochoanate condition, with the incomplete neochoanate palate as an intermediate stage of differentiation. In palaeochoanate lizards, the internal naris opens behind Jacobson's organ into a cleft extending between the maxilla laterally and the vomer and palatine medially: in *Sphenodon*

Fig. 7.9. (*opposite*) The formation of a secondary palate in the Chelonia. A. *Proganochelys*. B. *Chelydra serpentina*. C. *Caretta caretta*. D. *Chelonia mydas*. E. *Solnhofia parsoni*. F. *Erquelinnesia gosseletti*. Abbreviations: bo, basiocipital; bs, basisphenoid; in, internal naris (choana); m, maxilla; pl, palatine; pm, premaxilla; pt, pterygoid; q, quadrate; v, vomer. (A, redrawn after Gaffney and Meeker 1983, fig. 1; B, after Gaffney 1979, fig. 9; C, after A. Carr in Gaffney 1979, fig. 215; D, after A. Carr in Gaffney 1979, fig. 215; E, after Gaffney 1979, fig. 272; F, after R. Zangerl in Gaffney 1979, fig. 195)

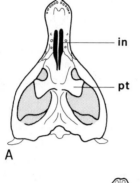

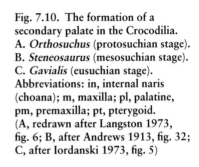

Fig. 7.10. The formation of a
secondary palate in the Crocodilia.
A. *Orthosuchus* (protosuchian stage).
B. *Steneosaurus* (mesosuchian stage).
C. *Gavialis* (eusuchian stage).
Abbreviations: in, internal naris
(choana); m, maxilla; pl, palatine,
pm, premaxilla; pt, pterygoid.
(A, redrawn after Langston 1973,
fig. 6; B, after Andrews 1913, fig. 32;
C, after Iordanski 1973, fig. 5)

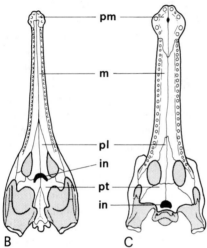

(fig. 7.11B) and such lizards as the Iguania, Gekkota (fig. 7.11C), and
some Anguimorpha, these two openings are not separated by bone. In the
neochoanate condition, the vomer establishes a sutural contact with the
maxilla behind the opening of Jacobson's organ, separating the latter from
the posterior internal naris. This condition is typical for some Scincomor-

Fig. 7.11. (*opposite*) The dermal palate in primitive reptiles and its modification
within the Squamata. A. *Eocaptorhinus laticeps*. B. *Spenodon punctatus*.
C. *Hemitheconyx caudicinctus*. D. *Dibamus novaeguineae*. E. *Varanus salvator*.
F. *Python sebae*. Abbreviations: ec, ectopterygoid; in, internal naris (choana);
ja, Jacobson's organ; ju, jugal; m, maxilla; pl, palatine; pm, premaxilla; pt, pterygoid;
q, quadrate; qj, quadratojugal; sm, septomaxilla; sof, suborbital fenestra; v, vomer.
(A, redrawn after Heaton 1979, fig. 2; B, after Starck 1979, fig. 200; C, after Rieppel
1984c, fig. 1; D, after Rieppel 1984a, fig. 1; E, after Rieppel 1980b, fig. 25; F, after
Frazzetta 1959, fig. 1)

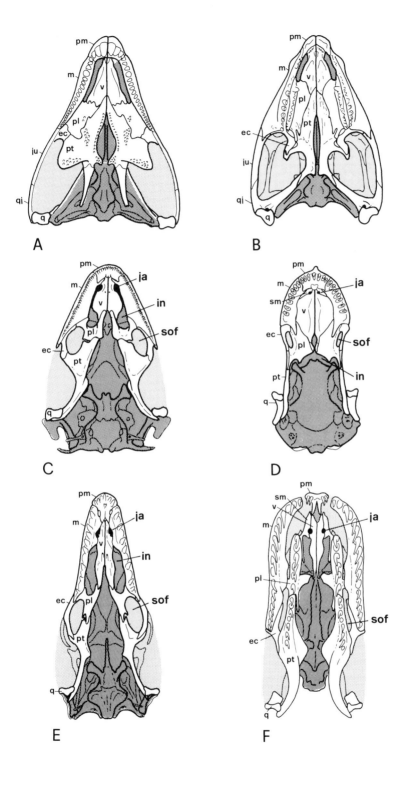

pha (fig. 7.11D), as well as for varanids (fig. 7.11E); in the incomplete neochoanate palate, the vomer merely overlaps the palatal shelf of the maxilla instead of establishing a true sutural contact.

Presch (1976) described the formation of a secondary palate in gymnophthalmid (microteiid) lizards: by this term he characterized the neochoanate palate of gymnophthalmids which, in addition, obliterated the interpterygoid vacuity by a contact of the pterygoid bones along the ventral midline of the skull.

Another group described as having a secondary palate are the Scincidae (Greer 1970). In the majority of the Scincidae, as well as in the genera *Anelytropsis* and *Dibamus* (Greer 1985), the palatine bones arch over the choanal tubes and enclose them with horizontal (palatal) shelves which extend medially below the choanal tubes: the internal nares thus open at the posterior end of scroll-like palatine bones (fig. 7.11D). Detailed functional interpretations for the formation of a secondary palate in burrowing scincomorph lizards are still lacking.

A tendency to form a secondary palate is also observed within the Amphisbaenia, the genus *Trogonophis* preserving the plesiomorph condition, comparable to the palate of the Gymnophthalmidae (Zangerl 1944; Gans 1978, 370–371). The most complete secondary palate, involving extensive palatal shelves of the maxillae and premaxillae, is observed in the genus *Monopeltis* (Kritzinger 1946).

KINETICS OF THE REPTILE SKULL

The lizard skull is known for its complex kinetic mechanism, involving a number of joints in addition to the palatobasal articulation. The quadrate is subject to streptostylic movement, i.e., rotation around its dorsal suspension. The braincase is movably suspended within the dermatocranium, a type of movement known as metakinesis (Versluys 1912). Mesokinesis permits the movement of the snout-complex relative to the parietal unit, and involves a number of joints in the dermatocranium, most notably a line of flexion passing through the frontoparietal suture and transversely through the palate (Versluys 1912).

Frazzetta (1962) has proposed a quadric crank-chain model for the functional analysis of cranial kinesis in lizards (fig. 7.12). The links in the chain are represented respectively by the snout complex (incorporating the upper jaw), the parietal unit (skull table and upper temporal arch), the quadrate bone, and the basal unit (pterygoid bone). Following Frazzetta's (1962, 1986) analysis, the snout complex would be raised and the upper jaw elevated relative to the resting position as the jaws are opened, whereas the snout complex and with it the upper jaw would be depressed during

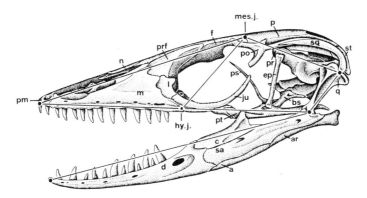

Fig. 7.12. Cranial kinesis in the lizard skull: the quadric crank chain exemplified in *Varanus salvator*. Abbreviations: a, angular; ar, articular; bs, basisphenoid; c, coronoid; d, dentary; ep, epipterygoid; f, frontal; hy.j, hypokinetic joint; ju, jugal; l, lacrimal; m, maxilla; mes.j, mesokinetic joint; n, nasal; p, parietal; pm, premaxilla; po, postorbital; pr, prootic; prf, prefrontal; ps, parasphenoid; pt, pterygoid; q, quadrate; sa, surangular; sq, squamosal; st, supratemporal. (Reproduced from Rieppel 1978d, with permission from Birkhäuser Verlag AG)

jaw closure. Various functional interpretations have been offered for this mechanism, among which Iordansky's proposal (1966) has gained considerable support: mesokinesis aligns the upper and lower jaws during jaw closure, thus exerting a balanced force on prey (see also Frazzetta 1986, 429).

Frazzetta's (1962) model has been questioned on the basis of experimental techniques: points at issue are the existence and degree of mesokinetic flexion, the pattern of intracranial movements during feeding, and the function of the jaw adductor musculature (e.g., Smith 1982; Throckmorton 1976, 1978; Throckmorton and Clarke 1981; de Vree and Gans 1987, 1989; Condon 1987, 1989). It appears that degree and patterns of movement vary within different taxonomic groups, perhaps with the age of the animals, and with varying food types. Rieppel (1979d) recorded distinct snout depression during jaw closure in juvenile specimens of *Varanus salvator*, and formulated a functional model (Rieppel 1978d) according to which the jaw adductors in a mesokinetic skull would form a self-reinforcing system: the stronger they contract, the more will the lower jaw be retracted and the more will the addutive force of the muscles increase. This amounts to a perfection of the static-pressure system characteristic of early reptiles (Olson 1961; Carroll 1969c). The model was criticized by Smith (1982) and Frazzetta (1986) for not explaining the protraction of the quadrate and correlated elevation of the upper jaw during mouth opening. However, protraction is easily understood as a consequence of the fact that a somewhat depressed upper jaw (flexion of the snout unit relative to the basal unit) is characteristic of the rest position in (juvenile) *Varanus* (Rieppel 1979d).

A case has been made to relate the splanchnocranium (of neural crest origin) to movements between skull bones (Rieppel 1978c). The mandibular joint in reptiles is formed by the quadrate and the articular, the bones representing ossifications in the mandibular arch. The basal process of the palatoquadrate becomes associated with the pterygoid bone, a prerequisite for the formation of a synovial palatobasal articulation. Where the palatobasal articulation has been lost (turtles, sauropterygians, crocodiles), this is due to secondary fusion of the expanded dermal palate to the basicranium. Turtles are particularly revealing in this respect, since the Triassic genus *Proganochelys* still preserves a palatobasal articulation (Gaffney 1983, 1990).

Other cranial movements may also involve synovial joints formed by cartilage derived from the splanchnocranium. Metakinesis depends on a movable support of the braincase via the paroccipital process on the medial aspect of the quadrate and of the dermal supratemporal bone. Here a synovial joint is developed by means of an intercalary cartilage of hyoid arch origin. Of particular interest is a juvenile specimen of *Varanus salvator* with the posterior tip of the dermal supratemporal capped by cartilage both at its articulation with the paroccipital process medially, and with the cephalic condyle of the quadrate ventrally (Rieppel 1978c).

Serial sections show that this cartilage becomes incorporated into the ossification of the supratemporal, which may explain why it is not observed in a serially sectioned head of an adult *Lacerta*. Serially sectioned embryos of *Podarcis sicula* show this cartilage to be most likely of splanchnic origin, derived from the quadrate process of the palatoquadrate: primary cartilage secondarily associated with a dermal element cannot be considered as adventitious cartilage, the occurrence of which is restricted to birds and mammals (Hall 1984; Hall and Hanken 1985b; Irwin and Ferguson 1986).

A splanchnic origin may also be hypothesized for the cartilage described by Oelrich (1956, 38) and covering the posterior medial surface of the quadrate ramus of the dermal pterygoid bone at its contact with the medial surface of the shaft of the quadrate in *Ctenosaura* (not confirmed for *Varanus:* Rieppel 1988). This joint is involved in streptostylic movements of the quadrate within the quadric crank chain. All other joints involved in mesokinesis are syndesmotic.

Snakes are characterized by an extraordinary mobility of their jaw bones (Gans 1961), which is not achieved by a further elaboration of synovial joints but rather by their obliteration. With the exception of the mandibular joint and the links in the sound-transmitting apparatus (Rieppel

1980d), there is no synovial joint in the snake head (Hall in Murray 1963; Hall 1984). Of particular interest is the palatobasal articulation (Rieppel 1980a): the pterygoid is only loosely connected to the basicranium by ligaments permitting rather unconstrained gliding along the antero-lateral wings of the basisphenoid-parasphenoid complex. "Basipterygoid processes" may develop, guiding the movements of the pterygoid bone, particularly in some booid snakes (Underwood 1976; Rieppel 1979b), but the homology of these processes with the basipterygoid processes of lizards requires closer study. The lizard basipterygoid process develops from the basitrabecular process, which becomes underlain by the parasphenoid. Presumed basitrabecular processes have been described in only a few booid snakes (Kamal and Hammouda 1965a; Genest-Villard 1966), and their role in the formation of basipterygoid processes remains unclear (Bellairs and Kamal 1981, 172).

HETEROCHRONY: THE TRANSITION FROM LIZARDS TO SNAKES

Heterochrony appears to have been an important agent in the modification of the reptilian skull, particularly in the reduction of the dermatocranium.

In an embryonic *Sphenodon* (stage R of Howes and Swinnerton 1901), the jugal has not yet established contact with the quadratojugal, suggesting that it ossifies from front to back. The embryonic *Sphenodon* closely resembles *Prolacerta* and other early diapsids with an incomplete lower temporal arch (fig. 7.8). If the lower temporal arcade in *Sphenodon* is considered plesiomorph, its loss in prolacertiforms, fossil Sphenodontida, thalattosaurs, and lepidosaurs may be explained by paedomorphosis. Alternatively, if the complete lower temporal arcade is considered a derived feature of *Sphenodon,* its completion may be interpreted as the result of terminal addition (hypermorphosis) to the ossification of the posterior ramus of the jugal (Whiteside 1986, 416).

The loss of the upper temporal arcade has also been explained by paedomorphosis (Rieppel 1984d). Among lizards, the upper temporal arch is incomplete in the Gekkonidae, Pygopodidae, most acontine skinks, *Anelytropsis, Dibamus,* the anguid genus *Anniella,* and the varonoid lizards *Heloderma* and *Lanthanotus.* In the acontine skinks, *Anelytropsis, Dibamus,* small and fossorial pygopodids, and *Anniella,* the loss of the upper temporal arcade is correlated with miniaturization of the skull (Rieppel 1984b). As the diameter of the skull is reduced in adaptation to fossorial habits, the neurocranium increases in size relative to the dermatocranium, owing to a relative size increase of the brain and of the labyrinth organs.

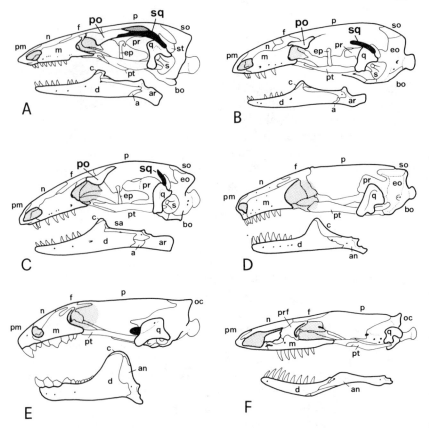

Fig. 7.13. The miniaturization of the lizard skull and the correlated reduction of the upper temporal arcade. Note the transition to the ophidian bauplan. A. *Typhlosaurus lineatus,* an acontine skink. B. *Typhlosaurus vermis.* C. *Typhlosaurus aurantiacus.* D. *Dibamus novaeguineae.* E. *Trogonophis wiegmanni,* an amphisbaenian genus. F. *Pseudotyphlops philippinus,* a uropeltid snake. Abbreviations: a, angular; an, angular complex; ar, articular; bo, basioccipital; c, coronoid; d, dentary; eo, exoccipital; ep, epipterygoid; f, frontal; m, maxilla; n, nasal; oc, occipital complex; p, parietal; pm, premaxilla; po, postorbital (postorbitofrontal); pr, prootic; prf, prefrontal; pt, pterygoid; q, quadrate; s, stapes; sa, surangular; so, supraoccipital; sq, squamosal; st, supratemporal. (A, redrawn after Rieppel 1981b, fig. 7; B, after Rieppel 1981b, fig. 9; C, after Rieppel 1981b, fig. 9; D, after Rieppel 1984a, fig. 1; E, after Rieppel 1981b, fig. 19; F, after Rieppel 1983, fig. 4)

No longer suspended within the dermatocranium, the neurocranium combines with the latter to form a closed cranial box (fig. 7.13): the posttemporal fossae are closed, and the lateral wall of the braincase is completed by hypermorphosis of the parietal bone (Rieppel 1984d) and by an extension of the anterior alar process of the prootic (Rieppel 1981b). The skull thus forms a supporting strut, from which the lower jaw is movably suspended by means of the streptostylic quadrate; the snout complex, incorporating the upper jaws, is suspended at the mesokinetic hinge, which shows a tendency toward immobilization, complete in *Dibamus* (Rieppel 1984a). These changes in skull structure are accompanied by a reduction of the upper temporal arcade. The acontine genus *Typhlosaurus* permits the construction of a morphocline (fig. 7.13A-C), illustrating a pattern of reduction which is suggestive of paedomorphosis (Rieppel 1984d). The squamosal and postorbitofrontal are reduced in a sequence reversing the pattern of ossification (see references in Rieppel 1984d; and personal observation; work on the development of the jaw adductor musculature and associated skull bones in the lizard *Podarcis sicula* indicates, however, that this interpretation may be too simplistic: Rieppel 1987b). The loss of the upper temporal arcade in miniaturized lizards permits an expansion of the area of origin of the jaw adductor musculature across the temporal region of the skull to the fasciae covering the epaxial neck muscles.

No such expansion of the jaw adductor is observed in other, nonfossorial lizards that have lost the upper temporal arcade. No functional explanation is available for the loss of the upper temporal arch in geckos. The Gekkonidae are paedomorphic with respect to many skeletal (Stephenson 1960; Bellairs and Kamal 1981, 82–83; Rieppel 1984c) and muscular (Rieppel 1984c, 1987b) characteristics. In this group, the loss of the upper temporal arcade may be just another aspect of paedomorphosis with no particular functional significance. It should be noted, however, that the hypothesis of paedomorphosis in the Gekkonidae still requires the test by comparison with developmental patterns in the sister group of the Gekkonidae, the Pygopodidae. (For an alternative view of gekkotan interrelationships see Kluge 1987.)

Paedomorphosis may also be responsible for the loosening of the contacts between palatal bones in the Gekkota (Rieppel 1984c). Combined with the loss of the upper temporal arch and with a flexible frontoparietal hinge, this permits a high degree of cranial kinesis. Patchell and Shine (1986) report adaptation to feeding on large prey in the pygopodid genus *Lialis*.

Another group adapted to feed on large prey are the snakes (Gans 1961). Iordansky (1978) was so impressed by similarities in the kinetics of the skull of gekkotan lizards and snakes, in particular with respect to the palate, that he suggested a common ancestry for the two groups (an unparsimonious hypothesis). Indeed, heterochrony also appears to have played a major role in the formation of the snake skull (Irish 1989). Immediate evidence for paedomorphosis in snakes comes from the anterior basicranium. A tropibasic skull, characterized by a fused trabecula communis, is plesiomorph at the level of the Reptilia, as is indicated by the narrow cultriform process on the parasphenoid in captorhinomorph reptiles (Prince 1935; Heaton 1979) and *Procolophon* (Carroll and Lindsay 1985). Snakes are the only extant reptiles with a platybasic skull characterized by the retention of paired trabeculae cranii (Bellairs 1949a): since all other lepidosaurs have a tropibasic skull, including *Sphenodon*, the snake condition must be interpreted as the result of paedomorphosis (Rieppel 1979e).

On the whole the *bauplan* of a snake skull (fig. 7.13F) is remarkably similar to that of miniaturized fossorial lizards such as acontine skinks (Brock 1941) or *Dibamus* (Gasc 1968). The neurocranium and the dermatocranium have combined to form a solid braincase involving hypermorphosis of the parietal. From it both the upper and lower jaws are movably suspended, the lower jaws by means of the streptostylic quadrate, the upper jaws (snout complex) at the prokinetic joint (Frazzetta 1959, 1966), located in front of the orbit, between nasal and frontal bones. In advanced snakes, the mobility of the jaw apparatus is further increased by a reduction of the contact between palatal elements, and between elements participating in the nasofrontal joint (Rieppel 1978b). The reduced contacts between dermal elements result from heterochronic changes affecting late stages of ossification (Irish 1989).

In snakes, the palate has become greatly modified into a system of loosely interconnected and therefore highly kinetic jaw arches (fig. 7.11F), performing movements during swallowing which Boltt and Ewer (1964) have characterized as "pterygoid walk." Cundall (1983, 1987) distinguishes a lateral prey-capturing device, the maxilla, from the medial swallowing unit, composed of the palatopterygoid arch. Within snakes, the successive perfection of the jaw apparatus, reflected in an increased prey ingestion ratio (Greene 1983), provides examples for terminal additions to ancestral ontogenies as a mode of structural change. In the anilioid snakes, the supratemporal is short and immovably intercalated in the temporal region of the braincase (fig. 7.14A). The quadrate is relatively short and vertically oriented. The mandibular joint lies in front of the occipital condyle. In the Macrostomata (fig. 7.3), including booids, acrochordids, and colubroids, the supratemporal is elongated and forms a free-ending posterior process (Underwood 1976). The quadrate, suspended from the posterior portion of the supratemporal, is elongated and rotated posteriorly. The mandibular joint is shifted to a position behind the occipital condyle (fig. 7.14B). As a consequence, the lower jaw ramus is elongated, and gape thereby increased. During ontogeny, the quadrate shows a rotation from an antero-ventrally inclined position in the early embryo through a vertical position, similar to the adult condition observed in aniloid snakes, to its final postero-ventrally inclined orientation (Kamal 1966). The supratem-

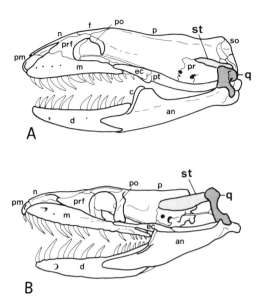

Fig. 7.14. The jaw suspension in anilioid (top) and macrostomatan (bottom) snakes.
A. *Cylindrophis rufus*. B. *Python sebae*. Abbreviations: an, angular complex;
c, coronoid; d, dentary; ec, ectopterygoid; f, frontal; m, maxilla; n, nasal; p, parietal;
pm, premaxilla; po, postorbital; pr, prootic; prf, prefrontal; pt, pterygoid;
q, quadrate; so, supraoccipital; st, supratemporal. (A, redrawn after B. Groombridge
in Parker and Grandison 1977, fig. 23; B, after B. Groombridge in Parker and
Grandison 1977, fig. 24)

poral is short in early macrostomatan embryos (e.g., Peyer 1912), and
grows posteriorly during later stages.

EXPERIMENTAL APPROACHES TO THE DEVELOPING SKULL

Whereas the morphology of the developing neurocranium is by now at
least partly known for a number of lizard and snake families (Bellairs and
Kamal 1981), the developmental pattern of the dermatocranium is very
poorly known. This is a serious gap of knowledge, since only a more complete sampling of developmental data will allow proper assessment of the
role of heterochrony in the differentiation and modification of the reptile
skull. A point should be made that different histological techniques, such
as clearing and staining versus serial sectioning, do not appear to provide
congruent results in all cases (Rieppel 1987b), perhaps because of different
staining methods and different scales of resolution. It might be worthwhile
to conduct a study addressing this issue in detail, before comparing the
results of a variety of authors over a broad taxonomic range.

Even more deficient is current knowledge of developmental interactions in the reptile skull. Bellairs and Kamal (1981, 8) quote pioneer work on the investigation of causal relationships between the formation of the otocyst and the otic placode, or between the nasal placode and nasal capsule; the influence of the developing eyes on the skull is another aspect of this wide field of future research. De Beer (1937, 377) suggested that the platybasic versus tropibasic condition of the anterior braincase may be developmentally correlated with the relative size of the eyeballs and of the brain at the level of the eyes, but Bellairs and Kamal (1981, 43) note the apparent absence of an influence of the developing eyes on the fusion of the interorbital cartilages in teratological lizard embryos with severe degrees of microphthalmia.

Experimental investigation should also focus on the development of the dermatocranium. Temporal fenestration and emargination is used with variable success in reptile classification, but there still is no true understanding of the causal mechanisms underlying the various patterns. The upper and lower temporal arches are reduced in different groups and following different patterns, but developmental and functional explanations offered for these observations continue to be simplistic. The same is true for the variable degrees of emargination observed in turtles. An experimental approach might be used to investigate the relation of ossification processes to developing muscles.

In mammals for example, the development of the coronoid process is dependent on its functional interaction with the developing jaw adductor musculature (Dullemeijer 1971; Hall 1978). In *Lacerta*, the development of the coronoid bone appears to be related to the differentiation of the bodenaponeurotic tendon in the developing jaw adductor musculature (Rieppel 1987b), but no experimental data are as yet available. The presence or absence of a coronoid bone has been used in snake classification ever since the contributions of Nopcsa (1923) and Underwood (1967), although there exist no data of its developmental interrelationships in that group.

Hall (1984, 162) suggests a search for secondary or adventitious cartilage in the dermatocranium of reptiles, either during normal development or experimentally induced, i.e., during fracture repair (see Irwin and Ferguson 1986, for an example). The reason is that amphibians do not form such cartilage (Hall and Hanken, 1985a), which is, however, present in endotherm mammals and birds (Hall 1984, 159; Hall and Hanken 1985a). Closer scrutiny in the study of reptiles might provide clues as to the developmental and evolutionary mechanisms which allowed secondary cartilage to be formed by pluripotential periost cells in birds and mammals.

REFERENCES

Andrews, C. W. 1913. *A Descriptive Catalogue of the Marine Reptiles of the Oxford Clay.* Vol 2. London: British Museum (National History).

Bäckström, K. 1931. Rekonstruktionsbilder zur Ontogenie des Kopfskelettes von *Tropidonotus natrix.* Acta zoologica, Stockholm 12: 83–143.

Baird, I. L. 1970. The anatomy of the reptilian ear. In *Biology of the Reptilia,* vol. 2, C. Gans and T. S. Parsons, eds. London: Academic Press, pp. 193–275.

Bartholomai, A. 1979. New lizard-like reptiles from the Early Triassic of Queensland. Alcheringa 3 (3): 225–234.

Bellairs, A. d'A. 1949a. The anterior braincase and interorbital septum of Sauropsida, with a consideration of the origin of snakes. Journal of the Linnean Society, Zoology 41 (281): 482–512.

———. 1949b. Orbital cartilages in snakes. Nature 163 (4133): 106.

———. 1958. The early development of the interorbital septum and the fate of the anterior orbital cartilages in birds. Journal of Embryology and Experimental Morphology 6 (1): 68–85.

Bellairs, A. d'A., and C. Gans. 1983. A reinterpretation of the amphisbaenian orbitosphenoid. Nature 302 (5905): 243–244.

Bellairs, A. d'A, and A. M. Kamal. 1981. The chondrocranium and the development of the skull in recent reptiles. In *Biology of the Reptilia,* vol. 11, C. Gans and T. S. Parsons, eds. London: Academic Press, pp. 1–263.

Benton, M. J. 1985. Classification and phylogeny of the diapsid reptiles. Zoological Journal of the Linnean Society 84 (2): 97–164.

Berman, D. S., and J. J. Regal. 1967. The loss of the ophidian middle ear. Evolution 21 (3): 641–643.

Boltt, R. E., and R. F. Ewer. 1964. The functional anatomy of the head of the puff adder, *Bitis arietans* (Merr.). Journal of Morphology 114 (1): 83–106.

Bramble, D. M., and D. B. Wake. 1985. Feeding mechanisms of lower tetrapods. In *Functional Vertebrate Morphology,* M. Hildebrand, D. M. Bramble, K. F. Liem, and D. B. Wake, eds. Cambridge: The Belknap Press of Harvard University Press, pp. 230–261.

Brock, G. T. 1929. On the development of the skull of *Leptodeira hotamboia.* Quarterly Journal of Microscopical Science 73 (290): 289–334.

———. 1941. The skull of *Acontias meleagris,* with a study of the affinities between lizards and snakes. Journal of the Linnean Society, Zoology 41 (277): 71–88.

Buffetaut, E. 1977. Eugène Eudes-Deslongchamps et le parallélisme entre formes et stades embryonnaires chez les Crocodiliens (1868). Histoire et nature 11: 81–94.

Carroll, R. L. 1964. The earliest reptiles. Journal of the Linnean Society, Zoology 45 (304): 61–83.

———. 1969a. A Middle Pennsylvanian captorhinomorph, and the interrelationships of primitive reptiles. Journal of Paleontology 43 (1): 151–170.

———. 1969b. Origin of reptiles. In *Biology of the Reptilia,* vol. 1, C. Gans and T. S. Parsons, eds. London: Academic Press, pp. 1–44.

————. 1969c. Problems of the origin of reptiles. Biological Reviews 44 (3): 393–432.

————. 1980. The hyomandibula as a supporting element in the skull of primitive Tetrapoda. In *The Terrestrial Environment and the Origin of Land Vertebrates*, A. L. Panchen, ed. London: Academic Press, pp. 293–317.

————. 1981. Plesiosaur ancestors from the Upper Permian of Madagascar. Philosophical Transactions of the Royal Society of London B 293 (1066): 315–383.

————. 1982. Early evolution of reptiles. Annual Review of Ecology and Systematics 13: 87–109.

————. 1985. A pleurosaur from the Lower Jurassic and the taxonomic position of the Sphenodontida. Palaeontographica A 189 (1–3): 1–28.

Carroll, R. L., and Dong Zhi-Ming. 1991. Hupehsuchus: An enigmatic aquatic reptile from the Triassic of China, and the problem of establishing relationships. Philosophical Transactions of the Royal Society of London B 331 (1260): 131–153.

Carroll, R. L., and P. Gaskill. 1985. The nothosaur *Pachypleurosaurus* and the origin of plesiosaurs. Philosophical Transactions of the Royal Society of London B 309 (1139): 343–393.

Carroll, R. L., and W. Lindsay. 1985. Cranial anatomy of the primitive reptile *Procolophon*. Canadian Journal of Earth Sciences 22 (11): 1571–1587.

Chatterjee, S. 1986. *Malerisaurus langstoni*, a new diapsid reptile from the Triassic of Texas. Journal of Vertebrate Paleontology 6 (4): 297–312.

Clark, J., and R. L. Carroll. 1973. Romeriid reptiles from the Lower Permian. Bulletin of the Museum of Comparative Zoology 144 (5): 353–407.

Colbert, E. H. 1955. *Evolution of the Vertebrates*. 1st ed. New York: John Wiley and Sons.

————. 1966. A gliding reptile from the Triassic of New Jersey. American Museum Novitates 2246: 1–23.

————. 1970. The Triassic gliding reptile *Icarosaurus*. Bulletin of the American Museum of Natural History 143 (2): 85–142.

Condon, K. 1987. A kinematic analysis of mesokinesis in the Nile monitor (*Varanus niloticus*). Experimental Biology, Berlin 42 (2): 73–87.

————. 1989. Kranial kinesis in the Nile monitor. In *Trends in Vertebrate Morphology*, H. Splechtna and H. Hilgers, eds. Progress in Zoology 35. Jena: Gustav Fischer, pp. 435–437.

Crompton, A. W., and K. K. Smith. 1980. A new genus and species of crocodilian from the Kayenta Formation (Late Triassic?) of Northern Arizona. In *Aspects of Vertebrate History*, L. L. Jacobs, ed. Flagstaff: Museum of Northern Arizona Press, pp. 193–217.

Cundall, D. 1983. Activity of head muscles during feeding by snakes: A comparative study. American Zoologist 23 (2): 383–396.

————. 1987. Functional morphology. In *Snakes: Ecology and Evolutionary Biology*, R. A. Seigel, J. T. Collins, and S. S. Novak, eds. New York: MacMillan, pp. 106–140.

De Beer, G. R. 1926. Studies on the vertebrate head. II. The orbitotemporal region of the skull. Quarterly Journal of Microscopical Science 70 (278): 263–370.

———. 1937. *The Development of the Vertebrate Skull*. Oxford: Clarendon Press.

de Vree, F., and C. Gans. 1987. Kinetic movements in the skull of adult *Trachydosaurus rugosus*. Zentralblatt für Veterinärmedizin, Reihe, C, 16 (3): 206–209.

———. 1989. Functional morphology of the feeding mechanisms in lower tetrapods. In *Trends in Vertebrate Morphology*, H. Splechtna and H. Hilgers, eds., Progress in Zoology 35. Jena: Gustav Fischer, pp. 115–127.

Dullemeijer, P. 1971. Comparative ontogeny and cranio-facial growth. In *Cranio-Facial Growth in Man*, R. E. Moyers and W. Krogman, eds. Oxford: Pergamon Press, pp. 45–75.

Estes, R. 1983. Sauria terrestria, Amphisbaenia. In *Encyclopedia of Paleoherpetology*, vol. 10A, P. Wellnhofer, ed. Stuttgart: Gustav Fischer.

Estes, R., T. H. Frazzetta, and E. E. Williams. 1970. Studies on the fossil snake *Dinilysia patagonica* Woodward. Part I. Cranial morphology. Bulletin of the Museum of Comparative Zoology 140 (2): 25–74.

Estes, R., K. de Queiroz, and J. A. Gauthier. 1988. Phylogenetic relationships within Squamata. In *Phylogenetic Relationships of the Lizard Families*, R. Estes and G. Pregill, eds. Stanford, Calif.: Stanford University Press, pp. 119–281.

Evans, S. E. 1980. The skull of a new eosuchian reptile from the Lower Jurassic of South Wales. Zoological Journal of the Linnean Society 70 (3): 203–264.

———. 1984. The classification of the Lepidosauria. Zoological Journal of the Linnean Society 82 (1 and 2): 87–100.

———. 1986. The braincase of *Prolacerta broomi* (Reptilia, Triassic). Neues Jahrbuch für Geologie und Paläontologie 173 (2): 181–200.

———. 1988. The early history and relationships of the Diapsida. In *The Phylogeny and Classification of the Tetrapods*, vol. 1, M. J. Benton, ed. Oxford: Clarendon Press, pp. 221–260.

Evans, S. E., and H. Haubold. 1987. A review of the Upper Permian genera *Coelurosauravus, Weigeltisaurus,* and *Gracilisaurus* (Reptilia: Diapsida). Zoological Journal of the Linnean Society 90 (3): 275–303.

Fraser, N. C. 1982. A new rhynchocephalian from the British Upper Trias. Palaeontology 25 (4): 709–725.

———. 1988. The osteology and relationships of *Clevosaurus* (Reptilia: Sphenodontida). Philosophical Transactions of the Royal Society of London B 321 (1204): 125–178.

Frazzetta, T. H. 1959. Studies on the morphology and function of the skull in the Boidae (Serpentes). Part 1. Cranial differences between *Python sebae* and *Epicrates cenchris*. Bulletin of the Museum of Comparative Zoology 119 (8): 453–472.

———. 1962. A functional consideration of cranial kinesis in lizards. Journal of Morphology 111 (3): 287–319.

———. 1966. Studies on the morphology and function of the skull in the Boidae (Serpentes). Part 2. Morphology and function of the jaw apparatus in *Python sebae* and *Python molurus*. Journal of Morphology 118 (2): 217–296.

———. 1968. Adaptive problems and possibilities in the temporal fenestration of tetrapod skulls. Journal of Morphology 125 (2): 145–158.

————. 1986. The origin of amphikinesis in lizards. In *Evolutionary Biology*, vol. 20, M. K. Hecht, B. Wallace, and G. T. Prance, eds. New York: Plenum Publishing Corp., pp. 419–461.

Frost, D. R., and R. Etheridge. 1989. A phylogenetic analysis and taxonomy of iguanian lizards (Reptilia, Squamata). University of Kansas Museum of Natural History Miscellaneous Publication 81: 1–65.

Gaffney, E. S. 1972. An illustrated glossary of turtle skull nomenclature. American Museum Novitates 2468: 1–33.

————. 1975. A phylogeny and classification of the higher categories of turtles. Bulletin of the American Museum of Natural History 155 (5): 387–436.

————. 1976. Cranial morphology of the European Jurassic turtles *Portlandemys* and *Plesiochelys*. Bulletin of the American Museum of Natural History 157 (6): 487–544.

————. 1979. Comparative cranial morphology of recent and fossil turtles. Bulletin of the American Museum of Natural History 164 (2): 65–376.

————. 1980. Phylogenetic relationships of the major groups of amniotes. In *The Terrestrial Environment and the Origin of Land Vertebrates*, A. L. Panchen, ed. London: Academic Press, pp. 593–610.

————. 1983. The basicranial articulation of the Triassic turtle, *Proganochelys*. In *Advances in Herpetology and Evolutionary Biology*, A. G. J. Rhodin and K. Miyata, eds. Cambridge, Mass.: Museum of Comparative Zoology, pp. 190–194.

————. 1990. The comparative osteology of the Triassic turtle *Proganochelys*. Bulletin of the American Museum of Natural History 194: 1–263.

Gaffney, E. S., and L. J. Meeker. 1983. Skull morphology of the oldest turtles: A preliminary description of *Proganochelys quenstedti*. Journal of Vertebrate Paleontology 3 (1): 25–28.

Gaffney, E. S., and P. A. Meylan. 1988. A phylogeny of turtles. In *The Phylogeny and Classification of the Tetrapods*, vol. 1, M. J. Benton, ed. Oxford: Clarendon Press, pp. 157–219.

Gans, C. 1961. The feeding mechanism of snakes and its possible evolution. American Zoologist 1 (2): 217–227.

————. 1978. The characteristics and affinities of the Amphisbaenia. Transactions of the Zoological Society of London 34 (4): 347–416.

Gans, C., and F. de Vree. 1987. Functional bases of fibre length and angulation in muscle. Journal of Morphology 192 (1): 63–85.

Gasc, J.-P. 1968. Contribution à l'ostéologie et à la myologie de *Dibamus novaeguineae* Gray (Sauria, Reptilia): Discussion systématique. Annales des sciences naturelles, Zoologie et biologie animale (12) 10 (2): 127–150.

Gaupp, E. 1900. Das Chondrocranium von *Lacerta agilis*. Ein Beitrag zum Verständnis des Amniotenschädels. Anatomische Hefte (1) 15 (49): 433–595.

Gauthier, J. A. 1982. Fossil xenosaurid and anguid lizards from the early Eocene Wasatch Formation, southeast Wyoming, and a revision of the Anguioidea. Contributions to Geology, University of Wyoming 21 (1): 7–54.

————. 1984. A cladistic analysis of the higher systematic categories of the Diapsida. Ph.D. diss., University of California, Berkeley.

————. 1986. Saurischian monophyly and the origin of birds. In *The Origin of*

Birds and the Evolution of Flight, K. Padian, ed. Memoirs of the California Academy of Sciences 8: 1–55. Berkeley: University of California Press.

Gauthier, J. A., R. Estes, and K. de Queiroz. 1988. A phylogenetic analysis of Lepidosauromorpha. In *Phylogenetic Relationships of the Lizard Families,* R. Estes and G. Pregill, eds. Stanford: Stanford University Press, pp. 15–98.

Gauthier, J. A., A. G. Kluge, and T. Rowe. 1988a. Amniote phylogeny and the importance of fossils. Cladistics 4: 105–209.

———. 1988b. The early evolution of the Amniota. In *The Phylogeny and Classification of the Tetrapods,* vol. 1, M. J. Benton, ed. Oxford: Clarendon Press, pp. 101–155.

Genest-Villard, H. 1966. Développement du crâne d'un boidé: *Sanzinia madagascariensis.* Mémoires du Muséum national d'histoire naturelle A 40 (5): 207–262.

Goodrich, E. S. 1930. *Studies on the Structure and Development of Vertebrates.* New York: Dover Editions. Reprinted 1958.

Gorniak, G. C., H. I. Rosenberg, and C. Gans. 1982. Mastication in the Tuatara, *Shpenodon punctatus* (Reptilia: Rhynchocephalia): Structure and activity of the motor system. Journal of Morphology 171 (3): 321–353.

Greene, H. W. 1983. Dietary correlates of the origin and radiation of snakes. American Zoologist 23 (2): 431–441.

Greer, A. E. 1970. A subfamilial classification of scincid lizards. Bulletin of the Museum of Comparative Zoology 139 (3): 151–184.

———. 1976. On the occurrence of a stapedial foramen in living non-gekkonid lepidosaurs. Copeia (3): 591–592.

———. 1985. The relationships of the lizard genera *Anelytropsis* and *Dibamus.* Journal of Herpetology 19 (1): 116–156.

Haas, G. 1955. The jaw musculature in *Protoceratops* and in other ceratopsians. American Museum Novitates 1729: 1–24.

Hall, B. K. 1978. *Developmental and Cellular Skeletal Biology.* London: Academic Press.

———. 1984. Developmental processes underlying the evolution of cartilage and bone. In *The Structure, Development, and Evolution of Reptiles,* M.-W. J. Ferguson, ed. London: Academic Press, pp. 155–176.

Hall, B. K., and J. Hanken. 1985a. Foreword to *The Development of the Reptile Skull,* by G. R. de Beer. Chicago: University of Chicago Press, pp. vii–xxvii.

———. 1985b. Repair of fractured lower jaws in the spotted salamander: Do amphibians form secondary cartilage? Journal of Experimental Zoology 233 (3): 359–368.

Haluska, F., and P. Alberch. 1983. The cranial development of Elaphe obsoleta (Ophidia, Colubridae). Journal of Morphology 178 (1): 37–55.

Heaton, M. J. 1979. Cranial anatomy of primitive captorhinid reptiles from the Late Pennsylvanian and Early Permian Oklahoma and Texas. Bulletin of the Oklahoma Geological Survey 127: 1–84.

———. 1980. The Cotylosauria: A reconsideration of a group of archaic tetrapods. In *The Terrestrial Environment and the Origin of Land Vertebrates,* A. L. Panchen, ed. London: Academic Press, pp. 497–551.

Heaton, M. J., and R. R. Reisz. 1986. Phylogenetic relationships of captorhino-morph reptiles. Canadian Journal of Earth Sciences 23 (3): 402–418.

Howes, G. B., and H. H. Swinnerton. 1901. On the development of the skeleton of the tuatara, *Sphenodon punctatus:* with remarks on the egg, on the hatching, and on the hatched young. Transactions of the Zoological Society of London 16 (1): 1–86.

Huxley, T. H. 1875. On *Stagonolepis Robertsoni* and the evolution of the crocodilia. Quarterly Journal of the Geological Society of London 31 (123): 423–438.

Iordansky, N. N. 1966. Cranial kinetism in lizards. Zoologicheskii zhurnal 45 (9): 1398–1410. (Translated by L. Kelso, Smithsonian Herpeological Information Services, 1968, no. 14)

———. 1973. The skull of the Crocodilia. In *Biology of the Reptilia,* vol. 4, C. Gans and T. S. Parsons, eds. London: Academic Press, pp. 201–262.

———. 1978. On the origin of snakes. Zoologicheskii Zhurnal 57 (6): 888–898.

Irish, F. J. 1989. The role of heterochrony in the origin of a novel bauplan: Evolution of the ophidian skull. Géobios, Mémoire spécial 12: 227–333.

Irwin, C. R., and M. W. J. Ferguson. 1986. Fracture repair of reptilian dermal bone: Can reptiles form secondary cartilage? Journal of Anatomy 146: 53–64.

Jaekel, O. 1910. Über das System der Reptilien. Zoologischer Anzeiger 35 (11): 324–341.

Kamal, A. M. 1966. On the process of rotation of the quadrate cartilage in Ophidia. Anatomischer Anzeiger 118 (1): 87–90.

———. 1971. On the fissura metotica in Squamata. Bulletin of the Zoological Society of Egypt 23 (1): 53–57.

Kamal, A. M., and H. G. Hammouda. 1965a. The chondrocranium of the snake *Eryx jaculus.* Acta zoologica, Stockholm 46: 167–208.

———. 1965b. The columella of the snake *Psammophis sibilans.* Anatomischer Anzeiger 116 (1): 124–138.

Kesteven, H. L. 1940. The osteogenesis of the base of the saurian cranium and a search for the parasphenoid bone. Proceedings of the Linnean Society of New South Wales 65 (4): 447–467.

Kilias, R. 1957. Die funktionell-anatomische und systematische Bedeutung der Schläfenreduktionen bei Schildkröten. Mitteilungen aus dem zoologischen Museum in Berlin 33 (2): 307–354.

Kluge, A. G. 1987. Cladistic relationships in the Gekkonoidea (Squamata, Sauria). Miscellaneous Publications, Museum of Zoology, University of Michigan 173: 1–54.

Kritzinger, C. C. 1946. The cranial anatomy and kinesis of the South African amphisbaenid *Monopeltis capensis* Smith. South African Journal of Science 42 (June): 175–204.

Kuhn-Schnyder, E. 1952. *Askeptosaurus italicus* Nopcsa. In *Die Triasfauna der Tessiner Kalkalpen,* vol. 17, B. Peyer, ed. Schweizerische Paläontologische Abhandlungen 69 (ser. zool. 117): 1–73. Basel: Birkhänser Verlag.

———. 1962. Ein weiterer Schädel von *Macrocnemus bassanii* Nopcsa aus der anisischen Stufe der Trias des Monte San Giorgio (Kt. Tessin, Schweiz). Paläontologische Zeitschrift, H. Schmid Festband: 110–133.

———. 1967. Das Problem der Euryapsida. Colloques internationaux du Centre national de la recherche scientifique 163: 335–348.

———. 1980. Observations on temporal openings of reptilian skulls and the classification of reptiles. In *Aspects of Vertebrate History*, L. L. Jacobs, ed. Flagstaff: Museum of Northern Arizona Press, pp. 153–175.

Lakjer, T. 1926. *Studien über die Trigeminus-versorgte Kaumuskulatur der Sauropsiden*. Copenhagen: C. A. Reitzel.

———. 1927. Studien über die Gaumenregion bei Sauriern im Vergleich mit Anamniern und primitiven Sauropsiden. Zoologische Jahrbücher, Abteilung für Anatomie und Ontogenie der Tiere 49 (1–2): 57–356.

Langston, W. 1973. The crocodilian skull in historical perspective. In *Biology of the Reptilia*, vol. 4, C. Gans and T. S. Parsons, eds. London: Academic Press, pp. 201–262.

Laurin, M. 1991. The osteology of a Lower Permian eosuchian from Texas, and a review of diapsid phylogeny. Zoological Journal of the Linnean Society 101 (1): 59–95.

Lull, R. S. 1908. The cranial musculature and the origin of the frill in the ceratopsian dinosaurs. American Journal of Science (4) 25 (149): 387–399.

Massare, J. A., and J. M. Callaway. 1990. The affinities and ecology of Triassic ichthyosaurs. Bulletin of the Geological Society of America 102 (4): 409–416.

Mazin, J.-M. 1982. Affinités et phylogénie des Ichthyopterygia. Géobios, Mémoire spécial 6: 85–98.

McDowell, S. B. 1967. Osteology of the Typhlopidae and Leptotyphlopidae: A critical review. Copeia (4): 686–692.

———. 1975. A catalogue of the snakes of New Guinea and the Solomons, with special reference to those in the Bernice P. Bishop Museum. Part II. Anilioidea and Pythoninae. Journal of Herpetology 9 (1): 1–79.

McGregor, J. H. 1902. The ancestry of the Ichthyosauria. Science, n.s., 16 (July 4): 27.

Merriam, J. C. 1905. The Thalattosauria, a group of marine reptiles from the Triassic of California. Memoirs of the California Academy of Sciences 5: 1–52.

Murray, P. D. F. 1963. Adventitious (secondary) cartilage in the chick embryo, and the development of certain bones and articulations in the chick skull. Australian Journal of Zoology 11 (3): 368–430.

Nick, L. 1912. Das Kopfskelett von *Dermochelys coriacea*. Zoologische Jahrbücher, Abteilung für Anatomie und Ontogenie der Tiere 33 (1): 1–238.

Nopcsa, F. 1923. *Eidolosaurus* und *Pachyophis:* Zwei neue Neocom-Reptilien. Palaeontographica 65 (4): 97–154.

Oelrich, T. M. 1956. The anatomy of the head of *Ctenosaura pectinata*. Miscellaneous Publications, Museum of Zoology, University of Michigan 94: 1–122.

Olsen, P. E. 1979. A new aquatic eosuchian from the Newark Supergroup (Late Triassic–Early Jurassic) of North Carolina and Virginia. Postilla 176: 1–14.

Olson, E. C. 1947. The family Diadectidae and its bearing on the classification of reptiles. Fieldiana Geology 11: 2–53.

———. 1961. Jaw mechanisms: Rhipidistians, amphibians, and reptiles. American Zoologist 1 (2): 205–215.

Ostrom, J. H. 1966. Functional morphology and evolution of the ceratopsian dinosaurs. Evolution 20 (3): 290–308.

Panchen, A. L., and T. R. Smithson. 1988. The relationships of the earliest tetrapods. In *The Phylogeny and Classification of the Tetrapods*, M. J. Benton, ed., vol. 1. Oxford: Clarendon Press, pp. 1–32.

Parker, H. W., and A. G. C. Grandison. 1977. *Snakes: A Natural History*. London: British Museum (Natural History).

Parker, W. S. 1879. On the structure and development of the skull in the common snake (*Tropidonotus natrix*). Philosophical Transactions of the Royal Society of London 169: 385–417.

Parrington, F. R. 1935. On *Prolacerta broomi* gen. et sp. nov., and the origin of lizards. Annals and Magazine of Natural History (10) 16 (92): 197–205.

Patchell, F. C., and R. Shine. 1986. Feeding mechanisms in pygopodid lizards: How can *Lialis* swallow such large prey? Journal of Herpetology 20 (1): 59–64.

Patterson, C. 1977. Cartilage bones, dermal bones, and membrane bones, or the exoskeleton versus the endoskeleton. In *Problems in Vertebrate Evolution*, S. M. Andrews, R. S. Miles, and A. D. Walker, eds. London: Academic Press, pp. 77–121.

Pehrson, T. 1945. Some problems concerning the development of the skull in turtles. Acta zoologica, Stockholm 26: 157–184.

Peyer, B. 1912. Die Entwicklung des Schädelskelettes von *Vipera aspis*. Morphologisches Jahrbuch 44 (4): 563–621.

Pratt, C. W. 1948. The morphology of the ethmoidal region in *Sphenodon* and lizards. Proceedings of the Zoological Society of London 118 (1): 171–201.

Presch, W. 1976. Secondary palate formation in microteiid lizards (Teiidae: Lacertilia). Bulletin of the Southern California Academy of Sciences 75 (3): 281–283.

Price, L. I. 1935. Notes on the brain case of *Captorhinus*. Boston Society of Natural History Proceedings 40: 377–385.

Reisz, R. R. 1980. The Pelycosauria: A review of phylogenetic relationships. In *The Terrestrial Environment and the Origin of Land Vertebrates*, A. L. Panchen, ed. London: Academic Press, pp. 553–592.

———. 1981. A diapsid reptile from the Pennsylvanian of Kansas. Special Publication of the Museum of Natural History, University of Kansas 7: 1–74.

Reisz, R. R., D. S. Berman, and D. Scott. 1984. The anatomy and relationships of the Lower Permian Reptile *Araeoscelis*. Journal of Vertebrate Paleontology 4 (1): 47–67.

Reisz, R. R., and M. Laurin. 1991. *Owenetta* and the origin of turtles. Nature 349: 324–326.

Ridgway, S. H., E. G. Wever, J. G. McCormick, J. Palin, and J. H. Anderson. 1969. Hearing in the giant sea turtle, *Chelonia mydas*. Proceedings of the National Academy of Sciences, U.S.A. 64 (3): 884–890.

Rieppel, O. 1976a. Die orbitotemporale Region im Schädel von *Chelydra serpentina* Linnaeus (Chelonia) und *Lacerta sicula* Rafinesque (Lacertilia). Acta anatomica 96 (3): 309–320.

————. 1976b. The homology of the laterosphenoid bone in snakes. Herpetologica 32 (4): 426–429.

————. 1978a. The braincase of *Anniella pulchra* Gray (Lacertilia, Anniellidae). Revue suisse de zoologie 85 (3): 617–624.

————. 1978b. The evolution of the naso-frontal joint in snakes and its bearing on snake origins. Zeitschrift für zoologische Systematik und Evolutionsforschung 16 (1): 14–27.

————. 1978c. The phylogeny of cranial kinesis in lower vertebrates, with special reference to the Lacertilia. Neues Jahrbuch für Geologie und Paläontologie, Abhandlungen 156 (3): 353–370.

————. 1978d. Streptostyly and muscle function in lizards. Experientia 34 (6): 776–777.

————. 1979a. The braincase of *Typhlops* and *Leptotyphlops*. Zoological Journal of the Linnean Society 65 (2): 161–176.

————. 1979b. The evolution of the basicranium in the Henophidia (Reptilia: Serpentes). Zoological Journal of the Linnean Society 66 (4): 411–431.

————. 1979c. The external adductor of amphisbaenids (Reptilia: Amphisbaenia). Revue suisse de zoologie 86 (4): 867–876.

————. 1979d. A functional interpretation of the varanid dentition (Reptilia, Lacertilia, Varanidae). Gegenbaurs morphologisches Jahrbuch 125 (6): 797–817.

————. 1979e. Ontogeny and the recognition of primitive character states. Zeitschrift für zoologische Systematik und Evolutionsforschung 17 (1): 57–61.

————. 1980a. The evolution of the ophidian feeding system. Zoologische Jahrbücher, Abteilung für Anatomie und Ontogenie der Tiere 103 (4): 551–564.

————. 1980b. The phylogeny of anguinomorph lizards. Denkschriften der schweizerischen naturforschenden Gesellschaft 94: 1–86.

————. 1980c. The skull of the Upper Jurassic cryptodire turtle *Thalassemys*, with a reconsideration of the chelonian braincase. Palaeontographica A 171 (4–6): 105–140.

————. 1980d. The sound-transmitting apparatus in primitive snakes and its phylogenetic significance. Zoomorphology 96 (1–2): 45–62.

————. 1980e. The trigeminal jaw adductor musculature of *Tupinambis*, with comments on the phylogenetic relationships of the Teiidae (Reptilia, Lacertilia). Zoological Journal of the Linnean Society 69 (1): 1–29.

————. 1981a. Die Funktion des Kragens der Ceratopsia. In *Paläontologische Kursbücher*, vol. 1, *Funktionsmorphologie*, W.-E. Reif, ed. Munich: Paläontologische Gesellschaft, pp. 205–216.

————. 1981b. The skull and the jaw adductor musculature in some burrowing scincomorph lizards of the genera *Acontias*, *Typhlosaurus*, and *Feylinia*. Journal of Zoology, London 195 (4): 493–528.

————. 1983. A comparison of the skull of *Lanthanotus borneensis* (Reptilia: Varanoidea) with the skull of primitive snakes. Zeitschrift für zoologische Systematik und Evolutionsforschung 21 (2): 142–153.

————. 1984a. The cranial morphology of the fossorial lizard genus *Dibamus* with a consideration of its phylogenetic relationships. Journal of Zoology, London 204 (3): 289–327.

————. 1984b. Miniaturization of the lizard skull: Its functional and evolutionary implications. In *The Structure, Development, and Evolution of Reptiles,* M.-W. J. Ferguson, ed. London: Academic Press, pp. 503–520.

————. 1984c. The structure of the skull and jaw adductor musculature in the Gekkota, with comments on the phylogenetic relationships of the Xantusiidae (Reptilia: Lacertilia). Zoological Journal of the Linnean Society 82 (3): 291–318.

————. 1984d. The upper temporal arcade of lizards: An ontogenetic problem. Revue suisse de zoologie 91 (2): 475–482.

————. 1985. The recessus scalae tympani and its bearing on the classification of reptiles. Journal of Herpetology 19 (3): 373–384.

————. 1987a. *Clarazia* and *Hescheleria:* A re-investigation of two problematical reptiles from the Middle Triassic of Monte San Giorgio (Switzerland). Palaeontographica A 195 (4–6): 101–129.

————. 1987b. The development of the trigeminal jaw adductor musculature and associated skull elements in the lizard *Podarcis sicula.* Journal of Zoology, London 212 (1): 131–150.

————. 1988. A review of the origin of snakes. In *Evolutionary Biology,* vol. 22, M. K. Hecht, B. Wallace, and G. T. Prance, eds. New York: Plenum Publishing, pp. 37–130.

————. 1989a. The closure of the lateral braincase wall in snakes. In *Trends in Vertebrate Morphology,* H. Splechtna and H. Hilgers, eds., Progress in Zoology 35. Jena: Gustav Fischer, pp. 409–411.

————. 1989b. A new pachypleurosaur (Reptilia: Sauropterygia) from the Middle Triassic of Monte San Giorgio, Switzerland. Philosophical Transactions of the Royal Society of London B 323 (1212): 1–73.

————. 1990. The structure and development of the jaw adductor musculature in the turtle *Chelydra serpentina.* Zoological Journal of the Linnean Society of London 98: 27–62.

Rieppel, O., and Gronowski, R. W. 1981. The loss of the lower temporal arcade in diapsid reptiles. Zoological Journal of the Linnean Society 72 (3): 203–217.

Robb, J. 1977. *The Tuatara.* Durham: Meadowfield Press.

Robinson, P. L. 1962. Gliding lizards from the Upper Keuper of Great Britain. Proceedings of the Geological Society of London 1601: 137–146.

————. 1973. A problematic reptile from the British Upper Trias. Journal of the Geological Society 129 (5): 457–479.

————. 1976. How *Sphenodon* and *Uromastyx* grow their teeth and use them. In *Morphology and Biology of Reptiles,* A. d'A. Bellairs and C. B. Cox, eds. London: Academic Press, pp. 43–64.

Romer, A. S. 1956. *The Osteology of the Reptiles.* Chicago: University of Chicago Press.

————. 1968a. An ichthyosaur skull from the Cretaceous of Wyoming. Contributions to Geology, University of Wyoming 7: 27–41.

————. 1968b. *Notes and Comments on Vertebrate Paleontology.* Chicago: University of Chicago Press.

————. 1971. Unorthodoxies in reptilian evolution. Evolution 25 (1): 103–112.

Romer, A. S., and L. W. Price. 1940. Review of the Pelycosauria. Geological Society of America Special Papers 28: 1–538.

Russell, D. A. 1967. Systematics and morphology of American mosasaurs. Peabody Museum of Natural History, Yale University, Bulletin 23: 1–240.

Säve-Söderbergh, G. 1946. On the fossa hypophyseos and the attachment of the retractor bulbi group in *Sphenodon, Varanus,* and *Lacerta.* Arkiv för Zoologi 38 (11): 1–24.

Schumacher, G.-H. 1973. The head muscles and hyolaryngeal skeleton of turtles and crocodilians. In *Biology of the Reptilia,* vol. 4, C. Gans and T. S. Parsons, eds. London: Academic Press, pp. 101–199.

Seeley, H. G. 1887. Researches on the structure, organization, and classification of the fossil Reptilia. I. On *Protorosaurus speneri* (von Meyer). Philosophical Transactions of the Royal Society of London 178: 187–213.

Shaner, R. F. 1926. The development of the skull of the turtle, with remarks on fossil reptile skulls. Anatomical Record 32 (4): 343–367.

Shiino, K. 1914. Studien zur Kenntnis des Wirbeltierkopfes. 1. Das Chondrocranium von *Crocodilus,* mit Berücksichtigung der Gehirnnerven und der Kopfgefässe. Anatomische Hefte (1) 50 (151): 253–381.

Shishkin, M. A. 1968. Cranial arteries of labyrinthodonts. Acta zoologica, Stockholm 49: 1–22.

Smith, K. K. 1982. An electromyographic study of the function of the jaw adducting muscles in *Varanus exanthematicus* (Varanidae). Journal of Morphology 173 (2): 137–158.

Starck, D. 1979. *Vergleichende Anatomie der Wirbeltiere auf evolutionsbiologischer Grundlage,* vol. 2. Berlin: Springer.

Stephenson, N. G. 1960. The comparative osteology of Australian geckos and its bearing on their morphological status. Journal of the Linnean Society, Zoology 44 (297): 278–299.

Sues, H.-D. 1987a. Postcranial skeleton of *Pistosaurus* and interrelationships of the Sauropterygia (Diapsida). Zoological Journal of the Linnean Society 90 (2): 109–131.

———. 1987b. The skull of *Placodus gigas* and the relationships of the Placodontia. Journal of Vertebrate Paleontology 7 (2): 138–144.

Tarsitano, S. 1982. A model for the origin of ichthyosaurs. Neues Jahrbuch für Geologie und Paläontologie, Abhandlungen 164 (1–2): 143–154.

———. 1983. A case for the diapsid origin of ichthyosaurs. Neues Jahrbuch für Geologie und Paläontologie, Monatsheft (1): 59–64.

Tarsitano, S., S. F. Frey, and J. Riess. 1989. On the method of tendon attachment to bone. I. Internationales Symposium des SFB 230 (3): 105–108.

Tarsitano, S., and B. W. Oelofson. 1985. The invasion of the periosteum. American Zoologist 25 (4): 44. Abstract

Throckmorton, G. 1976. Oral food processing in two herbivorous lizards, *Iguana iguana* (Iguanidae) and *Uromastyx aegyptius* (Agamidae). Journal of Morphology 148 (3): 363–390.

———. 1978. Action of the pterygoideus muscle during feeding in the lizard *Uromastyx aegyptius* (Agamidae). Anatomical Record 190 (2): 217–222.

Throckmorton, G., and L. K. Clarke. 1981. Intracranial joint movements in the agamid lizard *Amphibolorus barbatus.* Journal of Experimental Zoology 216 (1): 25–35.

Toerien, M. J. 1950. The cranial morphology of the Californian lizard—*Anniella pulchra* Gray. South African Journal of Science 46 (12): 321–342.

Underwood, G. 1967. *A Contribution to the Classification of Snakes.* London: British Museum (Natural History).

———. 1970. The eye. In *Biology of the Reptilia,* vol. 2, C. Gans and T. S. Parsons, eds. London: Academic Press, pp. 1–97.

———. 1976. A systematic analysis of snakes. In *Morphology and Biology of Reptiles,* A. d'A. Bellairs and C. B. Cox, eds. Linnean Society Symposium, ser. 3. London: Academic Press, pp. 151–175.

Versluys, J. 1912. Das Streptostylie-Problem und die Bewegungen im Schädel der Sauropsiden. Zoologische Jahrbücher, Abteilung für Anatomie und Ontogenie der Tiere, suppl. 15 (2): 545–716.

Werner, Y. L., and E. G. Wever. 1972. The function of the middle ear in lizards: *Gecko gecko* and *Eublepharis macularius* (Gekkonidae). Journal of Experimental Zoology 179 (1): 1–16.

Wever, E. G. 1978. *The Reptile Ear.* Princeton: Princeton University Press.

Wever, E. G., and C. Gans. 1972. The ear and hearing in *Bipes biporus.* Proceedings of the National Academy of Sciences, U.S.A. 69 (9): 2714–2716.

———. 1973. The ear and hearing in the Amphisbaenia (Reptilia): Further anatomical observations. Journal of Zoology, London 171 (2): 189–206.

Wever, E. G., and J. A. Vernon. 1956. Sound transmission in the turtle's ear. Proceedings of the National Academy of Sciences, U.S.A. 42 (5): 292–299.

Whetstone, K. N., and L. D. Martin. 1979. New look at the origin of birds and crocodiles. Nature 279 (5710): 234–236.

Whiteside, D. I. 1986. The head skeleton of the Rhaetian sphenodontid *Diphydontosaurus avonensis* gen. et sp. nov., and the modernizing of a living fossil. Philosophical Transactions of the Royal Society of London B 312 (1156): 379–430.

Wild, R. 1973. *Tanystropheus longobardicus* (Bassani) (Neue Ergebnisse). In *Die Triasfauna der Tessiner Kalkalpen,* vol. 23, B. Peyer and E. Kuhn-Schnyder, eds. Schweizerische Paläontologische Abhandlungen 95: 1–162.

Williston, S. W. 1914. The osteology of some American Permian vertebrates. Journal of Geology 22 (4): 364–419.

———. 1917. The phylogeny and classification of reptiles. Journal of Geology 25 (5): 411–421.

Yntema, C. L. 1968. A series of stages in the embryonic development of *Chelydra serpentina.* Journal of Morphology 125 (2): 219–252.

Zangerl, R. 1944. Contributions to the osteology of the skull of the Amphisbaenidae. American Midland Naturalist 31 (2): 417–454.

Zanon, R. T. 1990. The sternum of *Araeoscelis* and its implications for basal diapsid phylogeny. Journal of Vertebrate Paleontology 10 (suppl. to no. 3): 51A.

———. n.d. *Paraplacodus* and the diapsid origin of Placodontia. Journal of Vertebrate Paleontology. Forthcoming.

8

Patterns of Diversity in the Avian Skull

RICHARD L. ZUSI

INTRODUCTION

BIRDS ARE COMMON, conspicuous, taxonomically well known, and morphologically diverse. They are easily studied in the field, and they are well represented in osteological collections, at least at the generic level. Thus, birds would appear to be excellent subjects for the study of morphological evolution in the skull. Yet, their potential has been little realized for several reasons. Although patterns of evolutionary diversity are analyzed best in a phylogenetic context, avian systematics in the twentieth century has focused on the species and subspecies levels, emphasizing external morphology, rather than on comparative anatomy and phylogeny at higher levels. The current revolution in avian systematics brought about by biochemical techniques and the application of cladistic methods is only beginning to provide corroborated phylogenies. Furthermore, in recent decades research on avian anatomy has been displaced largely by studies of the living bird. In this context, I will present an introduction to morphological diversity of the avian skull, touching on comparative embryology and phylogeny, but emphasizing adaptation as one explanation of diversity. Patterns of covariation of skull structure, cranial kinesis, and jaw muscles will be examined, and guidelines for future work proposed.

As a convenience for readers unfamiliar with avian systematics, the orders of living birds are listed in table 8.1, and under each, the family of each species and genus mentioned in the text. Species, genera, and common names are cross-referenced to order or family when first mentioned in the text. Ordinal names (e.g., Anseriformes) may be anglicized (anseriforms). I shall refer frequently to the ostrich (Struthionidae), rheas (Rheidae), cassowaries (Casuariidae), emus (Dromaiidae), and kiwis (Apterygidae) as "ratites," and as "paleognaths" or "paleognathous birds" when including the tinamous (Tinamidae), without implying relationship; similarly, "neognathous birds" applies to all other living birds. Most avian families and subfamilies are widely regarded as monophyletic, but the composition

TABLE 8.1 Avian classification

Orders	Number of families and species	Cited families
Struthioniformes	1/1	Struthionidae
Rheiformes	1/2	Rheidae
Casuariiformes	2/5	Casuariidae
		Dromaiidae
Apterygiformes	1/3	Apterygidae
Tinamiformes	1/47	Tinamidae
Sphenisciformes	1/18	Spheniscidae
Gaviiformes	1/5	Gaviidae
Podicipediformes	1/20	Podicipedidae
Procellariiformes	4/104	Pelecanoididae
Pelecaniformes	6/62	Pelecanidae
		Sulidae
		Phalacrocoracidae
Ciconiiformes	5/114	Ardeidae
		Balaenicipitidae
		Ciconiidae
Phoenicopteriformes	1/6	
Anseriformes	2/150	Anatidae
Falconiformes	5/288	Accipitridae
Galliformes	4/269	Cracidae
		Phasianidae
Gruiformes	12/210	Gruidae
		Aramidae
		Otididae
Charadriiformes	16/329	Haematopodidae
		Charadriidae
		Scolopacidae
		Chionididae
		Laridae
		Rynchopidae
		Alcidae
Columbiformes	3/322	Columbidae
Psittaciformes	3/340	Loriidae
		Cacatuidae
		Psittacidae
Cuculiformes	2/147	
Strigiformes	2/146	Tytonidae
		Strigidae
Caprimulgiformes	5/105	Podargidae
		Nyctibiidae
		Caprimulgidae
Apodiformes	3/428	Trochilidae
Coliiformes	1/6	Coliidae
Trogoniformes	1/37	
Coraciiformes	10/200	Alcedinidae
		Upupidae
		Phoeniculidae
		Bucerotidae

TABLE 8.1   (*continued*)

Orders	Number of families and species	Cited families
Piciformes	6/383	Ramphastidae
		Picidae
Passeriformes	60/5273	Emberizidae
		Drepanididae
		Icteridae
		Fringillidae
		Estrildidae
		Sturnidae
		Callaeidae
		Corvidae

Notes: Based mainly on Bock and Farrand 1980. The first five orders constitute the paleognathous birds; the remainder are neognaths.

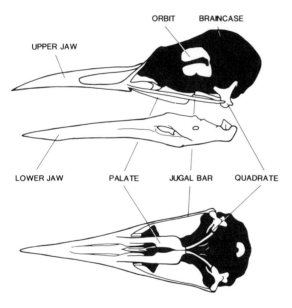

Fig. 8.1. Skull of *Gelochelidon nilotica* (Laridae). Above, left lateral view. Lower jaw separated from quadrate. Below, ventral view, lower jaw removed. Neurocranium solid; splanchnocranium open. (Modified from Zusi 1962)

of some orders is disputed (e.g., Pelecaniformes, Ciconiiformes, Falconiformes, Gruiformes, Coraciiformes, Piciformes).

Generally, I use the anatomical nomenclature proposed by Baumel et al. (1979), and the taxonomic nomenclature and classification of Morony et al. (1975). I use the following terminology for major features of the skull (fig. 8.1): the skull or cranium includes a neurocranium (braincase, orbit, and sensory capsules) and splanchnocranium (jaws, palate, and hyoid apparatus); the rostrum (mandibular rostrum or maxillary rostrum) is the anterior portion of the jaws making up the bill.

MORPHOLOGY OF THE AVIAN SKULL

Much of our knowledge of avian cranial structure comes from studies by comparative anatomists of the nineteenth and early twentieth centuries, such as H. Gadow, I. Geoffroy St. Hillaire, T. H. Huxley, H. Magnus, C. Nitzsch, T. J. Parker, W. K. Parker, W. P. Pycraft, and P. P. Sushkin. These authors provided detailed descriptions that are still useful, regardless of the quality of their conclusions on homology and systematics. Some important contributions to functional anatomy are those of H. Boker, W. Marinelli, and W. Moller. Perhaps the most comprehensive sources on diversity of the avian skull are the papers of Hofer (1945, 1949, 1950, 1952, 1953, 1955), in which different morphologies, their functional correlates, and homologies are emphasized. Hofer discussed cranial kinesis, palatal types and functions, ornamentation, skull types defined by cranial angles, and the relation of jaw muscles to cranial architecture, in addition to major variation in bones and processes. Many more recent references will be discussed in this chapter.

Several authors have undertaken single character studies in which a particular feature or region of the skull was surveyed in more or less morphological and taxonomic detail. Examples of such features are the bony labyrinth (Gray 1908; Turkewitsch 1936; Werner 1960), the quadrate (Walker 1888; Lowe 1926), the middle ear (Saiff 1988 and included references), the columella (Krause 1901; Feduccia 1975), the os opticus (Tiemeier 1939), the sclerotic ring (Lemmrich 1931), the occipital condyle (Goedbloed 1958), the palatine process of the premaxilla (Bock 1960a), the mandible (Lebedinsky 1920), the secondary articulation of the mandible (Bock 1960b), the lacrimal-ectethmoid complex (Cracraft 1968), the os uncinatum (Burton 1970), the nasal region (Technau 1936; Bang 1971), and pneumatization of the neurocranium (Winkler 1979). A series of studies of cranial structure as it relates to jaw and neck muscle attachment, covering various taxonomic groups, has been published by P. Dullemeijer and his students (see references in Dullemeijer 1974).

Systematic studies of particular taxa, both classical and recent, often contain data on osteology of the skull, but the data are sometimes difficult or impossible to use for other purposes because they are not comparable among studies and they may include only those features that are appropriate to a particular kind of analysis.

Description and Development

The neurocranium of adult birds consists of a bony box in which all bones are fused. Only in tinamous (Tinamidae) do sutures of the frontal bone persist. Loosely attached to the neurocranium is a scaffolding of movable bones, the splanchnocranium, comprised of the upper jaw or maxilla (not to be confused with the single bone by that name in other vertebrates), lower jaw or mandible, jugal bars, palate, and quadrates (fig. 8.1). The splanchnocranium connects with the neurocranium only by diarthroses of the quadrate and palate, and by a flattened elastic zone (craniofacial hinge) of the upper jaw. In a few species, even the craniofacial junction is represented by a syndesmosis (e.g., some parrots, Psittaciformes; frogmouths, Podargidae). Other bones associated with the skull are those of the tongue and hyoid apparatus, the columella, accessory bones of the eye (sclerotic ring, os opticus), the siphonium, the nuchal bone (cormorants, Phalacrocoracidae), and various sesamoids.

During embryonic development, cranial ossification is preceded by formation of a chondrocranium, which serves as a partial model for subsequent ossification of the skull by replacement of its cartilage (e.g., de Beer and Barrington 1934; de Beer 1937). Most bone and cartilage in the avian skull is of neural crest origin; the rest develops from mesoderm (Noden 1978). The upper jaw, much of the lower jaw, the palate, and much of the neurocranium are formed from membrane bones that constitute the dermatocranium. Secondary cartilages associated with membrane bones may ossify as extensions of the bones. The adult skull retains only fragments of the chondrocranium in the form of the nasal capsule, nasal septum, and nasal conchae (turbinals), and even these structures are ossified in some species. Ossified aponeuroses and ligaments may become integral parts of the adult skull in some taxa.

The development of individual cranial bones of the chicken (*Gallus,* Phasianidae) has been discussed by Erdmann (1940), Jollie (1957), and others; the brief account presented here follows Jollie, with some exceptions, and is illustrated by a species from the order Charadriiformes (*Uria lomvia,* Alcidae; fig. 8.2). Not all birds conform to this account, but only selected variants are mentioned. Bones that replace cartilage are designated by (c); those that replace condensed mesenchyme by (m).

Forming the rim of the foramen magnum and posterior wall of the braincase are the occipital bones—a dorso-medial supraoccipital (c), a ventro-medial basioccipital (c), and the lateral exoccipitals (c). In *Gallus* all but the first of these bones contribute to formation of the single occipital condyle, but the condyle may form from the basioccipital alone (e.g., *Rhea,* Rheidae; Müller 1963). In some anseriforms and charadriiforms the supraoccipital contains a pair of occipital fonticuli. Ventrolaterally, the exoccipital may be extended as a parotic (paroccipital) process (fig. 8.3c, e).

Closely associated with the occipitals but largely within the braincase are three otic bones (prootic, opisthotic, epiotic [c]), which fuse early in development and enclose the membranous labyrinth (fig. 8.2). They are represented by only one or two ossifications in the development of some

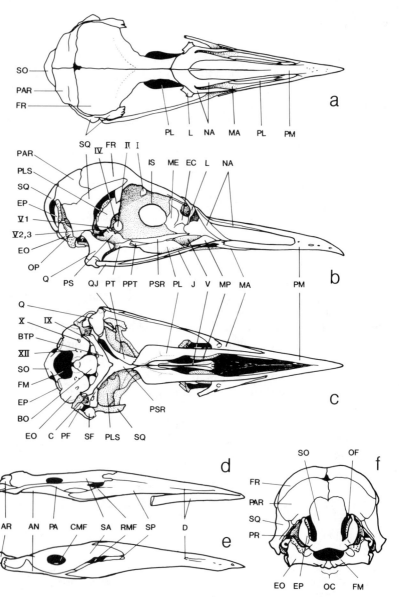

Fig. 8.2. Skull of juvenile *Uria lomvia* (Alcidae). Cranium in dorsal (a), lateral (b), and ventral (c) views; mandible in dorso-medial (d) and lateral (e) views; cranium in posterior view (f). AN, angular; AR, articular; BO, basioccipital; BTP, basitemporal plate; C, columella; CMF, caudal mandibular fenestra; D, dentary; EC, ectethmoid; EO, exoccipital; EP, epiotic; FM, foramen magnum; FR, frontal; IS, interorbital septum; J, jugal; L, lacrimal; MA, maxillary; ME, mesethmoid; MP, maxillopalatine; NA, nasal; OC, occipital condyle; OF, occcipital fonticulus; OP, opisthotic; PA, prearticular; PAR, parietal; PF, prootic facet; PL, palatine; PLS, pleurosphenoid; PM, premaxillary; PPT, pars palatina (pterygoid); PR, prootic; PS, parasphenoid; PSR, parasphenoidal rostrum; PT, pterygoid; Q, quadrate; QJ, quadratojugal; RMF, rostral mandibular fenestra; SA, supraangular; SF, squamosal facet; SO, supraoccipital; SP, splenial; SQ, squamosal; V, vomer. Roman numerals indicate foramina for cranial nerves.

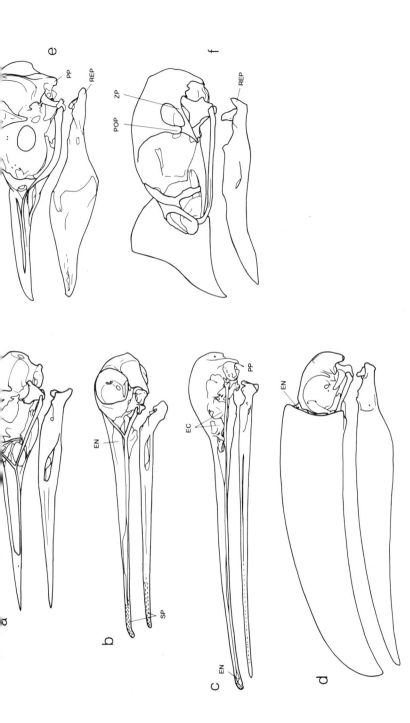

Fig. 8.3. Lateral view of cranium and lower jaw of (a) *Grus canadensis* (Gruidae), (b) *Scolopax rochussenii* (Scolopacidae), (c) *Apteryx australis* (Apterygidae), (d) *Ramphastos toco* (Ramphastidae), (e) *Eudyptes pachyrhynchus* (Spheniscidae), (f) *Crax mitu* (Cracidae). EC, ectethmoid; EN, external nares; NG, nasal gland depression; POP, postorbital process; PP, parotic process; REP, retroarticular process; SP, sensory pits; TF, temporal fossa; ZP, zygomatic process.

ratites (Webb 1957). The prootic includes an articular facet for the prootic (inner) condyle of the quadrate; the opisthotic is perforated by the cochlear fenestra (fenestra rotunda). These two bones are partially separated by the vestibular fenestra (fenestra ovalis), which houses the base of the columella.

The ventral portion of the neurocranium is composed of the basioccipital, the basisphenoid (c) and the parasphenoid (m). Protrusions from either side of the basisphenoid in some birds constitute the basipterygoid processes, which articulate with the pterygoids. The parasphenoid has many centers of ossification; when fully ossified it covers the basisphenoid (as the basitemporal plate), forms the postero-ventral portion of the orbit, and extends forward (parasphenoidal rostrum) as a support for the interorbital septum. The pharyngotympanic (eustachian) canals open near the anterior limit of the basitemporal plate, and the sella turcica is formed from the basisphenoid and the parasphenoid. This portion of the neurocranium is penetrated by rostral, caudal, and dorsal pneumatic sinuses, which open into the middle ear cavity; the dorsal pneumatic foramen separates the squamosal and prootic articular facets for the quadrate in neognathous birds.

Additional elements of the neurocranium are the parietals (m) and frontals (m) forming its roof and dorso-lateral sides, the squamosal (m) constituting its lateral wall, and the pleurosphenoid (c) contributing to the orbit. In some birds a small orbitosphenoid (c) develops antero-medial to the pleurosphenoid (Hogg 1978). (The pleurosphenoid [Erdmann 1940; Müller 1963] was termed "orbitosphenoid" by Jollie 1957.) Two major processes associated with these bones are the postorbital process of the pleurosphenoid, squamosal, or frontal, and the zygomatic process of the squamosal. In addition, the squamosal is marked by the squamosal cotyla, which receives the squamosal (outer) condyle of the quadrate. In most neognathous birds the squamosal separates the pleurosphenoid from the parietal and contributes to the braincase (fig. 8.2), but in paleognaths and a few neognaths the squamosal is less extensive and the pleurosphenoid meets the parietal.

The anterior ends of the frontals and parasphenoidal rostrum are interconnected by the mesethmoid (c), a median bone that contributes to the orbit. It stands between the nasal septum anteriorly and the interorbital septum posteriorly. These septa may be ossified and fused with the mesethmoid to varying degree; a small anterior portion of the mesethmoid may be separated from the main bone below the craniofacial hinge. The interorbital septum of birds is highly variable, ranging from essentially unossified to thick and spongy (Zusi 1978), and the nasal septum is either complete or perforate. Ectethmoid bones (c) develop as lateral wings to the mesethmoid, further defining the orbit. In kiwis the mesethmoid and ectethmoids are massive, displacing the interorbital septum and adjoining the brain case. A lacrimopalatine (uncinate) bone of unknown homology is attached to the ventral border of the ectethmoid in a few groups of birds (Burton 1970). In many birds a lacrimal (m) lies lateral to the ectethmoid; it may be separate or fused with the ectethmoid or the nasal. (I use "lacrimal" rather than "prefrontal" because the bone transmits the lacrimal duct in some ratites and it reaches the jugal bar in many living birds, *Hesperornis*, and *Archaeopteryx;* see discussion in Müller 1963.)

External foramina for the cranial nerves occur in various parts of the braincase (Bubien-Waluszewska 1981; Butendieck and Wissdorf 1982), and their positions relative to each other and to cranial bones are somewhat variable. Those that transmit the hypoglossal (XII), accessory (XI), vagus (X), and glossopharyngeal nerves (IX) penetrate or border the exoccipitals. The prootic transmits the vestibulocochlear (VIII) and facial (VII) nerves. In the orbit, the optic nerve (II) leaves the braincase by a large foramen between the pleurosphenoid and the interorbital septum, and the oculomotor (III), trochlear (IV), abducens (VI), and ophthalmic ramus of the trigeminal (V) are transmitted by foramina near or confluent with the optic foramen. Maxillary and mandibular branches of the trigeminal pass through one or two foramina at the ventral border of the pleurosphenoid. The olfactory nerve (I) enters the orbit through a foramen at the anterior end of the braincase.

The upper and lower jaws of all modern birds lack teeth. Such names as "tooth-billed pigeon" (Columbidae) and "double-toothed kite" (Accipitridae) refer only to pointed projections of the keratinized skin of the rostrum (rhamphotheca) and of the premaxillary. The maxilla consists of the nasals (m), the premaxillaries (m), the maxillaries (m), and sometimes parts of the vomer and palatines, which form a more or less monolithic rostrum that is movable relative to the neurocranium at the craniofacial hinge. The nasal forms the posterior border of the bony nares and sends processes to the premaxillary, maxillary, and frontals, except in ratites, which lack a connection with the maxillary. Anteriorly, right and left premaxillaries fuse to produce a solid tip of the rostrum, and each sends a process posteriorly above and below the bony nares. The dorsal process flattens and fuses with the mesethmoid; together with the adjacent process of the nasal it forms the craniofacial hinge, which may or may not be demarked as a transverse axis. The ventral process meets the maxillary. In birds, the premaxillary is highly developed, constituting much of the upper jaw, whereas the maxillary is much reduced (especially in neognathous birds) and confined to the base of the upper jaw and part of the jugal bar. Each maxillary has a medial process (maxillopalatine) that is pneumatized by the maxillary portion of the antorbital sinus. The maxillopalatine process is highly variable in size and shape among taxa. Median fusion of the

paired processes is a defining feature of one of the major palatal configurations in birds (desmognathous palate).

The bony nares range from small to very large relative to the size of
the maxillary rostrum. During development, the nares may be variously
occluded by ossification of the nasal capsule and conchae, or even obliterated (boobies, Sulidae). In kiwis the nares open only near the tip of the
maxilla, and the nasal passages occupy the interior of the long, tubelike
rostrum (fig. 8.3).

A jugal bar is always present in birds. Usually a slender rod, it connects
the postero-ventro-lateral portion of the upper jaw with the quadrate. Its
anterior end is formed in part by the posterior portion of the maxillary;
the posterior portion is represented by the quadratojugal (m), articulating
with the quadrate (fig. 8.2). The jugal (m) broadly overlaps the maxillary
and quadratojugal, completing the middle portion of the bar. In some species the jugal is absent (e.g., Scolopacidae, some Charadriidae), and in
them the bar is completed by overlapping of the maxillary and quadratojugal (personal observation).

A second series of bones connects the base of the upper jaw with the
quadrate. The palatines (m) attach anteriorly on the maxillaries or premaxillaries and extend posteriorly to the pterygoids (m), which in turn
articulate with the quadrate. The vomers (m) are paired bones that fuse
early and are then referred to as the "vomer." The vomer is highly variable
in shape among birds; in many paleognaths it connects the premaxillary
or maxillary with the pterygoid, but in most neognaths it has no connection with the upper jaw beyond an association with the nasal septum or
conchae, and its posterior connection is with the palatine. The vomer may
be greatly reduced or absent (fig. 8.4f).

The palate, consisting of the palatine and pterygoid, and sometimes
the vomer, typically forms a sliding articulation with the parasphenoidal
rostrum. Birds with a functional basipterygoid process have a sliding articulation between that process and the pterygoid, and they may lack a
palatal contact with the rostrum. The pterygoid and palatine meet by a
suture that may disappear by fusion. In most neognathous birds, an articulation develops within the pterygoid in its anterior portion, and the
anterior segment (pars palatina, variously termed the anteropterygoid,
hemipterygoid, or mesopterygoid) becomes fused to the palatine in adults
(Pycraft 1901; Jollie 1958).

In all birds, the quadrate (c) is a movable link between the neurocranium and the upper jaw via the palate and jugal bars. The quadrate
articulates dorsally with the braincase, ventrally with the lower jaw, ventro-
laterally with the quadratojugal, and anteriorly with the pterygoid. In
most birds a prominent orbital process of the quadrate serves for muscle
attachment.

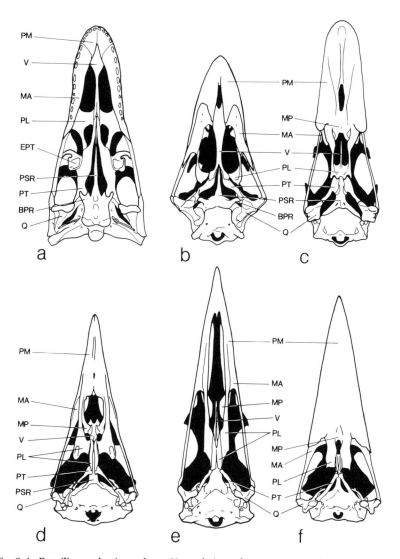

Fig. 8.4. Reptilian and avian palates. Ventral view of cranium. a. Coelurosaur
(*Dromaeosaurus albertensis*), modified from Colbert and Russell (1969).
b. Paleognathus palate (*Dromaius novaehollandiae*, Dromaiidae). c. Desmognathous
palate (*Asner albifrons,* Anatidae). d. Aegithognathous palate (*Corvus corax,*
Corvidae). e. Schizognathous palate (*Neotis cafra,* Otididae). f. Desmognathous palate
(*Dacelo novaeguinea,* Alcedinidae). BPR, basitemporal process; EPT, ectopterygoid;
MA, maxillary; MP maxillopalatine; PL, palatine; PM, premaxillary; PSR,
parasphenoidal rostrum; PT, pterygoid; Q, quadrate; V, vomer.

The mandible consists of six pairs of bones that are more or less fused (fig. 8.2). With few exceptions the anterior portions of the two dentaries (m) fuse medially in a symphysis that produces a monolithic, rostral tip, opposing that of the upper jaw. Each ramus of the mandible consists also of a dorsal supraangular (m), a ventral angular (m), a posterior articular (c), and two bones contributing to its medial surface—the splenial (m) and prearticular (m). At its posterior end, the ramus typically has a medial process and sometimes a retroarticular process.

Lying in the floor of the mouth and below the neurocranium are bones of the tongue and hyoid apparatus, consisting of an entoglossum in the base of the tongue, two median bones—the rostral basibranchial (basihyal) and caudal basibranchial (urohyal)—that often fuse in adults, and a pair of hyoid horns, each consisting of a ceratobranchial and epibranchial. Typically the hyoid horns are long and slender. Some of these elements may remain cartilaginous in the adult.

Ontogeny and Homology

Detailed descriptions of development of the chondrocranium and early ossification exist for a limited number of species (see references in Goldschmid 1972). These studies reveal phenomena that should be documented in more taxonomic groups. Examples are the variable relations of the squamosal to other bones of the braincase and the association of certain membrane bones (vomer, palatine) with cartilaginous elements that ossify and fuse with those bones (Parker 1878, 1879). Another example is the origin of the basipterygoid process, which in galliforms (Jollie 1957) and anseriforms (Hofer 1945) appears late in development as a pad of cartilage on the parasphenoidal rostrum and articulates with the anterior portion of the pterygoid. The basipterygoid process of ratites, tinamous, and various neognathous birds develops early as a cartilaginous projection of the basisphenoid, enclosed later by the parasphenoid; it articulates with the posterior portion of the pterygoid. The process in galliforms and anseriforms may not be homologous with the process from the basisphenoid. The ephemeral occurrence of a basipterygoid process of the basisphenoid in the embryo of many taxa is also of interest: it is known to occur in Spheniscidae, *Balaeniceps* (Balaenicipitidae), *Ciconia* (Ciconiidae), Otididae, Laridae, many Falconiformes, and Coliidae. In birds, loss of the process in the adult probably is derived relative to its presence in the adult; complete loss probably is derived relative to its presence only in the embryo.

The postorbital process in adult birds may be part of the pleurosphenoid, squamosal, or frontal. In development, however, the postorbital process of paleognaths (except *Struthio*, Struthionidae) and neognaths originates as a cartilaginous process of the pleurosphenoid, which may later ossify in the pleurosphenoid or be incorporated into the squamosal.

Thus the postorbital process is homologous in most birds as a cartilaginous projection of the pleurosphenoid (Müller 1964). In *Struthio* there is no postorbital process on the pleurosphenoid; instead it develops in the frontal.

Comparison with Reptiles

Modern birds differ from their reptilian relatives in proportions of the skull, reflecting an enlargement of the brain, eyes, and rostrum, and they lack certain bones and bony processes (figs. 8.4, 8.5). Among these are the postorbital, the postorbital process of the jugal, the squamosal process of the quadratojugal, the ectopterygoid, and the coronoid of the mandible, although a coronoid was identified in embryonic stages of *Taeniopygia* (Estrildidae) by Nemeschkal (1983). Loss of these bones (except the coronoid) and processes may relate to the development of a uniquely avian form of cranial kinesis (prokinesis), which depends on free movement of the quadrate, jugal bars, and palate. Anchoring of the jugal bar by the lacrimal in front of the eye, by the postorbital and jugal process behind the eye, and by firm connection between the quadratojugal and squamosal, would prevent kinesis of the avian type. Firm connection of the pterygoid and jugal bar by the ectopterygoid also could limit kinesis, but reduction of this bone may have been independent of the evolution of avian kinesis (Simonetta 1960).

Basic structure of the skull in *Archaeopteryx* is similar to that of coelurosaurian dinosaurs (Ostrom 1976; Gauthier 1986). Except for differences in shapes of bones, the palates of some living paleognathous birds (rhea, emu) also resemble those of some coelurosaurs (e.g., *Dromaeosaurus;* Colbert and Russell 1969), insofar as such reptilian palates have been reconstructed accurately (fig. 8.4). Bühler (1985) has shown that earlier reconstructions of the skull of *Archaeopteryx* were in error (e.g., Heilmann 1927), in that the brain housing is larger than typically shown, and

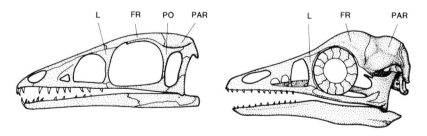

Fig. 8.5. Lateral view of skulls of a coelurosaur, *Compsognathus longipes* (left), and *Archaeopteryx lithographica* (right). Redrawn from Ostrom (1978) and Bühler (1985), respectively. FR, frontal; L, lacrimal; PAR, parietal; PO, postorbital.

a postorbital-jugal bar is lacking (fig. 8.5). He also suggested that avian prokinesis was present in *Archaeopteryx* (although poorly developed), based on an apparent craniofacial hinge and movable quadrate. Prokinesis was present also in the Cretaceous bird *Hesperornis* (Bühler et al. 1988). *Hesperornis* combines features typical of recent birds (quadrate morphology, slender jugal bar, lack of postorbital bar) with the presence of teeth.

PATTERNS OF DIVERSITY

Functional Anatomy, Covariation, and Adaptation

Bill Shape. Development of the rostrum (bill) as an independent, enlarged, and highly variable portion of the skull is characteristic of birds (fig. 8.3), and its shape and structure are highly correlated with foraging methods and food within phylogenetic lines. Many special adaptations (lamellae, hooked tip, crushing plates and ridges) are restricted to the rhamphotheca. The rostra of birds vary in size and shape, density of bone, flexibility, distribution of internal bony trabeculae, and ossification of associated nasal septa and chonchae. External bony nares vary from small (rarely absent) to very large. In the former case the rostrum is largely enclosed and filled with cancellous bone (Hesse 1907; Bignon 1889); in the latter it takes the form of three bars united anteriorly at the rostral symphysis, and closed posteriorly on each side by a postnarial bar (fig. 8.3a). Functional analysis of different bill shapes and internal structure has received some attention (e.g., Bock 1966; Bock and Kummer 1968; Bowman 1961; Guillet et al. 1985; Hofer 1945; Kripp 1935), but more detailed comparisons within monophyletic groups are needed.

Cranial Kinesis and Streptognathism. Manipulation of objects by the bill involves motion of both jaws. The jaws are not wholly independent because both depend on the pivotal quadrate, and they may be coupled further by ligaments or by the mandibular articulation (Bock 1964; Zusi 1967). Motion of the quadrates imparts motion to the jugal bars, palate, and upper jaw, which typically rotates upward or downward about its craniofacial hinge (fig. 8.6). This property—cranial kinesis—is probably universal in the avian skull, despite claims of akinesis in ratites (McDowell 1948), penguins (Spheniscidae; Reid 1835), colies (Coliidae; Schoonees 1963), toucans (Ramphastidae; Höfling and Gasc 1984), and the hawfinch (Fringillidae; Sims 1955). The extent of kinetic mobility of the upper jaw varies widely, and it is indeed limited in some of the above taxa. The most common, and probably ancestral, form of kinesis in birds is prokinesis, in which the upper jaw maintains its shape as it pivots about the craniofacial

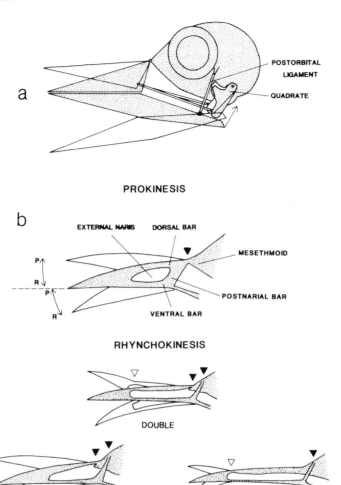

Fig. 8.6. Motion of the jaws in birds (diagrammatic). a. Coordination of jaw movement by force of M. depressor mandibulae (arrow) and shift of quadrate on mandible in presence of postorbital ligament. Modified from Zusi (1967).
B. Protraction (P) and retraction (R) of upper jaw in different forms of cranial kinesis. Solid triangles indicate craniofacial hinges; open triangles indicate other flexible zones. (Modified from Zusi 1984)

hinge (Hérissant 1752; Beecher 1951a; Bock 1964; Bühler 1981). Various forms of rhynchokinesis also occur (Nitzsch 1816, 1817; Hofer 1955; Bühler 1981; Zusi 1984); in all of them some portion of the upper jaw itself changes shape, and in most there are two bending axes in the craniofacial hinge (Zusi 1984; fig. 8.6). Although the basic mechanism of cranial kinesis is similar throughout birds, its permutations involve many differences in the form and occurrence of articulations and bony hinges, and in the shape of bones related to differences in size and attachments of jaw muscles and ligaments. Other modifications of the skull may serve as stops to limit jaw motion (Fisher 1955). The role of the jugal bars in kinesis must vary among birds because, in some, they are stout and in others, threadlike; in the latter, they may coordinate motion of the quadrates and, as tension rods, help to maintain contact between the palate and rostrum during kinesis (Zusi 1962).

The articulation between the quadrate and lower jaw (both of which are movable relative to the neurocranium) typically is a complicated one that permits the lower jaw to rotate dorso-ventrally and latero-medially and to slide back and forth on the quadrate. This articulation tends to promote coordinated motion of the lower jaw and quadrate, synchronizing motion of both jaws; the articulation is specialized for this coupling function in some species (e.g., herons, Ardeidae; some pelecaniform birds; the shoebill, Balaenicipitidae; and frogmouths, Podargidae). Accessory articulations between the mandible and the ectethmoid (Bock and Morioka 1971), basitemporal plate (Bock 1960b), and quadrate (Zusi 1987) occur in some birds.

Many birds display latero-medial flexibility of the lower jaw (streptognathism) in the region of the junction of the dentary and splenial on the one hand, and of the supraangular, angular, and prearticular on the other (Yudin 1961). A mandibular fenestra is often present at this junction. Lateral bowing of the lower jaw requires flexibility of the ramus near the mandibular symphysis as well (fig. 8.7). Streptognathism is well developed in those birds that swallow large objects and that feed their young with the chick's head inside their mouth. Streptognathism reaches its highest specialization in certain aerial insect-eaters whose opened mouth takes the form of a cylinder and serves as a net while feeding. In *Caprimulgus* (Caprimulgidae; Bühler 1970) and *Nyctibius* (Nyctibiidae), for example, the anterior and posterior portions of the rami are strongly differentiated and joined by a well-defined, obliquely oriented hinge, and the symphysis is minute (fig. 8.7b). Upon opening, the pneumatic, inflexible posterior portions spread laterally and rotate, springing the nonpneumatic, flexible distal portion into a bow. Frogmouths, also in the order Caprimulgiformes, lack streptognathism completely (fig. 8.7c), and are not habitual aerial foragers (Serventy 1936). The mandible of pelicans (Pelecanidae) may expand greatly by spreading at the base and bowing of at least the distal half of each ramus, but it lacks the well-defined hinge and the rotation seen in *Caprimulgus*.

The jaw mechanism of birds is powered by the jaw muscles and directed by the articulations, ligaments, and flexible, bony hinges. Not surprisingly, variations of the kinetic mechanism constitute a major source of

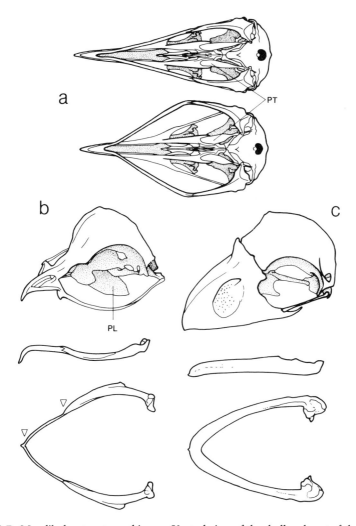

Fig. 8.7. Mandibular streptognathism. a. Ventral view of the skull and part of the pterygoideus muscle of *Larus argentatus* (Laridae) with mandible relaxed (above) and spread (below); redrawn from Yudin (1961). b. Antero-dorso-lateral view of the cranium, and lateral and dorsal views of the mandible of *Nyctibius griseus* (Nyctibiidae). c. *Podargus strigioides* (Podargidae [streptognathism absent]). Triangles indicate bending zones. PL, palatine; PT, M. pterygoideus.

diversity in the avian skull. Various hypotheses on the biological signifi-cance of cranial kinesis in birds have been offered, but few have been tested. Hypotheses include shock absorbing, stabilizing the central axis between the jaws as they open and close, increasing the speed of closing, and increasing the variety of ways in which the jaws may be opposed. One aspect of the latter function is an enhanced capability for grasping at the tip of the bill—a matter of special importance in slender, rhynchokinetic bills (Zusi 1984).

Support and Protection. Much of the basic structure of the cranium relates to its role as a protective package for the brain and associated sense organs, and as a support for the maxillary rostrum. The brain and membranous labyrinth are firmly embedded in a rigid, bony case, but the orbits are more open and less confining for the movable eyes. Among closely related birds, thickness of the orbital septum is inversely related to eye size relative to neurocranial size. Ossification in ligaments, aponeuroses, and membranes that bound and protect the eye may form new configurations such as the suborbital arch (parrots; snipe and woodcock, Scolopacidae) and supraorbital bones (e.g., tinamous). The large eyes of certain aerial insect eaters (Caprimulgiformes) are protected by greatly expanded palatines from the impact of insects on the roof of the opened mouth (fig. 8.7b).

Bones of the skull of birds are pneumatized to varying degrees by airsacs that invade them from the middle ear and nasal regions (Bignon 1889; Witmer 1990). Pneumatic bones are hollow, with walls supported by bony trabeculae (fig. 8.8a). The process of pneumatization, especially in the frontals, may continue long after fledging, providing an indication of immaturity in incompletely pneumatized individuals of some, but not all, species (Winkler 1979). Inflated bones may be uniformly spongy, or they may consist of multiple, thin sheets separated by trabeculae (Bühler 1972); soft structures such as semicircular ducts, nerves, and blood vessels that penetrate cancellous bone are sheathed in bony tubes. Inflation of neurocranial bones provides a high degree of independence in the conformation of their internal and external surfaces. For example, the brain cavity conforms closely to the shape of the brain, but the external surface of the cranium may assume various shapes in support of jaw muscles and ligaments (fig. 8.8). On the other hand, pneumaticity may be essentially absent, presumably reducing bouyancy and increasing resistance to pressure in certain aquatic birds that swim and forage underwater (e.g., penguins, loons [Gaviidae], grebes [Podicipedidae], diving petrels [Pelecanoididae], cormorants, mergansers [Anatidae], alcids [Alcidae]).

Many organs are supported on the surface of the skull and leave their mark on it (glands, integumentary sense organs, blood vessels, nerves, muscles, ligaments, and the hyoid apparatus). Striking examples are depressions of nasal glands in the supraorbital rim or orbit (Bock 1958; Siegel-Causey 1990), prominence of the temporal fossae and associated crests and processes as they relate to development of jaw muscles (Klaauw 1963), and pits that house tactile sense organs at the tip of the rostrum (Clara 1925; Bolze 1968; fig. 8.3b). The hyoid horns of most woodpeckers

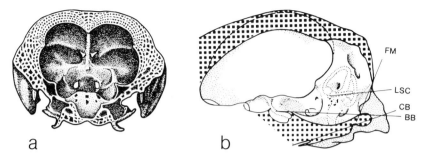

Fig. 8.8. Internal features of the avian skull. a. Transverse section through neurocranium of *Asio otus* (Strigidae), posterior view (redrawn from Gadow and Selenka 1891), showing spongy bone. b. Neurocranium of *Ara macao* (Psittacidae) sectioned midsagittally, left view; lines show angular relationships of base of brain (BB), base of cranium (CB), foramen magnum (FM), and lateral semicircular canal (LSC). Outline of membranous labyrinth dotted. Sectioned bone diagrammatic. (Modified from Werner 1963)

(Picidae) and hummingbirds (Trochilidae) are greatly elongated, curving dorsally and anteriorly over the neurocranium. They enter the bony nares on one side of the maxilla in certain hummingbirds, causing asymmetry of the base of the maxilla (Graves and Zusi 1990). In some species of penguins, an unusually thick and fleshy tongue is associated with an enlarged mouth cavity formed by deep mandibular rami (Zusi 1975; fig. 8.3e).

Orientation of the Skull and Its Parts. The position or angle of one portion of the skull relative to another is highly variable among birds (Duijm 1951; fig. 8.8b). Such comparisons have led some workers (Pycraft 1908; Cobb 1959) to claim that the ear of the woodcock lies uniquely anterior to the eye (fig. 8.3b); this conclusion follows if comparisons are made with the long axis of the bill horizontal. Thompson (1907), Marinelli (1928), and others have pointed out that other baselines provide a more meaningful comparison; the ear of the woodcock (*Scolopax*) lies behind the eye as in other birds, and the bill tilts downward, when the basitemporal plate is horizontal. Duijm (1951) provided a biological basis for the importance of certain baselines, supporting Marinelli's idea. He found that birds in an alert stance hold their heads with the lateral semicircular canals roughly parallel to the horizon and that the plane of the basitemporal plate approximates that of the lateral canals; by contrast, the angle of the bill to the horizon differs greatly in different species.

The topic (and terminology) of angular relationships of cranial parts and their significance has become increasingly complicated since Marinelli (1928) proposed the term "streckschadel" for birds whose bill was in line with the base of the brain, and "knickschadel" for those with the bill angled downward. Hofer (1945), Duijm (1951), Barnikol (1952), Lang (1952), Starck (1955), Werner (1963) and others have added variables, proposed more skull types, and debated the influence on cranial morphology of eye size, eye position and orientation, brain size and shape, orientation of the foramen magnum, position of the bill in foraging, development of jaw muscles, and allometry. Functional interpretations among distantly related groups are obscured by differences that have no adaptive explanation, but that reflect different ancestries.

Cranial Ornamentation. Birds respond to visual cues provided by the appearance of other individuals of their own and related species. Such cues include variation in plumage (structure, pattern, and color), exposed skin (structure and color), and probably differences in shape of the bill and head. The latter may be supported by bone in the form of cranial casques (cassowary), projections on the maxilla (currasows, Cracidae; hornbills, Bucerotidae) or highly inflated rostra marked with striking color patterns (toucans). Most of these enlargements (fig. 8.3d, f) consist of spongy bone and are extremely light. One exception is the more heavily ossified and cornified casque of the helmeted hornbill (*Rhinoplax vigil:* Bucerotidae). Modifications of the upper jaw or neurocranium, no matter how extensive, are always structured to preserve cranial kinesis (Hofer 1955).

Allometry. Allometric changes in size and shape are a pervasive aspect of vertebrate development. Adult members of a single population or of related species also may show size-related patterns in their proportions. A few examples of allometry in the avian skull are presented here.

Using skull length as an index of size in crows and jays (Corvidae), Schuh (1968) found a positively allometric lengthening of the bill and a negative allometry of brain volume among species. He also found intraspecific differences: a larger skull had a disproportionately longer bill and relatively reduced length, depth, and width of the neurocranium. In the Corvidae, Anatidae, and other groups, size of the occipital condyle relative to width of the foramen magnum and neurocranial dimensions varies allometrically, but the coefficients differ considerably among groups (Werner 1962). Werner (1963) also noted a positive allometry in amount of bone tissue of the braincase and its internal partitions. Deviations of certain cranial features from general allometric patterns in woodpeckers may be adaptations for increased force of pounding (Rüger 1972).

In the Galapagos finch genus *Geospiza* (Emberizidae), beak size varies allometrically with body size between and within some species. Bill dimensions (three measurements) vary isometrically within populations, but bill shape differs considerably (length/width) between species, partly because of differences in growth rates of those bill dimensions in different species.

Allometric patterns within populations do not necessarily parallel interspecific allometry (Grant 1986).

Phylogeny

Morphological diversity may be analyzed to produce phylogenetic trees that represent approximations of a true, branching sequence of evolutionary events. Although an accurate phylogenetic framework would be the best basis for interpreting patterns of diversity in the avian skull, well-corroborated phylogenies are rare.

The primary bases for present classifications of extant birds are the monographic works on avian anatomy by Fürbringer (1888) and Gadow and Selenka (1891). These works describe morphological variation among avian orders, families, and subfamilies, but despite the great range in size and shape of bird skulls, few characteristics grouped birds at the ordinal and familial levels (Gadow 1892). Most useful were the shape and extent of the posterior border of the narial opening (holorhinal versus schizorhinal nares), the presence or absence of a solid nasal septum (impervious versus pervious septum), presence or absence of the basipterygoid process, the presence of a single or double neurocranial articulation of the quadrate, and the type of palate. It was apparent, however, that similar states of these features were not necessarily homologous throughout birds. Convergent and parallel evolution as well as evolutionary reversal continue to impede efforts to construct phylogenetic patterns from the analysis of morphological features.

Studies on avian phylogeny based on DNA hybridization by C. G. Sibley and J. E. Ahlquist, beginning in 1980 and summarized in Sibley and Ahlquist (1990), attempted to circumvent the problem of convergence, but their techniques were subject to criticisms (Cracraft 1987; Houde 1987; Sarich et al. 1989). Nevertheless, some of their phylogenetic hypotheses and some molecular and anatomical studies by other workers provide frameworks in which evolution of the skull could be studied. In addition, recent works on Jurassic, Cretaceous, and early Tertiary birds and their reptilian relatives are providing data for out-group comparisons with recent birds (e.g., Ostrom 1976; Martin 1983; Cracraft 1986; Gauthier 1986; Bühler et al. 1988; Houde 1988; Witmer 1990; Elzanowski 1991; Elzanowski and Galton 1991). Unfortunately the gains in this field are tempered by controversy resulting from poor preservation of fossil material and serious gaps in the fossil record.

An ambitious attempt to find patterns in cranial morphology as a basis for avian classification was T. H. Huxley's classic study of the bony palate (Huxley 1867). He distinguished four types of palate—dromaeognathous (paleognathous), schizognathous, desmognathous, and aegithognathous (fig. 8.4). Pycraft (1900) included ratites with the tinamous under the dromaeognathous palate and renamed it "paleognathous." These types continue to influence avian classification. Raikow (1982) listed the aegithognathous palate as a synapomorphy of the Passeriformes, and Bock (1963) used an expanded concept of the paleognathous palate to support monophyly of the ratites and tinamous. Nevertheless, all but the first of Huxley's major taxa defined largely by the palate are now rendered polyphyletic by traditional classification and by Sibley and Ahlquist (1990), and monophyly of the paleognathous birds is disputed. The paleognathous palate has received more scrutiny than the others because the ratites and tinamous are a special problem in avian classification (Olson 1985). The major phylogenetic questions are whether or not they are sister taxa to all other extant birds, and whether or not they are monophyletic.

Huxley (1867) defined the paleognathous (dromaeognathous) palate as follows: (1) vomer broad and separating the palatine and pterygoid from articulation with the parasphenoidal rostrum, (2) basipterygoid process from basisphenoid articulates with caudal portion of pterygoid, (3) single cranial articular head of quadrate. Pycraft (1900) added the lack of segmentation of the pterygoid and its union with the vomer (except in *Struthio*) to the definition. McDowell (1948) studied the paleognathous palate, emphasizing differences among the several families of ratites, and concluded that many features were too diverse to permit its definition. After redefining the paleognathous palate, Bock (1963) concluded on the basis of its complexity and associated features that it was homologous among paleognathous birds and that they were monophyletic. He suggested that the paleognathous palate evolved from a neognathous one as an adaptation to an unknown feeding method.

Clearly, the paleognathous palate has been defined somewhat differently by almost every author who has studied it. If the palate is to support a hypothesis of monophyly of ratites and tinamous, its features must be analyzed separately and some must be found synapomorphous for the group. This conclusion would require a knowledge of relevant out-groups (Maddison et al. 1984), which, according to Sibley and Ahlquist (1990) would be among extant birds. But if paleognaths are sister taxa to all other living birds, the relevant out-groups are extinct and may be unknowable.

Despite a recent resurgence of interest in avian phylogeny and systematics, some of the best comparative and functional anatomical studies are of taxa that lack highly corroborated phylogenies. Nevertheless, I shall use a few such examples to illustrate factors other than phylogeny that influence patterns of avian diversity.

Divergence and Parallelism

The 14 species of Galapagos finches (Emberizidae) endemic to the Galapagos archipelago and Cocos Island apparently diverged from a common ancestor no more than five million years ago, and probably much more recently (Grant 1986). The finches now include three genera on the archipelago and one monotypic genus on Cocos Island (Paynter 1970), and they have evolved some striking differences in cranial shape (fig. 8.9). Bowman's analysis of morphological variation within the Galapagos finches (or Darwin's finches) provides a basis for discussion of divergence and parallelism in shape of the bill and cranium at the generic and specific levels (Bowman 1961). Similarities in plumage, behavior, and morphology unite the Galapagos finches and separate them from finches on the New World mainland. The Galapagos finches are not ideal subjects for analysis of evolutionary radiation because their sister taxon is disputed, phylogenies of the group vary, and even some species limits are not clear. Nevertheless, we can safely say that the patterns of morphological diversity in two genera of this monophyletic group are remarkably similar (fig. 8.9).

Figure 8.10 illustrates morphoclines in cranial attributes of nine species of finch representing three genera: four species of *Geospiza,* four of *Camarhynchus* (including *Platyspiza* and *Cactospiza*), and *Certhidea olivacea.* The genera are distinguished by plumage pattern and color, by subtle aspects of bill shape (Lack 1947), and by genetic distance based on protein electrophoresis (Yang and Patton 1981). The shape of the bill in *Geospiza* is typically conical, with relatively straight dorsal and ventral profiles, and a deep base. That of *Camarhynchus* is more parrotlike, with more decurved dorsal and recurved ventral profiles, and a moderately deep base. *Geospiza scandens* and *Camarhynchus pallida* have relatively long bills, but the subtle differences in curvature persist; *Certhidea* has a slender and slightly decurved bill. Within *Geospiza* and *Camarhynchus* the species differ in size and stoutness of bill (figs. 8.9, 8.10). In both genera, species with more massive (relatively deeper) jaws also have larger jaw muscles, stronger bony processes and crests, a relatively larger skull, relatively smaller eyes, a more down-angled bill, a more posteriorly situated quadrate, and a thicker interorbital septum (Bowman 1961). As a small, slender-billed species, *Certhidea olivacea* represents an extreme in the opposite direction.

Diversity at the generic and specific levels correlates with feeding habits, and this correlation has a basis in functional anatomy. *Certhidea* eats soft foods and uses its slender bill as a forceps and for probing vegetation and cracks in bark. The long-billed *Geospiza scandens* eats moderately hard seeds, soft plant tissues, and nectar. *Camarhynchus pallida* often obtains insects by probing with a stick or spine. In general, *Geospiza* crushes hard seeds at the base of the bill, whereas *Camarhynchus* bites with the tip into woody tissues of trees and shrubs in search of insects; the deep base of the former and the curved profile of the latter reduce the fracture risk of the bill under different stresses. Within the stout-billed genera, larger-billed species can crush harder seeds or manipulate harder substrates

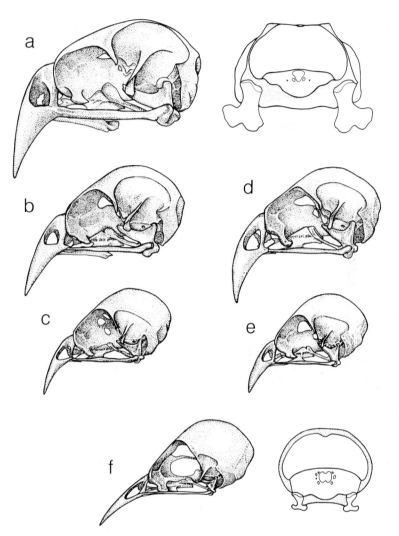

Fig. 8.9. Cranial diversity in Galapagos finches (Emberizidae). a. Lateral view of *Geospiza magnirostris* (and semidiagrammatic transverse section on right). b. *G. fortis*. c. *G. fuliginosa*, d. *Camarhynchus crassirostris*. e. *C. parvulus*. f. *Certhidea olivacea* (semidiagrammatic transverse section on right). (a) and (f) represent extremes in cranial differentiation; (b-c) and d-e) show parallel morphologies. (a-e) drawn to same scale, (f) enlarged. (Redrawn from Bowman 1961).

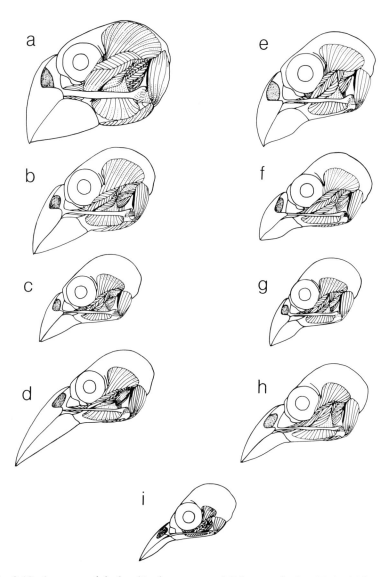

Fig. 8.10. Anatomy of the head in three genera of Galapagos finches (Emberizidae).
a. *Geospiza magnirostris*. b. *G. fortis*. c. *G. fuliginosa*. d. *G. scandens*.
e. *Camarhynchus crassirostris*. f. *C. psittacula*. g. *C. parvulus*. h. *C. pallida*.
i. *Certhidea olivacea*. All drawings to same scale. (Redrawn from Bowman 1961)

(Bowman 1961; Abbott et al. 1977). Boag and Grant (1981) showed that deeper-billed individuals of *G. fortis* survived better during drought years when hard seeds predominated.

In the Galapagos finches, divergent evolution within sister genera has produced similar patterns of complex cranial changes associated with size of the bill and jaw muscles. These patterns eventually may be explained in part by allometric growth. However, parallelism in morphoclines does not imply similar directions of evolution, and it may obscure true branching patterns. A phylogeny of *Geospiza* and *Camarhynchus* by Schluter (1984) indicates that neither genus underwent a simple phylogenetic progression from small to large bill.

A somewhat similar, but intraspecific, variation has been found in African seed eaters of the genus *Pyrinestes* (Estrildidae). A small-billed and a large-billed morph occur in each of three species, independent of sex or age. In one species "large-billed morphs readily crack large, hard seeds while small-billed morphs do so with difficulty and prefer not to feed on them" (Smith 1987, 718). Many differences in cranial structure accompany differences in bill size within the species (R. Zusi, personal observation).

Multiple Evolutionary Solutions and Nonadaptive Changes

Different morphological adaptations to the same biological role may be found within an order, and even within a subfamily. This is exemplified by skull structure in owls (Strigiformes). Owls are mostly crepuscular and nocturnal foragers that rely on their ears as well as their eyes for locating prey. Their eyes are oriented forward, increasing binocularity of vision. The broad, flattened postorbital process is expanded laterally and ventrally to extend the orbit as protection for the eye (fig. 8.11). The quadrate and external auditory meatus lie between the postorbital process and the tympanic wing of the exoccipital and squamosal. In more specialized forms, these wings curve antero-laterally and expand dorsally to form a shell around the posterior portion of the ear opening. The integumentary ear opening is modified by preaural and postaural folds, each supporting fans of specialized feathers. These modifications serve to collect and focus sound waves into the external auditory meatus. Further specialization of the external ear includes bilateral asymmetry in some species, which improves vertical sound location based on binaural intensity comparison (Norberg 1978).

Norberg (1977) studied species from nine genera—all of those known to have bilaterally asymmetrical external ears. Soft structures that exhibited bilateral asymmetry in size, shape, or position were the borders of the ear apertures, preaural skin folds, and an intraaural dermal septum. In the skull, the two ear apertures differed in shape and orientation owing to differences in the tympanic wings (*Aegolius*, Strigidae) or in the tympanic wings and postorbital processes (*Strix nebulosa,* Strigidae). Asymmetry was restricted to soft structures in seven genera and most species of another (*Strix*); it included soft structures and the skull in two other species of *Strix,* and affected only the skull in *Aegolius.* Variation in soft tissue asymmetry occurred in three different patterns plus several subpatterns. Norberg concluded that ear asymmetry is in a phase of rapid evolution and experimentation in *Strix,* and that it is stabilized in other genera. He recognized at least five cases of independent origin of asymmetry in owls, and at least three separate instances of intergeneric convergence, each involving a different asymmetric configuration.

Norberg's analysis was made in the context of a classification based on external features, especially the relative size of ear openings (Peters 1940), which might invalidate his conclusions about evolution of the ear. However, another classification based on comparison of the entire skeleton (Ford 1967) agreed essentially with that of Peters (1940), but included *Ciccaba* with *Strix,* and *Rhinoptynx* and *Pseudoscops* with *Asio*—changes that do not affect Norberg's major conclusions.

Modification of the tympanic wing affects the configuration of the temporal portion of the adductor mandibulae externus muscle (fig. 8.12). In less specialized owls, as in many other birds, the muscle originates in a temporal fossa and passes between the postorbital and zygomatic processes to its insertion on the mandible (fig. 8.12a, b). In the temporal region its fibers converge on a long, central aponeurosis that becomes a tendon toward its insertion. Dorsal and anterior expansion of the tympanic wing encroaches on the muscle, compressing it dorsad such that it changes direction abruptly in its midportion (*Athene,* Strigidae; Barnikol 1952). In *Aegolius* the wings encroach further, enclosing part of the muscle in a foramen. The muscle originates as a small belly from the temporal fossa of the cranium, passes through the foramen as a tendon, and abruptly angles ventrad. A second, larger belly supplies the tendon behind the broad, crescentic postorbital processes (Norberg 1978). The digastric form of this muscle in certain owls is unique among birds, and it is functionally related to passage through a foramen and abrupt change in direction. The muscle is further reduced in *Asio* (Strigidae) and *Tyto* (Tytonidae), where it consists of a single slender belly lying behind the postorbital process (Barnikol 1952; Starck and Barnikol 1954). In these genera the tympanic wing forms a vertical flange that isolates the external auditory meatus from the postero-lateral wall of the braincase.

The precise evolutionary pathways of morphological change in the external ear and adductor muscle of owls are not known, but asymmetry of the ear is probably adapted to a common function. Changes in the adductor muscle may be essentially nonadaptive, and explainable mainly as side effects of evolutionary experimentation in the external ear.

Evolutionary Novelty

In this section I shall consider the evolution of new structures in the skull of parrots, their relation to major innovations in jaw musculature, and the reciprocal effect of muscle innovations on the skull.

Parrots have a highly distinctive cranial morphology, unique among birds (fig. 8.13); the maxillary rostrum is deep and decurved; the mandible

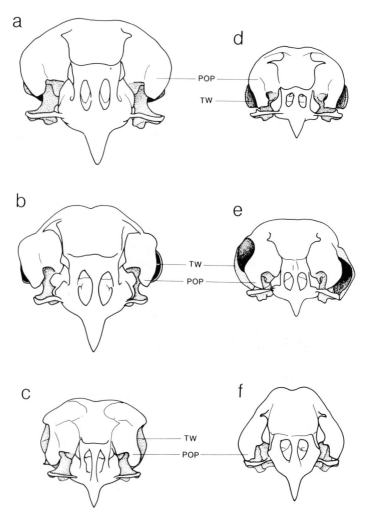

Fig. 8.11. Crania of owls (Strigiformes) in anterior view. a. *Bubo virginianus*. b. *Strix nebulosa*. c. *Asio otus*. d. *Athene noctua*. e. *Aegolius funereus*. f. *Tyto alba*. Note diverse shapes of postorbital processes (POP); bilateral asymmetry occurs predominantly in tympanic wings (TW).

is deep, broader than the maxilla, and strongly truncate and scoop-shaped; the palatines are large, bladelike, vertically oriented, and produced ventrally; the mandibular articulation of the quadrate is a single, semicircular articular condyle; and the foot of the lacrimal (suborbital process) projects posteriorly beneath the eye. In addition, they have a unique jaw muscle, the ethmomandibularis, that extends from the ethmoid portion of the interorbital septum ventrad to the mandible (fig. 8.13a, b, g). Cranial kinesis is highly developed, and all attachments of the upper jaw (cranial, jugal, palatal) are represented by well-developed syndesmoses or elastic zones. Although parrots eat a variety of soft fruits and some eat nectar, virtually

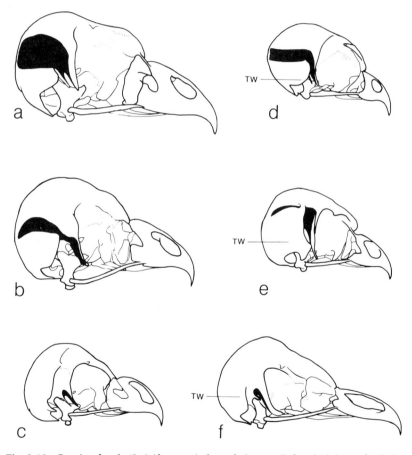

Fig. 8.12. Crania of owls (Strigiformes) in lateral view. a. *Bubo virginianus*. b. *Strix nebulosa*. c. *Asio otus*. d. *Athene noctua*. e. *Aegolius funereus*. f. *Tyto alba*. Attachment of M. adductor mandibulae externus, rostralis temporalis, shaded. TW, tympanic wing.

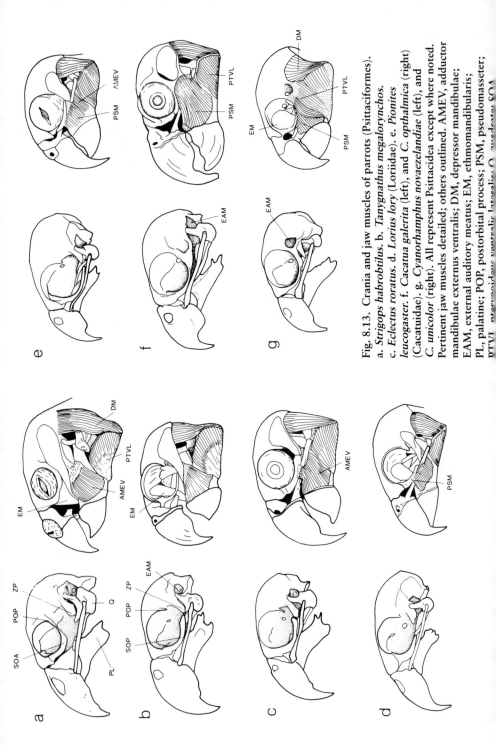

Fig. 8.13. Crania and jaw muscles of parrots (Psittaciformes). a. *Strigops habroptilus*. b. *Tanygnathus megalorynchos*. c. *Eclectus roratus*. d. *Lorius lory* (Loriidae). e. *Prioniturus leucogaster*. f. *Cacatua galerita* (left), and *C. opthalmica* (right) (Cacatuidae). g. *Cyanorhamphus novaezelandiae* (left), and *C. unicolor* (right). All represent Psittacidea except where noted. Pertinent jaw muscles detailed; others outlined. AMEV, adductor mandibulae externus ventralis; DM, depressor mandibulae; EAM, external auditory meatus; EM, ethmomandibularis; PL, palatine; POP, postorbital process; PSM, pseudomasseter; PTVL, pterygoideus ventralis lateralis; Q, quadrate; SOA

all of them shell seeds with the anterior edge of the mandibular rostrum while the seed is wedged against a ridge of the maxillary rostrum and manipulated by the tongue.

Many variations in cranial structure occur within the Psittaciformes (Thompson 1899; Smith 1975; fig. 8.13). In some species the suborbital process of the lacrimal is long, supporting the eye from below; in others it fuses with an elongate postorbital process, forming an orbital fenestra bounded by a complete suborbital arch that is positioned lateral or dorsolateral to the jugal bar. In the most specialized species, the zygomatic process fuses with the suborbital arch, producing a temporal fenestra. These bony arches are essentially ossifications of ligamentous sheets found in other species. Orbital and temporal fenestrae are unusual in birds, and their ossified boundaries provide a new configuration for muscle attachment in parrots.

The suborbital arch has evolved repeatedly in different phyletic lines of parrots (Thompson 1899; Smith 1975). In some it serves for muscle attachment and in others it does not. In *Strigops, Tanygnathus,* and *Psittacula* (Psittacidae), as in most birds, the adductor mandibulae externus ventralis muscle (= adductor externus medius) extends from the zygomatic process of the squamosal to the lateral surface of the mandibular ramus (Hofer 1945, 1953; Dubale and Rawal 1965). The jugal bar presses against the lateral surface of this muscle. Some of the dorsal fibers of the muscle may attach on the suborbital arch medial to the jugal bar (*Eclectus,* Psittacidae; fig. 8.13c). In other parrots, an aponeurotic sheet from the ventral edge of the suborbital process or arch meets the lateral surface of the aponeurosis of origin of the adductor mandibulae externus ventralis, forming a sling around the jugal bar. Anterior fibers of that muscle extend their dorsal attachment via the aponeurotic sheet to the suborbital process or arch, lateral to the jugal bar (*Lorius,* Loriidae; *Pionites,* Psittacidae; fig. 8.13d, e). The new belly, often called "pseudomasseter," is large, well defined, and separate from the parent muscle in various parrots (e.g., *Pionites; Cacatua,* Cacatuidae; Hofer 1950). Its attachments provide a more anterior origin and insertion than that of adductor mandibulae externus ventralis. In *Cacatua* and *Probosciger* (Cacatuidae) fusion of the zygomatic process with the suborbital arch provides additional attachment for the pseudomasseter, which expands posteriorly onto the zygomatic process (Gadow and Selenka 1891; Hofer 1950; fig. 8.13f). The muscle matches its progenitor in size but lies wholly lateral to the jugal bar, which now passes through a tunnel of muscle tissue.

A second "new" muscle attaches on the posterior portion of the orbital arch and zygomatic process in *Cyanorhamphus* (Psittacidae; Hofer 1950; Burton 1974c). It represents an anterior belly of pterygoideus ventralis lateralis, a muscle that, in other parrots, passes ventrad from the palatine around the postero-ventral edge of the mandibular ramus to its postero-lateral surface. The new belly in *Cyanorhamphus* extends beyond the mandible to the suborbital arch and zygomatic process, forming a sling under the mandibular ramus (fig. 8.13g). Burton (1974c) reported a similar innovation in the tooth-billed pigeon (*Didunculus*), a species that lacks a suborbital arch, but in which the postorbital and zygomatic processes are fused.

In some parrots the cranial attachment of a deep portion of the depressor mandibulae expands anteriorly, encroaching on the external auditory meatus (e.g., *Neophema; Psephotus; Platycercus,* Psittacidae). *Cyanorhamphus* is further derived in that the region of the external auditory meatus is covered by muscles, and the meatus walled over with bone, creating a tube and shifting the bony meatus uniquely dorsal to the quadrate (fig. 8.13).

These osteological experiments include the evolution of new bony bars, cranial fenestrae, and a tubular auditory meatus that opens in a unique location. New osteological configurations allow opportunistic shifts of muscle attachment in the adductor, the pterygoideus, and the depressor muscles, which probably influence further osteological modification. The new muscles, including the ethmomandibularis, constitute major deviations from typical avian jaw musculature, extending the surfaces of attachment of several muscles. Except for the depressor mandibulae, all of the changes produce greater torque for adducting the mandible because of their distal attachments and favorable angles of pull. The pseudomasseter may also pull the mandible forward (Burton 1974a), a function limited to parts of the pterygoideus complex in other birds. Novelties of the skull and jaw muscles of parrots remain within the functional requirements of traditional avian prokinesis, although they may promote unusual independence of jaw action. To judge from current classifications of parrots (Forshaw and Cooper 1973; Smith 1975; Homberger 1980), evolution of similar osteological and myological novelties has occurred repeatedly within the order, but the details of the evolutionary pattern must await a robust phylogeny of parrots.

Convergence: Case 1

Convergent evolution occurs between orders and families of birds, and it is frequent at lower taxonomic levels where it blends with parallelism. Similar adaptations for forceful opening of the jaws against resistance evolved repeatedly within the Passeriformes and within the Charadrii. The behavior, known as gaping, is used in foraging to part the substrate and reveal hidden prey. It correlates highly with a well-defined functional complex of the skull that includes a powerful mechanism for protracting the upper jaw and depressing the lower, a bill that effectively penetrates and

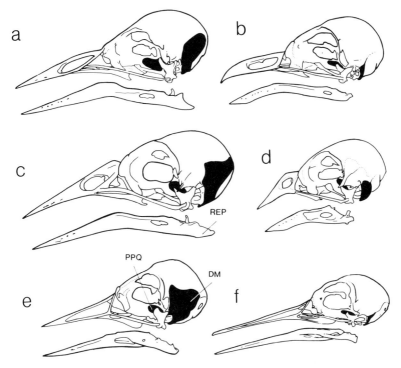

Fig. 8.14. Skulls of gapers (left) and nongapers (right). a. *Sturnus vulgaris*. b. *Aplonis metallica* (Sturnidae). c. *Sturnella neglecta*. d. *Dolichonyx oryzivorus* (Icteridae). e. *Arenaria interpres*. f. *Actitis macularia* (Scolopacidae). Attachments of depressor mandibulae and protractor pterygoidei et quadrati shaded. DM, depressor mandibulae; PPQ, protractor pterygoidei et quadrati; REP, retroarticular process.

moves the substrate, and an orientation of the eyes that increases binocularity at close range (Oehme 1962). Close binocular vision requires a narrow antorbital region of the skull. Parting the substrate is accomplished best by a bill that is at least moderately long, somewhat conical, and has straight dorsal and ventral profiles (fig. 8.14). A shield at the base of the bill may extend the dorsal profile of the maxilla. Depression of the mandible is effected by the depressor mandibulae muscle acting on the retroarticular process of the mandible, and raising of the maxilla is effected by the protractor pterygoidei et quadrati muscle, which connects the quadrate and pterygoid with the interorbital septum. A long retroarticular process and extensive muscle scar on the braincase indicate an enlarged depressor muscle; an enlarged scar of the protractor on the septum and a strong process for its attachment on the pterygoid reflect enlargement of the protractor (fig. 8.14). However, an inference of gaping from skull structure is complicated by the dual role of the depressor mandibulae (Zusi 1967;

Bock 1968; Zweers 1974)—depressing the lower jaw and raising the upper. Anterior extension of the origin of the depressor on the lateral side of the cranium in some species appears to enhance its role in raising the upper jaw by changing the direction of its force on the mandible (Zusi 1967). Some species with this form of the muscle have a relatively unmodified protractor; those without it may have a much enlarged protractor.

Gaping as a foraging technique has evolved in several passerine phyletic lines: Thraupinae (Emberizidae; Beecher 1951b; Zusi 1967), Drepanididae (Richards and Bock 1973), Callaeidae (Burton 1974a), Sturnidae (Lorenz 1949; Beecher 1978), Corvidae (Goodwin 1986; Zusi 1987), and many genera of Icteridae (Beecher 1951a). All of these birds are prokinetic. In the Icteridae (American blackbirds, orioles, meadowlarks, oropendolas, caciques, etc.), the adaptation is widespread in the subfamily and may have evolved early in the phyletic line. Gaping serves icterids variously to part the soil and grass, separate leaves of bromeliads and other plants, open curled leaves, moss, plant debris, and loose bark, pry open wood, and open flowers and fruits; as such it serves as a basis for adaptive radiation in the subfamily (Beecher 1951a). Outside the Passeriformes, strong gaping is found in the prokinetic hoopoes (Upupidae) and woodhoopoes (Phoeniculidae; Burton 1984), and in certain rhynchokinetic shorebirds (Scolopacidae, Haematopodidae; Burton 1974b).

As explained above, two configurations of the protractor and depressor muscles serve to increase the force of gaping: enlarged depressor/normal protractor, and enlarged depressor/enlarged protractor (Zusi 1959). Examples of the former are *Icterus* (Icteridae), *Heterolocha* (Callaeidae), and *Arenaria* (Scolopacidae), and of the latter, *Sturnus* (Sturnidae), *Phoeniculus* (Phoeniculidae), and *Limnodromus, Gallinago,* and *Scolopax* (Scolopacidae). Evolution of the complex has produced many similar features in the skulls of unrelated groups, and two basic configurations of the jaw muscles. Individual features of the gaping complex have evolved in nongapers for other purposes (e.g., enlarged protractor muscle and straight profile of the jaws in woodpeckers; enlarged depressor mandibulae muscle and retroarticular process of the mandible in parrots).

Convergence: Case 2

Garrod (1873) described two types of narial openings—holorhinal and schizorhinal—and applied them to the higher-level classification of birds. Holorhiny was defined by a rounded posterior border of the nares that stopped short of the craniofacial hinge and of the posterior limit of the nasal process of the premaxillary. Schizorhinal nares typically end in a narrow fissure that reaches back to or beyond the posterior limit of the nasal process and beyond the medial portion of the craniofacial hinge

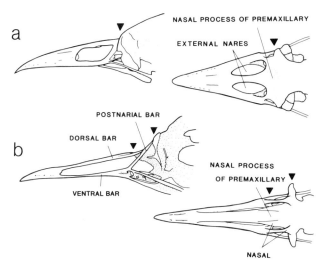

Fig. 8.15. Holorhiny and schizorhiny. a. Holorhinal nares (*Cyanocitta stelleri,* Corvidae). b. Schizorhinal nares (*Pluvialis squatarola,* Charadriidae). Lateral views are on the left and dorsal views on the right. Solid triangles show position of craniofacial hinge. (Modified from Zusi 1984)

(fig. 8.15). Functional analysis has shed light on the biological significance of holorhiny and schizorhiny.

The extended nares of schizorhiny separate the maxillary and premaxillary processes of the nasal such that the maxillary process can rotate about its neurocranial attachment independent of the premaxillary process. This property was noted by Hofer (1955), Marinelli (1928), and others, and linked to rhynchokinesis, which requires independent movement of the ventral bar of the maxilla as a means of changing the shape of the upper jaw. By contrast, the holorhinal construction maintains the dorsal and ventral bars in a constant relationship during prokinesis. An important consequence of schizorhiny is the presence of two transverse bending axes in the region of the craniofacial hinge (fig. 8.15b; Zusi 1984). Apparently this results from an evolutionary anterior shift of the medial portion of the craniofacial hinge.

The presence of two hinge axes imposes requirements on the kinetic structure of the upper jaw; the maxilla must be flexible in one or more additional places to facilitate kinesis, and limits are placed on the number and position of bony hinges in the upper jaw. Within these limitations, different hinge patterns produce different forms of rhynchokinesis (Bühler 1981; Zusi 1984; fig. 8.6). Each form has functional properties that can be related to foraging behavior. Double rhynchokinesis is most suitable for

bill-tip grasping during forceps feeding or shallow probing; distal rhynchokinesis is most suitable for deep probing and is restricted to shorebirds
(Scolopacidae; Haematopodidae) and kiwis; proximal rhynchokinesis permits a variety of forceful feeding methods such as pounding and manipulating hard prey and is thus more widespread than distal rhynchokinesis
(Zusi 1984). There is little doubt that distal rhynchokinesis evolved repeatedly from double rhynchokinesis within Charadriiformes, and that
proximal rhynchokinesis evolved from double rhynchokinesis in a variety
of orders and families (fig. 8.16e–h). Convergence in the hinge pattern of
proximal rhynchokinesis is easily overlooked because of its association
with widely divergent forms of the maxilla in unrelated birds. An explanation of proximal rhynchokinesis in each case must include its evolutionary history; explanations based on functional anatomy alone would be
incomplete because the species involved could probably feed as efficiently
with a prokinetic maxilla.

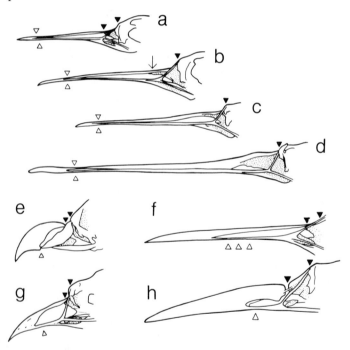

Fig. 8.16. Hinge patterns of rhynchokinesis. Double rhynchokinesis (a, *Actitis
macularia*, Scolopacidae); distal rhynchokinesis (b, *Philomachus pugnax*; c, *Calidris
alpina*; d, *Limnodromus griseus*, Scolopacidae); proximal rhynchokinesis
(e, *Didunculus strigirostris*, Columbidae; f, *Aramus guarauna*, Aramidae; g, *Chionis
alba*, Chionididae; h, *Rynchops niger*, Rynchopidae). Solid triangles show position
of craniofacial hinge; open triangles show other flexible zones. (Modified from
Zusi 1984)

Functional-Morphological Constraints

Configurations of bony hinges in the rhynchokinetic maxilla are limited to those that would not block kinesis or cause useless jaw motions. Evolution of distal rhynchokinesis by a gradual shift of a bony hinge from the base of the maxilla toward its tip has been suggested by several workers. However, such a shift would produce unacceptable kinetic consequences at certain stages—downward rotation of the bill tip during protraction of the upper jaw, upward rotation during retraction, or both. Instead, evolution probably occurred by simple loss of hinges from a generalized hinge pattern (fig. 8.16a–d; Zusi 1984).

Many avian jaw muscles are "two-joint muscles," in which the movable quadrate lies between their origin and insertion; as a result these muscles tend to move both jaws. The presence of a postorbital ligament and the configuration of the jaw articulation tend to couple the action of the jaws (Bock 1964; Zusi 1967; fig. 8.6a). Hypothetical configurations of the jaw mechanism differing little from those found in birds would neutralize the action of the depressor mandibulae, such that its contraction would be isometric—stressing, but not moving, the kinetic mechanism and mandible. Other hypothetical configurations would produce meaningless jaw motions such as simultaneous raising of both jaws (Zusi 1967). Such constraints on morphological variation in birds have been little studied.

FUTURE DIRECTIONS

In this chapter I have presented several patterns of morphological diversity of the avian skull. Conclusions concerning adaptation from these examples are limited in their precision by the absence of detailed phylogenetic hypotheses (Coddington 1988), but they serve to illustrate the prevalence of divergent, parallel, and convergent evolution of morphological features at various taxonomic levels. This in turn may explain why Fürbringer and Gadow found so few cranial features by which to define the major groups of birds.

Patterns of morphological diversity do not address directly the process or mechanism of diversification. Studies of pattern and process approach each other most closely at lower taxonomic levels when focused on the earliest stages of differentiation—birds of common parentage in studies of heritability, and local populations in the estimation of gene flow and morphological differentiation. Comprehensive analyses of variation in skull structure at these levels have not been done.

Limited aspects of morphological diversity have been used to address such topics as community structure (Hespenheide 1973; Ricklefs and Travis 1980), competition and character displacement (Schluter et al.

1985), adaptive variation in species populations (Johnson and Selander 1971), and morphological diversity in birds and mammals (Wyles et al. 1983; Hafner et al. 1984). These studies usually emphasize bill measurements and tell us little about cranial diversity, but they address important questions and offer hypotheses. The hypotheses should be tested against a wider range of pertinent morphological data.

The analysis of patterns of diversity at higher taxonomic levels depends on a good understanding of the phylogenetic relationships of most avian orders. The avian skull could play a major role in phylogenetic analysis if new characters and anatomical evidence for homology of their states were found. To this end we need further data on features of the skull in relation to their associated organs. Important topics for investigation are: the nasal region, the base of the neurocranium, the brain cavity, the ear region, the quadratomandibular articulation, the palate, and patterns of pneumaticity. The adult skeleton alone, however, may offer an insufficient data base for phylogenetic hypotheses at higher taxonomic levels. Unfortunately, our knowledge of ontogeny of the skull rests largely on an assortment of separate studies on single species. Broader taxonomic coverage and a more comparative approach would reveal the variation in developmental patterns among taxa that we need for phylogenetic analysis (de Queiroz 1985).

Recent studies of phylogeny within genera and families provide a new opportunity for the analysis of skull structure in a phylogenetic context (e.g., Livezey 1986, 1991, for Anseriformes). By comparing sister taxa, morphometric studies of the skull, combined with field and laboratory studies of the live birds, would further our understanding of the evolution of adaptation.

Advances in all these areas will depend ultimately on the availability of anatomical specimens. Museum curators should add cleared and stained specimens of developmental stages, and tissue samples, to their specimen collections. Preservation of juveniles as skeletons has been sadly neglected. Worldwide inventories of anatomical specimens make it possible to be selective and efficient in developing our collections for maximum benefit to science (Zusi et al. 1982; Wood and Schnell 1986).

Our first challenge for the future is to reconstruct the phylogeny of birds. We will then be able to define the most fruitful problems in the evolution of avian cranial diversity.

ACKNOWLEDGMENTS

Jonathan Becker, Peter Cannell, and Andrzej Elzanowski read early drafts of the manuscript, making many valuable suggestions; they also discussed various aspects of the chapter and suggested references. However, the author claims sole responsibility for any errors of fact, interpretation, logic, citation, or omission. S. Renner and A. Elzanowski generously helped with translations. Original drawings were made by the author using a dissecting microscope and drawing tube or an opaque projector; D. Roney drew the final illustrations from original drawings or published materials. I thank the authors and publishers cited in figure captions for permission to redraw published illustrations.

REFERENCES

Abbott, I., L. K. Abbott, and P. R. Grant. 1977. Comparative ecology of Galapagos ground finches (*Geospiza* Gould): Evaluation of the importance of floristic diversity and interspecific competition. Ecological Monographs 47: 151–184.

Bang, B. G. 1971. Functional anatomy of the olfactory system in twenty-three orders of birds. Acta anatomica 79 (suppl.): 1–76.

Barnikol, A. 1952. Korrelationen in der Ausgestaltung der Schädelform bei Vögeln. Gegenbaurs morphologisches Jahrbuch 92: 373–414.

Baumel, J. J., A. S. King, A. M. Lucas, J. E. Breazile, and H. E. Evans, eds. 1979. *Nomina anatomica avium*. London: Academic Press.

Beecher, W. J. 1951a. Adaptations for food-getting in the American blackbirds. Auk 68 (4): 411–440.

———. 1951b. Convergence in the Coerebidae. Wilson Bulletin 63: 274–346.

———. 1978. Feeding adaptations and evolution in the starlings. Bulletin of the Chicago Academy of Sciences 11 (8): 269–298.

Bignon, F. 1889. Contribution à l'étude de la pneumaticité chez les oiseaux. Mémoires de la Société zoologique de France 2: 260–320, plates X–XIII.

Boag, P. T., and P. R. Grant. 1981. Intense natural selection in a population of Darwin's finches (Geospizinae) in the Galapagos. Science 214 (4516): 82–84.

Bock, W. J. 1958. A generic review of the plovers (Charadriinae, Aves). Bulletin of the Museum of Comparative Zoology 118 (2): 27–97.

———. 1960a. The palatine process of the premaxilla in the Passeres. Bulletin of the Museum of Comparative Zoology 122 (8): 361–488.

———. 1960b. Secondary articulation of the avian mandible. Auk 77 (1): 19–55.

———. 1963. The cranial evidence for ratite affinities. In *Proceedings, Thirteenth International Ornithological Congress,* vol. 1. American Ornithologists' Union, pp. 39–54.

———. 1964. Kinetics of the avian skull. Journal of Morphology 114 (1): 1–41.

———. 1966. An approach to the functional analysis of bill shape. Auk 83 (1): 10–51.

———. 1968. Mechanics of one- and two-joint muscles. American Museum Novitates 2319: 1–45.

Bock, W. J., and J. Farrand, Jr. 1980. The number of genera and species of recent birds: A contribution to comparative systematics. American Museum Novitates 2703: 1–29.

Bock, W. J., and B. Kummer. 1968. The avian mandible as a structural girder. Journal of Biomechanics 1: 89–96.

Bock, W. J., and H. Morioka. 1971. Morphology and evolution of the ectethmoid-mandibular articulation in the Meliphagidae (Aves). Journal of Morphology 135 (1): 13–50.

Bolze, G. 1968. Anordnung und Bau der Herbstschen Körperchen in Limicolenschnäbeln im Zusammenhang mit der Nahrungsfindung. Zoologischer Anzeiger 181 (5/6): 313–355.

Bowman, R. I. 1961. Morphological differentiation and adaptation in the Galapagos finches. University of California Publications in Zoology 58: 1–326.

Bubien-Waluszewska, A. 1981. The cranial nerves. In Form and Function in Birds, vol. 2, A. S. King and J. McLelland, eds. London: Academic Press, pp. 385–438.

Bühler, P. 1970. Schädelmorphologie und Kiefermechanik der Caprimulgidae (Aves). Zeitschrift für Morphologie der Tiere 66: 337–399.

———. 1972. Sandwich structures in the skull capsules of various birds: The principle of lightweight structures in organisms. Information of the Institute for Lightweight Structures, Stuttgart 4: 39–50.

———. 1981. Functional anatomy of the avian jaw apparatus. In Form and Function in Birds, vol. 2, A. S. King and J. McLelland, eds. London: Academic Press, pp. 439–468.

———. 1985. On the morphology of the skull of Archaeopteryx. In The Beginnings of Birds: Proceedings of the International Archaeopteryx Conference, Eichstatt 1984, M. K. Hecht, J. H. Ostrom, G. Viohl, and P. Wellnhofer, eds. Eichstatt: Freunde des Jura-Museums Eichstatt, pp. 135–140.

Bühler, P., L. D. Martin, and L. M. Witmer. 1988. Cranial kinesis in the late Cretaceous birds Hesperornis and Parahesperornis. Auk 105 (1): 111–122.

Burton, P. J. K. 1970. Some observations on the os uncinatum in the Musophagidae. Ostrich 8 (suppl.): 7–13.

———. 1974a. Anatomy of the head and neck in the Huia (Heteralocha acutirostris) with comparative notes on other Callaeidae. Bulletin of the British Museum (Natural History), Zoology 27 (1): 1–48.

———. 1974b. Feeding and the Feeding Apparatus in Waders: A Study of Anatomy and Adaptations in the Charadrii. London: Trustees of the British Museum (Natural History).

———. 1974c. Jaw and tongue features in Psittaciformes and other orders with special reference to the anatomy of the Tooth-billed pigeon (Didunculus strigirostris). Journal of Zoology, London 174: 255–276.

———. 1984. Anatomy and evolution of the feeding apparatus in the avian orders Coraciiformes and Piciformes. Bulletin of the British Museum (Natural History), Zoology 47 (6): 331–443.

Butendieck, E., and H. Wissdorf. 1982. Beitrag zur Benennung der Knochen des Kopfes beim Truthuhn (Meleagris gallopavo) unter Berücksichtigung der Nomina Anatomica Avium (1979). Zoologische Jahrbücher, Abteilung für Anatomie und Ontogenie der Tiere 107: 153–184.

Clara, M. 1925. Über den Bau des Schnabels der Waldschnepfe (Scolopax rusticola L.). Zeitschrift für mikroskopische-anatomische Forschung, Leipzig 3 (1/2): 1–108.

Cobb, S. 1959. On the angle of the cerebral axis in the American woodcock. Auk 76 (1): 55–59.

Coddington, J. A. 1988. Cladistic tests of adaptational hypotheses. Cladistics 4 (1): 3–22.

Colbert, E. H., and D. A. Russell. 1969. The small Cretaceous dinosaur *Dromaeosaurus*. American Museum Novitates 2380: 1–49.

Cracraft, J. 1968. The lacrimal-ectethmoid complex in birds: A single character analysis. American Midland Naturalist 80 (2): 316–359.

———. 1986. The origin and early diversification of birds. Paleobiology 12 (4): 383–399.

———. 1987. DNA hybridization and avian phylogenetics. In *Evolutionary Biology*, vol. 21, M. K. Hecht, B. Wallace, and G. T. Prance, eds. New York: Plenum Press, pp. 47–96.

de Beer, G. 1937. *The Development of the Vertebrate Skull*. New York: Oxford University Press.

de Beer, G., and E. J. E. Barrington. 1934. The segmentation and chondrification of the skull of the duck. Philosophical Transactions of the Royal Society of London, ser. B, 223: 411–467, plates 46–52.

de Queiroz, K. 1985. The ontogenetic method for determining character polarity and its relevance to phylogenetic systematics. Systematic Zoology 34 (3): 280–299.

Dubale, M. S., and U. M. Rawal. 1965. A morphological study of the cranial muscles associated with the feeding habit of Psittacula krameri (Scopoli). Indian Journal of Ornithology 3 (1): 1–13.

Duijm, M. 1951. On the head posture in birds and its relation to some anatomical features. I–II. Proceedings, Koninklijke Nederlandse Akademie van Wetenschappen, ser. C, Biological and Medical Sciences 54: 202–271.

Dullemeijer, P. 1974. *Concepts and Approaches in Animal Morphology*. Assen: Van Gorcum and Co. B. V.

Elzanowski, A. 1991. New observations on the skull of *Hesperornis* with reconstructions of the bony palate and otic region. Postilla 207.

Elzanowski, A., and P. M. Galton. 1991. Braincase of *Enaliornis*, an early Cretaceous bird from England. Journal of Vertebrate Paleontology 11 (1): 90–107.

Erdmann, K. 1940. Zur Entwicklungsgeschichte der Knochen im Schädel des Huhnes bis zum Zeitpunkt des Ausschlüpfens aus dem Ei. Zeitschrift für Morphologie und Ökologie der Tiere 36: 315–400.

Feduccia, A. 1975. Morphology of the bony stapes (columella) in the Passeriformes and related groups: Evolutionary implications. University of Kansas Museum of Natural History, Miscellaneous Publication 63: 1–34.

Fisher, H. I. 1955. Some aspects of the kinetics in the jaws of birds. Wilson Bulletin 67 (3): 175–188.

Ford, N. 1967. A systematic study of the owls based on comparative osteology. Ph.D. diss., University of Michigan.

Forshaw, J. M., and W. T. Cooper. 1973. *Parrots of the World*. Melbourne: Lansdowne Press.

Fürbringer, M. 1888. *Untersuchungen zur Morphologie und Systematik der Vögel, zugleich ein Beitrag zur Anatomie der Stütz- und Bewegungsorgane*. 2 vols. Amsterdam: Van Holkema.

Gadow, H. 1892. On the classification of birds. Proceedings of the Zoological Society of London: 229–256.

Gadow, H., and E. Selenka. 1891. Vögel. In *Klassen und Ordnungen des Thierreichs*, H. G. Bronn, ed., vol. 6, pt. 4. Leipzig: C. F. Winter'sche Verlagshandlung.

Garrod, A. H. 1873. On the value in classification of a peculiarity in the anterior margin of the nasal bones of certain birds. Proceedings of the Zoological Society of London: 33–38.

Gauthier, J. 1986. Saurischian monophyly and the origin of birds. In *The Origin of Birds and the Origin of Flight*, K. Padian, ed. Memoirs of the California Academy of Sciences no. 8. San Francisco: California Academy of Sciences.

Goedbloed, E. 1958. The condylus occipitalis in birds I–III. Proceedings, Koninklijke Nederlandse Akademie van Wetenschappen, ser. C, Biological and Medical Sciences, 61 (1): 36–65.

Goldschmid, A. 1972. Die Entwicklung des Craniums der Mausvögel (Coliidae, Coliiformes, Aves). Gegenbaurs morphologisches Jahrbuch 118 (4): 553–569.

Goodwin, D. 1986. *Crows of the World.* 2d ed. London: British Museum (Natural History).

Grant, P. R. 1986. *Ecology and Evolution of Darwin's Finches.* Princeton: Princeton University Press.

Graves, G. R., and R. L. Zusi. 1990. An intergeneric hybrid hummingbird (*Heliodoxa leadbeateri* X *Heliangelus amethysticollis*) from Northern Colombia. Condor 92 (3): 754–760.

Gray, A. A. 1908. *The Labyrinth of Animals, Including Mammals, Birds, Reptiles, and Amphibians.* Vol. 2. London.

Guillet, A., W. S. Doyle, and H. Ruther. 1985. The combination of photogrammetry and finite elements for a fine grained functional analysis of anatomical structures. Zoomorphology 105.

Hafner, M. S., J. V. Remsen, Jr., and S. M. Lanyon. 1984. Bird versus mammal morphological diversity. Evolution 38 (5): 1154–1156.

Heilmann, G. 1927. *The Origin of Birds.* New York: D. Appleton and Co.

Hérissant, F. D. 1752. Observations anatomiques sur les mouvements du bec des oiseaux. Mémoires de l'Académie de l'Institut de France, Paris, Sciences mathématiques et physiques: 345–386.

Hespenheide, H. A. 1973. Ecological inferences from morphological data. Annual Review of Ecology and Systematics 4: 213–229.

Hesse, E. 1907. Über den inner knöchernen Bau des Vogelschnabels. Journal für Ornithologie 55 (2): 185–248.

Hofer, H. 1945. Untersuchungen über den Bau des Vogelschädels, besonders über den der Spechte und Steisshühner. Zoologische Jahrbücher, Abteilung für Anatomie und Ontogenie der Tiere 69 (1): 1–158.

―――. 1949. Die Gaumenlücken der Vögel. Acta zoologica 30: 209–248.

―――. 1950. Zur Morphologie der Kiefermuskulatur der Vögel. Zoologische Jahrbücher, Abteilung für Anatomie und Ontogenie der Tiere 70 (4): 427–556.

―――. 1952. Der Gestaltwandel des Schädels der Säugetiere und Vögel, mit besonderer Berücksichtigung der Knickungstupen und der Schädelbasis. Verhandlungen der Anatomischen Gesellschaft, Jena 50: 102–113.

————. 1953. Die Kiefermuskulatur der Papageien als Evolutionsproblem. Biologisches Zentralblatt 72 (5/6): 225–232.

————. 1955. Neuere Untersuchungen zur Kopfmorphologie der Vögel. In *Acta XI Congressus internationalis ornithologici*, A. Portmann and E. Sutter, eds. Basel: Birkhauser Verlag, pp. 104–137.

Höfling, E., and J.-P. Gasc. 1984. Biomécanique du crâne et du bec chez *Ramphastos* (Ramphastidae, Aves). Gegenbaurs morphologisches Jahrbuch 130 (2): 235–262.

Hogg, D. A. 1978. The articulations of the neurocranium in the postnatal skeleton of the domestic fowl (*Gallus gallus domesticus*). Journal of Anatomy 127 (1): 53–63.

Homberger, D. G. 1980. Funktionell-morphologische Untersuchungen zur Radiation der Ernährungs- und Trinkmethoden der Papageien (Psittaci). Bonner Zoologische Monographien 13.

Houde, P. 1987. Critical evaluation of DNA hybridization studies in avian systematics. Auk 104 (1): 17–32.

————. 1988. Paleognathous birds from the early Tertiary of the Northern Hemisphere. Publications of the Nuttall Ornithological Club 22: 1–148.

Huxley, T. H. 1867. On the classification of birds; and on the taxonomic value of the modifications of certain of the cranial bones observable in that class. Proceedings of the Zoological Society of London: 415–472.

Johnston, R. F., and R. K. Selander. 1971. Evolution in the house sparrow. II. Adaptive differentiation in North American populations. Evolution 25 (1): 1–28.

Jollie, M. T. 1957. The head skeleton of the chicken and remarks on the anatomy of this region in other birds. Journal of Morphology 100 (3): 389–436.

————. 1958. Comments on the phylogeny and skull of the Passeriformes. Auk 75 (1): 26–35.

Klaauw, C. J. van der. 1963. Projections, deepenings, and undulations of the surface of the skull in relation to the attachment of muscles. Koninklijke Nederlandse Akademie van Wetenschappen, Verhandelingen Afdeling Natuurkunde 55 (2): 1–246.

Krause, G. 1901. *Die Columella der Vögel (Columella auris avium): ihr Bau und dessen Einfluss auf die Feinhörigkeit.* Berlin: Friedlander und Sohn.

Kripp, D. v. 1935. Die mechanische Analyse der Schnabelkrümmung und ihre Bedeutung für die Anpassungsforschung. Gegenbaurs morphologisches Jahrbuch 76: 448–494, 1 table.

Lack, D. 1947. *Darwin's Finches.* Cambridge: Cambridge University Press.

Lang, C. T. 1952. Über die Ontogenie der Knickungsverhaltnisse beim Vögelschadel. Verhandlungen der Anatomischen Gesellschaft, Jena 50: 127–136.

Lebedinsky, N. G. 1920. Beiträge zur Morphologie und Entwicklungsgeschichte des Unterkiefers der Vögel. Verhandlungen der Naturforschenden Gesellschaft in Basel 3: 39–112, plates IV–VI.

Lemmrich, W. 1931. Der Skleralring der Vögel. Jenaische Zeitschrift für Naturwissenschaft 65: 513–586.

Livezey, B. C. 1986. A phylogenetic analysis of Recent anseriform genera using morphological characters. Auk 103 (4): 737–754.

———. 1991. A phylogenetic analysis and classification of Recent dabbling ducks (Tribe Anatini) based on comparative morphology. Auk 108 (3): 471–507.

Lorenz, K. Z. 1949. Über die Beziehungen zwischen Kopfform und Zirkelbewegung bei Sturniden und Ikteriden. In *Ornithologie als biologische Wissenschaft*, E. Mayr and E. Schuz, eds. Heidelberg: Carl Winter, Universitatsverlag, pp. 153–157.

Lowe, P. R. 1926. More notes on the quadrate as a factor in avian classification. Ibis: 152–188, plate II.

McDowell, S. 1948. The bony palate of birds: Part I the paleognathae. Auk 65 (4): 520–549.

Maddison, W. P., M. J. Donoghue, and D. R. Maddison. 1984. Outgroup analysis and parsimony. Systematic Zoology 33 (1): 83–103.

Marinelli, W. 1928. Über den Schadel der Schnepfe. Palaeobiologica 1: 135–160, 1 plate.

Martin, L. D. 1983. The origin and early radiation of birds. In *Perspectives in Ornithology*, A. H. Brush and G. A. Clark, Jr., eds. Cambridge: Cambridge University Press, pp. 291–338.

Morony, J. J., Jr., W. J. Bock, and J. Farrand, Jr. 1975. *Reference List of the Birds of the World*. New York: American Museum of Natural History.

Müller, H. J. 1963. Die Morphologie und Entwicklung des Craniums von *Rhea americana* Linné. II. Viszeralskelett, Mittelohr und Osteocranium. Zeitschrift für wissenschaftliche Zoologie. Leipzig 168: 35–116.

———. 1964. Morphologische Untersuchungen am Vogelschadel in ihrer Bedeutung fur die Systematik. Journal für Ornithologie 105 (1): 67–77.

Nemeschkal, H. L. 1983. Zum Nachweis eines Os coronoidenm bei Vögeln—Ein Beitrag zur Morphologie des Sauropsiden-Unterkiefers. Zoologische Jahrbücher, Abteilung für Anatomie und Ontogenie der Tiere 109: 117–151.

Nitzsch, C. L. 1816. Ueber die Bewegung des Oberkiefers der Vögel. Deutsches Archiv für die Physiologie 2: 361–380.

———. 1817. Zweiter Nachtrag zu Nitzsch's Abhandlung über die Bewegung des Oberkiefers der Vögel. Deutsches Archiv für die Physiologie 3: 384–388.

Noden, D. M. 1978. The control of avian cephalic neural crest cytodifferentiation. 1. Skeletal and connective tissues. Developmental Biology 67: 296–312.

Norberg, R. A. 1977. Occurrence and independent evolution of bilateral ear asymmetry in owls and implications on owl taxonomy. Philosophical Transactions of the Royal Society of London, ser. B, Biological Sciences 280 (973): 375–408.

———. 1978. Skull asymmetry, ear structure and function, and auditory localization in Tengmalm's owl, *Aegolius funereus* (Linne). Philosophical Transactions of the Royal Society of London, ser. B, Biological Sciences 282 (991): 325–410.

Oehme, H. 1962. Das Auge von Mauersegler, Star und Amsel. Journal für Ornithologie 103 (2/3): 187–212.

Olson, S. L. 1985. The fossil record of birds. In *Avian Biology*, vol. 8, D. S. Farner, J. R. King, and K. C. Parkes, eds. Orlando: Academic Press, pp. 79–256.

Ostrom, J. H. 1976. *Archaeopteryx* and the origin of birds. Biological Journal of the Linnean Society 8: 91–118.

————. 1978. The osteology of *Compsognathus longipes* Wagner. Zitteliana Abhandlungen der Bayerischen Staatssammlung für Palaontologie und historische Geologie 4: 78–118, plates 7–14.

Parker, W. K. 1878. On the skull of the aegithognathous birds, part II. Transactions of the Zoological Society of London 10, pt. 6: 251–314, plates XLVI–LIV.

————. 1879. On the structure and development of the bird's skull. Transactions of the Linnean Society of London, ser. 2, Zoology 1: 99–154, plates 22–27.

Paynter, R. A., ed. 1970. *Check-List of the Birds of the World*. Vol. 13. Cambridge: Harvard University Press.

Peters, J. L. 1940. *Check-List of the Birds of the World*. Vol. 4. Cambridge: Harvard University Press.

Pycraft, W. P. 1900. On the morphology and phylogeny of the palaeognathae (Ratitae and Crypturi) and neognathae (Carinatae). Transactions of the Zoological Society of London 15, pt. 5, no. 6: 149–290, plates XLII–XLV.

————. 1901. Some points in the morphology of the palate of the neognathae. Journal of the Linnean Society of London 28: 343–357.

————. 1908. On the position of the ear in the woodcock (*Scolopax rusticola*). Ibis, ser. 9, 2 (8): 551–558.

Raikow, R. J. 1982. Monophyly of the Passeriformes: Test of a phylogenetic hypothesis. Auk 99 (3): 431–445.

Reid, J. 1835. Anatomical description of the Patagonian penguin. Proceedings of the Zoological Society of London 3: 132–148.

Richards, L. P., and W. J. Bock. 1973. *Functional Anatomy and Adaptive Evolution of the Feeding Apparatus in the Hawaiian Honeycreeper Genus* Loxops (*Drepanididae*). Ornithological Monographs 15. Lawrence: Allen Press and American Ornithologists' Union.

Ricklefs, R. E., and J. Travis. 1980. A morphological approach to the study of avian community organization. Auk 97 (2): 321–338.

Rüger, A. 1972. Funktionell-anatomische Untersuchungen an Spechten. Zeitschrift für wissenschaftliche Zoologie, Leipzig 184 (1/2): 63–163.

Saiff, E. 1988. The anatomy of the middle ear of the Tinamiformes (Aves: Tinamidae). Journal of Morphology 196: 107–116.

Sarich, V. M., C. W. Schmid, and J. Marks. 1989. DNA hybridization as a guide to phylogenies: A critical analysis. Cladistics 5 (1): 3–32.

Schluter, D. 1984. Morphology and phylogenetic relations among the Darwin's finches. Evolution 38 (5): 921–930.

Schluter, D., T. D. Price, and P. R. Grant. 1985. Ecological character displacement in Darwin's finches. Science 227: 1056–1059.

Schoonees, J. 1963. Some aspects of the cranial morphology of Colius indicus. Annale Universiteit van Stellenbosch 38, ser. 7, no. 7: 215–246.

Schuh, J. 1968. Allometrische Untersuchungen über den Formenwandel des Schädels von Corviden. Zeitschrift für wissenschaftliche Zoologie, Abteilung A, 177 (1/2): 97–182.

Serventy, D. L. 1936. Feeding methods of Podargus. Emu 36: 74–90.

Sibley, C. G., and J. E. Ahlquist. 1990. *Phylogeny and Classification of Birds: A Study in Molecular Evolution*. New Haven: Yale University Press.

Siegel-Causey, D. 1990. Phylogenetic patterns of size and shape of the nasal gland depression in Phalacrocoracidae. Auk 107 (1): 110–118.

Simonetta, A. 1960. On the mechanical implications of the avian skull and their bearing on the evolution and classification of birds. Quarterly Review of Biology 35 (3): 206–220.

Sims, R. W. 1955. The morphology of the head of the hawfinch (*Coccothraustes coccothraustes*). Bulletin of the British Museum (Natural History), Zoology 2 (13): 371–393.

Smith, G. A. 1975. Systematics of parrots. Ibis 117 (1): 18–68.

Smith, T. B. 1987. Bill size polymorphism and intraspecific niche utilization in an African finch. Nature 329: 717–719.

Starck, D. 1955. Die endokraniale Morphologie der Ratiten, besonders der Apterygidae and Dinornithidae. Gegenbaurs morphologisches Jahrbuch 96: 14–72.

Starck, D., and A. Barnikol. 1954. Beiträg zur Morphologie der Trigeminus-muskulatur der Vögel (besonders der Accipitres, Cathartidae, Striges und Anseres). Gegenbaurs morphologisches Jahrbuch 94 (1–2): 1–64.

Technau, G. 1936. Die Nasendrüse der Vögel: Zugleich ein Beitrag zur Morphologie der Nasenhöhle. Journal für Ornithologie 84 (4): 511–616, plates IV–VI.

Thompson, D'Arcy W. 1899. On characteristic points in the cranial osteology of the parrots. Proceedings of the Zoological Society of London: 9–46.

———. 1907. The position of the ear in the woodcock. Field: The Country Gentleman's Newspaper. Nov. 16, no. 2864: 887.

Tiemeier, O. W. 1939. A preliminary report on the os opticus of the bird's eye. Zoologica: New York Zoological Society 24 (19): 333–338.

Turkewitsch, B. G. 1936. Ein Versuch zur Systematik der Vögel und Säugetiere auf Grund der anatomischen Struktur ihres knocheren Labyrinths. Archivio zoologico italiano 22: 79–122, 1 plate.

Walker, M. L. 1888. On the form of the quadrate bone in birds. Studies from the Museum of Zoology in University College, Dundee 1 (1): 1–18.

Webb, M. 1957. The ontogeny of the cranial bones, cranial peripheral and cranial parasympathetic nerves, together with a study of the visceral muscles of *Struthio*. Acta zoologica 38 (2/3): 81–203.

Werner, C. F. 1960. *Das Gehörorgan der Wirbeltiere und des Menschen*. Leipzig: Veb Georg Thieme.

———. 1962. Allometrische Grossenunterschiede und die Wechselbeziehung der Organe (Untersuchungen am Kopf der Vögel). Acta anatomica 50: 135–157.

———. 1963. Schädel-, Gehirn- und Labyrinthtypen bei den Vögeln. Gegenbaurs morphologisches Jahrbuch 104 (1): 54–87.

Winkler, R. 1979. Zur Pneumatisation des Schädeldachs der Vögel. Der ornithologische Beobachter 76 (2/3): 49–118.

Witmer, L. M. 1990. The craniofacial air sac system of Mesozoic birds (Aves). Zoological Journal of the Linnean Society 100: 327–378.

Wood, D. S., and G. D. Schnell. 1986. *Revised World Inventory of Avian Skeletal Specimens, 1986*. Norman: American Ornithologists' Union and Oklahoma Biological Survey.

Wyles, J. S., J. G. Kunkel, and A. C. Wilson. 1983. Birds, behavior, and anatomical evolution. Proceedings of the National Academy of Sciences, U.S.A. 80: 4394–4397.

Yang, S. Y., and J. L. Patton. 1981. Genic variability and differentiation in the Galapagos finches. Auk 98 (2): 230–242.

Yudin, K. A. 1961. [On the mechanism of the jaw in Charadriiformes, Procellariiformes and some other birds]. Academy of Sciences of USSR, Trudy Zoologicheskogo Instituta 29: 257–302. In Russian.

Zusi, R. L. 1959. The function of the depressor mandibulae muscle in certain passerine birds. Auk 76 (4): 537–539.

———. 1962. Structural adaptations of the head and neck in the black skimmer *Rynchops nigra* Linnaeus. Publications of the Nuttall Ornithological Club 3.

———. 1967. The role of the depressor mandibulae muscle in kinesis of the avian skull. Proceedings of the United States National Museum 123 (3607): 1–28.

———. 1975. An interpretation of skull structure in penguins. In *The Biology of Penguins,* B. Stonehouse, ed. London: Macmillan Press, pp. 59–84.

———. 1978. The interorbital septum in cardueline finches. Bulletin of the British Ornithologists' Club 98 (1): 5–10.

———. 1984. A functional and evolutionary analysis of rhynchokinesis in birds. Smithsonian Contributions to Zoology 395: 1–40.

———. 1987. A feeding adaptation of the jaw articulation in the New World jays (Corvidae). Auk 104 (4): 665–680.

Zusi, R. L., D. S. Wood, and M. A. Jenkinson. 1982. Remarks on a world-wide inventory of avian anatomical specimens. Auk 99 (4): 740–757.

Zweers, G. A. 1974. Structure, movement, and myography of the feeding apparatus of the mallard (*Anas platyrhynchos* L.): A study in functional anatomy. Netherlands Journal of Zoology 24 (4): 323–467.

9

Patterns of Diversity in the Mammalian Skull

MICHAEL J. NOVACEK

INTRODUCTION

IN HIS EXTRAORDINARY COMPILATION, de Beer (1937) summarized the major aspects of ontogenetic variation of the mammalian skull, but expressed some doubt over the use of this evidence in reconstructing phylogeny. For example, he remarked, "The problem of the relative affinities of various orders of placental mammals is one on which the study of the development of the skull can unfortunately throw but little light, and when it comes to attempt a grouping of various Orders *inter se,* grave difficulties are encountered" (1937, 468). While some persistent problems lend credence to de Beer's conservative outlook (Novacek 1980, 1986), considerable progress has been made in discriminating general trends and patterns of variation of the mammalian cranium. Unlike de Beer's coverage, much of this modern work focuses on comparative study of later stages of development and incorporates adult cranial data from a diversity of fossil as well as living taxa. Such analyses have been applied with variable effectiveness to phylogenetic problems. Although many questions remain, we now know significantly more about the diversification of mammalian cranial features than we did at the time de Beer's work was first published. This new information pertains not only to refined studies of ontogeny, but to a more explicit mapping of characters required for new approaches to systematic analysis.

It would be presumptious in a short chapter to attempt to match the scope and detail of de Beer's (1937) coverage on the mammalian skull. My contribution can be thought of as a footnote, modifying or amending certain aspects of that monumental treatise in order to account for more recent studies. To fulfill this purpose, I first present a brief survey of the mammalian skull and its components. My treatment here also draws on some excellent summaries of chondrocranial and osteocranial development (Starck 1967; Kuhn 1971; Moore 1981; Maier 1987a; Zeller 1987). The recent output of the modern community of German anatomists is particularly useful in this regard. This work echoes a long history of outstanding quality and importance (e.g., Gaupp 1902; Weber 1904) often poorly acknowledged in English-language publications. Descriptions of variation in later development and comparative adult structure are based on de Beer (1937) and Moore (1981) as well as a number of recent comparative monographs (e.g., MacPhee 1981; Novacek 1986).

The second part of this chapter highlights problems that have drawn much attention in phylogenetic studies. Obviously, the range of such topics greatly exceeds those mentioned here, but the areas discussed rank high on the list. Included is a review of work on auditory structure, with special reference to bullar architecture, ossicle morphology, and carotid circulation (McDowell 1958; MacPhee 1981; Novacek 1986; Wible 1987). Also considered is the substantial literature on the mammalian jaw joint and its relation to the "reptilian-mammalian transition" (Watson 1948; Parrington 1955; Crompton and Hotton 1967; Barghusen 1968; Kemp 1972, 1979; Allin 1975; Crompton and Jenkins 1979; Crompton and Sun 1985). Other regions (e.g., the orbital mosaic) have been less thoroughly treated, but offer problems with broad phylogenetic implications.

Terminology: Anatomical

It is important to try to clarify certain terms of varying usage. For example, there are different conventions for designating the turbinals and paranasal sinuses; this treatment follows the numeric system devised by Paulli (1900a, b, c). Discussions on the development of the chondocranium use terminology found in more recent studies by Kuhn (1971) and Zeller (1987). Other problems in terminology actually reflect different views on homology (the composition of the secondary braincase wall; see discussion below). In cases where alternative terms for the same feature are frequently encountered, the synonyms are given (e.g., sphenorbital fissure as used here [fig. 9.8] equals sphenoidal fissure or foramen lacerum anterius of other sources). Useful glossaries of terms for cranial features can be found in McDowell (1958) and MacPhee (1981).

Terminology: Taxonomic

A major problem in discussions of features of mammals is casting this group in the context of a proper classification and developing a terminology that reflects this classification. Many of the sources for this treatment, for example, refer to the conditions in "reptiles" versus mammals. Clearly, "Reptilia" in this sense refers to a paraphyletic group, as it includes the synapsid sister group of mammals as well as living turtles, lizards, crocodilians, and many fossil lineages. The term "Sauropsida" seems more appropriate because it traditionally refers to the suite of nonmammalian and nonsynapsid amniotes (including birds) as a monophyletic group. Gauthier et al. (1988) suggest the name "Reptilia" to denote a monophyletic group comprising all amniotes other than synapsids and mammals. Such usage, however, would engender confusion, since the term "Reptilia" is so commonly used in a different (and paraphyletic) sense.

Here, the terms "reptiles" and "reptilian" appear in quotation marks to indicate their problematic implications. More frequently, these paraphyletic associations are referred to as nonmammalian amniotes.

Following Gauthier et al. (1988), I recognize Synapsida as a major taxon including the following hierarchy:

Synapsida
  Therapsida
    Cynodontia
    Mammalia

Hence, Mammalia are actually members of Synapsida. Cynodonts (including Mammalia) include such taxa as *Exaeretodon, Diademodon, Thrinaxodon, Bienotherium, Cynognathus, Diarthrognathus,* and *Procynosuchus.* Noncynodont therapsid groups include Therocephalia (e.g., *Scylacosaurus*), Dicynodontia, Gorgonopsia, Dinocephalia, and Biarmosuchia. Nontherapsid synapsids include Sphenacodontinae, *Edaphosaurus, Ophiacodon, Casea,* and *Dimetrodon.* The latter five taxa are often collectively associated with others as "pelycosaurs," but again this term unfortunately denotes a paraphyletic group.

Gauthier et al. (1988) adopt a convention recognizing Mammalia as containing only extant and fossil taxa that stem from the last common ancestor of all living clades (monotremes, marsupials, and eutherians). This, of course, would exclude commonly recognized Mesozoic triconodonts, such as *Morganucodon.* The important point is not whether *Morganucodon* is a member of Mammalia (sensu stricto), but that it is more closely related to the latter than are the cynodont taxa mentioned above. Another triconodont in this category is *Sinoconodon.* Other Mesozoic taxa referred to here, including *Kuhneotherium, Amphitherium,* and Multituberculata are more closely associated with Mammalia, although their positions relative to Theria and Monotremata are a matter of debate (see McKenna 1975; Rowe 1988).

Readers should be acquainted with the basic groups of mammals, but confusion may arise with reference to certain categories (e.g., Eutheria, Euprimates, Glires, etc.). Here, in hierarchical array, are my definitions of the higher mammalian categories. Reference is also made to the placement of certain generic-level taxa (e.g., *Tachyglossus, Lepus, Myotis*) whose cranial structures are noted with some frequency in this and related papers.

Mammalia
  Monotremata

Theria
  Metatheria
  Eutheria

Monotremata include the living echidna (*Tachyglossus*) and duck-billed platypus (*Ornithorynchus*) and some fossil forms. An equivalent ranking is bestowed on the Theria, which comprises the Metatheria (or marsupials) and the Eutheria ("placental" mammals). Rowe (1988), along with certain other authors, has advocated the recognition of Eutheria in place of Theria and the recognition of Placentalia instead of Eutheria, in order to reflect the original use of these terms in some late nineteenth-century classifications. However, the application of Eutheria in this paper follows most later and well-known classifications.

The marsupial groups frequently referred to here include the didelphids ("opossums," e.g., *Didelphis*). Other marsupials cited here are the Australian dasyurids, the marsupial mole *Notoryctes,* and the gliding possum, *Petaurus.*

Eutherian examples given here represent most of the major extant orders as well as some fossil higher categories not assignable to these orders. Skull traits in the following groups are mentioned in text and figures:

Pholidota: pangolins (Manidae, e.g., *Manis*).

Edentata: sloths (Bradypodidae), armadillos (Dasypodidae), anteaters (Myrmecophagidae).

Insectivora: Noted here to include some archaic eutherians (e.g., *Leptictis*), as well as the lipotyphlan insectivorans, the group comprising shrews (Soricidae), moles (Talpidae), solenodons (*Solenodon*), tenrecs (Tenrecidae), golden moles (Chrysochloridae), hedgehogs (Erinaceidae).

Carnivora: cats (Felidae), dogs (Canidae), bears (Ursidae), raccoons (Procyonidae), weasels, skunks and others (Mustelidae), civets and mongooses (Viveriidae), seals, sea lions, walruses (Pinnipedia).

Tubulidentata: aardvarks (*Orycteropus*).

Scandentia: tree shrews (Tupaiidae).

Primates: lemurs (Lemuridae); also fossil adapids (e.g., *Notharctus, Adapis*), fossil omomyids, cheirogalines, indriids, New World monkeys (Cebidae), Aye-ayes (Daubentoniidae), Old World Monkeys (Cercopethicidae), Tarsiidae, great apes, and humans (Hominoidea).

Dermoptera: flying lemurs (Galeopithecidae).

Chiroptera: Old World "fruit bats" (Megachiroptera) and microchiropterans.

Macroscelidea: elephant shrews.

Rodentia: The most diverse mammalian order, including rats, mice, cavis, porcupines, squirrels, etc., comprising many families. Genera frequently cited here are *Mus, Cavia, Sciurus.*

Lagomorpha: rabbits, pikas.

Artiodactyla: pigs (Suiidae), Hippopotamidae, Camelidae, deer (Cervidae), sheep, cows, African antelopes and other bovids (Bovidae), American antelopes (Antelocapridae), Tragulidae, Moschidae.

Perissodactyla: tapirs (Tapiridae), horses (Equidae), and rhinoceros (Rhinocerotidae).

Cetacea: baleen whales, toothed whales (Odontoceti), porpoise and dolphins.

Hyracoidea: hyraxes.

Proboscidea: elephants and their relatives, and the Tertiary genus *Moeritherium*.

Sirenia: sea cows, manatees.

Although higher categories for these orders are controversial, a few such groupings have been proposed. These include: (1) Archonta, associating Primates, Chiroptera, Dermoptera, and Scandentia (McKenna 1975; Novacek and Wyss 1986a); (2) Glires (for Lagomorpha and Rodentia, see Novacek and Wyss 1986a); (3) Tethytheria (for Proboscidea and Sirenia, see McKenna 1975); (4) Paenungulata (for tethytheres and hyracoids, see Novacek and Wyss 1986a). There is also a recent argument for a grouping including the Xenarthra (New World edentates) and Pholidata (Novacek 1986; Novacek and Wyss 1986a). Cranial evidence bearing on some of these categories is mentioned in the text.

Aside from *Leptictis*, a few of the fossil eutherians cited here have problematic affinities with other orders. These include the Late Cretaceous genera *Asioryctes* and *Kennalestes* from Mongolia (see McKenna 1975), and the archaic taxa most often grouped with Primates (e.g., *Plesiadapis*, *Microsyops*, and *Plesiolestes*) but excluded from a clade that would contain all extant lineages and their last common ancestor, commonly referred to as Euprimates (see Wible and Covert 1987).

THE MAMMALIAN SKULL: A GENERAL DESCRIPTION

Ethmoidal Region

The ethmoidal region comprises the rostral and facial areas of the skull anterior to the orbit. Included therein is the nasal cavity and its complex osseous and cartilaginous components. The floor of the nasal cavity is formed by the hard palate and the roof by anterior extension of the cribriform plate of the ethmoid, part of the frontal, and the nasal bones. In early synapsids (fig. 9.1E) the nasal cavity is simple in structure, and represents the basic amniote condition: it consists of small (cartilaginous) capsules with external nares at the antero-dorsal edge of the rostrum

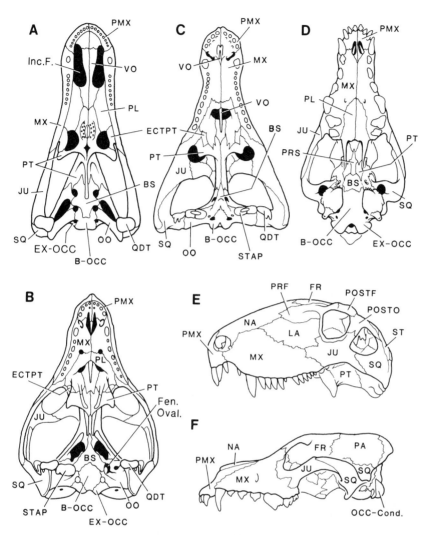

Fig. 9.1. Ventral views of skulls of (A) *Scylacosaurus* (a therocephalian),
(B) *Thrynaxodon* (a cynodont), (C) *Cynognathus* (a cynodont), (D) *Canis* (domestic
dog). Lateral views of skulls of (E) *Dimetrodon* (a synapsid) and (F) *Canis*. For
labeling see list of abbreviations. (After Moore 1981)

and internal nares that open into the anterior oral cavity. The nasal cavity
of later synapsids, including various (more primitive) therapsid lineages
(fig. 9.1B, C), is greatly enlarged and its posterior openings (internal nares)
are shifted far backward with the development of the secondary palate (see
review in Moore 1981).

The latter feature is a major innovation in the phylogeny of the Synapsida. An incipient secondary palate, for example, occurs in therocephalians (fig. 9.1A), where marginal dermal elements of the palate fold ventrally and then medially to produce palatine processes below the primary palate. In later cynodonts (fig. 9.1B, C) the palatine processes fuse at the midline to form a complete bony palate. This important modification results in the isolation of the airway from the first part of the alimentary passage. Above the secondary palate a medium septum, probably formed from the vomers, splits the airway into right and left tunnels. The homology of the mammalian vomers with the nonmammalian amniote "vomer" is, however, subject to debate (see below). The pterygoid bones, which in early synapsids and archosaurs are primitively the longest elements of the palate, are in cynodonts and mammals small flanges forming the roof and the sidewall of the most posterior part of the nasal passage.

Chondrocranial Developments. The ethmoidal region of the developing mammalian chondrocranium comprises primarily the nasal capsules as well as parts of the trabeculae cranii. The latter element is an ancient embryonic structure in vertebrates, which in tropybasic (high-vaulted) skulls, typical of amniotes, becomes a median plate formed by the fusion of the paired trabeculae. The anterior extensions of the trabeculae lie within the nasal capsules and contribute to the median nasal septum (fig. 9.2C; see also Moore 1981, 33).

During ontogeny, ventral flexion of the nasal skeleton, or klinorhynchy (Hofer 1952), decreases and the nasal capsules shift from an embryonic position beneath the projection of the brain to an adult position anterior to the brain (Spatz 1964). The early flexion represents the accommodation of embryonic cranial shape to a relatively large brain (Starck 1967).

The Nasal Cartilages. The development of the nasal cartilages (with special reference to the tree shrew, *Tupaia*) is clearly summarized by Zeller (1987), and only highlights of this discussion are mentioned here. Other important studies include descriptions of morphogenesis in the domestic cat, *Felis* (Terry 1917), the bat, *Myotis* (Frick 1954), and the echidna, *Tachyglossus* (Kuhn 1971). Generally in mammals, the rostrum nasi does not reach its definitive shape until late in ontogeny. Development of the rostrum nasi (figs. 9.2, 9.3) involves the chondrification of (1) the paries nasi, which constitute the uniform lateral wall of the nasal capsules; (2) the cupula nasi, which borders the nasal capsule rostro-ventrally; (3) the processus alaris superior, which supports the external nasal aperture from the lateral side; (4) the tectum nasi, which roofs the rostral portion of the nasal capsule; (5) the lamina cribrosa and lamina infracribrosa, which roof the caudal portion of the nasal capsule; (6) the nasal floor

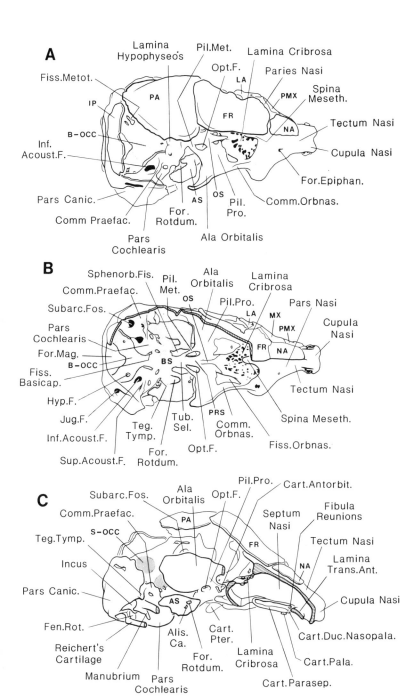

Fig. 9.2. Cranium of *Tupaia belangeri*. A. Dorsal view, day 34. B. Dorsal view, neonate. C. Right lateral view, day 34. Not to scale. Endochondral ossifications are indicated by uniform stipple. Dermal bones are reconstructed on left side only, with exception of the unpaired interparietal in (A) and the unpaired vomer and interparietal in (C). Most of right nasal capsule removed in (C) and Meckel's cartilage not shown in (A) and (C). For labeling see list of abbreviations. (After Spatz 1964 and Zeller 1987).

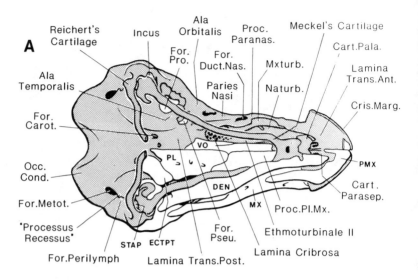

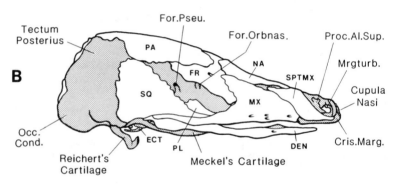

Fig. 9.3. Ventral (A) and right lateral (B) views of cranium of a pouch-young (53 mm crown-rump length) of *Tachyglossus aculeatus*. Endochondral elements are represented by uniform stipple. In ventral view, dermal elements are removed from right side of cranium. For labeling see list of abbreviations. (After Kuhn 1971)

(solum nasi) formed by the lamina transversalis anterior, cartilago paraseptalis, lamina transversalis posterior, cartilago ductus nasopalatini, cartilago papillae palatinae, and cartilago palatini.

These different components of the rostrum nasi show a mosaic of developmental trends. For example, in *Tupaia* the paries nasi caudal to the cupula nasi is completely chondrified by day 28, but, from day 37 on, the paries is resorbed and a longitudinal opening, the fenestra nasi superior (Spatz 1964), appears on the rostral portion of the nasal side well. This reduction of the paries proceeds through postnatal stages yielding a system of cartilaginous rods (Zeller 1987). In contrast, the cupula nasi postnatally retains its size and form and supports the rhinarium. During ontogeny, muscles arising from the paries stabilize the increasingly mobile rostrum (Maier 1980). Other components of the nasal rostrum develop quite late, for example, the lamina cribrosa in *Tupaia* and other mammals is generally not fully chondrified until the neonate stage.

According to Gaupp (1900), Starck (1967), Kuhn (1971), and others, the lamina cribrosa (fig. 9.2) is a mammalian neomorph, being part of the secondary floor of the braincase in the ethmoidal region. Zeller (1987, 24) has summarized the interrelationships between the development of this feature and that of the brain. A small space, the recessus supracribrosus, houses the olfactory bulbs, the ethmoidal nerve, and the filia olfactoria and separates the lamina cribrosa from the dura mater.

Elements of the Naso-Palatine Duct. The lamina transversalis anterior (fig. 9.2C), forming the anterior floor of the naso-palatine duct, is a primitive element, homologous with the rostral trabeculae cranii (de Beer 1937). This lamina also develops vertically, forming part of the sidewall of the nasal capsule (Sturm 1936). The lamina transversalis anterior appears to arise from the paries nasi (fig. 9.2B) in *Tupaia* (Spatz 1963, 1964; Zeller 1987), a pattern that is also found in other reference taxa (*Didelphis, Oryctolagus, Rousettus;* see Kuhn 1971). Later contact is made with the nasal septum (septum nasi), the vertical wall of cartilage longitudinally dividing the nasal capsule (fig. 9.2C).

Posterior to the naso-palatine duct, the cartilago paraseptalis forms as an elongated trough, somewhat C-shaped in cross section, in order to accommodate the vomeronasal, or Jacobson's organ (figs. 9.2C, 9.3A). Later in ontogeny, the cartilago paraseptalis is roofed, in part, by the fibula reuniens (fig. 9.2C), or the "outer bar," sensu Broom (1896). This latter structure is thought to be homologous with a turbinal which develops in monotremes from the lateral wall of the paraseptal cartilage and lies dorsal and lateral to the Jacobson's organ (Toeplitz 1920; contra Broom 1896). The fibula thus seems a remnant of the paraseptal cartilage (reviewed in Starck 1941), and is primitively present in therians (Starck 1975a) and separated from the nasal septum. The fibula and the nasal septum fuse secondarily in some forms (e.g., *Talpa,* some microchiropterans, *Canis;* see Kuhn 1971). In its primitive condition, the paraseptal cartilage extends from the lamina transversalis anterior to the lamina transversalis posterior, forming an elongated floor for the Jacobson's organ (e.g., Marsupialia, Rodentia, *Oryctolagus, Alouatta, Trichecus, Bradypus;* see Starck 1941; Schneider 1955). However, the caudal portion of the paraseptal cartilage is reduced, likely owing to expansion of the vomer, in most mammals (Toeplitz 1920).

Lamina Transversalis Posterior. The naso-palatine duct is also associated with three other small cartilages, the cartilago ductus nasopalatini (fig. 9.2C), the cartilago papillae palatinae, and the cartilago palatini (fig. 9.2C). The cartilago papillae palatinae is an appositional cartilage and likely a primitive element in the mammalian skull (de Beer 1937; Kuhn 1971; Zeller 1987). The cartilago palatini, which lies posterior to the naso-palatine duct below the anterior portion of the cartilago paraseptalis in the plane of the secondary palate, is regarded as the homologue of the cartilago ectochoanalis of sauropsids (Gaupp 1908b; de Beer 1937).

The lamina transversalis posterior (fig. 9.3A) seems to be a phylogenetic derivative of the antorbital wall that shifted horizontally with the expansion of the ethmoturbinal recess (Kuhn 1971). This lamina is secondarily lost in some mammals, including *Ornithorynchus* (Watson 1916), *Tarsius* (Wünsch 1975), and *Pan* (Starck 1960). When present, the lamina transversalis posterior is medially attached (but not fused) with the nasal septum and fused with the secondary cartilage of the lateral edge of the vomer (Zeller 1987).

The Cartilaginous Turbinals. The interior of the nasal capsule is dissected by the maxillo- and naso-turbinals, the pars lateralis, and the ethmoturbinalis. These elements are, in turn, divided into additional turbinals whose numbers and form vary markedly among mammalian taxa. The cartilaginous turbinals typically form relatively late during ontogeny. In *Tupaia* they are all chondrified by day 34, and undergo only minor changes before birth (day 44). In postnatal development, however, the turbinals are markedly extended by appositional formation of periosteal bone (Zeller 1987).

Formation of the Anterior Dermal Bones. In most mammals, the anterior dermal bones (premaxilla, maxilla, palatine, and frontal) are the first of the cranial bones to form, and even predate the complete chondrification of the rostral part of the nasal skeleton (Erdmann 1933; Frick 1954; Nesslinger 1956; Müller 1968, 1972; Maier 1987a; Zeller 1987). This early stabilization of the nasal rostrum by the dermal bones has adaptive implications in monotremes and marsupials. The premaxilla, for example, is the first dermal element to develop in monotremes and it carries the eggtooth (Gaupp 1908b; de Beer 1937). However, this adaptation is not at all relevant to eutherians, where early development of the rostral dermal bones is simply thought to represent the persistence of the plesiomorphous mammalian ontogeny (Zeller 1987).

With the exception of the ethmoid itself, the bones of the ethmoidal region are dermal in origin. Some general trends in the development of these elements can be noted. The nasals develop in *Tupaia* and other mammals somewhat later than the other rostral dermal bones (Zeller 1987). They form an elongate bone on the roof of the rostrum (figs. 9.2A, B; 9.3; 9.4; 9.5; 9.6; 9.14). The shape of this bone varies considerably, although the expanded posterior contact between it and the frontal (fig. 9.4A; cf. 9.5B) is the likely plesiomorphous condition for mammals (Butler 1956; McDowell 1958; Novacek 1986). The nasals are also variously retracted in many mammals (figs. 9.9A, B; 9.14C), especially where some develop-

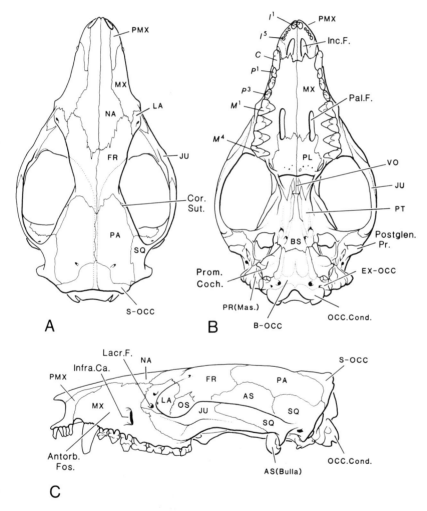

Fig. 9.4. Dorsal (A), ventral (B), and left lateral (C) views of skull at the American Museum of Natural History, Department of Mammalogy (A.M.) 130516 *Monodelphis brevicaudata* (a didelphid marsupial). For labeling see list of abbreviations.

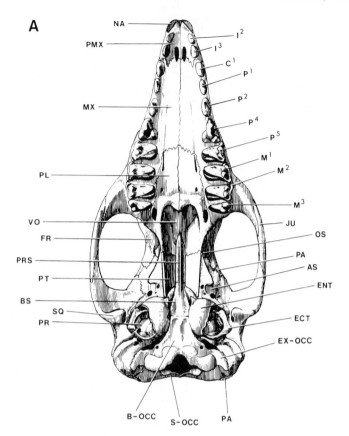

Fig. 9.5. Ventral (A), dorsal (B), and left lateral (C) views of skull of *Leptictis dakotensis* (an early eutherian mammal). For labeling see list of abbreviations. (From Novacek 1986)

ment of a mobile proboscis occurs (e.g., macroscelidids, tupaiids, tenrecids, elephants, tapirs, sirenians, and many extinct ungulate groups).

The premaxilla is usually a small element that primarily forms the anterior lateral wall of the nasal cavity (figs. 9.1–9.6). The postero-dorsal exposure of the premaxilla is usually limited, a primitive condition that occurs in monotremes, marsupials, and many eutherians (figs. 9.3–9.6). Secondarily, the postero-dorsal process shows expansion in some mammals, and may nearly or completely contact the frontals. This expansion is either accompanied by nasal retraction (e.g., fig. 9.9A, B; proboscideans, sirenians) or occurs even where such retraction is not evident (fig. 9.14B; Rodentia, Lagomorpha). Reduction of the premaxilla in certain mammals (e.g., fig. 9.6D–F; Chiroptera) correlates well with concomitant reduction or loss of upper incisors, increased surface area for facial muscles, and

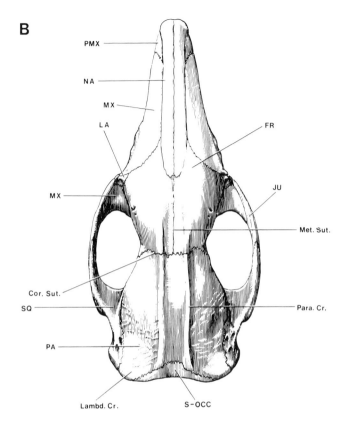

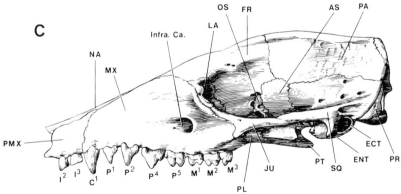

Fig. 9.5. *(continued)*

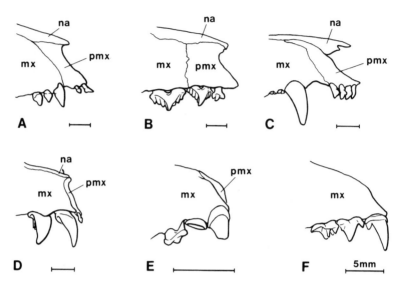

Fig. 9.6. Lateral views of right skull rostrum. A. The Eocene euprimate *Notharctus osborni* (AMNH 11466). B. The dermopteran *Cynocephalus* sp. (CA 3633). C. The marsupial *Didelphis marsupialis* (AM 2394). D. The megachiropteran *Dobsonia moluccensis* (AM 198750). E. The emballonurid microchiropteran *Taphozous flaviventrus* (AM 107759). F. The megadermatid microchiropteran *Macroderma gigas* (AM 162673). Scale bars equal 5 mm. Note marked development of premaxilla in A and B, and marked reduction in D–F. A small nasal process of the premaxilla is present in F, but is not visible in lateral view. For labeling and institutional acronyms see list of abbreviations.

enlargement of the canine (Novacek 1986). Likewise, the size of the incisive foramina (figs. 9.4B; 9.5A; 9.7) on the palate varies considerably. In lagomorphs and rodents these are elongated in relation to the marked expansion of the Jacobson's organs (Novacek 1985, fig. 1).

The maxilla is a complex bone associated with both the ethmoidal and orbitotemporal region of the skull. Typically this element is pierced on the lateral naso-facial eminence by an infraorbital canal (fig. 9.4C, 9.5C), which normally transmits the infraorbital nerve (trigeminal nerve, branch II), artery, and vein. The elongated canal seems a plesiomorphic condition for mammals (Muller 1934), since this feature is common to many therapsids (Broom 1915). Butler (1956) attributed the shortening of the infraorbital canal in several insectivoran groups (e.g., shrews, tenrecs) to emargination of the facial musculature.

Also well exposed on the lateral maxilla is the antorbital fossa (figs. 9.4C, 9.5C), an excavation for the attachment of the snout muscles (levator alae nasi) and muscles of the supralabial vibrissal pad (levator labii

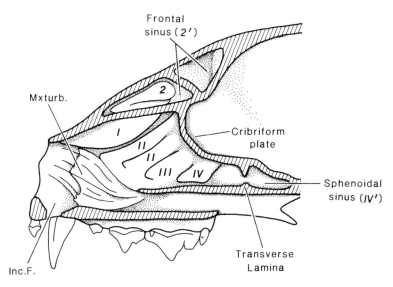

Fig. 9.7. Semidiagrammatic sagittal section of a domestic cat (*Felis catus*) showing right lateral wall of the nasal cavity, endoturbinals (roman numerals), ectoturbinals (arabic numerals), and sinuses, as discussed in text. For additional labeling see list of abbreviations. (After Moore 1981)

superioris). This excavation varies in development, being large in animals with well-developed snout muscles and a mobile proboscis (e.g., macroscelideans). The maxilla typically contributes to a large portion of the secondary palate (figs. 9.1B–D, 9.4B, 9.5A), although its contribution can be notably reduced with the enlargement of the premaxilla and incisive foramina and the forward displacement of the choanae (e.g., lagomorphs). The ventral exposure of the palatine is affected in a similar fashion.

In many mammals (e.g., *Tupaia*), the vomer ossifies relatively later than other dermal elements (figs. 9.1D, 9.1–9.5; Zeller 1987, table II). Posteriorly, the vomer, the cribriform plate, and the remaining ethmoid typically form a transverse lamina that isolates the choanae from the more dorsal olfactory chamber (fig. 9.2C). Anteriorly, the vomer forms a splint-like vertical plate that sagittally divides the ventral nasal capsule (fig. 9.3A). It supports the ventral border of the nasal septum and its posterior portion has a shelflike projection, the ala vomeris, which contributes to support of the ethmoturbinal. The vomer is commonly claimed to be homologous with the sauropsid parasphenoid (which underlies the trabecular segment of the cranial base), with the corollary that the mammalian vomer is not the homologue of the nonmammalian prevomer (de Beer 1937). The prevomer, as de Beer argued, may be retained in some mammals as a small anterior element (e.g., *Ornithorynchus*) or a paraseptal process of the premaxilla (Lagomorpha, *Sus*). This conclusion was disputed by Green and Presley (1978) and Presley and Steel (1978), who claimed that the small anterior element in *Ornithorynchus* is, at least in early stages, continuous with the premaxilla. These authors note that this small element found in several mammals represents the remnant of the anterior parasphenoid, which is an element separate from the vomer in the primitive synapsids. They thus equate the mammalian vomer with the fused platelike vomers (fig. 9.1C) or "prevomers" in the cynodont skull (see review in Moore 1981).

The Nasal Septum. The nasal septum is an anteriorly cartilaginous and posteriorly osseous plate that sagittally divides the nasal cavity (fig. 9.2C). The ossified nasal septum is a complex region, comprising contributions from the infolding of the paired nasals, the mesethmoid, and the presphenoid, and occasionally minor contributions from the frontal, sphenoidal, and maxillary. The components vary taxonomically. The large mesethmoid contribution to this septum does not occur in monotremes, marsupials, and many eutherians, suggesting that the mesethmoid contribution seen in pholidotans, tubulidentates, hyracoids, rodents, insectivores, chiropterans, dermopterans, carnivorans, and primates is a derived mammalian condition (de Beer 1937). The bony portion of the mesethmoid—also called the perpendicular plate (lamina perpendicularis) of the ethmoid bone—combines with the cartilaginous septum nasi and the presphenoid to form the posterior nasal septum. Where the ossified mesethmoid is absent or weakly developed, the entire bony portion of this septum in mammals is homologous with the tetrapod presphenoid (de Beer 1937).

The Bony Turbinals. The scroll-like turbinate bones which intrude the nasal cavity have a complex structure (figs. 9.7, 9.17). Ventrally, the maxilloturbinal (= inferior turbinate bone = concha nasalis inferior) is a finely ridged structure supported by the maxilla and the premaxilla (figs. 9.3A, 9.7). More dorsally positioned is an anterior naso-turbinal (fig. 9.7). The remaining ethmoturbinals consist of a system of branching lamellae. Morphology of this region is particularly elaborate in mammals with a well-developed olfactory sense. The ethmoturbinals are typically arrayed into two or more rows; the more lateral rows are denoted as ectoturbinals and those of the more medial rows as endoturbinals (fig. 9.17). In sagittal view the endoturbinals form large, obliquely oriented rows in the posterior nasal cavity (fig. 9.7).

There is some confusion in the terminology for the ethmoturbinals.

Endoturbinals are usually noted by roman numerals. However, endoturbinal I is the naso-turbinal which develops partly from the ethmoid, while the more ventral and posterior endoturbinals II, III, IV, etc., do not. There is also some variation in the use of the numbering system for the ectoturbinals, although it is common to designate these with arabic numerals (figs. 9.7, 9.17; Moore 1981, 243–244). Related to this system is a series of paranasal sinuses (figs. 9.7, 9.17, 9.18) developed as evaginations of the areas between the basal lamellae of the ethmoturbinals. Paulli's (1900a) convention designates these sinuses according to the ethmoturbinals lying immediately above them (e.g., sinus I opens below endoturbinal I, and sinus 1 opens below ectoturbinal 1). It is, however, also standard practice to name these sinuses after the bones they excavate (e.g., "frontal" sinus or "sphenoidal" sinus). To complicate this problem, there is an extreme amount of variation in the number, relative size, and branching patterns of the ethmoturbinal complex. Gregory (1910) and others attempted to develop a transformation scheme explaining this variation, but with limited success and moot phylogenetic implications. A useful review of the variety of ethmoturbinal architecture is provided by Moore (1981).

The Septomaxilla. A final component of interest in the ethmoidal region is the septomaxilla. This bone has been identified in many sauropsids and in certain mammals (monotremes, edentates) as a dermal bone lying behind the external narial aperture and projecting inward as a plate (fig. 9.3B) overlying Jacobson's organ (de Beer 1937). The presence of a septomaxilla in edentates is intriguing because it suggests that these taxa have retained a primitive sauropsid element lost in all other eutherians (McKenna 1975; Novacek 1982). However, this conclusion rests on ambiguous evidence. The septomaxilla is absent in all marsupials and several edentate lineages, leaving open the possibility that a new element is independently derived in those edentates where it occurs (Novacek and Wyss 1986a).

Orbitotemporal Region

The orbitotemporal region is that area of the developing cranium between the nasal and otic capsules. This region essentially represents the housing (the floor and the lateral wall) of the primary cranial cavity. In contrast to other amniotes, mammals have an additional or secondary wall lateral to a space called the cavum epiptericum, which houses certain cranial nerves and blood vessels (Gaupp 1902, 1905). Because these latter structures lie outside the skull in the primitive amniote condition, their shift "inside" the mammalian cranium through development of the secondary wall represents a dramatic modification (see also section below on the braincase wall).

Chondrocranial Development. Earliest stages of chondrification commonly involve the formation of the trabecular plate and the lamina hypophyseos (fig. 9.2A), which floor the primary cranial cavity. Other structures are variably developed. The interorbital portion of the trabecular plate sometimes forms a high, interorbital septum. More posteriorly, the hypophyseal plate may be associated with a cartilaginous, and later ossified, dorsum sellae (fig. 9.11B). The latter feature is present in some lagomorphs, carnivorans, bats, and many primates, including *Homo,* but it is absent in several other groups, including the tree shrew, *Tupaia* (Terry 1917; Starck 1943; Zeller 1987). A processus alaris (probably homologous to the basitrabecular process of other amniotes; Voit 1909; de Beer 1937) arises from the lateral edge of the hypophyseal plate.

Development of the Primary Wall of the Braincase. As noted above, the lateral wall of the primary cranial cavity in mammals shows dramatic reduction. Ventrally this reduction results in the fusion of openings for cranial nerves II–VII which are, to a varying extent, separate in the braincase of other amniotes. This extensive ventral fenestration is interrupted only by a series of narrow pillars (pila praeoptica, metoptica, and antotica, and commissura praefacialis; figs. 9.2, 9.19), some of which are variably lost in monotremes, marsupials, and eutherians (Kuhn and Zeller 1987; and discussion below). Above these pillars are platelike commissures (fig. 9.2). One of these dorsal cartilages, the ala orbitalis (fig. 9.2), becomes associated and later fused with the orbitosphenoid through appositional and endochondral bone formation (Zeller 1984). Another dorsal cartilage, the commissura orbitoparietalis, connects the expanding ala orbitalis (fig. 9.2A, B) with the parietal lamina of the otic capsule. The development of this commissure is, however, variable. It is large and persistent in monotremes, marsupials, some insectivorans (*Erinaceous, Talpa*), and the armadillo (*Dasypus*) (Fischer 1901; Fawcett 1918a; Toeplitz 1920; Reinbach 1952; Kuhn 1971), but it is ephemeral or virtually lacking in the tree shrew (*Tupaia,* fig. 9.2A, B), sloths (*Bradypus*), lagomorphs (*Oryctolagus*), the flying lemur (*Cynocephalus*), and many primates, including *Homo* (Matthes 1921a; Henckel 1927a, b, 1929; Frick and Heckmann 1955; Schneider 1955; Schliemann 1966; Halbsguth 1973; Wünsch 1975; Starck 1975a; Zeller 1987). The orbitoparietal commissure is reduced in many mammals apparently because its growth is outstripped by the expanding brain (Kuhn 1971; Kuhn and Zeller 1987). Only in some Cetacea and Carnivora (DeBurlet 1914; Schreiber 1916; Fawcett 1918b) does the dorsal part of the primary wall expand laterally to accommodate the increase in brain size. It is also possible that the alleged absence of the commissura orbitoparietalis in primates is an artifact of deficient ontogenetic sampling, and its ephemeral presence might be detected, as in *Tupaia*, with more complete developmental series (Zeller 1987).

Secondary Braincase Wall. Eutherians typically show a wide gap below the commissura orbitoparietalis (figs. 9.19, 9.20), the sphenoparietal fenestra, and here the presence of the primary braincase wall is indicated only by the dura mater. A secondary braincase wall is formed more laterally (fig. 9.20), incorporating nerves outside the braincase in other amniotes into the braincase of mammals. The reduced primary and the secondary braincase wall are separated by a space called the cavum epiptericum (Gaupp 1902, 1905), which contains the trigeminal ganglion, segments of cranial nerves III–VI, and the internal carotid artery (Voit 1909; Kuhn 1971; Zeller 1987).

The lateral wall of the cavum epiptericum is initially formed by the ascending lamina of the ala temporalis (figs. 9.3A, 9.20, 9.21). This element, which in most therians chondrifies independently of other structures, is of considerable phylogenetic interest (Zeller 1987; Maier 1987a; and comments below). In *Tupaia*, as in marsupials, carnivorans, and primates, the ala temporalis eventually surrounds the maxillary nerve, so that this nerve exits the cavum epiptericum through the foramen rotundum. Also, in Theria the lamina ascendens of the ala temporalis is partly ossified as the alisphenoid (fig. 9.2A). Subsequently the alisphenoid increases in size by appositional bone growth. Typically, in neonatal therians, the alisphenoid is broadly developed (fig. 9.2B) rostrally, laterally, and caudally and it also forms the floor of the supracochlear cavity between the tegmen tympani and the otic capsule (Zeller 1987).

The Osseous Orbital Wall. Aside from the endochondral alisphenoid, ethmoid, and orbitosphenoid, several dermal bones—the lacrimal, frontal, parietal, maxilla, palatine, and pterygoid—make variable contributions to the orbital wall (figs. 9.3–9.5; 9.8A, 9.11B, 9.22, 9.23). Both endochondral and dermal components in the orbitotemporal wall form a complex mosaic whose varying patterns are often difficult to interpret phylogenetically (Muller 1934; Novacek 1980; table 3 in Novacek 1986). The maxilla is generally poorly exposed in the orbit, although lipotyphlan insectivorans and some primates are exceptional in having a strong orbital process of the maxilla (Butler 1956; McDowell 1958; Cartmill 1975; Novacek 1986). The palatine, on the other hand, is primitively well developed in the orbital wall (e.g., monotremes, marsupials, many eutherians) to the extent that it may directly contact the antero-dorsal lacrimal and isolate the weak maxilla from contact with the frontal (fig. 9.22, in part). The proportions of the alisphenoid and orbitosphenoid vary according to some of the ontogenetic interactions discussed above. Many of these mosaic patterns, however, are obscured in adult and even juvenile skulls by fusion of the orbital elements (e.g., soricids, talpids, tenrecids, chiropterans).

Adding to the complexity of the orbitotemporal region are several foramina that convey nerves and blood vessels. Terminology for these foramina is often confused, and an understanding of basic patterns of variation is very poor (for good critical descriptions of these foramina see McDowell 1958; Wahlert 1974). In primitive therians the orbital wing of the palatine grows around two clusters of openings, a small, circular, dorsal palatine foramen (for the descending palatine artery and nerve) and an elliptical sphenopalatine foramen (for the sphenopalatine nerve, artery, and vein). In some taxa (leptictids, lipotyphlans, rodents) these foramina are well separated (fig. 9.8A), in others (macroscelidids, tupaiids, many marsupials) they are closely apposed or fused (Novacek 1986).

The lacrimal usually shows a large foramen whose position may vary from within the orbit (fig. 9.8A) to the antorbital rim (fig. 9.2C). To some extent this variation is also related to the construction of the lacrimal itself. It is likely that in primitive therians, the lacrimal had a prominent facial process (didelphid marsupials: fig. 9.2A, C; tupaiines, some macroscelidids, fossil plesiadapid "primates"). However, the loss or marked reduction of this facial process appears in many groups and is likely to have arisen on multiple occasions (Gregory 1920; Muller 1934; Novacek 1986).

The orbitosphenoid often shows a trio of foramina (fig. 9.8A), the optic, the suboptic, and the sphenorbital fissure (equals sphenorbital foramen [Butler 1956], foramen lacerum anterius [McDowell 1958], and sphenoidal fissure [Wahlert 1974]). The last fissure, which conveys cranial nerves III, IV, V (variably V_2) and VI, is the lateral opening of the developing cavum epiptericum. It can be regarded as a fissure at the contact between the posterior orbitosphenoid and the anterior rim of the alisphenoid (fig. 9.2B). Lateral to the sphenorbital fissure on the surface of the alisphenoid there may be a separate foramen rotundum (fig. 9.2A, B) for passage of the maxillary division of the trigeminal nerve and a (variably) transverse vein. In many taxa, however, the foramen rotundum is confluent with the sphenorbital fissure (e.g., didelphid marsupials, leptictids [fig. 9.8A], lipotyphlan insectivorans, dermopterans, chiropterans, carnivorans, pholidotans, and many others). The distinct separation of the foramen rotundum is most characteristic of edentates, tupaiids, and euprimates (Novacek 1986, table 3). Further laterally and posteriorly there is sometimes an alisphenoid canal (fig. 9.8A) for passage of the first part of the internal maxillary artery and its accompanying vein; though, again, the presence or absence of this canal, and its relative length, vary considerably (Butler 1956; Novacek 1985, 1986). In addition to one or two other small

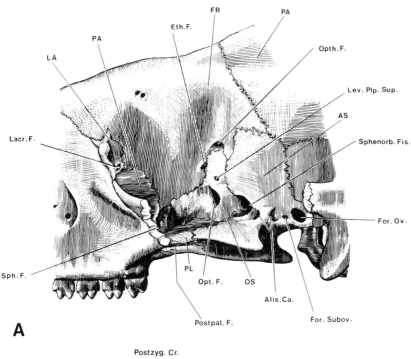

A

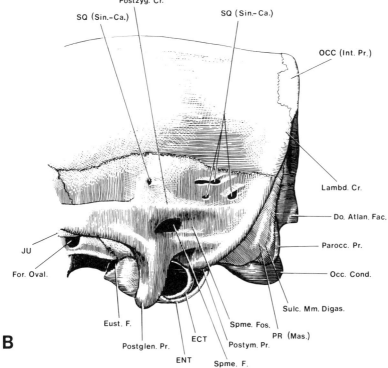

B

Fig. 9.8. Lateral views of left orbital (A) and squamosal (B) regions of *Leptictis dakotensis.* For labeling see list of abbreviations. (From Novacek 1986)

foramina variably present, the posterior alisphenoid surrounds a large, ventral opening, the foramen ovale (figs. 9.8A, B; 9.10), which normally transmits the mandibular branch of the trigeminal (V_3) nerve as well as other structures (fig. 9.11A). The foramen ovale is completely surrounded by the alisphenoid bone in most eutherians but seems to lie between the alisphenoid and periotic in monotremes, marsupials, edentates, and pholidotans (Novacek and Wyss 1986a).

The Zygomatic Arch. Lateral to the orbital wall is the zygomatic process formed anteriorly by the maxilla, posteriorly by the squamosal, and intermediately by the jugal (figs. 9.1F, 9.4, 9.5). The most widely distributed and plesiomorphous condition in therians is a well-developed continuous jugal (figs. 9.4C, 9.5C), but this element is greatly reduced or absent in some eutherians (soricids, tenrecids, pholidotans: figs. 9.14D, 9.15C; chiropterans). This reduction is surely independent in several lineages (Wible and Novacek 1988), although the virtual loss of the jugal and the interruption of the zygomatic arch is probably a shared derived condition of soricids and tenrecids (McDowell 1958). Where present, the jugal is variably developed. In certain eutherians (proboscideans, hyracoids) its ventral flange extends far backward on the zygomatic arch (fig. 9.9E, F) so that it terminates just lateral to the glenoid fossa for the jaw articulation (Novacek and Wyss 1986a). Although this condition is found in marsupials (fig. 9.9C), and even in some therapsids (Crompton and Sun 1985), it is likely an independently derived therian trait of uncertain function. The zygoma is also secondarily expanded through dorso-ventral thickening of the maxillary and squamosal contributions (e.g., sirenians, proboscideans: fig. 9.9A, B). These and other modifications of the zygomatic arch often relate to the development and rearrangement of the masseter muscles (Turnbull 1970).

The Skull Base. The pterygoid (figs. 9.1, 9.3–9.5, 9.10) is a dermal bone exposed at the base of the orbitotemporal region that often fuses early with the adjacent presphenoid, alisphenoid, and basisphenoid. The pterygoid forms the lateral roof of the interpterygoid fossa, which allows passage of the pharyngeal nerve, artery, and vein between the tuba auditiva and the sphenopalatine foramen (fig. 9.11A). The pterygoid sometimes develops medial entopterygoid crests which, together with the ectopterygoid crests of the alisphenoid, confine the sites of origin for the internal pterygoid muscles to an ectopterygoid fossa (fig. 9.10). While this fossa is well excavated in some early eutherians (e.g., leptictids) as well as solenodontids and erinaceids, it is weak or absent in macroscelidiids, tupaiids, and primates. The latter condition is related to the forward and dorsal migration of the pterygoid muscles to attach to the palatine in front of the optic

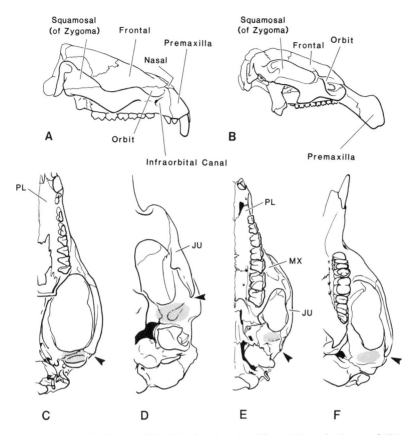

Fig. 9.9. Right side of the skull in (A) a fossil proboscidean, *Moeritherium*, and (B) a sirenian, *Trichechus*. Ventral views of left side of the skull in (C) a marsupial, *Didelphis*, (D) *Trichechus*, (E) a hyracoid, *Procavia*, and (F) a proboscidean, *Elephas*. Not to scale. Arrows in C–F indicate contact between the jugal and squamosal. Uniform stipple indicates glenoid region for jaw articulation. For other labeling see list of abbreviations. (From Novacek and Wyss 1986a)

foramen (Butler 1956). It is difficult to ascertain whether this condition or the marked excavation of the ectopterygoid fossa is derived for therians. It should be noted that the demarcation of the ectopterygoid fossa can be independent of the prominence of the ectopterygoid crests of the alisphenoid (e.g., macroscelideans, tupaiids, dermopterans, chiropterans, and others), which serve as the attachment site for the external pterygoid muscles.

Also forming the posterior base of the orbitotemporal region is the basisphenoid (figs. 9.1, 9.2, 9.4, 9.5). The intracranial surface of this element is marked by an elongate, raised sella turcica and a hypophyseal fossa for the pituitary gland (fig. 9.11B). In some mammals, the posterior

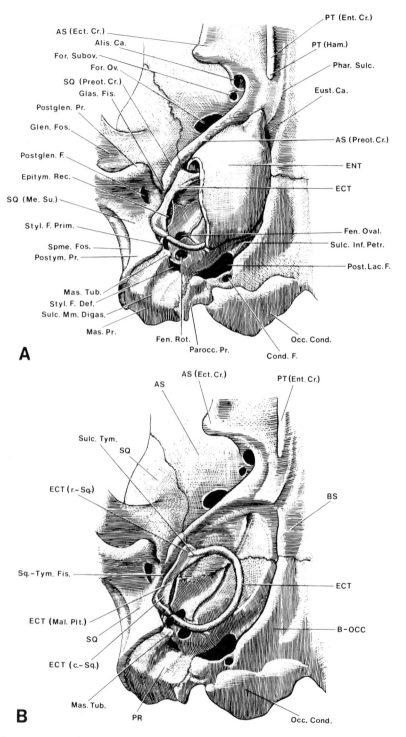

Fig. 9.10. Ventral views of right basicranium of the early eutherian mammal *Leptictis dakotensis*. A. Auditory bulla included, but lateral portion partly dissected. B. Auditory bulla not included. For labeling see list of abbreviations. (From Novacek 1986)

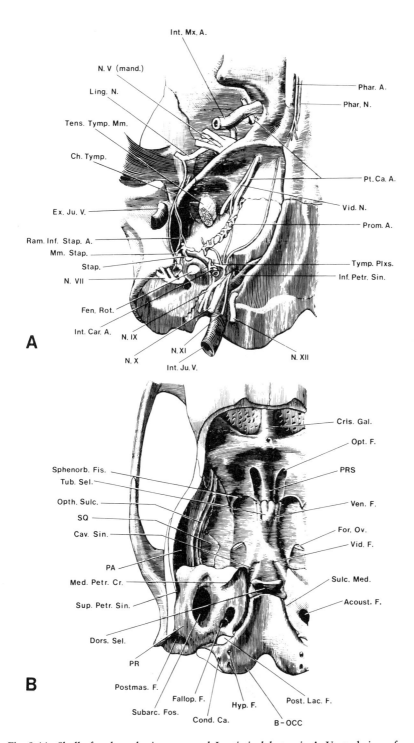

Fig. 9.11. Skull of early eutherian mammal *Leptictis dakotensis*. A. Ventral view of right basicranium with bulla and ectotympanic removed and major nerves and blood vessels reconstructed. B. Dorsal view of internal braincase with skull roofing bones removed. For labeling see list of abbreviations. (From Novacek 1986)

border of the hypophyseal fossa is developed into a prominent, semivertical dorsum sellae whose dorsal eminence is expanded into a posterior clinoid process. This feature is present in tupaiids and the extinct leptictids as well as in chiropterans, carnivorans, tubulidentates, and some euprimates. It has been argued (McDowell 1958) that an expanded dorsum sellae is a primitive therian condition even though it is absent in monotremes, didelphid marsupials, and many other mammalian groups.

Otic Region

The otic region represents an area of great interest in mammalian phylogenetics. Many otic components are important to an understanding of mammalian origins, and these features are cited also as evidence for higher-level patterns within Mammalia. Perhaps more modern studies of mammalian skull diversification have focused on this region (e.g., MacPhee 1981; Zeller 1985b; Wible 1986) than on any other.

At early developmental stages, the otic region of the chondocranium comprises the posterior section of the parachordal plate, the otic capsules, the braincase wall dorsal to these structures, and the commissura praefacialis (fig. 9.2A). The parachordal plate is the first element of the skull in *Tupaia* (Zeller 1987), and other mammals generally, chondrifying in the mesenchyme surrounding the chorda dorsalis (notochord). The position of the plate in relation to the chordal dorsalis is variable. The hypochordal position of the parachordal plate is probably plesiomorphous; it is the condition in monotremes, as well as in the shrew *Suncus* (de Beer 1937; Kuhn 1971).

Differentiation of the Otic Capsule. The developing otic capsule differentiates into two main parts (figs. 9.2, 9.12), the pars canalicularis (for the semicircular canals and the utriculus) and the pars cochlearis (for the sacculus and the cochlear duct). Chondrification is independent of that of the parachordal plate in most therians, including tupaiids, insectivorans, bats, and carnivorans. As development proceeds, the pars cochlearis is connected to the adjacent parts of the skull via six commissures (see Zeller 1987). A well-defined basicapsular fissure (fig. 9.2B) separates the cochlear capsule from the parachordal plate. In didelphid marsupials this fissure arises from resorption of cartilage connecting the otic capsule with the parachordal plate. Reduction or loss of all commissures bridging this fissure and other connections for the otic capsules sometimes occurs. This trend is extreme in Cetacea (DeBurlet 1914; Honigmann 1917) and Sirenia (Matthes 1921b) and is usually associated with special auditory requirements for hearing under water (Fleischer 1978). Many echolocating bats also show partial to extreme isolation of the otic capsule from surrounding elements (Novacek 1980), perhaps as a means of attenuating sounds transmitted through bone conduction (Henson 1970). It is likely that an ontogeny involving closure of the fissures and broad contact between the otic capsule and the parachordal plate is plesiomorphous for mammals (Toeplitz 1920; Kuhn 1971).

As skull elements grow, there is a general pattern of negative allometry for the otic capsule. A marked exception to this trend occurs in some adult mammals, where the ossified cochlea is relatively very large (e.g., Microchiroptera). During ontogeny the capsule shifts in position. The long axes of the canalicular portion of the capsule tend to diverge anteriorly with the broadening of the parachordal plate, although the vestibular part of the capsule does not notably shift. There is also a trend from a dorsal position relative to the parachordal plate to a ventral position wherein the dorsal surface of the capsule is aligned with the plane of the parachordal plate. This trend is a common one, seen both in didelphid marsupials (Toeplitz 1920) and monotremes (Kuhn 1971), but there are divergent patterns wherein the cochlear capsules shift dorso-caudally (e.g., *Canis;* see Schliemann 1966). These patterns have been associated with development of the brain relative to the cranial elements in different mammals (Zeller 1987).

Chondrification of the medial pars vestibularis (fig. 9.12B) is in *Tupaia* and other mammals generally slower than chondrification of other areas of the capsule. Differentiation of the superior and inferior acoustic foramina for passage of various branches of cranial nerve VIII follows (Voit 1909; Zeller 1987).

Cochlear Fenestrae and Labyrinths. The latero-ventral surface of the cochlear portion of the otic capsule is pierced by two large fenestrations, the fenestra ovalis (figs. 9.10A, 9.12) and the perilymphatic foramen (fig. 9.12). Later in ontogeny (day 34 in *Tupaia*) the fenestra ovalis is well defined by the increased chondrification of the otic capsule. It pierces the lateral wall of the cochlear capsule and is closed by contact with the stapes and the annular ligament (fig. 9.11A).

The perilymphatic foramen is caudo-ventral to the fenestra ovalis. As development proceeds, the caudal ridge of the base of the cochlear capsules produces a horizontal cartilaginous plate, the processus recessus, which lies in a plane ventral to the perilymphatic foramen. This process eventually connects medially to the parachordal plate and the floor of the canalicular part of the otic capsule via a small process from the latter. The opening separating the ventral edge of the promontorium cochlea from the processus recessus is the fenestra rotunda (figs. 9.2C, 9.10, 9.11A, 9.12B), a feature homologous with the recessus scalae tympani of reptiles (Zeller 1985a, b). The perilymphatic spaces of the cochlear labyrinth (perilym-

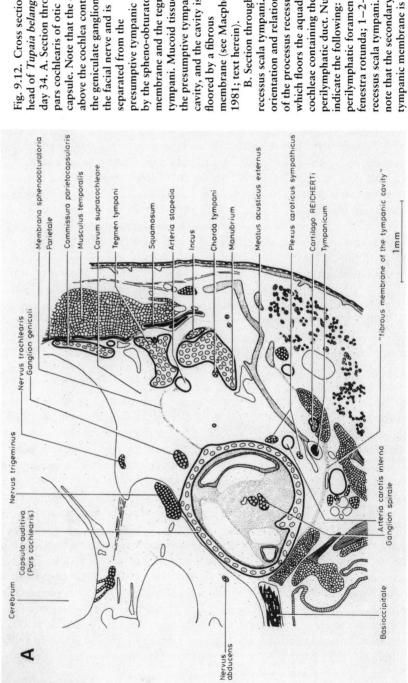

Fig. 9.12. Cross sections of head of *Tupaia belangeri*, day 34. A. Section through pars cochlearis of otic capsule. Note that the cavity above the cochlea contains the geniculate ganglion of the facial nerve and is separated from the presumptive tympanic cavity by the spheno-obturatory membrane and the tegmen tympani. Mucoid tissue fills the presumptive tympanic cavity, and the cavity is floored by a fibrous membrane (see Macphee 1981; text herein).

B. Section through recessus scala tympani. Note orientation and relationships of the processus recessus, which floors the aquaductus cochleae containing the perilymphatic duct. Numbers indicate the following: 1–2, perilymphatic foramen; 1–3, fenestra rotunda; 1–2–3, recessus scala tympani. Also note that the secondary tympanic membrane is

A

Cerebrum

Capsula auditiva (Pars cochlearis)

Nervus trigeminus

Nervus trochlearis

Ganglion geniculi

Membrana sphenoobturatoria

Parietale

Commissura parietocapsularis

Musculus temporalis

Cavum supracochleare

Tegmen tympani

Squamosum

Arteria stapedia

Incus

Chorda tympani

Manubrium

Meatus acusticus externus

Plexus caroticus sympathicus

Cartilago REICHERTi

Tympanicum

Arteria carotis interna

Ganglion spirale

Basioccipitale

Nervus abducens

"fibrous membrane of the tympanic cavity"

1mm

located medial to the
fenestra rotunda, and spans
the gap between the ventral
edge of the promontorium
and the septum
metacochleare in the plane of
the perilymphatic foramen
(1–2), and between the
septum metacochleare and
the lateral edge of the
processus recessus at the
lateral surface of the
perilymphatic duct. The
secondary tympanic
membrane thus forms the
medial boundary of the
fossula fenestrae rotundae,
which represents an
extension of the tympanic
cavity into the recessus scala
tympani. (From Zeller 1987)

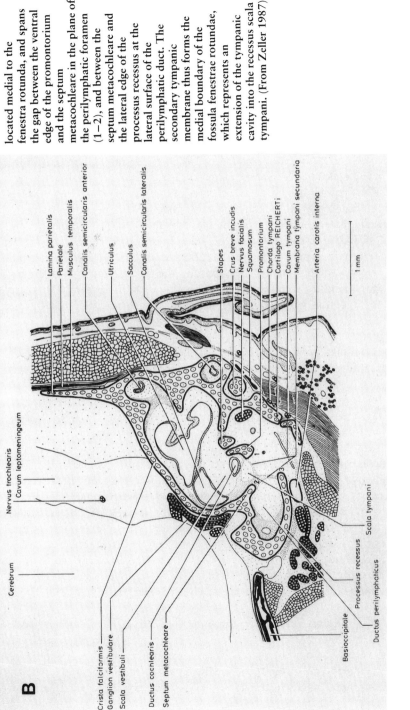

B

Cerebrum

Nervus trochlearis
Cavum leptomeningeum

Lamina parietalis
Parietale
Musculus temporalis
Canalis semicircularis anterior

Utriculus

Sacculus

Canalis semicircularis lateralis

Stapes
Crus breve incudis
Nervus facialis
Squamosum
Promontorium
Chorda tympani
Cartilago REICHERTi
Cavum tympani
Membrana tympani secundaria

Arteria carotis interna

Crista falciformis
Ganglion vestibulare
Scala vestibuli

Ductus cochlearis
Septum metacochleare

Basioccipitale

Ductus perilymphaticus

Processus recessus

Scala tympani

1 mm

phatic cistern, scala tympani, scala vestibuli, perilymphatic duct) develop in the mesenchyme between the membranous labyrinth and the otic capsule (fig. 9.12B).

The perilymphatic duct runs in a canal, the aqueaductus cochlea (Zeller 1985a, b), floored by the processus recessus. The aqueaductus cochlea is not present in *Ornithorhynchus* and the canal present in *Tachyglossus* is not homologous with that in therians, as it encloses the glossopharyngeal nerve (Kuhn 1971). The aqueaductus cochlea (sensu stricto) is thus a therian neomorph (J. Wible, personal communication). According to Kuhn (1971) and Zeller (1985a, b), the processus recessus is part of the parachordal plate which was shifted laterally together with the recessus scala tympani in mammalian phylogeny. The secondary tympanic membrane does not develop in the plane of the fenestra rotunda; it is instead located more medially at the lateral surface of the scala tympani and the proximal part of the perilymphatic duct (fig. 9.12B). The secondary tympanic membrane hence constitutes the medial boundary of the fossula of the fenestra rotunda, which is an extension of the tympanic cavity into the recessus scalae tympani of mammals (Frick 1952a, b; Zeller 1985a, b, 1987).

Pars Canalicularis and Subarcuate Fossa. The pars canalicularis is caudal, lateral, and dorsal to the pars cochlearis (figs. 9.2, 9.13), and its dorsal surface is usually excavated by a subarcuate fossa (figs. 9.2B, C; 9.11B). This fossa tends to deepen during development as it lodges the expanding cerebellar paraflocculus. However, the subarcuate fossa is poorly developed in some mammalian groups (e.g., *Tachyglossus*, edentates, pholidotans, tubulidentates, hyracoids, sirenians, proboscideans, and various ungulates). The transformational pattern here is ambiguous. Within some mammalian groups (e.g., Primates) there is a clearly documented relation between the size of the subarcuate fossa and the expansion of the petrosal lobule of the cerebellar paraflocculus (Gannon et al. 1988). Both features are small or absent in cercopithicids and even more notably in great apes and humans, suggesting an evolutionary trend toward reduction or loss within primates (Gannon et al. 1988). If this reflects a broader-scale trend, the reduction or loss of the subarcuate fossa occurred independently several times within therians (Novacek 1986; Novacek and Wyss 1986a).

Tegmen Tympani. The tegmen tympani (figs. 9.13B, 9.30), which constitutes part of the roof of the tympanic cavity, derives from the rostral wall of the vestibular part of the cochlear capsule. This feature has been regarded as a therian neomorph (van Kampen 1905; Starck 1941), as it is absent in monotremes (Kuhn 1971). In therians, the tegmen tympani con-

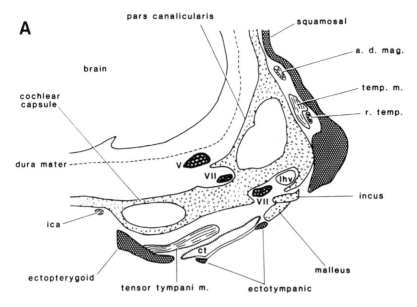

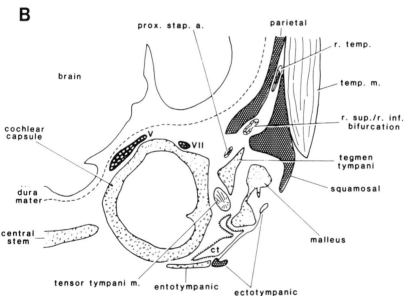

Fig. 9.13. Schematic cross sections through the middle tympanic regions in (A) 92 mm (crown-rump length) pouch young of the monotreme *Tachyglossus aculeatus,* (B) 93.5 mm (crown-rump length) fetus of the megachiropteran bat *Pteropus.* Open circles indicate elements preformed in cartilage. Cross-hatching indicates dermal bone. Note positions of the ramus temporalis (r. temp.), arteria diploetica magna (a. d. mag.), cavum tympani (ct), internal carotid artery (ica), temporalis muscle (temp. m.), and cranial nerves V and VII. In B, the bifurcation of the ramus superior/ramus inferior (r. sup/r. inf.) is above the tympanic roof formed by the tegmen tympani (see text discussion on carotid circulation). Note also that in B the tegmen tympani projects directly ventrad into the tympanic cavity, a feature unique to bats. (From Wible 1987)

tributes, along with the squamosal and the alisphenoid, to the secondary lateral wall of the braincase (de Beer 1937; Kuhn and Zeller 1987). The tegmen tympani varies in structure (cf. figs. 9.12A and 9.13B), and its vertical orientation and composite development are especially peculiar in chiropterans (figs. 9.13B, 9.30B).

The Tympanic Cavity. The otic region is replete with structures contained within the tympanic cavity or contributed by adjacent bony elements. Ossification of the petrosal clearly defines many of the above noted fenestra. In addition, there is in many mammals an elongate groove on the antero-lateral wall of the tympanic cavity, the glaserian fissure (fig. 9.10A). This groove appears early in ontogeny as the aperture for Meckel's cartilage, which eventually disappears. Thereafter, the channel is occupied by the chorda tympani (figs. 9.11A, 9.12) and occasionally the ramus inferior of the stapedial artery (van der Klaauw 1931). It is uncertain whether or not the presence of the glaserian fissure denotes a plesiomorphous condition, as its form varies distinctly among different groups (Novacek 1986).

The lateral edge of the tympanic roof is typically excavated by a deep epitympanic recess (figs. 9.10A, 9.13B). The recess is, however, poorly excavated in monotremes (fig. 9.13A) and only moderately excavated in most didelphid marsupials; these likely represent more conservative mammalian conditions. The epitympanic recess lodges the incudomalleolar articulation, so its development reflects the size of these ossicles. Hence, the recess is very large in burrowing forms (e.g., *Chrysochloris*) with large, loosely articulated ossicles suited for low-frequency impedance matching (Fleischer 1973). In living mammals, the membranous lateral wall of the epitympanic recess is dorsal to the level of the tympanic membrane and so is formed by the membrana Shrapnelli (Bondy 1907). The composition of the bony lateral wall of this recess varies notably in mammals. A major contribution by the squamosal occurs in many therians (Novacek 1986). Alternative contributions to the epitympanic recess are diverse, variably involving the ectotympanic, tegmen tympani, and the mastoid process (van Kampen 1905; Bondy 1907; van der Klaauw 1931).

Postero-lateral to the fenestra rotunda is a deep pit, the foramen stylomastoideum definitivum (fig. 9.10A), for exit of the facial nerve (fig. 9.11A). This fossa is continuous anteriorly with the facial canal. In some mammals this area may be obscured ventrally by a well-developed mastoid tubercle (fig. 9.10), which incorporates the tympanohyal, the most cranial element of the hyoid apparatus. In late developmental stages the tympanohyal often fuses with the petrosal (de Beer 1937; MacPhee 1981). The mastoid tubercle is particularly well developed in archaic leptictids, lipotyphlan insectivorans, tubulidentates, and some perissodactyls (Novacek 1986). This condition seems secondary, since the mastoid tubercle is very weakly developed in most mammals, including monotremes and marsupials.

Another prominent feature of the tympanic region is the system of grooves or canals associated with the branching pattern of the internal carotid artery (figs. 9.10, 9.11A, 9.28–9.30). The variation in this system has received much attention in higher phylogenetic inquiries (Szalay 1975; Novacek 1980, 1986; MacPhee 1981; and especially Wible 1986, 1987).

The posterior lacerate foramen separates the postero-medial petrosal from the basioccipital (fig. 9.10). In cases where there is no separate jugular foramen the posterior lacerate foramen conveys the internal jugular vein as well as cranial nerves IX, X, and XI (fig. 9.11A).

Aside from its contributions to the epitympanic wall, the squamosal serves as the lateral and anterior rim of the tympanic cavity. Anteriorly it develops a shallow fossa (the glenoid fossa) for the mandibular articulation (figs. 9.9, 9.10) bounded posteriorly by the postglenoid process (figs. 9.8, 9.9, 9.10). The latter feature is variably developed in mammals. A derived condition involves the great reduction or loss of the postglenoid process and the development of a more medial process (the "pseudopostglenoid process") in lipotyphlans (McDowell 1958). Behind the postglenoid process is a (usually) large postglenoid foramen (fig. 9.10) for the external jugular vein (fig. 9.11A). In mammals with a very specialized craniomandibular joint (e.g., Rodentia, Lagomorpha) this foramen is shifted laterally and dorsally.

Occipital Region

In mammals, the early components of the occipital region include the posterior parachordal plate and the pilae occipitalis. The more dorsal tectum posterius is either an occipital or an otic element (Gaupp 1906). The pilae occipitalis are produced by the caudo-lateral corners of the parachordal plate, and the junction between these two structures is indicated by the hypoglossal (or condylar) foramen for cranial nerve XII (figs. 9.10, 9.11A). In adult eutherian skulls there is usually only one hypoglossal foramen on each side of the basicranium (e.g., marsupials, insectivorans, tupaiids, various ungulates). However, some eutherians (lagomorphs, rodents) and many marsupials are distinguished by two or three closely spaced foramina in this region (Novacek 1985, 1986).

Development proceeds with the upward growth and more vertical orientation of the occipital arches and their fusion with the tectum posterius, which begins ossification relatively early as the supraoccipital (fig. 9.2C). The increasingly vertical orientation of the tectum posterius (fig. 9.3B) is probably due to the enlargement of the cerebellum (Zeller 1987).

The occipital condyles are outgrowths of the pilae occipitalis. Primitively the condyles articulate with the vertebral column in a monocoelic fashion, a feature found in monotremes, many Insectivora, Carnivora, and lemuriform primates (Gaupp 1907b, 1908a; Starck 1979). The foramen magnum is bounded dorsally by the ventral edge of the posterior tectum, laterally by the medial borders of the pilae occipitalis, and rostrally by the posterior edge of the parachordal plate. An indentation on the ventral side of the tectum posterius, the incisura occipitalis superior, is first closed by the membrana atlantooccipitalis posterior and subsequently sealed by appositional bone from the supraoccipital. This closure does not occur in monotremes, where the incisura is retained in adults (Kuhn 1971).

The development of the supraoccipital is variable in mammals; it ossifies from a single unpaired center in *Felis*, *Sus*, and *Homo*, but from paired centers in *Bos* and *Canis* (de Beer 1937). There is no basic pattern to this variation and it is likely that ossification of the supraoccipital is fairly homoplastic at various taxonomic levels.

Between the supraoccipitals and parietals there forms in many mammals a membranous interparietal bone (fig. 9.2). The distribution of this condition is of interest (fig. 9.14). Although the interparietal is discriminated in some adult skulls (fig. 9.14A, B), it is very often fused with the supraoccipitals at late juvenile and adult stages (e.g., *Homo, Canis, Bos, Felis*). Presence of the interparietal is thought to be the primitive mammalian condition, and this element is regarded as a homologue of the sauropsid postparietal (de Beer 1937). The interparietal is allegedly absent in monotremes (de Beer 1937; Kuhn 1971), but there is some ambiguity concerning this condition (Novacek and Wyss 1986a). The interparietal is also absent in marsupials and edentates (fig. 9.14E) and certain genera of ungulates (e.g., *Sus*). Pholidotans (fig. 9.14D) have also been cited as lacking an interparietal (Gregory 1910), but this element is clearly demarcated in neonatal and certain fossil pangolins (Starck 1941; Emry 1970; Novacek and Wyss 1986a, addendum).

An interesting aspect of the adult occiput is its relation to the invasive petromastoid. The mastoid process is clearly exposed on the ventro-lateral surface of the posterior occiput in many mammals (fig. 9.15A, B, E). A more derived "amastoid" condition may be attained either by reduction of the mastoid process or overgrowth of the supra- and exoccipitals and the squamosal (fig. 9.15C, D, F). It is clear that amastoidy then is not necessarily attained in the same fashion among different mammals and any homology statement should be suspect without further inquiry. However, certain ungulate clades (hyracoids, proboscideans, sirenians, and desmostylians) do share a common type of amastoidy (Novacek and Wyss 1986a).

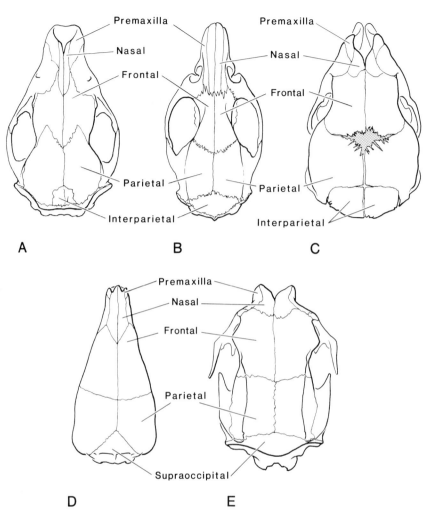

Fig. 9.14. Dorsal views of skulls in (A) an insectivoran (*Erinaceus*), (B) a rodent (*Rattus*), (C) a microchiropteran (*Rhinolophus*), (D) a pholidotan (*Manis*), and (E) an edentate (*Bradypus*). Note the marked backward extension of the premaxilla in *Rattus,* and marked reduction of these elements in *Rhinolophus*. In the adult *Manis* (D) the interparietal exposed in fetal skulls is obscured by its fusion with adjacent elements. The interparietal is lacking in *Bradypus* and other edentates. (From Novacek and Wyss 1986a)

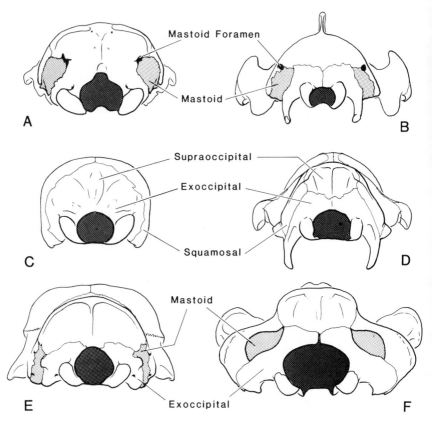

Fig. 9.15. Posterior views of skulls in (A) a tubulidentate (*Orycteropus*), (B) a marsupial (*Didelphis*), (C) a pholidotan (*Manis*), (D) a hyracoid (*Procavia*), (E) an edentate (*Choloepus*), and (F) a sirenian (*Trichechus*). Exposure of the mastoid process of the petrosal on the occiput is extensive in A and B, weak in E, and absent in C and D. In F the exposure is clearly secondary, as the mastoid is below a large gap in the occiput and does not extend continuously from the vertical occipital plane to the horizontal basicranial plane, as in A, B, and E. (From Novacek and Wyss 1986a)

Visceral Skeleton

The visceral skeleton involves both elements comprising the adult jaw and the ectotympanic and ossicles incorporated in the basicranium. Primordial structures of this system include the following derivatives:

Mandibular arch (first visceral arch):
    Meckel's cartilage
    Cartilaginous anlage of the malleus
    Palatoquadrate and derivative incus

Hyoid arch (second visceral arch):
  Reichert's cartilage
  Stapes
Third to fifth visceral arches:
  Hyobranchial skeleton (hyoid apparatus, etc.)

Ontogeny and Homology of the Auditory Ossicles. Meckel's cartilage generally forms early in ontogeny when the neurocranial endoskeleton is blastemal. Caudally this cartilage extends to form the anlage of the malleus (fig. 9.3A, 9.16). Somewhat later the dentary (dentale) covers the lateral surface of Meckel's cartilage (fig. 9.16) and eventually the latter is lodged in a longitudinal groove on the median side of the dentary. Ossification of Meckel's cartilage occurs by endochondral replacement through invasive action of the dentary (Spatz 1967). This is also accompanied by reduction of Meckel's cartilage at paranatal stages. Postnatally the remnant of Meckel's cartilage typically separates from the anlage of the malleus (fig. 9.16). The latter element undergoes endochondral ossification, initiated in later fetal stages, in direct contact with the membranous goniale. The malleus is therefore a mosaic element formed by the membranous goniale and the endochondral articular. The goniale gives rise to the anterior folian process of the malleus.

The palatoquadrate is no longer retained in mammals as the primitive component in the upper jaw of gnathostomes. Instead this vestigial element gives rise to the incus (fig. 9.16), the antorbital cartilage, the pterygoid cartilage, and the ala temporalis (Kuhn 1971; Zeller 1987). The incus derives from the pars quadrate of the palatoquadrate. The stapes is derived from the dorsal end of the hyoid arch. Where a stapedial artery develops,

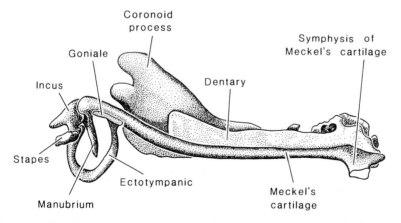

Fig. 9.1 ✶. *Tupaia belangeri*, day 34, showing development of the dermal elements of the lower jaw, Meckel's cartilage, and the incus and stapes. (After Zeller 1987)

the stapes chondrifies as a perforated triangle around this vessel (Goodrich 1930). Variation in formation of the stapes is, however, clearly evident (Novacek and Wyss 1986b). Reichert's cartilage (figs. 9.2, 9.3, 9.12B), which also develops from the hyoid arch, gives rise, in part, to the cornu minus of the hyoid bone.

Floor of the (Secondary) Tympanic Cavity. The ossicles (malleus, incus, and stapes) remain outside the tympanic cavity during prenatal stages. In the adult, these elements are encased in muco-periosteal tissue, derived from the mucoid tissue that originally filled the epithelial-lined primary tympanic cavity. Resorption of mucoid tissue and pneumatization of the primary tympanic cavity lead to the development of the secondary tympanic cavity (van Kampen 1905). The floor of the latter is composed of a dense fibrous membrane (fig. 9.12; van Kampen 1905; van der Klaauw 1931; Novacek 1977; MacPhee 1981), within which some mammals develop a neomorphic cartilage, the entotympanic (fig. 9.13B). This process occurs usually at early postnatal stages. Entotympanics may then ossify through cartilage replacement. In certain mammals, the entotympanic bone comprises nearly all (e.g., fig. 9.10A, *Leptictis;* tupaiids) or part (macroscelidians) of the floor of the tympanic cavity or auditory bulla. Composition of the bulla is, however, exceptionally variable, since contributions may come from the ectotympanic, alisphenoid, basisphenoid, and petrosal, as well as the entotympanic (figs. 9.24, 9.25; van Kampen 1905; van der Klaauw 1931; Novacek 1977; MacPhee 1981). In monotremes and in some Cretaceous mammals, there is no bulla and the ectotympanic ring lies nearly horizontally against the tympanic cavity (figs. 9.24, 9.25; Novacek 1977). This fact, coupled with the observation that the ectotympanic attains a progressively more vertical orientation in the ontogeny of bullate mammals (Kuhn 1971; Hunt 1974), suggests that the monotreme condition is primitive for mammals (Gregory 1910; Novacek 1977). It has therefore been argued that a tympanic floor or bulla was necessary to seal off the tympanic cavity exposed by vertical orientation of the ectotympanic (Kuhn 1971). The bony composition of the bulla has been applied, with mixed success, to the higher phylogenetics of mammals (see reviews in Novacek 1977, 1980; MacPhee 1981).

Ectotympanic. The ectotympanic is a membrane bone that forms as a dorsally open, horseshoe-shaped element (figs. 9.13, 9.16). In later stages the ectotympanic may also form a simple, complete ring (figs. 9.8, 9.10B), or may develop flanges that laterally form an external auditory tube or medially form part or nearly all of the auditory bulla (figs. 9.24, 9.25). Parts of the ectotympanic may also contribute to the lateral wall of the epitympanic recess. As noted above, the ectotympanic may shift during ontogeny from a more horizontal to a more vertical position (van der Klaauw 1931; Hunt 1974). The pattern is, however, more complicated than usually portrayed. In some adult mammals, the semihorizontal orientation of the ectotympanic is retained, with the effect that the tympanic membrane actually functions as partial floor of the tympanic cavity (Novacek 1977). It is also noteworthy that the anular ectotympanics in some adult mammals (e.g., tree shrews, lemurs) are the result of an anomalous cessation of bone growth around the time of birth, and thus the simple ring-shaped structure of the ectotympanic may in some cases be a specialized condition derived from a somewhat broader ectotympanic at an earlier developmental stage (MacPhee 1981). At a general level, however, it seems valid to claim that a narrow anular or horseshoe-shaped ectotympanic is the primitive mammalian condition.

SELECTED PROBLEMS

Nasal Turbinals and Paranasal Sinuses

As noted above, the scroll-like nasal turbinal bones often form a complex structure in mammals. The turbinals increase the surface area for the nasal mucosa and thus enhance thermoregulatory, respiratory, and olfactory function. The more anterior maxilloturbinal (figs. 9.3, 9.7) is usually covered with respiratory ciliated and stratified squamous epithelium. The more postero-dorsal ethmoturbinals (figs. 9.7, 9.17) are associated with a specialized olfactory epithelium. In some nonmammalian amniotes (for example, crocodiles) there is also a complex system of olfactory scrolls or concha, apparently homologous to the mammalian maxilloturbinal. This system does not, however, compare with the elaborate ethmoturbinals of some mammals. Such elaboration is most extreme in forms where the nasal cavity and its structures are markedly developed in correspondence with the expansion of the rhinencephalon and an emphasis on olfaction.

Earlier studies (Gregory 1910; Weber 1904) stressed a correspondence between turbinal variation and phylogenetic pattern. However, this relationship is appreciably complicated by the obvious correlation between structure and respiratory and olfactory function in different mammalian taxa. *Tachyglossus,* with seven endoturbinals, contrasts with *Ornithorhyncus,* where there are only three endoturbinals. The primitive condition in marsupials, thought to be characterized by didelphids, is a complex with five endoturbinals (Gregory 1910).

Despite the marked diversity of turbinals within eutherians, several orders share a basic pattern. Insectivorans, chiropterans, hyracoids, some primates, many rodents, and many carnivorans have an extensive ethmoid with four endoturbinals (figs. 9.7, 9.17A, B). There is also a row of two

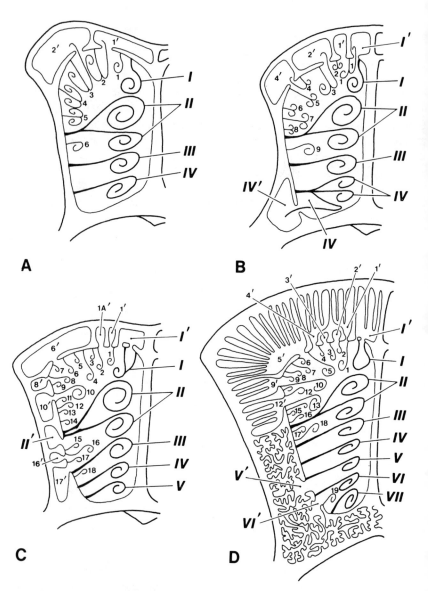

Fig. 9.17. Schematic representations of coronal sections parallel to the cribriform plate through the nasal cavities of (A) a dog (*Canis*), (B) a bear (*Ursus arctos*), (C) a cow (*Bos*), (D) an African elephant (*Loxodonta*). Endoturbinals are indicated by roman numerals; ectoturbinals, by arabic numerals; sinuses, by a prime (accent) and the number referring to the corresponding turbinal, e.g., 1′ = sinus for ectoturbinal 1. (After Paulli 1900 b, c; Moore 1981)

(or three) small ectoturbinals. The olfactory region with its complex of ethmoturbinals extends posteriorly into the presphenoid, influencing the form of adjacent elements. Various modifications of the anterior orbital region in insectivorans are related, for example, to the expansion of the ethmoidal complex (see discussion below).

Paulli (1900a, b, c) proposed that this general pattern represents the primitive one for eutherians and that the four endoturbinals are homologous in the above listed orders. Another shared feature of this system is the marked division of lamellae of endoturbinal II, to the extent that two nearly independent olfactory scrolls are found (figs. 9.7, 9.17). An increase in the number of olfactory scrolls seen in some bears, mustelids, procyonids, and many of the ungulate groups (artiodactyls, perissodactyls, proboscideans, and others) seems derived from the splitting of the posterior endoturbinals (usually IV) in addition to endoturbinal II (fig. 9.17C, D). Even greater complexity occurs in aardvarks and in myrmecophagid edentates (anteaters), where as many as nine endoturbinals indicate extreme olfactory specialization associated with termite feeding. Gregory (1910, 427) claimed that Paulli's (1900a, b, c) study confirmed his own view of mammalian higher relationships, although this character information contributes little to the resolution among the various eutherian orders.

Another interesting aspect of Paulli's (1900c) argument is that the four endoturbinals in "primitive" eutherians actually represent a reduction from the primitive number of five in marsupials through fusion of the second and third lamellae in the marsupial row. This is an intriguing, if only tentative proposal, for it suggests a complex transformation involving fusion and reduction in the eutherian ancestor and subsequent phases for either (1) further reduction (e.g., anthropoids and cetaceans) or (2) a reversal in this trend with elaboration of the ethmoturbinals (e.g., ungulates and tubulidentates). An updated comparative study would be most welcome here. Moore (1981) provides a detailed accounting of the turbinals and describes their adaptive implications in anthropoids, cetaceans, and selected mammalian groups.

Also associated with the nasal cavity is the development of the paranasal sinuses (figs. 9.7, 9.17, 9.18). Paulli's (1900c) classic study revealed that such pneumatization was absent in monotremes and in representative genera of didelphid, dasyurid, and macropodid marsupials. Among eutherians, the only paranasal sinus present in insectivorans and bats is the maxillary sinus. Since this sinus is also present in most placental orders (fig. 9.18), it likely represents a primitive eutherian feature (Paulli 1900b, c; Moore 1981). Noteworthy is Kemp's (1979) suggestion that this sinus may have been present in some cynodonts. Further consideration of the homology of the maxillary sinus will require broad comparative study of sectioned skulls of both Recent and fossil mammals.

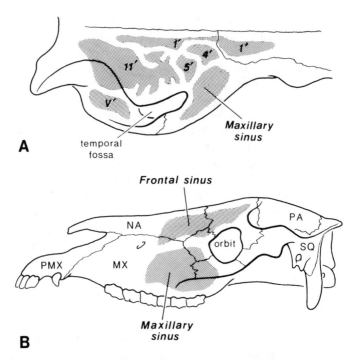

A

temporal fossa

Maxillary sinus

B

Maxillary sinus

Frontal sinus

Fig. 9.18. A. Dorsal view of the skull of a pig (*Sus*) showing paranasal sinuses. Conventions for numbers are described in figure 9.17 and text. B. Left lateral views of skull of a horse (*Equus*) showing frontal and maxillary sinuses. (After Paulli 1900b and Moore 1981)

Although, as noted above, the maxillary sinus is usually present in placental mammals, there are departures from the typical insectivoran condition. The sinus is absent in certain small bats (e.g., *Vesperugo*). Within carnivorans its consistent presence is somewhat disputable, partly because of discrepancies in terminology (Negus 1958, contra Paulli 1900b, c; see Moore 1981). The sinus is extensive only in bears, where it extends far into the frontal and into the nasal bone. In ungulate groups, the maxillary sinus is usually quite large and it may invade many of the bony elements of the rostrum and anterior orbital region. For example, *Equus* (fig. 9.18B) shows the extension of the maxillary sinus from the maxilla into the lacrimal, jugal, naso-turbinal, palatine, sphenoid, and frontal (Paulli 1900b). The sinus is notably large and complicated in elephants. The aquatic pinnipeds, cetaceans, and sirenians show an opposite trend, where this sinus is either completely lacking or rudimentary. Aside from this basic pattern of occurrence, there is a relationship between the degree of development of the maxillary sinus and head and overall body size.

Additional paranasal sinuses, most notably the "sphenoidal" (IV′) and "frontal" (2') sinuses (sensu Paulli 1900a, b, c), occur in many mammalian groups (fig. 9.7, 9.17B). The sinuses are expectedly associated with the bones of the same name, but they may also invade several other adjacent elements. These and other sinuses develop as expanding pneumatic areas in the interstices between the basal lamellae of the ethmoturbinals (fig. 9.17) and accordingly they nearly always number fewer than the number of intervals between the lamellae.

Development of the sphenoidal and frontal and adjacent sinuses is usually variable not only at higher taxonomic levels but also among individuals of species and even between either side of an individual skull. Nevertheless, the distribution of these lacunae mirrors, to some extent, the basic trends seen with regard to the elaboration of the maxillary sinus (Moore 1981). The sinus are absent in mammals where pneumatization of the naso-facial region is otherwise moderate (insectivores and bats) or lacking (aquatic mammals). Development of the sinuses is particularly extensive in the large ungulates, including proboscideans (fig. 9.17C, D). In several orders development of these sinuses is markedly variable. Within Carnivora the frontal sinus system is most extensive in bears (fig. 9.17B), moderately developed in felids (fig. 9.7), hyaenids, and mustelids, and very poorly developed or absent in procyonids. Many rodents and lagomorphs have virtually no frontal or sphenoidal sinuses, but additional sinuses are found in the porcupine, capybara, and other larger rodents. The edentate sloths have two or three accessory sinuses, but in armadillos and anteaters the frontal sinuses are absent. Primitively, primates show very poor development of any openings besides the maxillary sinus, but African apes and humans have a distinctive series involving the ethmoidally derived frontal sinus and a large, irregular sphenoidal sinus containing a labyrinth of thin-walled cavities. Despite the complex structures involved, the detailed resemblance of the paranasal sinuses among hominoids is striking (Cave and Haines 1940).

The functional or adaptive significance of the paranasal sinuses is uncertain. The most popular notions are discussed by Moore (1981). The sinuses certainly reduce the weight of the skull, an advantage seen most clearly in the larger perissodactyls, artiodactyls, and in the elephants. (As noted above, there is a general but by no means perfect correlation between sinus development and skull size.) Another view is that the paranasal sinuses accommodate expansion of the ethmoturbinals and thus augment the olfactory system. This relationship is limited, however, to only a few of the mammalian groups (e.g., carnivorans) that show extensive pneumatization. Other suggestions are that the sinuses act as sound resonators, or prevent heat loss from the nasal cavity. Finally, it has been argued that the paranasal sinuses have no function at all, but are simply incidental to the architecture of the mammalian skull (Weidenreich 1941).

TABLE 9.1 Skeletal elements contributing to the braincase wall in mammals (see also figs. 9.19–9.21)

	Ornithorhynchus	Tachyglossus	Therians
Primary braincase wall (principal structures)	Commissura orbitonasalis, Ala orbitalis, Pila praeoptica, Pila antotica (later reduced leaving only base), Commissura preafacialis. Pila metoptica absent leaving common foramen for exit of nerves II, III	Expanded Commissura orbitoparietalis, reduction of other elements through resorption at juvenile stages (e.g., upper Pila antotica, posterior Pila praeoptica, Commissura parietoorbitalis). Pila metoptica absent leaving common foramen for nerves II–III	Ala orbitalis, Commissura orbitonasalis, Commissura orbitoparietalis (ephemeral or absent in some forms), Commissura praefacialis Pila praeoptica, Pila metoptica, Pila antotica (= Pila postoptica) absent in eutherians, leaving common foramen III –VI; Pila antotica and Pila metoptica absent in marsupials, leaving common exit for nerves II–VI
Secondary braincase wall			
Early ontogeny	Small Ala temporalis Spheno-obturator membrane	Small Ala temporalis Spheno-obturator membrane	Ala temporalis with lamina ascendens (variably developed and persistent), Spheno-obturator membrane
Late ontogeny	Lamina obturans (intra-membranous ossification within spheno-obturator membrane), alisphenoid forms only floor of the cavum epiptericum	Lamina obturans (ossifies later than in Ornithorhynchus), anterior process of periotic, ectopterygoid, squamosal, secondary lateral lamella of orbitosphenoid (preformed by cartilage of pila praeoptica), temporal wing of the palatine	Ascending lamina of alisphenoid, squamosal, tegmen tympani

Under this view, the sinuses can be regarded as merely the spaces between the necessary bony struts and pillars. As in the case of many cranial features, the paranasal sinuses suggest many possible functions but elude a single satisfactory explanation.

The Braincase Wall and Cavum Epiptericum

The distinctive aspect of the mammalian braincase wall involves, as noted above, (1) marked reduction of the ventral lateral wall of the primary cranial cavity, (2) formation of a secondary, more lateral wall, and (3) persistence of space between the primary and secondary braincase walls, the cavum epiptericum (fig. 9.20), which houses the trigeminal ganglion and other neural and vascular structures.

Although these basic features were first contrasted with the "reptilian" condition by Gaupp (1900, 1902), active research on this anatomical problem continues. Critical here are recent findings on the variation in the ontogeny of the primary and secondary lateral braincase walls in monotremes and marsupials (Kuhn 1971; Kuhn and Zeller 1987; Maier 1987a), which underscore the basic differences between monotremes and therians emphasized by Watson (1916), de Beer (1937), and others. Such differences have led workers to suggest patterns of evolution of the mammalian braincase wall that also account for various conditions in Mesozoic mammals (e.g., Kermack 1963; Kermack and Kielan-Jaworowska 1971). These interpretations cannot be judged, however, without a clear notion of the ontogenetic sequences known in living mammals.

Table 9.1 summarizes the basic aspects of these developmental sequences for both the primary and secondary braincase walls in the echidna *Tachyglossus*, the platypus *Ornithorhynchus,* and therians. The reduction pattern of the primary braincase wall notably varies in these groups (Gaupp 1902; de Beer 1937; Kuhn 1971; Kuhn and Zeller 1987). In monotremes (fig. 9.19B) the vertical cartilaginous pillar, the pila metoptica, is absent. As a result, the openings for the optic (II) and oculomotor (III) nerves coalesce to form a common foramen, the foramen pseudoopticum (fig. 9.3A), sensu Kuhn and Zeller (1987). In eutherians (fig. 9.19D) the pila antotica is absent, leaving a common opening for the oculomotor (III), trochlear (IV), trigeminal (V), and abducens (VI) nerves. Marsupials (fig. 9.19C) show more marked reduction wherein both the pila antotica and pila metoptica are absent and there is a single large foramen for the exit of cranial nerves III–VI. The phylogenetic implications of this pattern of reduction are unclear. Nonetheless, assuming a trend involving reduction of the primary braincase wall in the transition from early cynodont taxa to mammals, the marsupial condition would seem the most derived (Kuhn and Zeller 1987).

One of the major issues concerning the cranial evidence for higher

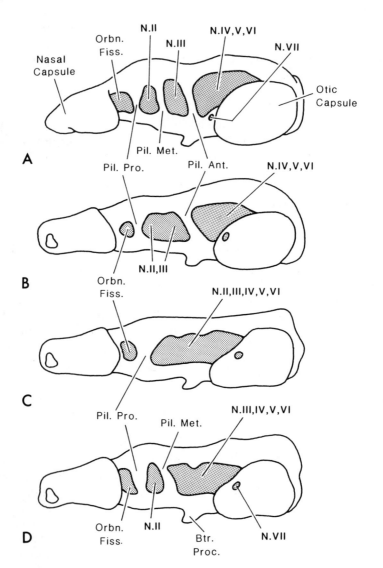

Fig. 9.19. Highly diagrammatic views of the sidewall of the primary braincase in chondrocrania of (A) nonmammalian tetrapods, (B) monotremes, (C) metatherians, (D) eutherians. Uniform stipple indicates openings for passage of cranial nerves. (After Moore 1981)

mammal phylogeny concerns the composition of the secondary lateral wall of the braincase. The primary elements of concern here are the alisphenoid, the ala temporalis, the spheno-obturator membrane, and a bone, the lamina obturans, closely associated with the latter membrane.

In monotremes, the ala temporalis occurs during early ontogeny along with the spheno-obturator membrane (fig. 9.3A). The alisphenoid is later formed through independent ossification at the rostro-ventral surface of the ala temporalis, and it may eventually give rise to a small rostro-lateral process of appositional bone (Kuhn and Zeller 1987). Nonetheless, the alisphenoid remains small throughout life and contributes only to the flooring of the cavum epiptericum (figs. 9.20, 9.21) in both *Tachyglossus* and *Ornithorhynchus* (Vandebroek 1964; Griffiths 1978; Kuhn and Zeller 1987). The secondary side wall is instead dominated by the lamina obturans, a bone forming within the spheno-obturator membrane (*Ornithorhynchus*), or a mosaic of elements including the lamina obturans and outgrowths of the periotic, ectopterygoid, squamosal, orbitosphenoid, and palatine (*Tachyglossus;* table 9.1).

Therians show a substantially greater contribution of the ascending lamina of the alisphenoid to the secondary lateral wall (fig. 9.20), which also incorporates lesser contributions from the squamosal and the tegmen tympani (fig. 9.21). There is, however, marked variation in the formation of the alisphenoid within Theria. The ascending lamina may either secondarily fuse with the processus alaris of the skull base (Terry 1917; de Beer 1937; Starck 1967) or develop in primary connection to this process (e.g., *Talpa, Bos, Ovis;* de Beer 1937). There is also a basic difference between eutherians and some marsupials in the relations of the ala temporalis. In the former the ala temporalis usually remains small and ossifies through endochondral replacement as the alisphenoid, which subsequently expands through appositional bone formation (fig. 9.2). In this manner, the alisphenoid grows caudally and laterally to invade the spheno-obturator membrane. In some marsupials, however, the ala temporalis has a strong vertical flange that may even contact dorsally the commissura orbitoparietalis (e.g., *Monodelphis*, Maier 1987a). Hence, although this element has the same direction of growth in marsupials and eutherians, distinct differences pertain to the size of the initial cartilaginous element.

It is noteworthy that in didelphid and peramelid marsupials this ascending process of the ala temporalis differentiates into cartilage between the first and second branch of the trigeminal nerve, a topographic relation very like the ascending branch of the "reptilian" epipterygoid. Accordingly, Maier (1987a) suggested that at least some marsupials represent a link in the transformation from the vertical lamina of the epipterygoid in nonmammalian cynodonts to the primitive mammalian condition. Maier also stressed, however, an important caveat. The relation between the ala tem-

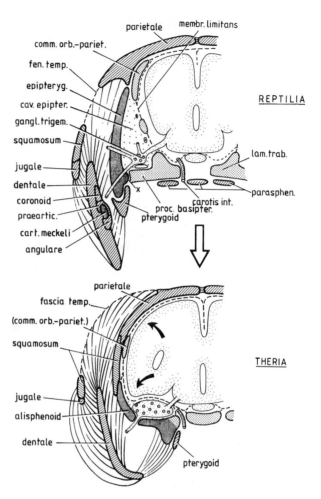

Fig. 9.20. Schematic cross sections in the orbitotemporal regions of a primitive synapsid and therian, showing the relations of the trigeminal ganglion to surrounding elements. Soft tissues in synapsid condition are inferred from comparisons with relevant living taxa. Dermal elements are indicated by diagonal hatching, endochondral elements by uniform stipple, ganglia by pattern with open circles. In the "primitive" synapsid condition, the ganglion lies outside the more extensive primary wall of the braincase and inside the epipterygoid. In therians and monotremes, the primary braincase wall is markedly reduced and the trigeminal ganglion is essentially enclosed within the braincase proper, occupying a space named the cavum epiptericum. In *Ornithorhynchus,* the ala temporalis (of the alisphenoid) is confined to the floor of the cavum epiptericum, whereas in therians (B) the alisphenoid ala temporalis forms an extensive lateral wall of the cavum epiptericum. The complex form of the secondary braincase wall in *Tachyglossus* also differs from the conditions shown here. (From Maier 1987a)

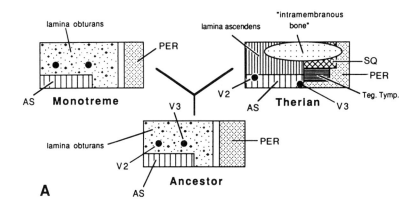

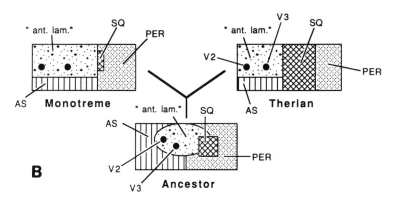

Fig. 9.21. Diagrams showing competing theories for origin of the secondary braincase wall in mammals. A. According to Kuhn and Zeller (1987), the alisphenoid is primitively a small element of the ventral sidewall and more dorsal intramembranous ossifications are not necessarily homologous in therians and in monotremes.
B. According to Presley and Steel (1976) and Kemp (1983), the lamina ascendens of the alisphenoid in therian mammals is actually completed by an intramembranous ossification representing the "anterior lamina" of the periotic in cynodonts and the ancestral mammal, which is retained in monotremes. The latter scheme thus suggests a basic homology of the secondary braincase wall between therians and monotremes not endorsed by Kuhn and Zeller (1987). For labeling see list of abbreviations. B is modified from Kemp (1983).

poralis and the trigeminal branches varies considerably among marsupials and it is not at all certain that the didelphid-peramelid condition is plesiomorphous for the group. Other marsupials resemble eutherians in that the ascending lamina of the ala temporalis lies between the second and third branches of the trigeminal nerve. This difference underlies Gaupp's

(1902) influential rejection of the homology between the ascending branch of the reptilian epipterygoid and the mammalian alisphenoid. Further skepticism is expressed by Kuhn and Zeller (1987), who note that if the ascending lamina of the ala temporalis is homologous with the epiptery-goid, it is curious that the former structure (1) is not incorporated into the secondary lateral wall of monotremes, (2) changes its topographic re-lationship with the maxillary branch of the trigeminal nerve in therians, (3) develops ontogenetically in a different manner from the ascending branch of the epipterygoid in nonmammalian amniotes, and (4) shows marked ontogenetic variability among therians. For these reasons, Kuhn and Zeller (1987, 65) postulated that the common ancestor of monotremes and therians had only a small basal alisphenoid and that the lamina ascen-dens of the alisphenoid is a therian neomorph.

Despite these conclusions, Maier's (1987a) cautious suggestion need not be abandoned altogether. Monotremes also show many anomalous, highly derived features, and the basally confined alisphenoid may not be exceptional in this regard. Moreover, a plastic ontogenetic relationship be-tween nerves and skeletal elements does not rule out homology for various components. As Maier (1987a, 85) appropriately remarks, peripheral nerves develop much earlier than the first skeletal structures and even ho-mologous cartilaginous and bony elements may develop topographically in different ways in order to accommodate the primary organization of other head organs.

A major issue also concerns the dominant element in the monotreme secondary side wall, the lamina obturans, and its possible homology with the elements of the secondary braincase wall in therians. In a highly influ-ential paper, Watson (1916) argued that the lamina obturans was simply the anterior outgrowth of the periotic. This led workers to argue for var-ious evolutionary patterns of the braincase wall, using as reference markers the foramina for the second and third branches of the trigeminal nerve. In many therians these foramina are associated with ascending lamina of the alisphenoid, whereas in monotremes they are allegedly notches on the ven-tral edge of the anterior lamina of the "periotic." A popular scheme sug-gests that the anterior periotic contribution to the sidewall is the more derived condition, and one shared by monotremes, multituberculates, and morganucodontid triconodonts (Kermack and Kielan-Jaworowska 1971).

A serious challenge to Watson's (1916) theory, and phylogenetic schemes based upon it, comes from more recent ontogenetic studies of monotremes. Presley and Steel (1976) and Presley (1981) found that the lamina obturans is an intramembranous ossification forming wholly within the spheno-obturator membrane; only later does it fuse with the periotic and other adjacent elements (see also Griffiths 1978). They further argued that this intramembranous bone was homologous in monotremes and therians, differing only with respect to its relative growth and pattern of fusion (fig. 9.21B). According to their view, this large intramembranous bone in monotremes eventually fuses with the periotic, whereas in therians it eventually fuses with the ventral alisphenoid (fig. 9.21B). Kemp (1983) used this argument to claim that the secondary sidewall of the braincase in monotremes and therians is homologous (see also Patterson 1980). The morganucodontid braincase secondary wall, which appears to have both a well-developed lamina obturans (fused to periotic in the adult skull) and an ascending lamina of the alisphenoid, was regarded by Kemp (1983) as a plesiomorphic mammal condition (fig. 9.21B) from which the mono-treme and therian conditions were divergently derived.

In recent ontogenetic studies of the monotreme braincase, Kuhn (1971) and Kuhn and Zeller (1987) acknowledge that the lamina obturans forms independently of the periotic, but dispute the above assertion that the monotreme and therian secondary lateral walls are strictly homologous (fig. 9.21A). These authors argue that ossifications within the spheno-obturator membrane of some therians (de Beer 1937; MacIntyre 1967; Griffiths 1978) are highly variable, appear very late in ontogeny, and differ from the lamina obturans of monotremes in topographic relations to nerves. Kuhn and Zeller (1987, 64–65) also noted that all skull elements are preceded by condensation of connective tissue during ontogeny. They accordingly reject homologies for the braincase secondary wall based simply on the common occurrence of an intramembranous ossification in therians and monotremes. The phylogenetic pattern favored by Kuhn and Zeller (1987) is one wherein the common ancestor of monotremes and therians had a small basal alisphenoid, similar to that in Recent mono-tremes. Subsequently, the secondary sidewall of the braincase evolved in-dependently in the following manner: (1) In monotremes the sidewall is formed primarily through intramembranous ossification of the lamina ob-turans, which later fuses with the periotic. This pattern is seen in *Ornitho-rhynchus* (fig. 9.21). The mosaic of elements contributing to the secondary sidewall in *Tachyglossus* (table 9.1) is a highly derived and anomalous condition. (2) In therians the sidewall is formed primarily through the os-sification of the lamina ascendens of the alisphenoid (fig. 9.20), a therian neomorph without a homologue in monotremes (fig. 9.21A). Other con-tributions to the sidewall are the squamosal and the tegmen tympani.

This scheme clearly contrasts with the one preferred by Presley and Steel (1976), Presley (1981), and Kemp (1983). However, the argument for independent evolution of the sidewall in monotremes and therians re-lies on distinctions of questionable weight. This proposal hinges on the assumption that an intramembranous ossification in the same general re-gion of the skull of both groups is not also homologous in both groups. In this respect, the above noted differences (Kuhn and Zeller 1987) for the ossification in question are of moot significance, since differences in topography and ontogenetic timing can apply to elements that are clearly homologous.

As noted in the above survey of the mammalian cranium, there is some variation among therians with respect to the exit of nerves from the cavum epeptericum. In most therians cranial nerves III, IV, and VI and ophthalmic and maxillary branches of V leave the cavum epeptericum through a large opening (fig. 9.20C), the sphenorbital fissure, which lies between the lateral posterior surface of the orbitosphenoid and the anterior edge of the alisphenoid (fig. 9.8A). In certain therians (*Tupaia*, some carnivorans, primates, edentates, pholidotans) a foramen rotundum conveying the maxillary branch of the trigeminal may be separated from the sphenorbital fissure by either cartilage or appositional bone arising from the alisphenoid. The latter condition seems to be secondary (Novacek 1986; Kuhn and Zeller 1987), although the occurrence of a foramen rotundum probably arose independently several times within Eutheria.

The Orbital Mosaic and the Postorbital Septum

A variety of bones, including the lacrimal, frontal, parietal, maxilla, palatine, pterygoid, alisphenoid, and orbitosphenoid may contribute to the complex pattern exposed in the lateral orbital wall. The relative proportions of these elements are influenced by many factors involved with allometric growth, function, and the concomitant emphasis on particular sensory organs. As expected, a good deal of unexplained variation can be found in mammals (fig. 9.22).

The problem of transformation of the orbital mosaic has not received a great deal of attention, although Muller (1934) provided a comprehensive survey of this region in insectivorans. The ontogeny of the orbital wall and its influence on pattern in adult taxa have been of particular concern in studies on insectivoran and primate relationships (Roux 1947; Butler 1956; McDowell 1958; Novacek 1980, 1986). From these investigations emerges a basic hypothesis concerning the quartet of elements occupying the anterior moiety of the mammalian orbit. In many mammals the orbital wing of the palatine is a large element that broadly contacts the frontal and, to a lesser extent, the lacrimal (fig. 9.22). By contrast, the orbital contribution of the maxilla is very weak and is excluded from contact with the frontal by the lacrimal-palatine bridge. This condition is widely found; it applies to morganucodontids, monotremes, the more "generalized" (polyprotodont) marsupials, tupaiids, macroscelidids, hyaenodontids, and some artiodactyls and carnivorans (Haines 1950; Butler 1956; Van Valen 1965; Kermack and Kielan-Jaworowska 1971). The marked orbital exposure of the palatine is therefore thought to be a primitive mammalian condition (Butler 1956; Novacek 1980, 1986).

Lipotyphlan insectivorans show a distinct departure from this pattern in that the maxilla makes a substantial contribution to the anterior orbit. The intrusion of this element is enough to effect broad contact with the frontal and exclude the palatine from a contact with the lacrimal (fig. 9.22). This pattern is not confined to lipotyphlan insectivorans—it is also found in some rodents, primates, edentates, and hyracoids—but the orbital expansion of the maxilla is particularly strong and the resulting mosaic pattern is particularly consistent within lipotyphlans. Muller (1934) surmised that the intrusion of the maxilla was a developmental pattern relating to the posterior expansion of the nasal capsule. It seems likely that the interplay of growth involving the eye, the neopallium, and the nasal capsule are all contributing factors (Novacek 1980, fig. 3).

This arrangement of these anterior orbital elements provides evidence for the monophyly of the lipotyphlan insectivorans (Butler 1956; McDowell 1958; Novacek 1986). It is not known, however, whether this derived condition is expressed in early fossil members of the group, where preservation of the orbitotemporal region is poor (Novacek 1982). An early group of eutherians, the leptictids, do show excellent preservation of cranial sutures, and provide some clues bearing on the origin of the insectivoran orbital mosaic. Leptictids are, for a variety of anatomical reasons, thought to be a close sister group of lipotyphlan insectivorans, but they are excluded from a grouping of all extant and many fossil lipotyphlan clades (Butler 1956; Novacek 1986). The orbital wall in leptictids (which is clearly known in at least the Eocene-Oligocene members of the group) shows a greater intrusion of the maxilla into the orbit than is typical of marsupials and many eutherians (fig. 9.22). This element is still excluded from contact with the frontal by a well-developed orbital wing of the palatine (fig. 9.8A; McDowell 1958; Novacek 1986). The acquisition of the derived "hyper-maxillary" orbital condition seems therefore restricted to the lipotyphlan insectivorans and does not apply to the alleged nearest relatives of this group. Other clades that show a relatively substantial contribution of the maxilla to the orbit (e.g., some edentates, rodents) are likely to have acquired this condition independently of lipotyphlans.

The only potential exception to this last generalization concerns the primates. The near affinities of primates continue to be elusive, but some have suggested a close relationship between this order and at least the living and fossil "hedgehogs" and related forms, the erinaceomorph insectivorans (Szalay 1975; Novacek 1982). In this light, it is intriguing that the expanded maxilla and the frontal-maxillary contact does occur in some primates (e.g., indriids, daubentoniids, adapids, *Plesiadapis*, cheirogalines, certain lemurs; fig. 9.22). Cartmill (1975) concluded that this condition is primitive for the order and that the expansion of the palatine in the orbit of certain primates is a secondary feature. By implication, the latter con-

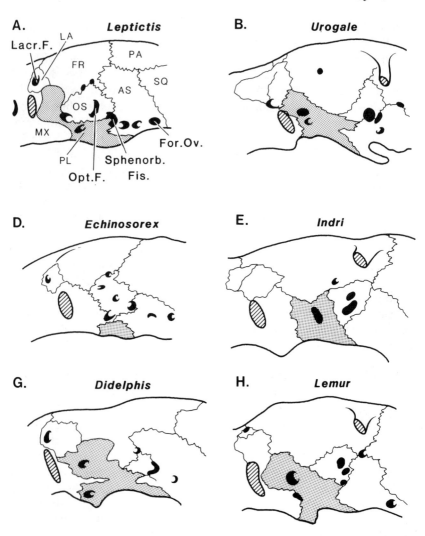

A. *Leptictis*
Lacr.F. LA
FR PA
AS SQ
OS
MX
PL Sphenorb.
Opt.F. Fis.
For.Ov.

B. *Urogale*

D. *Echinosorex*

E. *Indri*

G. *Didelphis*

H. *Lemur*

dition would represent a secondary reversal to a more primitive therian trait. The pattern favored by Cartmill (1975) also could be interpreted as evidence for a close affinity between primates and either lipotyphlans or erinaceomorph lipotyphlans (assuming that the basicranial similarities noted by Szalay [1975] are exclusive to primates and erinaceomorphs).

Such a conclusion, while compelling, would disrupt a popular notion that primates are more likely associated with tree shrews, flying lemurs, and chiropterans (Gregory's [1910] "superorder" Archonta) in a clade of very ancient origin that excludes the lipotyphlans (Szalay 1977; Novacek and Wyss 1986a). The case for close lipotyphlan-primate affinities, how-

C.

Manis

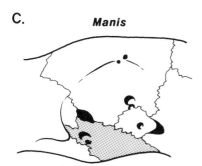

Fig. 9.22. Diagrams of the orbital mosaic in various mammals. For labeling see list of abbreviations.

F.

Marmota

I.

Orycteropus

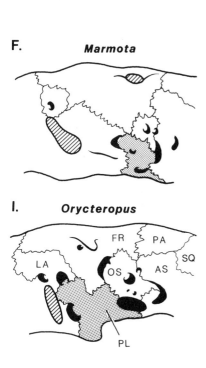

ever, seems to be weakening, as many alleged basicranial similarities between these groups (Szalay 1975) are either absent in fossil lipotyphlans or are of ambiguous phylogenetic significance (Novacek et al. 1983; MacPhee et al. 1988). Acknowledgment of this recent skepticism as well as the evidence for the Archonta grouping (Wible and Covert 1987), would lead one to conclude that the frontal-maxillary contact in some primates and lipotyphlans represents an interesting case of convergence.

The above discussion should not suggest that interesting phylogenetic questions bearing on the variation of the orbital mosaic are confined to insectivorans and primates. In passing, I note that the ventrally expanded frontal bone in the orbital wall of the edentates and pholidotans (fig. 9.22) is coincident with a number of other anatomical specializations that suggest a relationship between these groups (Novacek and Wyss 1986a). Moreover, the relation of the lacrimal to the nasal facial region as well as the orbit has elicited much discussion (Williston 1925; Salomon 1930; Muller 1934; Gregory 1920; Novacek 1980). In general, there has been less attention to the orbital mosaic than warranted and an updated, more comprehensive treatment is greatly needed.

A final aspect of the orbital mosaic demanding consideration here is the postorbital septum (fig. 9.23). Although confined only to some primates, this feature has attracted an unusual level of interest in both the systematic and anatomical literature. The septum also provides a useful example of an anatomical region examined for ontogenetic, functional, and phylogenetic influences. The postorbital septum is a concave area of the orbit that essentially walls off this region from the temporal fossa. The resultant structure is the cup-shaped eye socket unique to anthropoids and the bizarrely specialized *Tarsius* (fig. 9.23). The septum has been generally regarded as the key feature grouping all the anthropoids (New and Old World monkeys, great apes, hominids) and indicating close affinity between anthropoids and *Tarsius* within the "Haplorhini" (Pocock 1918; Jones 1929; Cartmill and Kay 1978; Luckett and Szalay 1978).

In more recent years, this argument has been challenged primarily from a paleontological perspective. The competing assertion is that *Tarsius* is closely related to Eocene "tarsioids" (lacking the septum), lemurs are more closely related to anthropoids, and anthropoids may indeed be a polyphyletic taxon (Simons and Russell 1960; Gingerich 1973; Cachel 1979; Schwartz et al. 1978). Under this arrangement, the postorbital septum would not likely be a homologous trait shared by anthropoids and *Tarsius*.

Cartmill (1980) has addressed this issue with a detailed examination of the septum and relevant functional and evolutionary factors. According to Cartmill, variation in relative contributions of the frontal, alisphenoid, and "zygomatic" (zygomatic process of the maxilla) to the septum within Haplorhini (fig. 9.23) does not justify the conclusion that the septum evolved independently in *Tarsius* and anthropoids. He also suggested that the platyrrhine condition, where the "zygomatic" makes a substantial contribution, is also common to hylobatids and therefore represents the primitive condition for anthropoids (fig. 9.23). Differences between *Tarsius* and anthropoids were ascribed to the less complete septum in the former. To explain this pattern, Cartmill (1980) interpreted the reduction of the inferior orbit through the development of large fissures in *Tarsius* as the result of the extraordinary enlargement of the eyes. This hypertrophy has restricted the area of attachment of the masticatory muscles, and the ptery-

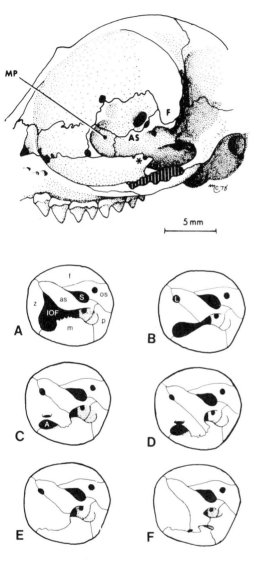

Fig. 9.23. Orbit of juvenile *Tarsius bancanus* (U.S. National Mus. 300916) showing relationships of alisphenoid (AS) and frontal (F) to the postorbital septum. Vertical hachure indicates broken surfaces. Asterisk denotes periorbital process of the maxilla. MP is center of semicircular fossa for origin of the periorbital head of the medial pterygoid muscle.

Architecture of the postorbital septum shown by diagrams of anterior views of the right orbits in (A) *Tarsius*, (B) *Aotus*, (C, D) variants of *Saimiri*, (E) *Ateles*, (F) *Alouatta*. Abbreviations are: A, anterior orbital fissure; IOF, inferior orbital fissure; L, lateral orbital fissure; S, superior orbital fissure. Bones: as, alisphenoid; f, frontal; m, maxilla; os, orbitosphenoid; p, palatine; z, zygomatic or jugal. (From Cartmill 1980)

goids are accordingly shifted back within the inferior orbital fissure. Under this interpretation, the postorbital septum of *Tarsius,* like its specialized retinal fovea, represents a significant departure, but one that was most likely derived from the primitive anthropoid condition. The postorbital septum in primitive haplorhines is thought to have served primarily to insulate the foveate retina of the enlarged eyes from contractions of temporalis muscles. However, a variety of other functions can also be correlated with different conditions of the septum (Cartmill 1980).

The Auditory Bulla

The floor of the tympanic cavity in adult mammals is usually occupied by one or more skeletal elements contributed by the bones adjacent to the cavity or by a mammalian neomorph, the entotympanic, which forms independently of other basicranial elements. The term "auditory bulla" (referring to its commonly inflated structure) is applied to this bony or cartilaginous floor.

The variation in structure and composition of the auditory bulla has been comprehensively treated in the literature on the mammalian skull. In some cases, there is an obvious relation between bullar structure and phylogenetic patterns (e.g., the petrosal bulla in euprimates), but there is also evidence that similar bullae were derived independently in several major lineages (van Kampen 1905; van der Klaauw 1931; Novacek 1977; MacPhee 1979, 1981). Early studies (e.g., Gregory 1910; McDowell 1958) stressing the phylogenetic importance of bullar structure should therefore be regarded with some caution.

As noted above, the tympanic cavity which is floored by the bulla is distinguishable from an "embryological tympanic cavity" or primary cavum tympani (fig. 9.12B). The latter is a space bounded by endoderm that differentiates from the first (and possibly second) pharyngeal pouch (van Kampen 1905; Bast and Anson 1949; MacPhee 1981). During prenatal ontogeny, the cavum tympani expands into the presumptive or secondary tympanic cavity, which takes form with the progressive resorption of the mucoid tissue initially filling it and with pneumatization of the surrounding basicranial elements. In the adult, the cavum tympani fills the entire (secondary) tympanic cavity, so the distinction between these two spaces pertains only to earlier ontogenetic stages.

As the secondary tympanic cavity develops, its ventral outlet is sealed with a fibrous membrane (fig. 9.12A). The membrane forms through proliferation of sheetlike cells and fibers within the mesenchyme surrounding the expanding cavum tympani. This process yields a structure referred to as a "tympanic floor of dense connective tissue" (Novacek 1977) or the "fibrous membrane of the tympanic cavity" (MacPhee 1981). The fibrous membrane is continuous with other connective tissue lining the basicranium. It also extends beneath the ventral surface of the ectotympanic (fig. 9.12A) without meeting the tympanic membrane (eardrum) at any point, to reach the auricular cartilages (MacPhee 1981).

The fibrous membrane of the tympanic cavity is an important feature because it relates directly to the question of transformation from primitive to derived bullar ontogenies. As MacPhee (1981) notes, the membrane seems to be a ubiquitous aspect of early basicranial development in mammals, and bony or cartilaginous bullar elements develop either adjacent to or within this membrane. The fibrous membrane therefore always precedes the appearance of bony floor elements. It is misleading to state, however, that the fibrous membrane is always replaced by these bony elements. The membrane persists as the outermost layer where bullae completely enclose the tympanic cavity. It becomes part of the definitive tympanic floor where the adult bulla is incompletely formed. Most interesting is that in some mammals (e.g., soricids, *Solenodon*, monotremes) osseous bullar structures are weak or essentially absent (fig. 9.24), and the tympanic cavity is "sealed off" by the fibrous membrane and the tympanic membrane (eardrum) of the semihorizontally inclined ectotympanic (Novacek 1977). Several archaic fossil groups in which bullae are not preserved (e.g., the Cretaceous *Kennalestes* and *Asioryctes* [Kielan-Jaworowska, 1969, 1975]) also show a highly inclined ectotympanic anulus very much like that of living shrews. In most mammalian ontogenies, the ectotympanic is progressively reoriented to a semivertical position (fig. 9.25), increasing the ventral outlet of the tympanic cavity medially to this structure (van Kampen 1905; Hunt 1974). Ontogenetic trends, comparisons among living taxa, and fossil evidence therefore agree with Gregory's (1910) claim that the "membranous structure" is a primitive feature of the mammalian tympanic floor. More explicitly, the primitive adult condition in the common ancestor of living mammals may have been one wherein the functional tympanic floor was a fibrous membrane retained throughout ontogeny, and ventral closure of the tympanic cavity was augmented by the horizontally inclined ectotympanic (fig. 9.27; and Novacek 1977). Such a condition may also apply to many abullate fossil skulls (MacPhee 1981).

In addition to the fibrous membrane, other nonosseous elements variably contribute to the tympanic floor. These are elongate cartilages associated with the auditory or eustachian tubes. The tubal cartilages are poorly studied and enigmatic in derivation; they are unlikely to be components of the visceral skeleton (Keibel 1912) and seem to represent a neomorphic feature of mammals (Werner 1960; MacPhee 1981).

The skeletal elements of the mammalian tympanic floor show an unusual diversity in composition and form (figs. 9.24, 9.25). These contributions are either (1) outgrowths of basicranial elements, called tympanic processes, or (2) developmentally independent endochondral elements, the entotympanics, which may secondarily contact the tympanic processes of basicranial elements. The distribution and development of these components were discussed in the classic treatments by van Kampen (1905) and van der Klaauw (1931). An updated review addressing some phylogenetic issues was provided by Novacek (1977), and more recent considerations of homology and ontogeny are found in MacPhee (1981) and Moore

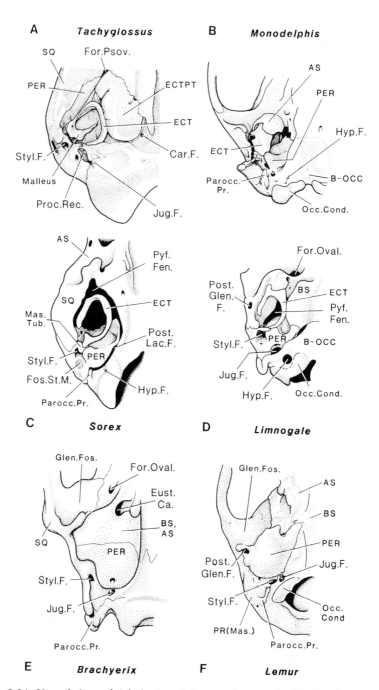

Fig. 9.24. Ventral views of right basicrania in several mammals, showing absence or variable development of the auditory bulla and its components. For labeling see list of abbreviations. (After McDowell 1958; Novacek 1977; Kuhn 1971; and Maier 1987b)

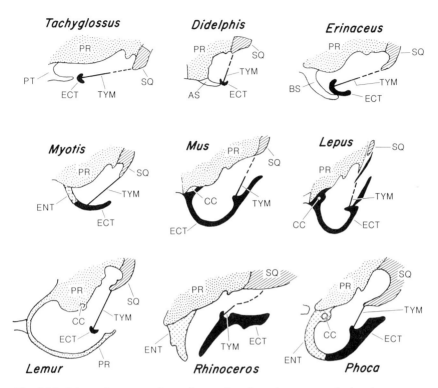

Fig. 9.25. Schematic cross sections of ear regions in various mammals showing relationships of the bullar elements, tympanic membrane (TYM) and carotid canal (CC). Dashed line indicates pars flaccida. For other labeling see list of abbreviations. (From Novacek 1985, based on Van Kampen 1905)

(1981). A summary of this information (table 9.2), reveals a general pattern. Although a large number of elements may contribute to the skeletal tympanic floor, dominant components in most taxa are either one or two of the following: petrosal, ectotympanic, basisphenoid, alisphenoid, or entotympanic. A major exception are the elephant shrews (Macroscelidea), where the bulla is an anomalous mosaic (fig. 9.27) with substantial contributions from rostral and caudal petrosal processes, rostral and caudal entotympanic, ectotympanic, alisphenoid, basisphenoid, pterygoid, and squamosal (MacPhee 1981). Moreover, the distribution of certain elements is quite limited. The petrosal is the dominant element only in euprimates (figs. 9.24, 9.25, 9.26), the basisphenoid only in certain lipotyphlan insectivorans (figs. 9.24, 9.25), and the alisphenoid only in marsupials (figs. 9.24, 9.25). The most widely distributed major bullar components are either outgrowths of the ectotympanic or independent (endochondral) ossifications of the entotympanics.

TABLE 9.2 Skeletal elements contributing to the tympanic floor (auditory bulla) of mammals

Element	Ontogenetic origin	Taxonomic distribution
1) Tympanic Processes (TyP)		
Petrosal	Rostral TyP periosteal outgrowth from pars cochlearis,[1] caudal TyP in cartilage from pars canalicularis	Major bulla element in Euprimates. Contributes in lipotyphlan insectivores
Ectotympanic	Medial outgrowths of annular or horseshoe-shaped ectotympanic	Major bullar element in several mammal orders.[2] Contributes in a majority of mammalian groups
Basisphenoid	Periosteal outgrowth of the margin of the basisphenoid near junction with auditory capsule	Major bullar element in certain lipotyphlan insectivorans (erinaceids, tenrecids). Contributes in other lipotyphlans and in Macroscelidea[3]
Alisphenoid	Periosteal outgrowth of posterior alisphenoid near the anterior edge of the tympanic cavity	Major bullar element in marsupials. Contributes in some lipotyphlans, macroscelideans, and the tree-shrew *Ptilocercus*
Squamosal	Periosteal continuation of entoglenoid process, usually ventrally overlaps other floor components	Contributes in lipotyphlans and other mammals
Exoccipital	Periosteal outgrowth	Rarely contributes (e.g., elephants)
Tympanohyal, anterior process of malleus, Spence's cartilage, pterygoid	various	minor components in many mammals[4]
2) Independent elements		
Entotympanic	Develops in cartilage rostrally (associated with tubal cartilage) caudally (posterior tympanic floor) entotympanics, or both. Cartilaginous bulla persists in some forms[5]	Major bullar element in Edentata, Scandentia (tree-shrews), Microchiroptera, Hyracoidea + Leptictida, some Rodentia and Carnivora. Contributes in Macroscelidea, others[5]

1. Complex variation in development, especially in the case of the caudal tympanic process of the petrosal (MacPhee 1981).
2. Artiodactyla, Perissodactyla, Cetacea, Rodentia, Lagomorpha, Proboscidea, as well as certain Carnivora, e.g. Ursidae, Pinnipedia, and lutrine and mephitine Mustelidae (van der Klaauw 1931; Hunt 1974; Novacek 1977; Mood 1981).
3. Small but present in talpids and chrysochlorids; *contra* van der Klaauw (1931). Also present in elephant shrew macroscelideans (Presley 1978; MacPhee 1981).
4. Distribution given in van der Klaauw (1931).
5. Carnivores show unusual variation, having either enlarged caudal entotympanic, enlarged rostral and caudal entotympanic (with ectotympanic), or primarily ectotympanic bullae (Hunt 1974). Cartilaginous entotympanics persist in some adults, such as megachiropterans, the edentate *Dasypus*, and the African Palm Civet *Nandinia* (Hunt 1974; Novacek 1977).

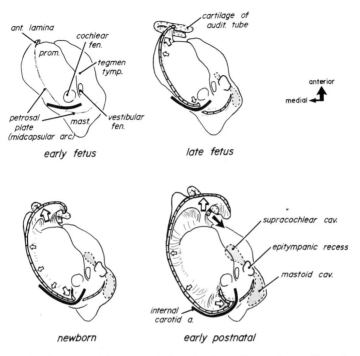

Fig. 9.26. Development of the tympanic floor in a lemuriform primate. Rostral and caudal tympanic processes of the petrosal coalesce early in ontogeny to form the petrosal plate. The plate expands by appositional growth along its leading edge and by pneumatization (remodeling). Outline arrows indicate relative degree of pneumatization. Stipple indicates specific pneumatic spaces in the dorsal aspect of the tympanic region. Black arrow represents pathway of the tubal canal and auditory tube. (From MacPhee et al. 1988, as modified from MacPhee and Cartmill 1986)

This complicated distribution of bullar types resists a simple transformational scheme. Entotympanics are broadly distributed (in living mammals) 'and are known to have existed in some archaic fossil eutherians (e.g., leptictids: McDowell 1958; Novacek 1986), leading to the conclusion that entotympanics were a primitive element of the mammalian bulla. This supposition, however, does not settle another issue; namely, whether a variety of bullar types were derived independently from the primitive abullate condition or whether derivation involved the incorporation of the entotympanic and its eventual fusion with (or replacement by) tympanic processes of the basicranial elements (fig. 9.27). The latter modification has been invoked, for example, in explanations of the origin of the petrosal-dominated bulla of euprimates or the basisphenoid bulla of some lipotyphlans (van Kampen 1905; McDowell 1958; Bown and Gingerich 1973).

The critical importance of the entotympanic in this regard reflects

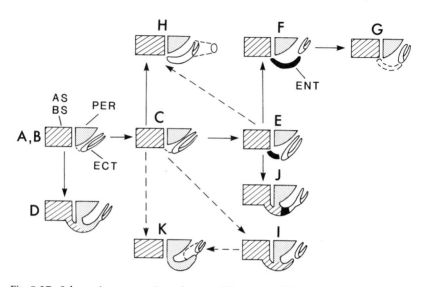

Fig. 9.27. Schematic cross sections showing different conditions for the auditory bulla in mammals and their possible derivation. Relevant elements are alisphenoid and basisphenoid (diagonal lines) petrosal (uniform stipple), entotympanic (solid), and other elements as labeled. A, B, C. Primitive mammalian, marsupial, and eutherian condition where bulla is absent and ectotympanic ring is inclined at a low angle to the horizontal plane of the skull. D. More derived marsupial condition with primarily alisphenoid bulla (lesser contributions from ectotympanic and petrosal). E. Leptictid condition with small entotympanic bulla. F. Eutherian condition with large entotympanic bulla (e.g., many carnivorans, edentates, ungulates; see table 9.2). G. Bulla retained in adults as cartilaginous (entotympanic) element (e.g., *Nandinia*, some Chiroptera). H. Eutherian condition with primarily ectotympanic bulla (e.g., rodents, some insectivorans, lagomorphs, some ungulates). I. Lipotyphlan insectivoran condition with composite structure dominated by basisphenoid and contributions from alisphenoid and petrosal processes. J. Macroscelidid condition with complex, composite bulla. K. Euprimate condition with primarily petrosal bulla. Dashed arrows indicate alternative pathways of derivation. It is unlikely that conditions H, I, and K are rooted in a condition where the entotympanic was present. (Modified from Novacek 1977)

some unclear notions concerning its occurrence. Van Kampen's (1905) influential comments on its existence in marsupials is not based on first-hand studies by him. There is, at present, no clear evidence for an entotympanic in any fossil or living marsupial (MacPhee 1979; Maier 1989). Moreover, the cited occurrence of entotympanics in a variety of fossil mammals is usually weakly based on either the supposition that absence of the bulla in these forms must have resulted from the loss of a loosely attached entotympanic, or that the bulla, where preserved, is likely to be an entotympanic. Without exquisitely fossilized basicrania, such as that known for leptictids (fig. 9.10), neither supposition can be tested (Novacek 1977; MacPhee

1979, 1981). Finally, the argument that the entotympanic is a primary, but perhaps ephemeral, element in the bullae of euprimates and lipotyphlans (e.g., van der Klaauw 1931; McDowell 1958; Bown and Gingerich 1973) is contradicted by detailed embryological studies (fig. 9.26; MacPhee 1979, 1981). The only controversial matter here is Starck's (1975a) description of a small cartilage in the petrosal plate of young tarsiers as an entotympanic. This interpretation fails to exclude, however, the possibility that *Tarsius*'s "entotympanic" is either a secondary cartilage or an endochondral remnant of the caudal tympanic process of the petrosal (MacPhee 1979; MacPhee and Cartmill 1986). Living primates, like marsupials and many fossil mammals, show no clear evidence of either a persistent or suppressed entotympanic.

One reason why the idea of an ancestral entotympanic has proved appealing is that the entotympanic does persist as a cartilaginous element in some adult mammals (e.g., megachiropterans, the carnivoran *Nandinia;* table 9.2). Such a condition has been viewed as a holdover from an ancestral mammalian ontogeny where the cartilaginous bulla was maintained in adults. Phylogenetic transformation of this cartilaginous bulla could then be effected through incorporation or suppression of the cartilaginous entotympanic with the development of various tympanic processes (McDowell 1958). Novacek (1977) considered this alternative and rejected the argument that the primitive mammalian condition involved a cartilaginous bulla. The rare persistence of cartilaginous entotympanics in a few adult placental mammals seems more likely a highly specialized condition where an embryological component (cartilage) is paedomorphically retained (fig. 9.27). Instead, the fibrous membrane was probably the major component of the primitive tympanic floor in mammals (Novacek 1977). The alisphenoid-dominated bullae in marsupials and the variety of eutherian bullae chiefly comprising either basisphenoid, ectotympanic, petrosal, or entotympanic (or combinations of these) were most likely independently derived from the ancestral condition involving a membranous floor of the tympanic cavity (fig. 9.27). Only in some cases (e.g., rodent-lagomorph common ancestry [Novacek 1985]) does a bulla of particular composition potentially indicate homology expressed above the ordinal level.

The foregoing concerns the contribution of bullar elements most often cited in the rather diverse literature on the subject. There are, however, contributions of small elements, whose significance to the problem of bullar transformation may be greater than originally acknowledged. Perhaps most notable among these is Reichert's cartilage, which Presley (1980) described as fusing with the promontorium in monotremes and contributing to the posterior osseous wall of the tympanic cavity. Presley argued that a similar ontogeny may account for the tympanic process of the petrosal in marsupials. The latter process is present in nearly all marsupials (J. Wible, personal communication), but Maier (1987b, 1989) found no evidence of a contact between the promontorium and Reichert's cartilage in the marsupial *Monodelphis*. Nonetheless, Presley (1980) did observe this contact in *Didelphis*, and the variation of the condition in marsupials warrants further inspection.

The independent origin of the auditory bulla likely indicates strong selection for the convergent development of this feature regardless of its bony composition. This implicates the bulla as an important functional component of the auditory region. Unfortunately, the functional significance of the bulla is not clearly understood. The most popular theory is that the bulla, especially where inflated, isolates a large volume of air space of the middle ear cavity from the surrounding skull and cranial tissues (see also Lombard and Hetherington, vol. 3 of this work). Since there is an inverse relation between middle ear volume and acoustic impedence (in the form of stiffness), a large middle ear cavity should enhance response to lower frequencies (Dallos 1970; Webster and Webster 1975). This is because lower frequencies are particularly attenuated by impedence due to stiffness. Although some experimental evidence in heteromyid rodents (Webster and Webster 1975) supports this relationship, there is no straightforward functional explanation for the presence of the bulla or its relative inflation. In this context, it is noteworthy that some mammals with relatively greater middle ear volume and more inflated bullae are not necessarily or always more sensitive to lower frequencies than are mammals in which these morphological traits are less emphasized. The relationship is complicated by the reality that many factors, including the shape of the middle ear cavity, the stiffness of the tympanic membrane, the design of ossicular ligaments and muscles, and a variety of other features, all influence the acoustic impedence of the middle ear system (Novacek 1977; MacPhee 1981; and see below).

Basicranial (Carotid) Arterial Circulation

Although the carotid arteries are just one of many soft anatomical systems associated with the mammalian skull, this system is singled out here because of its intimate relationship with the architecture of the mammalian basicranium and its great interest to students of mammalian systematics. Most issues concern variation of the internal carotid arteries. Highlights of a diverse literature on the subject (Grosser 1901; Tandler 1902; Fuchs 1905; Matthew 1909; Sicher 1913; Hafferl 1916; Goodrich 1930; Lindahl and Lundberg 1946; Bugge 1974; Wible 1983, 1984, 1986, 1987, 1990; Novacek 1986; MacPhee and Cartmill 1986) are only briefly discussed here.

The homologies of the internal carotids are the subject of recent controversy where, once again, embryological studies prove illuminating.

Matthew (1909) cited osseous structures (generally open grooves or sulci on the promontorium of the petrosal) in fossil carnivorans for his claim that the internal carotid in primitive eutherians had a trichotomous pattern consisting of a medial internal carotid and a more lateral internal carotid that splits into stapedial and promontorial branches. Embryological studies by Presley (1979) indicated, however, that no living mammal shows all three branches. Instead, Presley (1979) argued that the promontorial branch simply represents the lateral migration of the medial internal carotid to a position over the ventral promontorium of the cochlea. Hence, a revised terminology should apply only to the two main branches of the internal carotid, the stapedial artery and a second branch located either on the surface of the promontorium (fig. 9.28A) or near the medial boundary of the tympanic (fig. 9.29).

The primitive mammalian condition for the "more medial" branch of the internal carotid is another matter of controversy. The tendency of this vessel to migrate laterally during the ontogeny of mammals with the artery in "promontorial position" (Presley 1979) as well as the medial location of this vessel in monotremes, marsupials, and some eutherians, would suggest that the medial position is primitive (Novacek 1986). However, there is some variation with respect to this condition. In monotremes and marsupials the medially located internal carotid is excluded from the tympanic cavity by either the fibrous membrane of the tympanic floor or by the fibrous membrane and an osseous bulla (Wible 1983). By contrast, in eutherians where the artery is present in this medial position, it differentiates within the fibrous membrane and is either enclosed fully within the median bullar wall or is excluded from the tympanic cavity by the less completely developed bulla. Wible (1983) therefore suggested that the putative Mesozoic eutherians *Kennalestes* and *Asioryctes*, which show only a median sulcus on the basicranium and not a groove for a more lateral branch on the surface of the promontorium, developed a "medial" internal carotid in a eutherian rather than a marsupial-monotreme fashion. In a later study, Wible (1986) argued that the intermediate but "trans-promontorial" position of this branch of the internal carotid was primitive for mammals. Under this scheme, derived states are represented by either more medially or more laterally directed migrations of this vessel (fig. 9.29). The appeal of Wible's (1983) hypothesis is that it is consistent with the widespread occurrence in eutherians of this branch of the internal carotid in a lateral position (on the ventral surface of the promontorium), a feature that also pertains to many fossil skulls (Cifelli 1982; Novacek 1986; Wible 1986). The weakness of the hypothesis is that it fails to explain why this branch of the internal carotid is located medial to the tympanic cavity in the nearest eutherian out-groups, the monotremes and marsupials.

At the most general level, the above ambiguities do not plague the

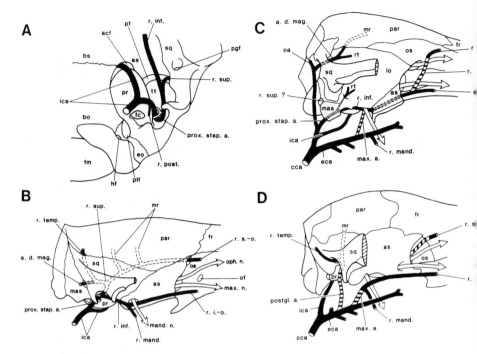

Fig. 9.28. Ventral (A) and lateral (B) views of the skull of a hypothetical eutherian ancestor and lateral views of the monotreme *Ornithorhynchus* (C) and the marsupial *Didelphis* (D) showing reconstruction of internal carotid and stapedial arteries. Dashed arteries run within the cranial cavity. Striped vessels are neomorphic anastomoses. Essentials of these differing patterns are outlined in the text. For further discussion of details of the diagrams, see Wible (1987). Abbreviations are: a. d. mag., arteria diploetica magna; as, alisphenoid; acf, anterior carotid foramen; bo, basioccipital; bs, basisphenoid; cca, common carotid artery; eca, external carotid artery; eo, exoccipital; fc, fenestra cochleae; fm, foramen magnum; fr, frontal; hf, hypoglossal foramen; ica, internal carotid artery; lo, lamina obturans; mas, mastoid portion of the petrosal; max. a., maxillary artery; max. n., maxillary nerve; mr, meningeal ramus; oa, occipital artery; of, optic foramen; oph. n., opthalmic nerve; os, orbitosphenoid; par, parietal; pf, piriform fenestra; pgf, postglenoid foramen; postgl. a., postglenoid artery; pr, promontorium of the petrosal; prox. stap. a., proximal stapedial artery; r. i.-o., ramus infraorbitalis; r. inf., ramus inferior; r. mand., ramus mandibularis; r. orb., ramus orbitalis; r. post., ramus posterior; r. s.-o., ramus supraorbitalis; r. sup., ramus superior; r. temp. *or* rt, ramus temporalis; sq, squamosal; tt, tegmen tympani. (From Wible 1987)

homology of the stapedial branch of the internal carotid artery (fig. 9.28). This vessel, also referred to as the orbital, temporal, or orbitotemporal, displays continuity throughout the Vertebrata, from selachians to mammals (Goodrich 1930). The stapedial artery is derived from the artery of the second branchial or hyoid arch (the second aortic arch) and diverges

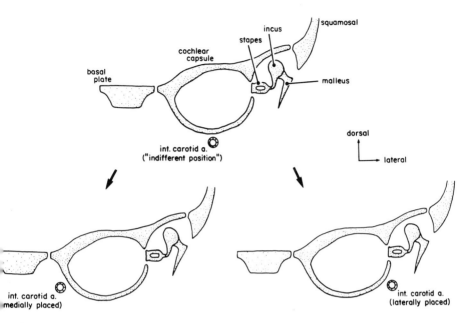

Fig. 9.29. Diagrammatic transverse sections through the tympanic region of mammalian embryos, showing Presley's (1979) descriptions of the relative migration during development of the internal carotid artery (int. carotid a.). Early stages are represented by the intermediate ("indifferent") position of this vessel directly below the cochlear capsule. At later stages, the internal carotid artery shifts either laterally or medially relative to the cochlear capsule. (From Wible 1986)

from the "common" internal carotid near the hyomandibular (in fish) or the stapes (in tetrapods). A spate of transformational theories for the mammalian stapedial arterial system (e.g., Bugge 1974; Szalay 1975; Archibald 1977) are less effective because detailed ontogenetic information for this vessel in relation to adjacent bony elements is known in only a small sampling of extant mammalian orders (Wible 1987, table 1).

The stapedial artery in eutherians exhibits a rather consistent branching pattern. A proximal stapedial artery diverges laterally from the internal carotid and courses through or around the stapes (figs. 9.11A, 9.28A). Distally the stapedial artery divides into a ramus inferior and a ramus superior. The ramus inferior usually runs anteriorly through the tympanic cavity and bifurcates into arteries that accompany the maxillary and mandibular nerves in the infraorbital and mandibular regions, respectively (fig. 9.28A-C). The ramus superior accompanies the ophthalmic nerve into the supraorbital region (fig. 9.28B). It is also noteworthy that three comm nly overlooked branches of the stapedial artery, the a. diploetica magna, ramus temporalis, and ramus posterior (fig. 9.28B–D) are probably primitive for Eutheria and Amniota (Wible 1987). In a recent review of petrosals in Cretaceous marsupials, Wible (1990) further proposed that both the lateral head vein and the stapedial artery run through the middle ear in the common ancestor of marsupials and eutherians, but in the former the artery is lost and in the latter the vein disappears.

With a few exceptions (e.g., aardvarks, cetaceans, perissodactyls, proboscideans, sirenians) this basic branching pattern appears at some point in the ontogeny of all eutherian orders (Wible 1987). The homology of the superior ramus, however, is perplexing. In sauropsids this vessel is extracranial in its route and lateral to the ascending process of the epipterygoid (Goodrich 1930; Hafferl 1933). In eutherians, the superior ramus exits the tympanic cavity and follows the intracranial surface of the alisphenoid (which some claim to be homologous with the nonmammalian epipterygoid; see above). As Wible (1987) states, this forces one to decide whether the ramus superior of the stapedial in mammals is homologous with the extracranial vessel in other amniotes that has been shifted endocranially, or whether the mammalian vessel is a neomorph. Unfortunately, the nearest extant eutherian out-groups, the monotremes and marsupials, only enhance the enigma. In all these forms, except *Ornithorhynchus*, the stapedial system is greatly reduced and its peripheral branches are annexed to the external carotid (fig. 9.28C, D). The lack of the superior ramus in the ontogeny of any of these taxa suggests that this artery is a eutherian neomorph. On the other hand, terminal branches of the stapedial system internal to the cranial wall present in some monotremes and marsupials (fig. 9.28C, D) might be viewed as remnants of a superior ramus common to all extant mammals (Wible 1987). At present, the issue simply cannot be resolved.

Wible's (1987) superb comparative study of the stapedial system also reveals some conditions with intriguing phylogenetic implications. In most mammals, the inferior ramus runs extracranially and forward along the ceiling of the tympanic cavity (figs. 9.28A, 9.30A) to exit the cavity either in or near the Glaserian fissure (e.g., some primates [MacPhee and Cartmill 1986]). Alternatively, this vessel distally degenerates and is annexed by the external carotid (several orders; Wible 1987, 122). In Lagomorpha, Rodentia, Macroscelidea, and Chiroptera, the inferior ramus branches from the proximal stapedial artery, exits through a posteriorly located foramen, and runs forward above the tympanic roof (figs. 9.13B, 9.30B; Wible 1987). There is some indirect evidence that this condition is also shared by fossil leptictids (fig. 9.11A; Novacek 1980, 1986).

Wible (1987) reasoned that this specialized pathway of the inferior ramus most likely involves the ventral shift of the tegmen tympani relative to the position of the inferior ramus. This hypothesis is consistent with Kuhn's (1971) important thesis that all or part of the tegmen tympani, as

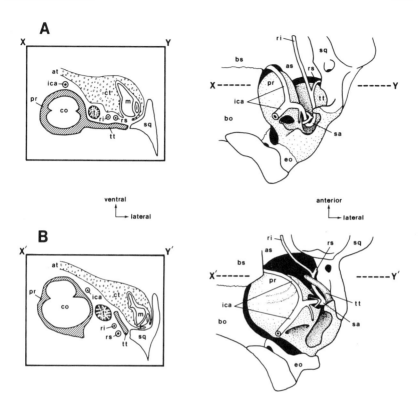

Fig. 9.30. Auditory regions in (A) the hypothetical eutherian ancestor and (B) the microchiropteran *Myotis myotis*. Both ventral (right) and cross-sectional (left) views are given. Bulla, middle ear ossicles, cavum tympani, tensor tympani and stapedius muscles, and various vessels and nerves are not included in ventral views. XY and X'Y' indicate planes for cross sections. Note the intracranial pathway of the stapedial artery above the tegmen tympani in B. Abbreviations are: at, auditory tube; co, cochlea; ct, cavum tympani; i, incus; m, malleus; ri, ramus inferior of the stapedial artery; rs, ramus superior of the stapedial artery; sa, stapedial artery; t, tensor tympani muscle. For other abbreviations, see fig. 9.28. (From Wible and Novacek 1988)

indicated by its highly variable morphogenesis, was added independently to the tympanic roof numerous times in mammals. Accordingly, Wible (1987) distinguished two different derived conditions for the intracranial pathway of the inferior ramus of the stapedial. In the macroscelidid-rodent-lagomorph (morphotypical) condition, the inferior ramus runs above a horizontal tegmen tympani that constitutes a major roofing element for the tympanic cavity. In chiropterans (fig. 9.30B), the inferior ramus runs above a tegmen tympani that is unique in its rodlike structure, its vertical projection into the tympanic cavity, and its development in continuity with the cartilage of the auditory tube (Wible 1984). The latter condition is of special significance because it is evidence for the monophyly of bats independent of wing structure (Wible and Novacek 1988). The endocranial position of the inferior ramus in fossil leptictids (Novacek 1986) seems more akin to that in macroscelidids, rodents, and lagomorphs (where the tegmen tympani is a horizontal flange), although the development of the tegmen tympani is obviously not ascertainable in these fossils.

The course of the internal carotid arteries is often marked by sulci, open grooves, and foramina. These tracings are useful, if sometimes misleading (Conroy and Wible 1978), clues to the carotid pathways of extinct mammals (e.g., Butler 1956; McDowell 1958; Novacek 1986; MacPhee et al. 1988). In a few mammals (e.g., some erinaceomorphs and primates) a varying proportion of the internal carotid arteries running within the tympanic cavity are enclosed in bony tubes (MacPhee 1981; MacPhee et al. 1988). Fleischer (1978) suggested that these bony canals dampen the noise produced by pulsations of the carotid arteries in animals particularly sensitive to lower-frequency sounds. A similar effect could also be achieved by reduction or loss of the internal carotid arteries. This thesis, however, fails to explain why osseous carotid canals or degenerate stapedial arteries occur in some mammals that are not unusually sensitive to lower frequencies (MacPhee 1981).

Auditory Ossicles and the Tympanic Membrane

Few aspects of the mammalian skull rival the auditory ossicles in dramatically revealing the divergence of mammals from the typical amniote plan. Indeed, the discovery that the mammalian malleus and incus were actually homologues of visceral elements of the "reptilian" jaw articulation (Meckel 1820; Reichert 1837) ranks as one of the milestones in the history of comparative biology. Refinement of this argument, which came to be known as Reichert's theory, was a critical contribution of classic reviews by Gaupp (1913) and Goodrich (1930). By the time of de Beer's (1937) volume on the vertebrate skull, the essentials of Reichert's theory were well established. This did not, however, preclude a steady flow of more recent publications on ossicle structure and relative otic features in mammals—a literature that cannot be comprehensively reviewed in this brief treatment. Discussion here will focus on the origins of the mammalian ossicles and the tympanic membrane, variation in ossicle structure, and some basic functional considerations.

In all jawed vertebrates (gnathostomes) except mammals, the articulation of the jaws lies between the quadrate region of the palatoquadrate above and the articular region of Meckel's cartilage below. Although there are many compelling aspects of the fossil evidence for modification of the synapsid articular and quadrate, the essential evidence for the origin and homology of the mammalian ossicles comes from embryology, not pale-ontology. Early stages of development in mammals mirror the basic patterns of differentiation common to all gnathostomes. Meckel's cartilage develops as a derivative of the mandibular arch and in close association with the medial surface of the dentary (fig. 9.16). At this stage, the caudal end of Meckel's cartilage is represented by the cartilaginous anlage of the malleus. As Meckel (1820) first discovered, the separation of the anlage of the malleus from the cartilage that bears his name is an unusually late ontogenetic event; in adult *Tupaia*, for example, it occurs twelve days after birth (Zeller 1987). Chondral ossification of the malleus begins some days earlier, when this element comes in contact with a relatively late-forming dermal bone, the goniale (fig. 9.16), adjacent to the posterior Meckel's cartilage. The malleus in adult mammals is thus a composite of the endo-chondral (articular) end of Meckel's cartilage and the dermal goniale. The latter comprises the anterior folian process of the malleus.

The incus is clearly derived from the quadrate region of the palato-quadrate. It generally chondrifies early in ontogeny (day 24 in *Tupaia*; Zeller 1987), and is distinguishable as a cartilaginous anlage well before the separation of the malleus from Meckel's cartilage (fig. 9.16). The homology of the incus with the quadrate and the malleus with the articular (and goniale) is reaffirmed by the common development and position of these elements in relation to the chorda tympani, the innervation patterns of muscles inserting on the ossicles (m. tensor tympani and m. stapedius), pathways of the internal carotid, and other aspects of basicranial structure (Goodrich 1930).

The third ossicle, the stapes, is clearly homologous with the stapedial portion of the columella auris in the otic region in nonmammalian tetra-pods (Goodrich 1930). The stapes, like the columella auris and the hyomandibular of the fishes, develops from the dorsal region of the hyoid arch. The extrastapedial elements, which in nonmammalian tetrapods link the columella auris with the tympanic membrane, are apparently lost in mammals, and the stapes is distally articulated with the incus (fig. 9.16).

The homology of additional elements allegedly related to the stapes has been the source of some debate. There are two diminutive cartilages—one in the tendon of the stapedius muscle ("the element of Paauw") and the other above the chorda tympani between the stapes and the hyoid cornu ("the element of Spence"). These cartilages have been interpreted as phylogenetic "remnants" of the extrastapedial region in nonmammalian tetrapods (van der Klaauw 1923, 1931; Westoll 1944). These claims were rejected by Shute (1956), who observed that cartilages of Spence and of Paauw develop very late in ontogeny and without continuity with the developing stapes. Presley (1984) has, however, implicated the element of Spence as a functional link between the stapes and tympanic membrane in the earliest mammals (see below). In a detailed ontogenetic study of the marsupial *Monodelphis*, Maier (1987b) suggested that the element of Spence was homologous with some aspect of the styloid process.

Another intriguing controversy relates to Noden's (1978) experimental evidence for the role of neural crest cells in the origin of the avian columella. These results imply that the mammalian ossicles are of neural crest origin (van de Water et al. 1980). The argument is here regarded as problematic, since there is little relevant evidence from mammalian development. However, first-arch elements do seem to derive from neural crest cells, indirectly supporting the argument that neural crest cells give rise to the malleus and incus (see Langille and Hall, chap. 3 in vol. 1).

The transformation from the early synapsid to the mammalian otic region is related to modification in the jaw articulation in the therapsid relatives of mammals. These changes, as well as the emergence of the squamosal-dentary jaw joint of mammals, are documented in an extraordinary series of studies that date back to Owen (1845) and carry on through the works of Broom (1911), Westoll (1943, 1944, 1945), Olson (1944), Parrington (1955), Hopson (1966), Crompton (1972), Allin (1975), Lombard and Bolt (1979), Crompton and Jenkins (1979), and Crompton and Sun (1985). The essentials of this transition are outlined here, and in a section to follow on the craniomandibular joint. With respect to the "ossicle problem" it suffices here to state that the primitive condition in therapsids is one where the postdentary elements (articular, surangular, angular, retroarticular process) are large and the articular contact with the quadrate of the skull lies on a plane roughly even with the tooth row (fig. 9.31A, B). More advanced states in therapsids are represented by marked expansion of the dentary to form a coronoid process and encroach upon the articular in the area of the jaw articulation (fig. 9.31C, D). Postdentary elements are concomitantly reduced. These trends are not simply components of a single line of evolution; many divergent expressions of this transition are found in various therapsid clades (Moore 1981; Kemp 1983).

At some stage after the establishment of the squamosal-dentary jaw joint, the quadrate-articular might have been redundant in articulation of the lower jaw. Nonetheless, both articulations persist even after the appearance of what are traditionally recognized as earliest mammals (e.g., the late Triassic triconodont, *Morganucodon*). This suggests that the quadrate and incus were incorporated within the otic region subsequent to the condition represented in *Morganucodon*. Unfortunately, aside from fragments of the stapes (Kermack et al. 1981) ossicles are very poorly known for Mesozoic mammals (Archibald 1977). The derivation of the modern mammalian ossicular chain from the condition in more advanced non-

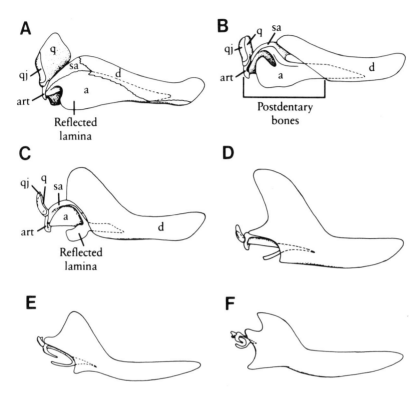

Fig. 9.31. Diagrams of lateral views of the jaws and postdentary elements showing modifications leading to the mammalian condition. Scheme essentially follows arguments of Allin (1975). A. The synapsid *Dimetrodon,* where all elements of the lower jaw are suturally attached and the angular bears a reflected lamina. B. A reconstructed therocephalian condition, where postdentary elements lose attachment with the dentary but remain large. C. *Thrinaxodon,* a cynodont. D. A more derived cynodont condition represented by *Probainognathus.* E. An early mammal relative, *Morganucodon.* Note the reduction of the postdentary elements in D and E. F. Hypothetical reconstruction of a Mesozoic mammal showing middle ear ossicles. Note the hiatus of information between stages E and F. Abbreviations are: a, angular; art, articular; d, dentary; q, quadrate; qj, quadratojugal; sa, surangular. (From Carroll 1988)

mammalian cynodonts and the earliest mammals must then rely on indirect evidence of basicranial and jaw structure.

A fundamental analysis in this regard is Hopson's (1966) assessment of otic structure in *Bienotherium, Thrinaxodon,* and other cynodonts. Applying the analogy of the ossicular condition in the echidna, *Tachyglossus,* Hopson (1966) suggested that the quadrate and articular in *Bienotherium,* while related primarily to mastication, is preadapted to become part of the

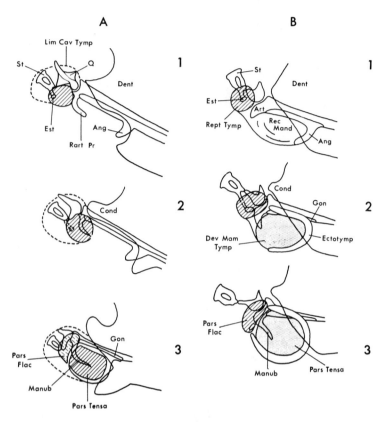

Fig. 9.32. Diagrams showing contrasting theories of the derivation of the mammalian middle ear. A. Hopson's (1966) reconstruction based on the cynodont *Bienotherium* (stage 1), *Morganucodon* (2), and inferred to be the stage for a Mesozoic mammal resembling *Amphitherium* (3). B. A simplified version of Westoll's (1945) theory, represented by three comparable stages. See text for explanation. Abbreviations are: Ang, angular; Art, articular; Cond, dentary condyle; Dent, dentary; Dev Mam Tymp, developing mammalian tympanum; Est, extrastapes; Gon, goniale; Lim Cav Tymp, limits of tympanic cavitiy; Manub, manubrium; Pars Flac, pars flaccida; Q, quadrate; Rart Pr, retroarticular process; Rec Mand, recessus mandibularis; Rept Tymp, reptilian tympanum; St, stapes. (From Hopson 1966)

sound-conducting mechanism of the middle ear (fig. 9.32A). The articular in this form bears resemblance to the malleus in *Tachyglossus*; its retroarticular, for example, is reminiscent of the recurved manubrium of the malleus. Hopson (1966) reasoned that the articular in *Bienotherium* could be transformed into a functional malleus if it were separated from the other postdentary bones and realigned to rotate around a new functional axis (fig. 9.32A, 1 and 2). A similar conversion would involve the quadrate.

Such changes would be accompanied by loss of the "extrastapes elements," which in living nonmammalian tetrapods form the functional link between the columella of the stapes and the tympanic membrane. Distal to the columella would now be the articulated quadrate and articular. The converted articular, particularly the retroarticular process, would thus contact the tympanic membrane and be the first osseous element to transmit sound vibrations affecting this membrane (fig. 9.32A, 2 and 3).

The nature of the contact between the tympanic membrane (eardrum) and the modified articular poses some problems for Hopson's (1966) arguments, as the homology of the mammalian tympanic membrane is uncertain. Westoll (1943, 1944, 1945) speculated that the mammalian tympanic membrane was a neomorph, derived from a ventral diverticulum from the tympanic cavity and originally distinct from the synapsid tympanic membrane (fig. 9.32B). The diverticulum was allegedly attached distally to the angular in the lower jaw. With its separation from the jaw, the angular was transformed into the incomplete annulus (the ectotympanic) supporting the mammalian eardrum. The synapsid tympanic membrane then migrated anteriorly to the postero-dorsal edge of the new functional drum, where it remains as the pars flaccida (fig. 9.32B, 2 and 3).

The series of assumptions required by Westoll's (1943, 1944, 1945) model also encounters several difficulties. Most important, Westoll's argument conflicts with the conventional notion that, at least in "primitive" therapsids, the angular notch was primarily the site for the insertion of the pterygoid musculature and therefore could not accommodate, in these early stages, attachment of the tympanic diverticulum. Hopson (1966) accordingly proposed that the mammalian tympanic membrane was derived from the antero-ventral expansion of the synapsid tympanic membrane, and that the reflected lamina of the angular moved caudally (along with the angle of the dentary) to surround this expanded membrane (fig. 9.32A). The site of pterygoid muscle insertion was thus transferred to the angle of the dentary, freeing the (detached) angular for support of the mammalian eardrum.

Hopson's (1966) intriguing hypothesis must be acknowledged with the caveat that there is no direct evidence for these transitions in therapsids and early fossil mammals. As expected, a number of conflicting views have surfaced. Kermack et al. (1973) rejected the homology between the manubrium of the mammalian malleus and the retroarticular process of the synapsid articular, equating the former instead with a downward projecting spur of the articular, the infraarticular process, found in some therapsids (e.g., *Cynognathus*). Moreover, Kermack et al. identify a boss or eminence of the surangular as a homologue of the retroarticular process. Like Watson (1951), Kermack et al. (1973) regarded the infraarticular process as a neomorph of "more advanced" therapsids that originally served as the insertion for the posterior pterygoid muscles. Parrington (1978), however, disputed these claims and homologized the infraarticular process with the more generalized synapsid retroarticular process. He also equated the surangular eminence with a surangular structure of similar location in the secondary jaw articulation of some cynodonts as described by Crompton (1972). Parrington's (1978) view that the surangular boss is not derived from the retroarticular process is more compatible with the general transition outlined by Hopson (1966).

A radical alternative to these views is Allin's (1975) argument that early therapsids lacked a tympanic membrane of the typical amniote condition and instead developed de novo a mammal-like tympanic membrane behind the angular notch. Allin also suggested that in all but the sphenacodont synapsids, the reflected lamina of the angular was the lateral boundary for an air-filled chamber derived from either a diverticulum of the tympanic cavity (fide Westoll 1943, 1945) or the pharynx. Hence, Allin (1975) disputed the conventional view that the angular in such forms served as an insertion site for the pterygoid muscles before its conversion to the ectotympanic. This scheme rejects some of the osteological evidence cited for the location of the tympanic membrane in some therapsids. Instead, Allin (1975) surmised that a functional eardrum, not homologous with the "reptilian" tympanic membrane, was represented by fibrous tissue in the gap between the medial retroarticular process and the more lateral reflected lamina. Sound vibrations picked up by this drum would then be transmitted by the postdentary bones, the quadrate and the stapes, to reach the inner ear. This emphasis on bone-transmitted sound conduction assumes that the quadrate at an early stage in therapsid phylogeny was a sound-conducting element. For this argument, Allin (1975) notes that the quadrate (as well as the stapes) is quite small and "more mobile" in many therapsid relatives of mammals. Nonetheless, the large size of these elements in comparison to the mammalian ossicle chain would suggest high efficiency only in conduction of lower-frequency sounds (Fleischer 1973, 1978; Moore 1981).

Complete resolution among these various perspectives has not been achieved. Allin's (1975) views on the origin of the therapsid and mammalian tympanic membrane are consistent with a comprehensive review of the tetrapod ear by Lombard and Bolt (1979). Moreover, the otic notch is absent in labyrinthodonts, and the stapes in these forms does not seem appropriate for contact with a tympanic membrane (Smithson 1982). These findings support the notion that there is no "primitive tetrapod" tympanic membrane, and the membranes in various extant tetrapods (e.g., lizards and mammals) were independently derived and thus are not strictly homologous (see also Tumarkin 1955; Barry 1963). Ironically, this recent trend vindicates an essential point in Gaupp's (1913) extraordinary treatise. Gaupp endorsed the view that the tympanic membranes of anurans, lizards and crocodilians, and mammals are not homologous because there is no embryological evidence to support this homology. This conclusion was rejected by Goodrich (1916, 1930), who claimed that Gaupp greatly exaggerated the differences between the reptilian and mammalian tympanic membranes. A recent embryological study by Presley (1984), however, emphatically supports Gaupp's (1913) argument for nonhomology of these structures. The growing consensus is that the mammalian tympanic membrane may be derived from an innovative therapsid condition, where a membrane, not homologous with that found in other tetrapods, was supported by the angular notch (Allin 1975; Lombard and Bolt 1979; Crompton and Jenkins 1979; Kermack et al. 1981; Kemp 1982, 1983; Presley 1984).

Such agreement does not extend to all aspects of Allin's (1975) theory. There is still great uncertainty as to whether the reduced quadrate functioned as a sound-transmitting element in certain therapsids and early mammals. Moreover, the retroarticular origin for the manubrium of the malleus is not clearly substantiated. Findlay (1944) suggested, for example, that the manubrium may be an isolated derivative of the element of Spence later incorporated into the malleus. Implicit here is the notion that the element of Spence is the vestige of the extrastapes connection between the stapes and the tympanic membrane. Presley (1984) speculated that in *Morganucodon* the skeletal chain for transmitting sound vibrations to the middle ear was a tympanohyal (derivative of the second hyoid arch) contacting the rear of the tympanic membrane, linked by the element of Spence to the distal end of the stapes and constrained by muscles homologous to the second-arch levator hyoidea. Such a condition bears a very general resemblance to ontogenetic stages of monotremes. Unfortunately, this reconstruction for *Morganucodon,* as Presley (1984) acknowledges, is untestable with fossil material.

Uncertainties also extend to the controversy over a single or dual origin for the mammalian ossicle chain. The debate is influenced by some fundamental differences noted in early studies (Gaupp 1908a) between the monotreme and therian otic regions. In both living monotremes the detrahens mandibulae muscle, innervated by the mandibular branch of the trigeminal nerve, is found in place of the posterior head of the digastric muscle of therians, which is innervated by the facial nerve. The detrahens mandibulae muscle, which runs from the paroccipital region, is sometimes compared with depressor mandibulae in living lizards and birds. However, the ontogeny of the detrahens is clearly different from that of the depressor mandibulae. Its orientation in newly hatched platypus suggests that initially it pulls anterior to the axis of the primary jaw joint (malleo-incudal) and hence serves in this stage as a jaw adductor. With allometric growth the dentary-squamosal joint moves dorsally and caudally in relation to the detrahens, transforming its action to that of a retractor and a very weak depressor of the jaw. The detrahens is therefore not a homologue of the depressor mandibulae, but is instead a unique specialization of mono-tremes (Presley 1984). Because the external auditory meatus lies below the detrahens mandibulae in monotremes and lies above the digastric in ther-ians, it has been argued (Hopson 1966) that the middle ear ossicles arose independently at least twice with respect to these nonhomologous muscles. However, Presley (1984) stressed that the course of the external auditory meatus of monotremes in relation to the ectotympanic and other cranial bones, the mandible, and the first- and second-arch musculature in the early ontogeny of monotremes, is very similar to that of other mammals. He therefore rejected the argument for independent origin of the middle ear among mammals, and cautioned against the reliance on adult structure in the highly specialized jaw apparatus of monotremes as evidence for such a pattern.

Another difference cited for the argument that the monotreme ossicle chain and middle ear arose independently is that the ectotympanic ring (tympanum) in this group lies semihorizontally, whereas the therian ecto-tympanic is tilted more vertically. An additional putative distinction is the vibration of the ectotympanic with the tympanic membrane in mono-tremes (Aitkin and Johnstone 1972), because of its fusion with the malleus. These alleged differences between monotremes and therians are, however, misleading. As noted in a preceding section, several extant and fossil therians show a nearly horizontal orientation of the ectotympanic resem-bling that of monotremes (Novacek 1977). Moreover, the fusion of the ectotympanic with the ossicular chain in monotremes is clearly present in many therian groups (Fleischer 1973, 1978; Kemp 1983).

Taken as a whole, I find the arguments that the middle ear ossicles were acquired independently in monotremes and therians unconvincing (see also Patterson 1980; Kemp 1983; Presley 1984). The basic similarity in this system for all extant mammals far outweighs the differences noted, especially when one considers that several alleged differences between monotremes and therians do not exist (Novacek 1977; Kemp 1983; No-vacek and Wyss 1986a). Moreover, a case for diphyletic origin of the os-sicles in mammals should not be built on Allin's (1975) claim that this system, through divergent modifications of therapsid postdentary bones, could easily be subject to parallel evolution. However compelling the tran-sition proposed by Allin, this functional theory does not predict parallel origin of the ossicles as a necessary outcome. As Kemp (1983, 377) notes, "One must of course accept that parallel evolution could have occurred, but unless overall phylogenetic analysis indicates that it had to occur, there is no reason to assume that it did." It thus seems likely that the three-ossicle chain is a shared-derived feature of modern therians and mono-tremes. This acquisition is not common to morganucodont triconodonts and the Mesozoic form *Kuhneotherium* (Kemp 1983), but it is now known in Paleocene multituberculates (Miao and Lillegraven 1986), suggesting that this extinct group, along with living mammals, forms a monophyletic clade that excludes those triconodonts known from postdentary and basicranial features.

Diversification of ossicle structure in mammals follows myriad pathways (figs. 9.33, 9.34), although the basic design in the system is maintained (Fleischer 1973, 1978). No modern treatment matches the scope of Doran's (1878) masterly comparative study of mammalian ossicles. The framework established by Doran in combination with basic embryological studies (Gaupp 1913) invites a modern investigation of ossicles in phylogenetic studies. For example, Wyss (1987) recently cited ossicle structure as evidence for the monophyly of pinnipeds (seals, sea lions, and walruses). A brief treatment here concerns the problem of ossicle variation in relation to (1) the structure of the stapes and (2) the basic types of ossicle systems in relation to functional problems (see also Fleischer 1973, 1978).

Early in ontogeny the cartilaginous anlage of the stapes forms around mesenchymal connective tissue for the proximal stapedial artery. As a result, the stapes in many mammals has a large foramen for passage of the stapedial artery (figs. 9.33, 9.34). Many therapsids as well as other tetrapods show a stapes with a large stapedial foramen. For this reason, Goodrich (1930) equated the horseshoe-shaped, perforated stapes seen in many mammals with the primitive mammalian condition. Goodrich's thesis implies that the imperforate or weakly perforate columellar stapes in monotremes, some marsupials, and some eutherians (figs. 9.33, 9.34) was secondarily derived. The columellar imperforate stapes is, however, also now known in extinct multituberculates (Miao and Lillegraven 1986), and the distribution of this condition (summarized by Novacek and Wyss 1986b) at least allows the alternative that such a stapes was the most primitive condition for therians or even mammals. Moreover, acceptance of Goodrich's (1930) hypothesis would not rule out transformation from an imperforate, columelliform stapes to a perforate (horseshoe-shaped) structure (or the reversal of this change), several times in mammalian phylogeny.

One objection to the more complex transformational scheme suggested by Novacek and Wyss (1986b) is that the ontogeny of the stapes in mammals generally shows only two basic patterns: (1) the persistence of the stapedial foramen, or (2) its progressive reduction and loss to form the imperforate columelliform stapes. There is no case in which the stapes appears as an imperforate column and later develops a stapedial foramen. The absence of this pattern may seem inconsistent with the view that the

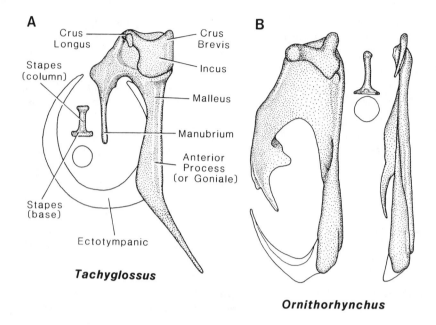

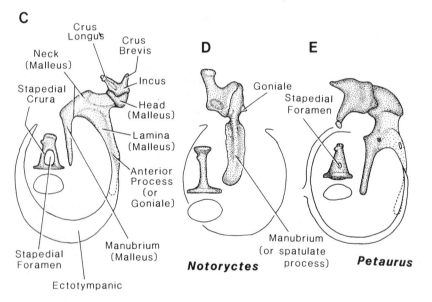

Fig. 9.33. Diagrams showing middle ear ossicles and ectotympanic in monotremes and marsupials. Oval outline represents shape of stapedial footplate. (After Fleischer 1973)

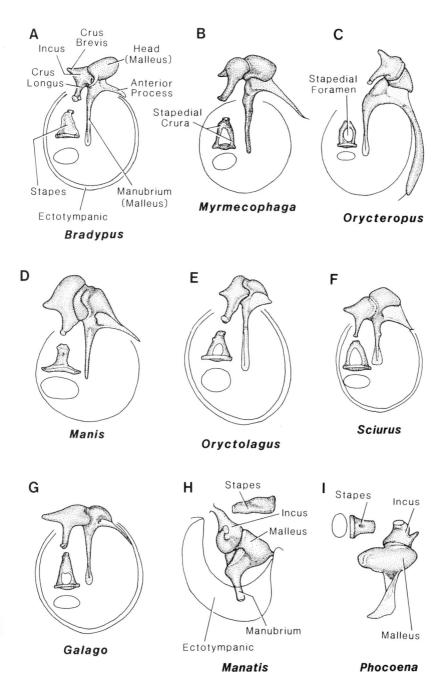

Fig. 9.34. Diagrams showing middle ear ossicles and ectotympanic in eutherian mammals. Oval outlines represent shape of the stapedial footplate. (After Fleischer 1973)

columnar stapes is primitive for mammals. However, it is noteworthy that the perforate stapes forms around the embryonic mesenchymal tissue for the proximal stapedial artery even in cases where this vessel never completely develops. Hence, the phylogenetic transformations that produce either columellar imperforate stapes or perforate (horseshoe-shaped) stapes could be most greatly influenced by ontogenetic changes involving the form, pathway, or loss of the stapedial artery (Novacek and Wyss 1986b). Subsequent development of stapes would merely be the consequence of these earlier ontogenetic changes. In cases where the stapedial artery is well developed and is located in the region of the stapes' attachment to the fenestra ovalis, a perforate or horseshoe-shaped adult stapes would develop. In cases where the stapedial artery is degenerate, absent, or markedly displaced in position, a columelliform imperforate stapes would develop. As Goodrich (1930) emphasized, the relation of the stapedial artery to the developing stapes can vary markedly even at lower taxonomic levels.

Variation in form of the stapes, as well as the malleus and incus (figs. 9.33, 9.34), is clearly correlated with function. The ossicle chain serves as an impedance transformer (Wever and Lawrence 1954; Dallos 1973; Webster and Webster 1975; Fleischer 1978). Sensitivity to certain frequencies will then depend on the overall design of the middle ear (Moore 1981). The ossicles have an intrinsic impedance relating to their mass, stiffness, and friction. The variation shown in figures 9.33 and 9.34 relates to these parameters (fig. 9.35) and to the great range of hearing adaptations ascribed to echolocation, burrowing, swimming, or other modes of life (Fraser and Purves 1960; Henson 1970; Fleischer 1973, 1978; Hunt and Korth 1980; and Lombard and Hetherington, vol. 3 of this work).

The Craniomandibular Joint (CMJ)
and the Masticatory Apparatus

As noted above, many therapsid lineages show modifications that foreshadow the mammalian jaw articulation (fig. 9.31). Primitively, synapsids have very prominent postdentary elements (articular, angular, surangular, and others). Some cynodont therapsids (e.g., *Procynosuchus, Thrinaxodon*) show an expansion of the dentary, with a more prominent coronoid process and the incipient development of a postero-ventral angular process. The postdentary bones in these cynodonts are not greatly reduced. Cynodonts with more derived jaw features (e.g., *Cynognathus*) show further expansion of the dentary and its encroachment on the postdentary elements. The coronoid process is very strongly projecting and occupies much of the temporal fossa, and the angle of the dentary is prominent. A longitudinal groove on the medial side of the dentary may indicate the position of Meckel's cartilage. The postdentary elements are lodged in this

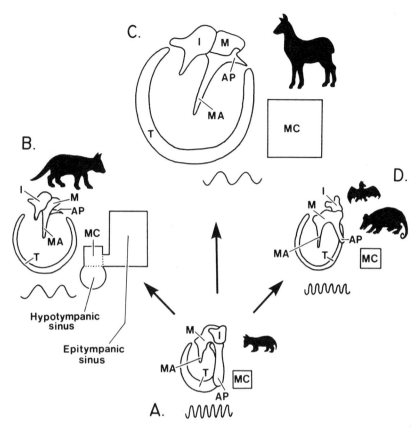

Fig. 9.35. Hypothesis for modifications of the middle ear system in mammals.
A. System with low mass and much stiffness (including attachment of malleus with
ectotympanic) suitable for high-frequency reception. B. System for small- to moderate-
size mammals where lower frequency reception is enhanced through detachment of the
malleus from the ectotympanic and through increase of middle ear volume with
inflated extratympanic sinuses. C. System in large mammals suitable for lower-
frequency reception showing modifications similar to those in B. Negative allometry
of the middle ear system limits mass so that it does not become a restrictive factor in
large mammals. D. System in some mammals (microchiropterans, marsupials) suitable
for high-frequency reception represented by only slight modification from the
primitive therian condition. A and D are of low mass and much stiffness. B is of
low mass and little stiffness. C has limited mass and little stiffness. Abbreviations
are: AP, anterior process of the malleus; I, incus; MA, manubrium of the malleus;
M, malleus; MC, middle ear cavity proper; T, ectotympanic. (After Hunt and Korth 1980)

groove and they partly obscure the cartilage from dorso-medial view. Even more extreme modifications are seen in *Diarthrognathus*, where the dentary extends to form a condylar (posterior) process which articulates with a ventrally concave surface on the squamosal. The quadrate-articular joint persists in *Diarthrognathus*, but both this and the squamosal-dentary joint lie well above the plane of the tooth row, a condition that contrasts strongly with the relatively lower (quadrate-articular) joint in theriocephalians, *Procynosuchus*, and *Thrinaxodon* (fig. 9.31).

Within synapsids and Mesozoic mammals, there is a rough correspondence between increasing jaw specializations and more recent geologic occurrence, but these patterns do not constitute a simple trend. Many therapsid lineages show divergent specializations. Moreover, the "progressive" reduction of the postdentary elements is not simply a transition that straddles the mammaliaform boundary. Although it has a well-developed squamosal-dentary articulation, the triconodont *Morganucodon* retains a strong quadrate-articular joint and is more conservative in reduction of the postdentary elements than is *Diarthrognathus* (e.g., Kermack et al. 1973). On the other hand, a basic series of modifications describes the common ancestral conditions of the jaw and the jaw articulation for mammals and their successively more remote sister lineages (Kemp 1983; Gauthier et al. 1988; Rowe 1988). Detailed accounts of morphological features can be found in Hopson and Crompton (1969), Barghusen (1968), Crompton (1972), and Kemp (1979, 1983), among many others.

The rearrangements of jaw musculature that accompanied the above-noted modifications are inferred from fossae, grooves, and surface ornamentation preserved in the relevant fossils. At a very general level, a pattern for change in therapsid jaw mechanics and the derivation of the mammalian mastication apparatus seems reasonably secure (fig. 9.36). The origin of the mammalian jaw apparatus (figs. 9.36, 9.37, 9.38) and its variation in design and function are discussed in numerous papers (e.g., Davis 1955; Parrington 1955; Schumacher 1961, 1985; Crompton and Hotton 1967; Barghusen 1968; Turnbull 1970; Kemp 1972, 1979; Crompton et al. 1977; Bramble 1978) and in other contributions to this work (see Herring, vol. 1; Smith, vol. 3; Weishampel, vol. 3; Russell and Thomason, vol. 3).

Secondary Cartilages

As in many other instances, Gaupp (1970a) was the first to discuss cogently the presence and implications of secondary cartilages on certain membrane bones of the mammalian skull. De Beer (1937, 502) distinguished these cartilages histologically from primary cartilages by their large cells and very thin extracellular matrix. More recent studies (Durkin 1972; Patterson 1977; Starck 1979; Zeller 1987) do not recognize this

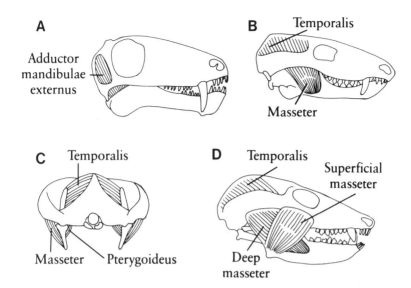

A

Adductor
mandibulae
externus

B

Temporalis

Masseter

C Temporalis

Masseter   Pterygoideus

D Temporalis

Superficial
masseter

Deep
masseter

Fig. 9.36. Diagrammatic scheme for transformation of the jaw-closing muscles.
A. Putative arrangement in the primitive therapsid condition. B, C. Differentiation of
masseter and temporalis in primitive cynodont condition. D. Further differentiation of
the masseter in a more specialized cynodont condition. Note diversification in fiber
orientation and thus vectors for muscle contraction. (From Carroll 1988)

histological distinction as significant and rely on the basic definition (also
in de Beer 1937) that secondary cartilages form after the initiation of ossification in membrane bones. By contrast, primary cartilages always appear before the related endochondral ossifications.

The occurrence of secondary cartilages varies greatly in mammals. In
Tachyglossus, for example, secondary cartilages appear only on the squamosal (Kuhn 1971). In the flying lemur, *Cynocephalus*, secondary cartilages form on the dentary, maxilla, palatine, squamosal, vomer, jugal, and
frontal (Gaupp 1907a). There is also ambiguity concerning the status of
certain cartilages. The pterygoid cartilage was regarded by de Beer (1929),
Frick (1954), and Starck (1967) as a secondary cartilage whose uncusto-
marily early appearance results from heterochronous ontogeny in response
to stresses exerted by the tensor veli palatini muscle (Starck 1967). Others,
however, note that pterygoid cartilage develops before the latter muscle,
and favor its recognition as a primary cartilage phylogenetically derived
from the palatoquadrate (see Zeller 1987). Confusion also stems from the
fact that some dermal bone may invade cartilages of the chondocranium
(e.g., the vomer invades lamina transversalis posterior, the dentary invades
Meckel's cartilage) and, histologically, these cartilages ossify endochondrally as well (Zeller 1987). These examples are important because they

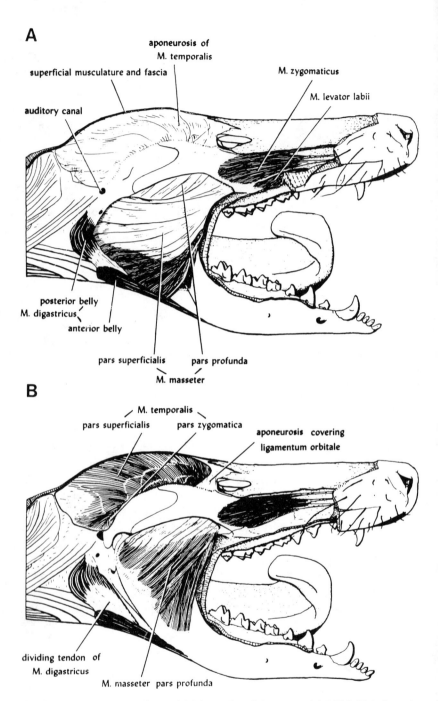

Fig. 9.37. Masticatory and naso-labial muscles of the marsupial *Didelphis* in lateral view. A. Superficial muscles. B. Temporal aponeurosis and M. masseter pars superficialis removed to expose deep musculature. (From Turnbull 1970)

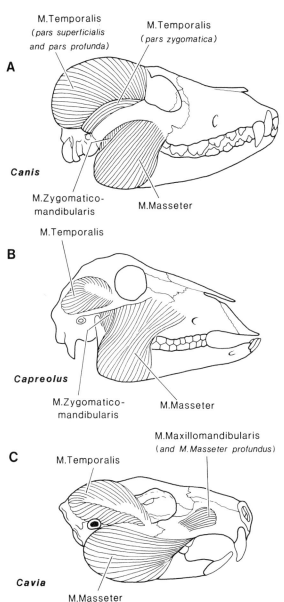

A

M.Temporalis
(pars superficialis
and pars profunda)

M.Temporalis
(pars zygomatica)

C

Canis

M.Zygomatico-
mandibularis

M.Masseter

B

M.Temporalis

Capreolus

M.Zygomatico-
mandibularis

M.Masseter

C

M.Temporalis

M.Maxillomandibularis
(and M.Masseter profundus)

Cavia

M.Masseter

Fig. 9.38. Diagrammatic representation of the masticatory musculature in (A) a domestic dog (*Canis familiaris*), (B) a Roe-deer (*Capreolus capreolus*), (C) a guinea pig (*Cavia porcellus*). All views are of right lateral side. Note the emphasis of temporalis mass and thus orthal shear in A. B and C represent more specialized systems emphasizing masseter and pterygoideus musculature mass and lateral and antero-posterior movement. See text for further explanation. (After Schumacher 1985)

demonstrate the limitations of simple morphological or histological comparisons in making homology statements. Thus homology statements reflecting this relationship can be achieved only with out-group comparison of structures and their relevant ontogenies (Gaupp 1913; Kuhn 1971; Starck 1975a, b; Zeller 1987).

Secondary cartilage, then, is not simply an unexplainable anomaly (Hall and Hanken 1985a). It most likely represents an adaptation to the functional demands of rapid growth and mechanical stress during on-togeny and the need for repair mechanisms (Hall 1968; Starck 1975a; Hall and Jacobson 1975; Beresford 1981). Secondary cartilages seem restricted to birds and mammals, and that they are apparently not present in other vertebrates offers intriguing questions concerning their origin and adaptation (Hall and Hanken 1985a).

CONCLUDING REMARKS

Viewed against the imposing early literature on the mammalian skull, even de Beer's (1937) volume might be regarded as a modern work. Knowledge of the major components of the skull reflects treatments of the early nineteenth century (Meckel 1820; Reichert 1837). These works were effectively synthesized and embellished in the classic studies of the early twentieth century (e.g., Gaupp 1913). Modern investigators, despite their sophisticated approaches, consistently pay homage to older discoveries. There is thus clearly a cyclic pattern to trends in this area of research. We have seen, for example, early concepts (Gaupp's 1913 distinction of tympanic membranes in various tetrapods) rejected at later stages (e.g., Goodrich's 1930 support for homology of the tympanic membranes in mammals and living "reptilian" groups) only to be resurrected in recent studies (Presley 1984). From this, one might wonder how much we have gained from such recent investigations in comparison to new lines of evidence for phylogeny (e.g., molecular systematics).

Long-standing traditions should not be equated, however, with a lack of progress or innovation. The accumulation of information on the mammalian skull is the subject of ongoing and future revision combined with first-hand analysis. It seems that in this respect certain avenues are particularly auspicious. The recent developments in systematic methods require a clearer rationale and more explicit presentation for homology statements (McKenna 1975; Patterson 1977; Novacek 1986). Characters for groups must be clearly described and assessed for the level at which homology statements apply to the monophyletic origin of groups. This involves a tabulating procedure characteristically shunned in much earlier work.

Related here is a more comprehensive and clearer tie-in between comparative ontogeny and adult structure (consider the exemplary work of the modern German morphologists, e.g., Zeller 1987). A major challenge in this area is to extend our sampling of ontogenies—a painstaking and time-consuming venture—to a much broader range of mammalian and vertebrate taxa. Paleontological studies also provide important information that may be missing in Recent taxa (Gauthier et al. 1988). Fossil evidence of the skull and other areas may radically overturn theories for relationships among Recent taxa, if such theories are initially based only on structures known in living forms (Novacek and Wyss 1986a; Gauthier et al. 1988). Finally, modern studies of functional morphology show a greater emphasis on analysis based on experimental observation, a broader comparative base, and a stronger anchoring in phylogenetic premises (Lauder 1981). This review of the mammalian skull is thus meant to be an interim report addressing the above-noted trends for this dynamic area of research.

ACKNOWLEDGMENTS

I am grateful to André Wyss, John Wible, Ross MacPhee, and the editors for their numerous and valuable comments on the manuscript. Artists Edward Heck and Lorraine Meeker contended adroitly with a large and complicated set of illustrations. Access to mammal specimens was provided by Guy Musser, Department of Mammalogy, American Museum of Natural History. The project was supported by the Frick Laboratory Endowment Fund.

LIST OF ABBREVIATIONS

Anatomical

Abbreviations in figures taken directly from other sources are explained in legends for those figures. Otherwise abbreviations for structures are as follows:

Teeth

C	canine
I	incisor
M	molar
P	premolar

Elements

AS (or as)	alisphenoid
BS (or bs)	basisphenoid
B-OCC (or bo)	basioccipital
DEN	dentary
ECT	ectotympanic
ECTPT,	ectopterygoid
EX-OCC (or eo)	exoccipital
FR	frontal
IP	interparietal
JU	jugal

LA	lacrimal
MX (or mx)	maxilla
NA (or na)	nasal
OO	opisthotic
OS (or os)	orbitosphenoid
PA	parietal
PER	periotic
PL	palatine
PMX (or pmx)	premaxilla
POSTF	postfrontal
POSTO	postorbital
PR (or pr)	petromastoid
PRF	prefrontal
PRS	presphenoid
PT	pterygoid
QDT	quadrate
QJT	quadratojugal
S-OCC	supraoccipital
SPTMX	septomaxilla
SQ (or sq)	squamosal
ST	supratemporal
STAP	stapes
VO	vomer

Foramina, Fossae, Sulci

Acoust. F	acoustic foramen
Alis. Ca.	alisphenoid canal
Antorb. Fos.	antorbital fossa
Car. F.	carotid foramen
Cond. Ca.	condyloid canal
Cond. F.	condyloid foramen
Epitym. Rec.	epitympanic recess
Eth. F.	ethmoidal foramen
Eust. Ca.	eustachian canal
Eust. F.	eustachian foramen
Fallop. F.	fallopian foramen
Fen. Oval.	fenestra ovalis
Fen. Rot.	fenestra rotunda
Fiss. Basicap.	fissura basicapsulas
Fiss. Metot.	fissura metotica
Fiss. Orbnas.	fissura orbitonasalis
For. Carot.	foramen caroticum
For. Duct. Nas.	foramen ductus nasolacrimalis
For. Epiphan.	foramen epiphaniale
For. Mag.	foramen magnum

For. Metot.	foramen metoticum
For. Orbtns.	foramen orbitonasale
For. Ov. (or For. Oval.)	foramen ovale
For. Perilymph.	foramen perilymphaticum
For. Pro.	foramen prooticum
For. Pseu.	foramen pseudoopticum
For. Psov.	foramen pseudovale
For. Rotdum.	foramen rotundum
For. Subov.	foramen subovale
Fos. St. M.	fossa for the stapedius muscle
Glas. Fis.	glaserian fissure
Glen. Fos.	glenoid fossa
Hyp. F.	hypoglossal foramen
Inc. F.	incisive foramen
Inf. Acoust. F.	inferior acoustic foramen
Infra. Ca.	infraorbital canal
Jug. F.	jugular foramen
Lacr. F.	lacrimal foramen
Lev. Plp. Sup.	pit for levator palpebrae superioris
Mx. Ant.	maxillary antrum
Opt. F.	optic foramen
Opth. F.	ophthalmic foramen
Opth. Sulc.	ophthalmic sulcus
Orbn. Fiss.	orbitonasal fissure
Phar. Sulc.	pharyngeal sulcus
Post. Glen. F.	postglenoid foramen
Post. Lac. F.	posterior lacerate foramen
Post. Vid. F.	posterior vidian foramen
Postmas. F.	postmastoid foramen
Postpal. F.	postpalatine foramen
Pyf. Fen.	pyriform fenestra
Sin. Can.	sinus canal
Sph. F.	sphenopalatine foramen
Sphenorb. Fis.	sphenorbital fissure
Spme. F.	suprameatal fissure
SQ. (Sin.-Ca.)	squamosal sinus-canal
Styl. F. Def.	stylomastoid foramen (definitivum)
Styl. F. Prim.	stylomastoid foramen (primitivum)
Subarc. Fos.	subarcuate fossa
Sulc. Med.	sulcus medialis (of petromastoid)
Sulc. Mm. Digas.	sulcus for the digastric muscle
Sup. Acoust. F.	superior acoustic foramen
Supr. F.	supraorbital foramina
Ven. F.	venous foramen
Vid. F.	vidian foramen

Processes, Sutures, Septa, Membranes, Cartilages

AS (Ect. Cr.)	ectopterygoid crest of the alisphenoid
AS (Preot. Cr.)	preotic crest of the alisphenoid
Btr. Proc.	basitrabecular process
Cart. Antorbit.	cartilago antorbitalis
Cart. Duc.	cartilago ductus
Nasopala.	nasopalatini
Cart. Pala.	cartilago palatini
Cart. Parasep.	cartilago paraseptalis
Cart. Pter.	cartilago pterygoidea
Com. Orbnas.	commissura orbitonasalis
Com. Praefac.	commissura praefacialis
Cor. Sut.	coronal suture
Cris. Gal.	crista galli
Cris. Marg.	crista marginalis
Do. Atlan. Fac.	dorsal atlantal facet
Dors. Sel.	dorsum sellae
Lambd. Cr.	lambdoidal crest
Lamina Trans. Ant.	lamina transversalis anterior
Lamina Trans. Post.	lamina transversalis posterior
Mas. Pr.	mastoid process
Mas. Tub.	mastoid tubercle (including tympanohyal)
Mrgturb.	marginoturbinale
Mxturb.	maxillaturbinale
Naturb.	nasalturbinale
Occ. Cond.	occipital condyle
OCC (Int. Pr.)	anterior orbital process of the palatine
Parocc. Pr.	paroccipital process
Pars. Canic.	pars canicularis
Pil. Ant.	pila antotica
Pil. Met.	pila metoptica
Pil. Pro.	pila praeoptica
Postglen. Pr.	postglenoid process
Postpal. Tor.	postpalatine torus
Postym. Pr.	posttympanic process
PR (Mas.)	mastoid exposure of petromastoid
PR (Mas. Pr.)	mastoid process (of petromastoid)
Proc. Al. Sup.	processus alaris superior
Proc. Paranas.	processus paranasalis
Proc. Pl. Max.	processus palatinus maxillaris
Proc. Rec.	processus recessus
PT (Ent. Cr.)	entopterygoid crest (of pterygoid)
PT (Ham.)	pterygoid hamulus
Postzyg. Cr.	postzygomatic crest

Spina Meseth.	spina mesethmoidalis
SQ (Me. Su.)	suprameatal surface of the squamosal
SQ (Preot. Cr.)	preotic crest of the squamosal
Teg. Tymp.	tegmen tympani
Tub. Sel.	tuberculum sellae
TYM	tympanic membrane

Nerves, Arteries, Veins, Muscles

Cav. Sin.	cavernosus sinus
Ex. Ju. V.	external jugular vein
Inf. Petr. Sin.	inferior petrosal sinus
Int. Car. A.	internal carotid artery
Int. Ju. V.	internal jugular vein
Int. Max. A.	internal maxillary artery
Ling. N.	lingual nerve
M. Stap.	stapedius muscle
N. I	olfactory nerve
N. II	optic nerve
N. III	oculomotor nerve
N. IV	trochlear nerve
N. V. (mand.)	mandibular branch of trigeminal nerve
N. VI	abducens nerve
N. VII	facial nerve
N. IX	glossopharyngeal nerve
N. X	vagus nerve
N. XI	spinal accessory nerve
N. XII	hypoglossal nerve
Pal. F.	palatine foramen
Phar. A.	pharyngeal artery
Phar. N.	pharyngeal nerve
Pt. Can. A.	artery of the pterygoid canal
Prom. A.	promontory artery
Ram. Inf.	ramus inferior of the stapedial artery
Stap. A.	stapedial artery
Sup. Petr. Sin.	superior petrosal sinus
Tymp. Plxs.	tympanic plexus
Vid. N.	vidian nerve
V_2	2d (maxillary) branch of trigeminal nerve
V_3	3d (mandibular) branch of trigeminal nerve

Institutional

| AMNH | Department of Vertebrate Paleontology, American Museum of Natural History |
| AM | Department of Mammalogy, American Museum of Natural History |

CA   Comparative Anatomy Collection, American Museum of Natu-
              ral History
US Natl. Mus. United States National Museum of Natural History, the Smith-
              sonian Institution

REFERENCES

Aitkin, I. M., and B. M. Johnstone. 1972. Middle ear function in a monotreme:
    The echidna (*Tachyglossus aculeatus*). Journal of Experimental Zoology 80:
    245–250.
Allin, E. F. 1975. Evolution of the mammalian middle ear. Journal of Morphology
    47: 403–437.
Archibald, J. D. 1977. Ectotympanic bone and internal carotid circulation of eu-
    therians in reference to anthropoid origins. Journal of Human Evolution 6:
    609–622.
Barghusen, H. R. 1968. The lower jaw of cynodonts (Reptilia, Therapsida) and the
    evolutionary origin of mammalian adductor musculature. Postilla 116: 1–49.
Barry, T. H. 1963. On the variable occurrence of the tympanum in Recent and
    fossil tetrapods. South African Journal of Science 59: 160–175.
Bast, T. H., and B. J. Anson. 1949. *The Temporal Bone and the Ear.* Springfield:
    Charles C Thomas.
Beresford, W. A. 1981. *Chondroid Bone, Secondary Cartilage, and Metaplasia.*
    Munich: Urban and Schwarzenberg.
Bondy, G. 1907. Beiträge zur vergleichenden Anatomie des Gehörorgans der Säu-
    ger (Tympanicum, Membrana Shrapnelli und Chordaverlauf). Anatomische
    Hefte 35: 293–408.
Bown, T. M., and P. D. Gingerich. 1973. The Paleocene primate *Plesiolestes* and
    the origin of the Microsyopidae. Folia primatologica 19: 1–18.
Bramble, D. M. 1978. Origin of the mammalian feeding complex: Models and
    mechanisms. Paleobiology 4: 271–301.
Broom, R. 1896. On the comparative anatomy of Jacobson's organ in marsupials.
    Proceedings of the Linnean Society of New South Wales 21: 591–623.
———. 1911. On the structure of the skull in cynodont reptiles. Proceedings of the
    Zoological Society of London: 893–925.
———. 1915. On the origin of mammals. Transactions of the Royal Society, Lon-
    don B206: 1–49.
Bugge, J. A. 1974. The cephalic arterial system in insectivores, primates, rodents,
    and lagomorphs, with special reference to the systematic circulation. Acta ana-
    tomica 87: 1–160.
Butler, P. M. 1956. The skull of *Ictops* and the classification of the Insectivora.
    Proceedings of the Zoological Society of London 126: 453–481.
Cachel, S. M. 1979. A functional analysis of the primate masticatory system and
    the origin of the anthropoid post-orbital septum. American Journal of Physical
    Anthropology 50: 1–18.
Carroll, R. L. 1988. *Vertebrate Paleontology and Evolution.* New York: W. H.
    Freeman and Co.

Cartmill, M. 1975. Strepsirhine basicranial structures and affinities of the Cheiro-galeidae. In *Phylogeny of the Primates: A Multidisciplinary Approach*, W. P. Luckett and F. S. Szalay, eds. New York: Plenum Press, pp. 313–354.

————. 1980. Morphology, function, and evolution of the anthropoid postorbital septum. In *Evolutionary Biology of New World Monkeys and Continental Drift*, R. L. Ciochon and A. B. Chiarelli, eds. New York: Plenum Press, pp. 243–274.

Cartmill, M., and R. F. Kay. 1978. Cranio-dental morphology, tarsier affinities, and primate sub-orders. In *Recent Advances in Primatology*, vol. 3, D. J. Chivers and K. A. Joysey, eds. London: Academic Press, pp. 205–214.

Cave, A. J. E., and R. W. Haines. 1940. The paranasal sinuses of the anthropoid apes. Journal of Anatomy 74: 493–523.

Cifelli, R. L. 1982. The petrosal structure of *Hyopsodus* with respect to that of some other ungulates, and its phylogenetic implications. Journal of Paleontology 56: 795–805.

Conroy, G. C., and J. R. Wible. 1978. Middle ear morphology of *Lemur variegatus:* Some implications for primate paleontology. Folia primatologica 29: 81–85.

Crompton, A. W. 1963. The evolution of the mammalian lower jaw. Evolution 17: 431–439.

————. 1972. The evolution of the jaw articulation of cynodonts. In *Studies of Vertebrate Evolution*, K. A. Joysey and T. S. Kemp, eds. Edinburgh: Oliver and Boyd, pp. 231–253.

Crompton, A. W., and N. H. Hotton. 1967. Functional morphology of the masticatory apparatus of two dicynodonts (Reptilia, Therapsida). Postilla 109: 1–51.

Crompton, A. W., and F. A. Jenkins. 1979. Origin of mammals. In *Mesozoic Mammals: The First Two-thirds of Mammalian History*, J. A. Lillegraven, Z. Kielan-Jaworowska, and W. A. Clemens, eds. Berkeley: University of California Press, pp. 59–73.

Crompton, A. W., and A. L. Sun. 1985. Cranial structure and relationship of the Liassic mammal *Sinocondon**. Zoological Journal of the Linnean Society 85: 99–119.

Crompton, A. W., A. J. Thexton, P. Parker, and K. M. Hiiemae. 1977. The activity of the jaw and hyoid musculature in the Virginian opossum, *Didelphis virginiana*. In *The Biology of Marsupials*, B. Stonehouse and D. Gilmore, eds. London: Macmillan Co.

Dallos, P. 1970. Low-frequency auditory characteristics: Species dependence. Acoustical Society of America Journal 48: 489–499.

————. 1973. *The Auditory Periphery Biophysics and Physiology*. New York: Academic Press.

Davis, D. D. 1955. Masticatory apparatus in the spectacled bear *Tremarctos ornatus*. Fieldiana: Zoology 37: 24–46.

De Beer, G. R. 1929. The development of the skull of the shrew. Philosophical Transactions of the Royal Society of London 217: 411–480.

————. 1937. *The Development of the Vertebrate Skull*. Oxford: Clarendon Press. Reprint. Chicago: University of Chicago Press, 1985.

DeBurlet, H. M. 1914. Zur Entwicklungsgeschichte des Walschädels. IV. Ueber das Primordialcranium eines Embryo von *Balaenoptera rostrata* (105 mm). Morphologisches Jahrbuch 49: 393–406.

Doran, A. 1878. Morphology of mammalian ossicula auditus. Linnean Society Transactions, Zoology (pt. 7): 371–497.

Durkin, J. F. 1972. Secondary cartilage: A misnomer? American Journal of Orthodontics 62: 15–41.

Emry, R. J. 1970. A North American Oligocene pangolin and other additions to the Pholidota. Bulletin of the American Museum of Natural History 142: 457–510.

Erdmann, K. 1933. Zur Entwicklung des knöchernen Skeletts von *Triton* und *Rana* unter besonderer Berücksichtigung der Zeitfolge der Ossifikationen. Zeitschrift für Anatomie und Entwicklungsgeschichte 101: 566–651.

Fawcett, E. 1918a. The primordial cranium of *Erinaceus europaeus*. Journal of Anatomy 52: 211–250.

———. 1918b. The primordial cranium of *Poecilophoca wedelli* (Weddell's seal), at the 27 mm C. R. length. Journal of Anatomy 52: 412–441.

Findlay, G. H. 1944. The development of the auditory ossicles in the elephant shrew, the tenrec, and the golden mole. Proceedings of the Zoological Society, London 114: 91–99.

Fischer, E. 1901. Das Primordialcranium von *Talpa europaea*. Anatomische Hefte 17: 467–548.

Fleischer, G. V. 1973. Studien am Skelett des Gehörorgans der Säugetiere, einschliesslich des Menschen. Säugetierkundliche Mitteilungen 21: 131–239.

———. 1978. Evolutionary principles of the mammalian middle ear. Advances in Anatomy, Embryology, and Cell Biology 55: 1–70.

Fraser, F. C., and P. E. Purves. 1960. Anatomy and function of the cetacean ear. Proceedings of the Royal Society, London 152: 62–77.

Frick, H. 1952a. Ueber die Aufteilung des Foramen perilymphaticum in der Ontogenese der Säugetiere. Zeitschrift für Anatomie und Entwicklungsgeschichte 116: 523–551.

———. 1952b. Zur Morphogenese der Fenestra rotunda. Verhandlungen der Anatomischen Gesellschaft 50: 194–203.

———. 1954. *Die Entwicklung und Morphologie des Chondrokraniums von Myotis Kaup.* Stuttgart: Thieme.

Frick, H., and U. Heckmann. 1955. Ein Beitrag zur Morphogenese des Kaninchenschädels. Acta anatomica 24: 268–314.

Fuchs, H. 1905. Zur Entwicklungsgeschichte des Wirbeltierauges. I. Ueber die Entwicklung der Augengefässer des Kaninchens. Anatomische Hefte 21: 1–251.

Gannon, P. J., A. R. Eden, and J. T. Laitman. 1988. The subarcuate fossa and cerebellum of extant primates: Comparative study of a skull-brain interface. American Journal of Physical Anthropology 77: 143–164.

Gaupp, E. 1900. Das Chondrocranium von *Lacerta agilis:* Ein Beitrag zum Verständnis des Amniotenschädels. Anatomische Hefte 15: 433–595.

———. 1902. Ueber die Ala temporalis des Säugerschädels und die Regio orbitalis einiger anderer Wirbeltierschädel. Anatomische Hefte 19: 155–230.

―――. 1905. Neue Deutungen auf dem Gebiete der Lehre vom Säugetierschädel. Anatomischer Anzeiger 27: 273–310.

―――. 1906. Ueber allgemeine und spezielle Fragen aus der Lehre vom Kopfskelett der Wirbeltiere. Verhandlungen der Anatomischen Gesellschaft 20: 21–73.

―――. 1907a. Demonstration von Präparaten, betreffend Knorpelbildung in Deckknochen. Verhandlungen der Anatomischen Gesellschaft 21: 251–252.

―――. 1907b. Hauptergebnisse der an dem Semonschen *Echidna*-Material vorgenommenen Untersuchungen der Schädelentwicklung. Verhandlungen der Anatomischen Gesellschaft 21: 129–141.

―――. 1908a. Ueber die Entwicklung und Bau der ersten Wirbel und der Kopfgelenke von *Echidna aculeata,* nebst allgemeine Bemerkungen über die Kopfgelenke der Amnioten. Semon, Zoologische Forschungsreisen in Australien. Denkschriften der medizinischen-naturwissenschaftlichen Gesellschaft zu Jena, pt. 2: 481–538.

―――. 1908b. Zur Entwicklungsgeschichte und vergleichenden Morphologie des Schädels von *Echidna aculeatea* var. *typica.* Semon, Zoologische Forschungsreisen in Australien. Denkschriften der medizinischen-naturwissenschaftlichen Gesellschaft zu Jena, pt. 2: 539–788.

―――. 1913. Die Reichertsche Theorie (Hammer-, Amboss- und Kieferfrage). Archiv für Anatomie und Entwicklungsgeschichte 1912: 1–416.

Gauthier, J., A. G. Kluge, and T. Rowe. 1988. Amniote phylogeny and the importance of fossils. Cladistics 4: 105–209.

Gingerich, P. D. 1973. Anatomy of the temporal bone in the Oligocene anthropoid *Apidium* and the origin of the Anthropoidea. Folia primatologica 19: 329–337.

Goodrich, E. S. 1916. The chorda tympani and middle ear in reptiles, birds, and mammals. Quarterly Journal of Microscopical Science 61: 137–156.

―――. 1930. *Studies on the Structure and Development of Vertebrates.* London: Macmillan Co. Reprint. Chicago: University of Chicago Press, 1986.

Green, H. L. H. H., and R. Presley. 1978. The dumb-bell bone of *Ornithorhynchus.* Journal of Anatomy 127: 216.

Gregory, W. K. 1910. The orders of mammals. Bulletin of the American Museum of Natural History 27: 1–525.

―――. 1920. Studies of the comparative myology and osteology, no. IV: A review of the evolution of the lacrimal in vertebrates with special reference to that of mammals. Bulletin of the American Museum of Natural History 42: 95–263.

Griffiths, M. 1978. *The Biology of the Monotremes.* London: Academic Press.

Grosser, O. 1901. Zur Anatomie und Entwicklungsgeschichte des Gefässsystems der Chiropteren. Anatomische Hefte 17: 203–424.

Hafferl, A. 1916. Zur Entwicklungsgeschichte der Aortenbögen und der Kopfarterien von *Tarsius spectrum.* Gegenbaurs Morphologisches Jahrbuch 50: 19–48.

―――. 1933. Das Arteriensystem. In *Handbuch der Vergleichenden Anatomie der Wirbeltiere,* vol. 6, L. Bolk, E. Göppert, E. Kallius, and W. Lubosch, eds., pp. 563–684. Reprint 1967, Amsterdam: Ascher.

Haines, R. W. 1950. The interorbital septum in mammals. Zoological Journal of the Linnean Society 41: 585–607.

Halbsguth, A. 1973. Das Cranium eines Foeten des Flattermaki *Cynocephalus volans* (*Galeopithecus volans*) (Mammalia, Dermoptera) von 63 mm SchStlg. Inaugural-Dissertation (Medizin), Johann Wolfgang Goethe Universität, Frankfurt.

Hall, B. K. 1968. The fate of adventitious and embryonic articular cartilage in the skull of the common fowl, *Gallus domesticus* (Aves: Phasianidae). Australian Journal of Zoology 16: 795–806.

Hall, B. K., and J. Hanken. 1985a. Foreword to G. R. de Beer, *The Development of the Vertebrate Skull,* Chicago: University of Chicago Press, pp. vii–xxviii.

———. 1985b. Repair of fractured lower jaws in the spotted salamander: Do amphibians form secondary cartilage? Journal of Experimental Zoology 233: 359–368.

Hall, B. K., and H. N. Jacobson. 1975. The repair of fractured membrane bones in the newly hatched chick. Anatomical Record 185: 55–70.

Henckel, K. O. 1927a. Das Primordialcranium der Halbaffen und die Abstammung der höheren Primaten. Verhandlungen der Anatomischen Gesellschaft 36: 108–116.

———. 1927b. Zur Entwicklungsgeschichte des Halbaffenschädels. Zeitschrift für Morphologie und Anthropologie 26: 365–383.

———. 1929. Die Entwicklung des Schädels von *Galeopithecus temmincki* Waterh. und ihre Bedeutung für die stammesgeschichtliche und systematische Stellung der Galeopithecidae. Morphologisches Jahrbuch (Mauerfestschrift part 1) 62: 179–205.

Hennig, W. 1966. *Phylogenetic Systematics.* Urbana: University of Illinois Press.

Henson, O. W. 1970. The ear and audition. In *Biology of the Bats,* vol. 2, W. A. Wimsatt, ed. New York: Academic Press.

Hofer, H. 1952. Der Gestaltwandel des Schädels der Säugetiere und Vögel mit besonderer Berücksichtigung der Knickungstypen und der Schädelbasis. Verhandlungen der Anatomischen Gesellschaft 50: 102–113.

Honigmann, H. 1917. Bau und Entwicklung des Knorpelschädels vom Buckelwal. Zoologica 27: 1–85.

Hopson, J. A. 1966. The origin of the mammalian middle ear. American Zoologist 6: 437–450.

Hopson, J. A., and A. W. Crompton. 1969. Origin of mammals. Evolutionary Biology 3: 15–72.

Hunt, R. M. 1974. The auditory bulla in Carnivora: An anatomical basis for reappraisal of carnivore evolution. Journal of Morphology 143: 21–76.

Hunt, R. M., and W. W. Korth. 1980. The auditory region of Dermoptera: Morphology and function relative to other living mammals. Journal of Morphology 164: 167–211.

Jones, F. W. 1929. *Man's Place among the Mammals.* London: E. Arnold.

Keibel, F. 1912. The development of the sense-organs. In *Manual of Human Embryology,* vol. 2, F. Keibel and F. P. Mall, eds. Philadelphia: Lippincott, pp. 180–290.

Kemp, T. S. 1972. Whaitsiid Therocephalia and the origin of cynodonts. Philosophical Transactions of the Royal Society B264: 1–54.

———. 1979. The primitive cynodont *Procynosuchus:* Functional anatomy of the skull and relationships. Philosophical Transactions of the Royal Society B285: 73–122.

———. 1982. *Mammal-like Reptiles and the Origin of Mammals.* London: Academic Press.

———. 1983. The relationships of mammals. Zoological Journal of the Linnean Society 77: 353–384.

Kermack, K.A. 1963. The cranial structure of the triconodonts. Philosophical Transactions of the Royal Society B246: 83–103.

Kermack, K. A., and Z. Kielan-Jaworowska. 1971. Therian and non-therian mammals. In *Early Mammals,* D. M. Kermack and K. A. Kermack, eds. Zoological Journal of the Linnean Society 50 (suppl. 1): 103–115. London: Academic Press.

Kermack, K. A., F. Mussett, and H. W. Rigney. 1973. The lower jaw of *Morganucodon.* Zoological Journal of the Linnean Society 53: 87–175.

———. 1981. The skull of *Morganucodon.* Zoological Journal of the Linnean Society 71: 1–158.

Kielan-Jaworowska, Z. 1969. Preliminary data on the Upper Cretaceous eutherian mammals from Bayn Dzak, Gobi Desert. Palaeontologica polonica 19: 171–191.

———. 1975. Preliminary description of two new eutherian genera from the late Cretaceous of Mongolia. Palaeontologica polonica 33: 5–13.

Kuhn, H.-J. 1971. Die Entwicklung und Morphologie des Schädels von *Tachyglossus aculeatus.* Abhandlungen der Senckenbergischen Naturforschenden Gesellschaft 528: 1–192.

Kuhn, H.-J., and U. Zeller. 1987. The cavum epeptericum in monotremes and therian mammals. In *Morphogenesis of the Mammalian Skull,* H.-J. Kuhn and U. Zeller, eds. Mammalia Depicta, Heft 13: 51–70. Hamburg: Verlag Paul Parey.

Lauder, G. V. 1981. Form and function: Structural analysis in evolutionary analysis. Paleobiology 7: 430–442.

Lindahl, P. E., and M. Lundberg. 1946. On the arteries in the head of *Procavia capensis* Pall and their development. Acta zoologica 27: 1–53.

Lombard, R. E., and J. R. Bolt. 1979. Evolution of the tetrapod ear: An analysis and reinterpretation. Biological Journal of the Linnean Society 11: 19–76.

Luckett, W. P., and F. S. Szalay. 1978. Clades versus grades in primate phylogeny. In *Recent Advances in Primatology,* vol. 3, D. J. Chivers and K. A. Joysey, eds. New York: Academic Press, pp. 227–235.

MacIntyre, G. T. 1967. Foramen pseudoovale and quasi-mammals. Evolution 21: 834–841.

MacPhee, R. D. E. 1979. Entotympanics, ontogeny, and primates. Folia primatologica 31: 23–47.

———. 1981. Auditory regions of primates and eutherian insectivores: Morphology, ontogeny, and character analysis. In *Contributions to Primatology,* F. S. Szalay, ed. Basel: S. Karger, pp. i–xv + 1–282.

MacPhee, R. D. E., and M. Cartmill. 1986. Basicranial structures and primate systematics. In *Comparative Primate Biology*, vol. 1, *Systematics, Evolution, and Anatomy*, D. R. Swindler and J. Erwin, eds. New York: Alan R. Liss, pp. 219–275.

MacPhee, R. D. E., M. J. Novacek, and G. Storch. 1988. Basicranial morphology of early Tertiary erinaceomorphs and the origin of primates. American Museum Novitates 2921: 1–42.

Maier, W. 1980. Nasal structures in Old and New World primates. In *Evolutionary Biology of the New World Monkeys and Continental Drift*, R. L. Ciochon and A. B. Chiarelli, eds. New York: Plenum Press, pp. 219–241.

————. 1987a. The ontogenetic development of the orbito-temporal region in the skull of *Monodelphis domestica* (Didelphidae, Marsupialia), and the problem of the mammalian alisphenoid. In *Morphogenesis of the Mammalian Skull*, H. J. Kuhn and U. Zeller, eds. Mammalia Depicta, Heft 13: 71–90. Hamburg: Verlag Paul Parey.

————. 1987b. Der processus angularis bei *Monodelphis domestica* (Didelphidae; Marsupialia) und seine Beziehungen zum Mittelohr: Eine ontogenetische und evolutions-morphologische Untersuchung. Gegenbaurs Morphologisches Jahrbuch 133: 123–161.

————. 1989. Morphologische Untersuchungen am Mittelohr der Marsupialia. Zeitschrift für Zoologische Systematik und Evolutionsforschung 27: 149–168.

Matthes, E. 1921a. Neuere Arbeiten über das Primordialcranium der Säugetiere. Ergebnisse der Anatomie und Entwicklungsgeschichte 23: 669–912.

————. 1921b. Zur Entwicklung des Kopfskeletts der Sirenen. II. Das Primordialcranium von *Halicore dugong*. Zeitschrift für Anatomie und Entwicklungsgeschichte 60: 1–306.

Matthew, W. D. 1909. The Carnivora and Insectivora of the Bridger Basin, middle Eocene. Memoirs of the American Museum of Natural History 9: 291–567.

McDowell, S. B. 1958. The Greater Antillean insectivores. Bulletin of the American Museum of Natural History 115: 113–214.

McKenna, M.C. 1975. Toward a phylogenetic classification of the Mammalia. In *Phylogeny of the Primates: A Multidisciplinary Approach*, W. P. Luckett and F. S. Szalay, eds. New York: Plenum Press, pp. 21–46.

Meckel, J. F. 1820. *Handbuch der Menschlichen Anatomie*. Halle.

Miao, D., and J. A. Lillegraven. 1986. Discovery of three ear ossicles in multituberculate mammals. National Geographic Research 2: 500–507.

Moore, W. J. 1981. *The Mammalian Skull*. Cambridge: Cambridge University Press.

Müller, F. 1968. Methodische Gesichtspunkte zum Studium der Evolution der Säuger-Ontogenesetypen. Revue suisse de zoologie 75: 63–643.

————. 1972. Zur stammesgeschichtlichen Veränderung der Eutheria-Ontogenesen. Versuch einer Uebersicht aufgrund vergleichend morphologischer Studien an Marsupialia und Eutheria. Revue suisse de zoologie 79: 1–97.

Muller, J. 1934. The orbitotemporal region in the skull of the Mammalia. Archives neerlandaises de zoologie 1: 118–259.

Negus, V. 1958. *The Comparative Anatomy and Physiology of the Nose and Paranasal Sinuses.* Edinburgh: Livingstone.

Nesslinger, C. L. 1956. Ossification centers and skeletal development in the postnatal Virginia opossum. Journal of Mammalogy 37: 382–394.

Noden, D. W. 1978. The control of avian cephalic neural crest cytodifferentiation. I. Skeletal and connective tissues. Developmental Biology 67: 296–312.

Novacek, M. J. 1977. Aspects of the problem of variation, origin, and evolution of the eutherian auditory bulla. Mammal Review 7: 131–149.

———. 1980. Cranioskeletal features in tupaiids and selected eutherians as phylogenetic evidence. In *Comparative Biology and Evolutionary Relationships of Tree Shrews,* W. P. Luckett, ed. Advances in Primatology 4. New York: Plenum Press, pp. 35–93.

———. 1982. Information for molecular studies from anatomical and fossil evidence on higher eutherian phylogeny. In *Macromolecular Sequences in Systematic and Evolutionary Biology,* M. Goodman, ed. New York: Plenum Press, pp. 3–41.

———. 1985. Cranial evidence for rodent affinities. In *Evolutionary Relationships among Rodents,* W. P. Luckett and J.-L. Hartenberger, eds. New York: Plenum Press, pp. 59–81.

———. 1986. The skull of leptictid insectivorans and the higher-level classification of eutherian mammals. Bulletin of the American Museum of Natural History 183: 1–111.

Novacek, M. J., M. C. McKenna, N. A. Neff, and R. L. Cifelli. 1983. Evidence from the earliest known erinaceomorph basicranium that insectivorans and primates are not closely related. Nature 306: 238–244.

Novacek, M. J., and A. R. Wyss. 1986a. Higher-level relationships of the recent eutherian orders: Morphological evidence. Cladistics 2: 257–287.

———. 1986b. Origin and transformation of the mammalian stapes. Contributions to Geology, University of Wyoming, Special Paper 3: 35–53.

Olson, E. C. 1944. Origin of mammals based upon cranial morphology of the therapsid suborders. Bulletin of the Geological Society of America, Special Papers 55: 1–136.

Owen, R. 1845. Description of certain fossil crania discovered by A. G. Bain, Esq., in the sandstone rocks at the southeastern extremity of Africa, referable to different species of an extinct genus of Reptilia (*Dicynodon*) and indicative of a new tribe of Sauria. Transactions of the Geological Society, London 2: 59–84.

Parrington, F. R. 1955. On the cranial anatomy of some gorgonopsids and the synapsid middle ear. Proceedings of the Zoological Society of London 125: 1–40.

———. 1978. A further account of the Triassic mammals. Philosophical Transactions of the Royal Society B282: 177–204.

Patterson, C. 1977. Cartilage bones, dermal bones, and membrane bones, or the exoskeleton versus the endoskeleton. In *Problems in Vertebrate Evolution,* S. M. Andrews, R. S. Miles, and A. D. Walker, eds. New York: Academic Press, pp. 77–121.

———. 1980. Methods of paleobiogeography. In *Vicariance Biogeography: A Cri-*

tique, G. J. Nelson and D. E. Rosen, eds. New York: Columbia University Press, pp. 446–500.

Paulli, S. 1900a. Ueber die Pneumaticität des Schädels bei den Säugethieren. I. Ueber den Bau des Siebbeins. Ueber die Morphologie des Siebbeins der Pneumaticität bei den Monotremen und den Marsupialiern. Morphologisches Jahrbuch 28: 147–178.

———. 1900b. Ueber die Pneumaticität des Schädels bei den Säugethieren. II. Ueber die Morphologie des Siebbeins und die Pneumaticität bei den Ungulaten und Probosciden. Morphologisches Jahrbuch 28: 179–251.

———. 1900c. Ueber die Pneumaticität des Schädels bei den Säugethieren. III. Ueber die Morphologie des Siebbeins und die Pneumaticität bei den Insectivoren, Hyracoideen, Chiropteren, Carnivoren, Pinnipedien, Edentates, Rodentiern, Prosimien und Primaten. Morphologisches Jahrbuch 28: 483–564.

Pocock, R. I. 1918. On the external characters of the lemurs and of *Tarsius*. Proceedings of the Zoological Society, London: 19–53.

Presley, R. 1979. The primitive course of the internal carotid artery in mammals. Acta anatomica 103: 238–244.

———. 1980. The braincase in Recent and Mesozoic therapsids. Memoirs de la Société géologique de France 139: 159–162.

———. 1981. Alisphenoid equivalents in placentals, marsupials, monotremes, and fossils. Nature 294: 668–670.

———. 1984. Lizards, mammals, and the primitive tetrapod tympanic membrane. Symposium of the Zoological Society, London 52: 127–152.

Presley, R., and F. L. D. Steel. 1976. On the homology of the alisphenoid. Journal of Anatomy 121: 441–459.

———. 1978. The pterygoid and ectopterygoid in mammals. Anatomy and Embryology 154: 95–100.

Reichert, C. 1837. Ueber die Visceralbogen der Wirbelthiere im Allegemeinen und deren Metamorphosen bei den Vögeln und Säugethieren. Archiv für Anatomie, Physiologie, und wissenschaftliche Medizin, Leipzig: 120–122.

Reinbach, W. 1952. Zur Entwicklung des Primordialcraniums von *Dasypus novemcinctus* Linné (*Tatusia novemcincta* Lesson). I. Zeitschrift für Morphologie und Anthropologie 44: 375–444. II. Zeitschrift für Morphologie und Anthropologie 45: 1–72.

Roux, G. 1947. The cranial development of certain Ethiopian "insectivores" and its bearing on the mutual affinities of the group. Acta zoologica 28: 165–397.

Rowe, T. 1988. Definition, diagnosis, and origin of Mammalia. Journal of Vertebrate Paleontology 8: 241–264.

Salomon, M. I. 1930. Considerations sur l'homologie de l'os lachrymal chez les Vertébrés supérieurs. Acta zoologica 11: 151–183.

Schliemann, H. 1966. Zur Morphologie und Entwicklung des Craniums von *Canis lupus* f. *familiaris* L. Morphologisches Jahrbuch 109: 501–603.

Schneider, R. 1955. Zur Entwicklung des Chondrocraniums der Gattung *Bradypus*. Morphologisches Jahrbuch 95: 209–301.

Schreiber, K. 1916. Zur Entwicklungsgeschichte des Walschädels. Das Primordialcranium eines Embryos von *Globicephalus melas* (13,3 cm). Zoologisches Jahrbuch, Abteilung für Anatomie und Ontogenie der Tiere 39: 201–236.

Schumacher, G. H. 1961. *Funktionelle Morphologie der Kaumuskulatur.* Jena: Fischer.

———. 1985. Comparative functional anatomy of jaw muscles in reptiles and mammals. In *Functional Morphology in Vertebrates,* H. R. Duncker and G. Fleischer, eds., Fortschritte der Zoologie 30. Stuttgart: Gustav Fischer Verlag, pp. 203–212.

Schwartz, J. H., I. Tattersall, and N. Eldredge. 1978. Phylogeny and classification of the primates revisited. Yearbook of Physical Anthropology 21: 95–133.

Shute, C. C. D. 1956. The evolution of the mammalian eardrum and tympanic cavity. Journal of Anatomy 90: 261–281.

Sicher, H. 1913. Die Entwicklungsgeschichte der Kopfarterien von *Talpa europaea.* Gegenbaurs Morphologisches Jahrbuch 44: 465–487.

Simons, E. L., and D. E. Russell. 1960. Notes on the cranial anatomy of *Necrolemur.* Breviora 127: 1–14.

Smithson, T. R. 1982. The cranial morphology of *Greererpeton burkemorani* Romer (Amphibia: Temnospondyli). Zoological Journal of the Linnean Society 76: 29–90.

Spatz, W. B. 1963. Zur Entwicklung des Nasenskeletts bei Säugetieren. Naturwissenschaften 50: 454.

———. 1964. Beitrag zur Kenntnis der Ontogenese des Cranium von *Tupaia glis* (Diard 1820). Morphologisches Jahrbuch 106: 321–416.

Spatz, W. E. 1967. Zur ontogenese der Cartilago Meckeli und der Symphysis mandibularis bei *Tupaia glis* (Diard 1820). Die distal Verknöcherung des Meckelschen Knorpels als funktionelle Anpassung an den Saugakt. Folia primatologica 4: 26–50.

Starck, D. 1941. Zur Morphologie des Primordialkraniums von *Manis javanica* Desm. Morphologisches Jahrbuch 86: 1–122.

———. 1943. Ein Beitrag zur Kenntnis der Morphologie und Entwicklungsgeschichte des Chiropterencraniums: Das Chondrocranium von *Pteropus semindus.* Zeitschrift für Anatomie und Entwicklungsgeschichte 112: 588–633.

———. 1960. Das Cranium eines Schimpansenfetus (*Pan troglodytes,* Blumenbach, 1799) von 71 mm Scheitel-Steiss Länge, nebst Bemerkungen über die Körperform von Schimpansenfeten. Morphologisches Jahrbuch 100: 599–647.

———. 1967. Le crâne des Mammifères. In *Traité de Zoologie,* vol. 16, P. P. Grassé, ed. Paris: Masson, pp. 405–549.

Starck, D. 1975a. The development of the chondrocranium in primates. In *Phylogeny of the Primates: A Multidisciplinary Approach,* W. P. Luckett and F. S. Szalay, eds. New York: Plenum Press, pp. 127–155.

———. 1975b. *Embryologie.* Stuttgart: Thieme.

———. 1979. *Vergleichende Anatomie der Wirbeltiere auf Evolutionsbiologischer Grundlage,* vol. 2. Berlin: Springer.

Sturm, H. 1936. Die Entwicklung des praecerebralen Nasenskeletts beim Schwein (*Sus scrofa domestica*) und beim Rind (*Bos taurus*). Zeitschrift für wissenschaftliche Zoologie 149: 161–220.

Sues, H.-D. 1985. The relationships of the Tritylodontidae (Synapsida). Zoological Journal of the Linnean Society 85: 205–217.

Szalay, F. 1975. The origin of primate higher categories: An assessment of basi-cranial evidence. In *Phylogeny of the Primates: A Multidisciplinary Approach*, W. P. Luckett and F. S. Szalay, eds. New York: Plenum Press, pp. 91–125.

———. 1977. Phylogenetic relationships and a classification of the eutherian Mammalia. In *Major Patterns in Vertebrate Evolution*, M. K. Hecht, P. C. Goody, and B. M. Hecht, eds. New York: Plenum Press, pp. 315–374.

Tandler, J. 1902. Zur Entwicklungsgeschichte der Kopfarterien bei den Mammalia. Gegenbaurs Morphologisches Jahrbuch 30: 275–373.

Terry, R. J. 1917. The primordial cranium of the cat. Journal of Morphology 29: 281–433.

Toeplitz, C. 1920. Bau und Entwicklung des Knorpelschädels von *Didelphis mar-supialis*. Zoologica 27: 1–84.

Tumarkin, A. 1955. On the evolution of the auditory conducting apparatus: A new theory on functional considerations. Evolution 9: 119–140.

Turnbull, W. D. 1970. Mammalian masticatory apparatus. Fieldiana: Geology 18: 149–356.

Vandebroek, G. 1964. Recherches sur l'origine des mammifères. Annales de la Société royale zoologique de Belgique 94: 117–160.

Van der Klaauw, C. J. 1923. Die Skelettstücke in der Sehne des musculus stapedius und nahe dem Ursprung der Chorda tympani. Zeitschrift für Anatomie und Entwicklungsgeschichte 69: 32–83.

———. 1931. The auditory bulla in some fossil mammals, with a general intro-duction to this region of the skull. Bulletin of the American Museum of Natu-ral History 62: 1–352.

Van de Water, T. R., F. A. Maderson, and T. F. Jaskoll. 1980. The morphogenesis of the middle and external ear. Birth Defects: Original Article Series 16: 147–180.

Van Kampen, P. N. 1905. Die Tympanalgegend des Säugetier-schädels. Morpho-logisches Jahrbuch 34: 321–722.

Van Valen, L. 1965. Treeshrews, primates, and fossils. Evolution 19: 137–151.

Voit, M. 1909. Das Primordialcranium des Kaninchens unter Berücksichtigung der Deckknochen. Anatomische Hefte 38: 425–616.

Wahlert, J. H. 1974. The cranial foramina of protrogomorphous rodents: An ana-tomical and phylogenetic study. Bulletin of the Museum of Comparative Zo-ology 146: 363–410.

Watson, D. M. S. 1916. The monotreme skull: A contribution to mammalian mor-phogenesis. Philosophical Transactions of the Royal Society, London B207: 311–374.

———. 1948. *Dicynodon* and its allies. Proceedings of the Zoological Society, London 118: 823–877.

———. 1951. *Paleontology and Modern Biology*. New Haven: Yale University Press.

Weber, M. 1904. *Die Säugetiere: Einführung in die Anatomie und Systematik der Recenten und Fossilen Mammalia*. 8 vols. Jena.

Webster, D. B., and M. Webster. 1975. Auditory systems of Heteromydiae: Func-tional morphology and evolution of the middle ear. Journal of Morphology 146: 343–376.

Weidenreich, F. 1941. The brain and its role in the phylogenetic transformation of the human skull. American Philosophical Society 31: 321–442.

Werner, C. F. 1960. *Das Gehörorgan der Wirbeltiere und des Menschen: Beispiel für eine Vergleichende Morphologie der Lagesbeziehungen.* Leipzig: Thieme.

Westoll, T. S. 1943. The hyomandibular of *Eusthenopteron* and the tetrapod middle ear. Proceedings of the Royal Society, London B131: 393–414.

―――. 1944. New light on the mammalian ossicles. Nature 154: 770–771.

―――. 1945. The mammalian middle ear. Nature 155: 114–115.

Wever, E. G., and M. Lawrence. 1954. *Physiological Acoustics.* Princeton: Princeton University Press.

Wible, J. R. 1983. The internal carotid artery in early eutherians. Acta palaeontologica polonica 28: 281–293.

―――. 1984. The ontogeny and phylogeny of the mammalian cranial arterial system. Ph.D. diss., Duke University.

―――. 1986. Transformation in the extracranial course of the internal carotid artery in mammalian phylogeny. Journal of Vertebrate Paleontology 6: 313–325.

―――. 1987. The eutherian stapedial artery: Character analysis and implications for superordinal relationships. Zoological Journal of the Linnean Society 91: 107–135.

―――. 1990. Petrosals of late Cretaceous marsupials from North America, and a cladistic analysis of the petrosal in therian mammals. Journal of Vertebrate Paleontology 10: 183–205.

Wible, J. R., and H. H. Covert. 1987. Primates: Cladistic diagnosis and relationships. Journal of Human Evolution 16: 1–22.

Wible, J. R., and M. J. Novacek. 1988. Cranial evidence for the monophyletic origin of bats. American Museum Novitates 2911: 1–19.

Williston, S. W. 1925. *The Osteology of the Reptilia.* Cambridge, Mass.

Wünsch, D. 1975. Zur Kenntnis der Entwicklung des Craniums des Koboldmaki, *Tarsius bancanus boreanus,* Horsfield, 1821. (Beiträge zur Kenntnis des Primaten-Craniums no. IV) Selbstverlag des Zentrums der Morphologie, Frankfurt am Main.

Wyss, A. R. 1987. The walrus auditory region and the monophyly of pinnipeds. American Museum Novitates 2871: 1–31.

Zeller, U. 1984. Die Ontogenese und Morphologie der Cartilage antorbitalis (Reinbach) am Schädel von *Tupaia belangeri.* Verhandlungen der Anatomischen Gesellschaft 78: 251–253.

―――. 1985a. The morphogenesis of the fenestra rotunda in mammals. In *Functional Morphology in Vertebrates,* H.-R. Duncker and G. Fleischer, eds., Fortschritte der Zoologie 30. Stuttgart: Fischer Verlag, pp. 153–157.

―――. 1985b. Die Ontogenese und Morphologie der fenestra rotunda und des Aquaeductus cochlea von *Tupaia* und anderen Säugern. Morphologisches Jahrbuch 131: 179–204.

―――. 1987. Morphogenesis of the mammalian skull with special reference to *Tupaia.* In *Morphogenesis of the Mammalian Skull,* H.-J. Kuhn and U. Zeller, eds., Mammalia Depicta, Heft 13: 17–50. Hamburg: Verlag Paul Parey.

LIST OF CONTRIBUTORS

William A. Beresford
Department of Anatomy
School of Medicine
West Virginia University
Morgantown, West Virginia 26506
U.S.A.

Carl Gans
Department of Biology
University of Michigan
Ann Arbor, Michigan 48109–1048
U.S.A.

Brian K. Hall
Department of Biology
Dalhousie University
Halifax, Nova Scotia B3H 4J1
Canada

James Hanken
Department of Environmental, Population, and Organismic Biology
University of Colorado
Boulder, Colorado 80309–0334
U.S.A.

Philippe Janvier
Institut de Paléontologie
Muséum National d'Histoire Naturelle
8, rue Buffon
75005 Paris
France

Michael J. Novacek
Department of Vertebrate Paleontology
American Museum of Natural History
Central Park West at 79th Street
New York, New York 10024-5192
U.S.A.

Olivier Rieppel
Department of Geology
Field Museum of Natural History
Roosevelt Road at Lake Shore Drive
Chicago, Illinois 60605–2496
U.S.A.

Hans-Peter Schultze
Museum of Natural History and
Department of Systematics and Ecology
University of Kansas
Lawrence, Kansas 66045–2454
U.S.A.

Keith Stewart Thomson
Academy of Natural Sciences
1900 Benjamin Franklin Parkway
Philadelphia, Pennsylvania 19103–1195
U.S.A.

Linda Trueb
Museum of Natural History and
Department of Systematics and Ecology
University of Kansas
Lawrence, Kansas 66045–2454
U.S.A.

Richard L. Zusi
Department of Vertebrate Zoology
National Museum of Natural History
Smithsonian Institution
Washington, D.C. 20506
U.S.A.

INDEX

Acanthodactylus boskianus, neurocranium of, fig. 7.4

Acanthodes
cranial morphology, 215–217, figs. 5.4, 5.5, 5.6, 5.7, 5.8
development, 217

Acanthodii, monophyly and phylogenetic relationships of, 215–216

Acanthopsis choirorhynchus, mucoid chondroid in, table 3.6

Acontias, sound-transmitting apparatus of, 356

Acontophiops, sound-transmitting apparatus of, 356

Actinopterygii, monophyly and phylogenetic relationships of, 221–222

Actitis macularia, cranial morphology and kinesis in, figs. 8.14, 8.16

Adapis, phylogenetic relationships of, 441

Adventitious cartilage. *See* Cartilage, secondary

Aegolius
adductor mandibulae externus muscle, 417
cranial morphology and asymmetry, 416–417, figs. 8.11, 8.12

Albanerpeton, phylogenetic relationships of, 257

Allometry
in birds, 410–411
in crossopterygians, 242
in mammals, 465
in teleosts, 224

Alouatta, naso-palatine duct of, 447

Ambystoma
adaptive zone, 287
cranial morphology, 288, 297, figs. 6.11–6.12
hyoid apparatus, tongue, and feeding behavior, 306–307, fig. 6.13

Amia calva
development, fig. 5.11
dentine in, 109

Amphibamus, phylogenetic relationships of, 257

Amphioxides, as vertebrate ancestor, 4

Amphioxus. See *Branchiostoma*

Amphisbaena
cranial morphology, fig. 7.5
sound-transmitting apparatus, 357

Amphistyly, in elasmobranchs, 208

Amphitherium
auditory region, 513
phylogenetic relationships, 440

Amphiuma
cranial morphology, 297, 300
plectral apparatus, 289

Anaspida, cranial morphology of, 159–161

Andrias
adaptive zone, 287
jaw and hyoid movements during prey capture, 307

Aneides, hyoid apparatus of, fig. 6.13

Anelytropsis
effects of miniaturization, 373
secondary palate, 370

Anniella
  effects of miniaturization, 373
  sound-transmitting apparatus, 356–
    357
Anser albifrons, palate of, fig. 8.4
Aparasphenodon, cranial morphology
  of, 322
Apateon
  cranial morphology, fig. 6.2
  dentition, 333
  phylogenetic relationships, 256–
    257, fig. 6.1
Aplonis metallica, cranial morphology
  of, fig. 8.14
Apteryx australis, cranial morphology
  of, fig. 8.3
Ara macao, cranial morphology of,
  fig. 8.8
Araeoscelis gracilis, temporal fenestration of dermatocranium in, 364–
    365, fig. 7.7
Aramus quarauna, cranial kinesis in,
  fig. 8.16
Arandaspis
  cranial morphology, 153–154
  fossil record, 152
Arapaima, exoskeleton of, 223
Archaeopteryx lithographica, cranial
  morphology and kinesis in, 399,
  403–404, fig. 8.5
Arenaria interpres, cranial morphology of, 424, fig. 8.14
Ascaphus, cranial morphology and
  hypo-ossification in, 313, 326,
  332, figs. 6.18–6.19
Asio otus
  adductor mandibulae externus
    muscle, 417
  cranial morphology, figs. 8.8, 8.11,
    8.12
Asioryctes
  auditory bulla, 497
  basicranial arterial circulation, 505
  phylogenetic relationships, 442
Askeptosaurus, temporal fenestration
  of dermatocranium in, 364

Aspidin, in fossil jawless craniates,
  154, 159, fig. 4.21
Astatotilapia elegans
  types of bone, 101, figs. 3.9, 3.18
  joints between cartilages, fig. 3.10
Astraspis
  cranial morphology, 153
  fossil record, 152
  reconstruction, fig. 4.8
Asymmetry
  in birds, 416–417
  in flatfishes, 224
Athene
  adductor mandibulae externus
    muscle, 417
  cranial morphology, figs. 8.11, 8.12
Auditory bulla, in mammals, 496–
  504
Auditory ossicles, in mammals, 474–
  476, 510–522. *See also* Otic region, Plectral apparatus
Axocranium. *See* Braincase, in
  hagfishes

Balaeniceps, basipterygoid process in,
  402
Balaenoptera physalus, dentine in,
  109
Bandringa, rostral process in, 208
Barbourula, cranial morphology of,
  321, figs. 6.18–6.19
Basicranial arterial circulation, in
  mammals, 471, 504–510, 519,
  522
Basicranial series, in hagfishes, 135–
  136
Batrachuperus
  adaptive zone, 287
  cranial morphology, 301–303, fig.
    6.2
  feeding behavior, 307
Bdellostoma. See *Eptatretus*
Belonaspis, cranial morphology of,
  fig. 4.15
Benneviaspis, cranial morphology of,
  fig. 4.15

Bienotherium
  otic region, 513–514
  phylogenetic relationships, 440
Bipes, sound-transmitting apparatus
  in, 357
Bolitoglossa subpalmata, cranial development in, 308
Bombina, skull and hyobranchial
  morphology in, 322, 329, fig. 6.20
Bone
  endosteum, 106
  evolutionary origin, 7–8, 10–11,
    14, 17
  histology and types, 75–81, 100, 345
  marrow, 106
  periosteum, 102–103
  vasculature, 106
  See also Aspidin, Ossification, Os-
    teoblasts, Osteoclasts
Boreaspis, cranial morphology of, fig.
  4.13
Bos, cranila morphology of, 472, 485,
  fig. 9.17
Botia horae, fibrohyaline-cell cartilage
  in, fig. 3.13
Brachycephalus, hyperossification in,
  322, 332
Brachyerix, auditory bulla in, fig. 9.24
Bradypus, cranial morphology of,
  447, 456, figs. 9.14, 9.33
Braincase
  in hagfishes, 135
  in lampreys, 143
  in mammals, 456–457, 483–490,
    table 9.1
*Branchial skeleton. See Viscero-
  cranium*
Branchiosaurus, phylogenetic relationships of, 256, fig. 6.1
Branchiostoma, as vertebrate ancestor, 4–6, 9–10, 12–15, 17, 23,
  25–26
Brookesia, effects of miniaturization,
  357
Bubo virginianus, cranial morphology
  of, figs. 8.11, 8.12

Bufo
  cranial morphology and hyperossifi-
    cation, 309, 332
  hyobranchial skeleton, fig. 6.20

Cacatua, skull and jaw muscles of,
  421, fig. 8.13
Cactospiza. See Camarhynchus
Caecilia albiventris, cranial morphology of, figs. 6.6–6.7
Calcification
  in Devonian fishes, 242–243
  origin of, in vertebrates, 14, 18,
    113–114
  See also Cartilage, calcified
Calidris alpina, cranial kinesis in, fig.
  8.16
Camarhynchus, cranial morphology
  of, 413, figs. 8.9, 8.10
Canis
  cranial morphology, 447, 472, figs.
    9.1, 9.17
  masticatory musculature, fig. 9.38
Capreolus capreolus, masticatory
  musculature in, fig. 9.38
Caprimulgus, cranial kinesis in, 406
Caretta caretta
  secondary cartilage, 86
  secondary palate, fig. 7.9
Carotid artery. *See* Basicranial arterial
  circulation
Cartilage
  calcified, 98–100, 143, 153, 203,
    243
  histology and types of, 81–87
  origin of, in vertebrates, 10–11
  perichondrium, 103
  secondary, 83–86, 93–97, 372,
    378, 503, 524–528
  See also Chondroblasts, Mucocarti-
    lage, Skeletal tissues, chordoid
    and chondroid
Casea, phylogenetic relationships of,
  440
Caspiomyzon, phylogenetic relationships of, 141

Casquing, of anuran skull, 322–323, 326–327, 332–333
Caudiverbera, cranial morphology and hyperossification in, 332
Cavia
    masticatory musculature, fig. 9.37
    phylogenetic relationships, 441
Cavum epiptericum. See Braincase, in mammals
Cementum, histology of, 75–76
Cephalaspidomorphi, monophyly of, 178–179
Ceratobatrachus, cranial morphology of, 327
Ceratophrys, cranial morphology and hyperossification in, 322, 328, 332
Certhidea olivacea, cranial morphology of, 413, figs. 8.9, 8.10
Chamaeleo, effects of miniaturization in, 357
Cheirolepis, exocranium and dentition in, 221–222
Chelonia mydas
    cranial morphology, figs. 7.6, 7.9
    sound-transmitting apparatus, 357
Chelydra, cranial morphology of, 354, 362, fig. 7.9
Chioglossa, hyoid apparatus of, 308
Chionis alba, cranial kinesis in, fig. 8.16
Chirodipterus australis, cranial morphology of, figs. 5.3, 5.4, 5.5, 5.7
Choloepus, cranial morphology of, fig. 9.15
Chondrichthyes
    classification, table 5.2
    monophyly and phylogenetic relationships, 203–205
Chondroblasts, and evolutionary origin of the skull, 111
Chondrocranium
    development in mammals, 444, 456
    in birds, 395
    See also Endocranium, Neurocranium, Viscerocranium
Chrysemys concinna, cranial morphology of, fig. 7.6

Chrysochloris, tympanic cavity in, 470
Ciconia, basipterygoid process in, 402
Cirrhitus rivulatus, lipid in skull of, 108
Cladodus, cranial morphology of, 205
Clarazia, temporal fenestration of dermatocranium in, 364
Clevosaurus, temporal fenestration of dermatocranium in, 364
Cobitis taenia, chondroid cartilage in, table 3.5
Coelurosaurus, temporal fenestration of dermatocranium in, 364
Collagen, types of, 72–73
Compsognathus longipes, cranial morphology of, fig. 8.5
Conodonts, and vertebrate origins, 25–29
Co-ossification, of anuran skull, 323
Corvus corax, palate of, fig. 8.4
Coryodorus paleatus, chondroid cartilage in, table 3.5
Corythomantis, cranial morphology and hyperossification in, 322, 326
Cosmine, in sarcopterygians, 230
Cottus gobio, chondroid cartilage in, table 3.5
Craniomandibular joint, in mammals, 522–524
Crax mitu, cranial morphology of, fig. 8.3
Crocodylus porosus, neurocranium of, fig. 7.4
Crossopterygii, monophyly and phylogenetic relationships of, 237–238
Crotaphatrema, cranial morphology of, 283–284, figs. 6.6–6.7
Cryptobranchus
    skull and hyobranchial morphology, 289, 300, 303, figs. 6.11–6.12, 6.13
    jaw and hyoid movements during prey capture, 307
Ctenosaura, cartilage development in, 372
Culmacanthus, exocranium in, 214

Cyanocitta stelleri, holorhinal nares in, fig. 8.15

Cyanorhamphus, skull and jaw muscles of, 421–422, fig. 8.13

Cylindrophis rufus, jaw suspension of, 376, fig. 7.14

Cynocephalus
cranial morphology, 456, fig. 9.6
secondary cartilage, 525

Cynognathus
cranial morphology, 515, 522, fig. 9.1
phylogenetic relationships, 440

Cyprinus carpio, chondroid cartilage in, table 3.5

Dacelo novaeguinea, palate of, fig. 8.4

Dasypus
cranial morphology, 456, table 9.2
dentine in, 109

Dentine
evolutionary origin, 7, 10, 17, 28, 69, 113
histology, 75–76
in extant species, 108–109
in thelodonts, 175

Dentition
in hagfishes, 138
in lampreys, 145
in lissamphibians, 267, 280, 304, 329
See also Cementum, Dentine, Enamel, Enameloid

Dermatocranium
and head segmentation, 36–68
in birds, 394–402
in gnathostomes, 49–59
in mammals, 448–454
in reptiles, 358–365, 377–378
See also Exocranium, Exoskeleton

Dermophis mexicanus, cranial morphology of, 278, figs. 6.6–6.7

Development
in acanthodians, 217
in actinopterygians, 227–230
in chondrichthyans, 209–213
in crossopterygians, 242

in dipnoans, 236–237
in placoderms, 203

Desmognathus quadramaculatus, cranial morphology of, figs. 6.11–6.12

Diabolepis, cranial morphology of, 231–232, 234–235, 237–238

Diademodon, phylogenetic relationships of, 440

Diarthrognathus
craniomandibular joint and masticatory apparatus, 522
phylogenetic relationships, 440

Dibamus
effects of miniaturization, 373–376, fig. 7.13
secondary palate, 370, fig. 7.11
sound-transmitting apparatus, 356

Dicamptodon
adaptive zone, 287
skull and hyobranchial morphology, 285, 297, 304, 306–307, table 6.2A
phylogenetic relationships, fig. 6.9

Dicksonosteus arcticus, cranial morphology of, figs. 5.3, 5.4, 5.7

Didelphis
masticatory musculature, fig. 9.37
phylogenetic relationships, 441
cranial morphology, 447, 504, figs. 9.6, 9.9, 9.15, 9.22, 9.25, 9.28

Didunculus
cranial kinesis, fig. 8.16
skull and jaw muscles, 422

Digestion, and vertebrate origins, 8–9, 15

Dikenaspis, cranial morphology of, fig. 4.10

Dimetrodon
cranial morphology, figs. 9.1, 9.31
phylogenetic relationships, 440

Diphydontosaurus, temporal fenestration of dermatocranium in, 364

Diplacanthus, exocranium in, 214

Dipnoi, monophyly and phylogenetic relationships of, 233–234

Dipnorhynchus, cranial morphology of, 220, 231, 234

Discoglossus, cranial morphology of, 321
Dobsonia, cranial morphology of, fig. 9.6
Doleserpeton, phylogenetic relationships of, 257
Dolichonyx oryzivorus, cranial morphology of, fig. 8.14
Doryaspis, dermal head armor in, 158, fig. 4.11
Dromaeosaurus albertensis, palate of, 403, fig. 8.4
Dromaius novaehollandiae, palate of, fig. 8.4
Duyunolepis, cranial morphology of, fig. 41.7

Ear. *See* Auditory bulla, Auditory ossicles, Otic region, Plectral apparatus
Echeneis naucates, perichondrium in, 104
Echinosorex, orbital region in, fig. 9.22
Echinotriton andersoni, cranial morphology of, 302
Eclectus roratus, skull and jaw muscles of, 421, fig. 8.13
Ectotympanic, in mammals, 476–477
Edaphosaurus, phylogenetic relationships of, 440
Edops, dermatocranium of, fig. 2.8
Eglonaspis, cranial morphology of, 159, figs. 4.9, 4.11
Electroreception, and vertebrate origins, 6–7, 17–18, 112–113
Elephas, cranial morphology of, fig. 9.9
Elpistostege, dermatocranium of, 53
Emargination, of dermatocranium, in reptiles, 361–362, 378
Empedaspis, cranial morphology of, fig. 4.9
Emydura, orbitotemporal ossifications in, 351
Emys orbicularis, neurocranium of, fig. 7.4

Enamel
evolutionary origin, 17, 28
in sarcopterygians, 221, 230
Enameloid, evolutionary origin of, 7, 14, 28
Endeiolepis, phylogenetic relationships of, 159
Endocranium
of acanthodians, 216
of actinopterygians, 224–225
of anaspids, 159
of anurans, 312–322, 327–329
of gymnophionans, 269–274, 278–280
of chondrichthyans, 205–208
of crossopterygians, 239–241
of dipnoans, 235
of gnathostomes, 191
of lissamphibians, 260–263, 265–266
of osteichthyans, 219–221
of placoderms, 199
of sarcopterygians, 231–232
of teleostomes, 214
of urodeles, 288–297, 302–304
Eocaptorhinus
cranial morphology, 365, figs. 7.7, 7.11
sound-transmitting apparatus, 356
Eopneumatosuchus, basicranium of, 350
Epicrionops
skull and hyobranchial morphology, 281, figs. 6.2, 6.5, 6.8
microhabitat, 268
Eptatretus
cranial morphology, 135, 140, fig. 4.2
ontogeny, 140
Equus, paranasal sinuses in, fig. 9.18
Erinaceus, cranial morphology of, 456, figs. 9.14, 9.25
Eriptychius
calcified cartilage, 153
fossil record, 152
Erpetoichthys, phylogenetic relationships of, 221

Erquelinnesia gosseletti, secondary palate in, fig. 7.9

Errivaspis waynensis, cranial morphology of, 154, fig. 4.9

Eryx, orbitotemporal ossifications in, 353

Ethmoidal region, in mammals, 442–455

Eudontomyzon, phylogenetic relationships of, 141

Eudyptes pachyrhynchus, cranial morphology of, fig. 8.3

Eugaleaspis, cranial morphology of, 173, fig. 4.18

Euphanerops, skull and phylogenetic relationships of, 159, 161, fig. 4.12

Eurycea, cranial morphology of, 301, 304

Eusthenopteron
cranial morphology, 50, 52–53, 57, 59, 236, 241, figs. 2.7, 2.8, 5.3, 5.4, 5.5, 5.6, 5.7, 5.8, 5.10
development, 242

Evolution, convergent, of bird skull, 422–426

Evolutionary rate, in coelocanths, 239

Exaeretodon, phylogenetic relationships of, 440

Excretion, and vertebrate origins, 8–9, 14–15

Exocranium
in acanthodians, 216
in actinopterygians, 222–224
in chondrichthyans, 205
in crossopterygians, 238–239
in dipnoans, 234–235
in gnathostomes, 191–195
in lissamphibians, 263–266, 274–280, 297–304, 322–329
in osteichthyans, 218–219
in placoderms, 196–199
in sarcopterygians, 231
in teleostomes, 214
See also Dermatocranium, Exoskeleton

Exoskeleton
in jawless craniates, 152–175, fig. 4.21
See also Dermatocranium, Exocranium

Exostosis, of anuran skull, 323, 333

Felis, cranial morphology of, 444, 472, fig. 9.7

Fenestration, of dermatocranium, in reptiles, 361–362, 373–375, 378

Function, role of, in dermal bone patterning, 60–62

Gabreyaspis, cranial morphology of, fig. 4.9

Galago, auditory ossicles and ectotympanic in, fig. 9.33

Galeaspida, cranial morphology of, 169–173

Gallinago, skull and jaw muscles of, 424

Gallus, cranial development in, 395

Ganoine, in actinopterygians, 221, 230

Gas exchange, and vertebrate origins, 5, 13

Gasterosteus aculeatus, atypical cartilage in, table 3.5

Gastrotheca
cranial morphology, 313
dentition, 329

Gavialis, secondary palate in, fig. 7.10

Gegeneophis carnosus, microhabitat of, 268

Gelochelidon nilotica, cranial morphology of, fig. 8.1

Geomyda mouhotii, cranial morphology of, fig. 7.6

Geospiza
allometry, 410–411
cranial morphology, 413, figs. 8.9, 8.10

Geotria, phylogenetic relationships of, 141

Geotrypetes seraphini, cranial morphology of, figs. 6.6–6.7

Gephyrosaurus, temporal fenestration of dermatocranium in, 364, fig. 7.8

Gilpichthys greeni, phylogenetic relationships and reconstruction of, 141, fig. 4.3

Gnathonemus petersi, mucoid chondroid in, table 3.6

Grandisonia alternans, cranial morphology of, figs. 6.6–6.7

Griphognathus whitei, viscerocranium of, 236, fig. 5.8

Grus canadensis, cranial morphology of, fig. 8.3

Gustavaspis, cranial morphology of, 168, fig. 4.16

Gymnophis, hyobranchial skeleton of, fig. 6.8

Gyrinocheilus aymonieri, elastic hyaline-cell cartilage in, fig. 3.14, table 3.6

Hagfishes
and vertebrate origins, 25–26
cranial morphology, 135–141
ontogeny, 140

Hanyangaspis, cranial morphology of, 172, 175, fig. 4.18

Hapalemur griseus, calcified cartilage in, 99

Hardistiella
cranial morphology, 149–150, fig. 4.7
phylogenetic relationships, 141

Head, evolution of the, in vertebrates, 1–2, 12

Heleioporus albopunctatus, hyobranchial skeleton of, fig. 6.20

Heloderma, loss of upper temporal arcade in, 373

Hemichromis bimaculatus, chondroid bone in, 101

Hemiphractus
cranial morphology, 309, 322, 327, 332, figs. 6.18–6.19
dentition, 329

Hemitheconyx caudicinctus, palate in, fig. 7.11

Hescheleria, temporal fenestration of dermatocranium in, 364

Hesperornis, cranial morphology and kinesis in, 399, 404

Heterochrony, in reptiles, 367, 373–378. *See also* Hypermorphosis, Neoteny, Paedogenesis, Paedomorphosis

Heterolocha, skull and jaw muscles of, 424

Heterostraci, cranial morphology of, 154–159

Hirella, cranial morphology of, fig. 4.13

Hoelaspis, cranial morphology of, 169, fig. 4.16

Holonema westolli, cranial morphology of, fig. 5.6

Holoptychius, dermatocranium of, 50, 59, fig. 2.7

Holorhiny, of avian skull, 424–425

Holostyly, in holocephalans, 208

Homeobox genes, 24

Homo, cranial morphology of, 456, 472

Homology
criteria for evaluating, 37–40, 48–60, 151–152, 527–529
of skull in agnathans and gnathostomes, 176–178, 190
of skull in birds, 402–403
of skull in Recent jawless craniates, 150–152

Howittacanthus kentoni, development of, 217

Hupehsuchus, temporal fenestration of dermatocranium in, 365

Hybodus, cranial morphology of, 209, figs. 5.6, 5.8

Hylonomus, sound-transmitting apparatus of, 356

Hymenochirus, skull and hyobranchial morphology of, 326, 329, 331

Hynobius
metapterygoid, 303
phylogenetic relationships, fig. 6.9

Hyobranchial apparatus, of lissam-
  phibians, 267, 280–281, 304–
  308, 329–331
Hyostyly, in elasmobranchs, 208
Hypermorphosis, in miniaturized liz-
  ards and *Sphenodon*, 373–374,
  376. *See also* Hyperossification
Hyperoartia. *See* Lampreys
Hyperossification, in anurans, 322–
  323, 327–328, 332–333
Hyperotreti. *See* Hagfishes
Hypogeophis, jaw morphology in,
  278
Hypo-ossification, in anurans, 322,
  332
Hypostomus, Zellknorpel in, fig. 3.16
Hypotic arch complex, in hagfishes,
  136

Icarosaurus, temporal fenestration of
  dermatocranium in, 364
Ichthyomyzon
  cranial morphology, 150
  phylogenetic relationships, 141
Ichthyophis glutinosus
  microhabitat, 268, 282
  skull and hyobranchial morphology,
    260–261, figs. 6.4, 6.8
Ichthyostega, 55, 57
Icterus, skull and jaw muscles of, 424
Indri, orbital region in, fig. 9.22

Jamoytius
  cranial morphology, 159, 161, fig.
    4.12
  phylogenetic relationships, 159
Jaws, origin of, 176–178, 190
Jordanella floridae, Zellknorpel in, fig.
  3.17

Kadimakara, temporal fenestration of
  dermatocranium in, 363
Kansasiella eatoni, cranial morphology of, fig. 5.4
Karaurus, phylogenetic relationships
  of, 257, figs. 6.1, 6.9

Kennalestes
  auditory region, 497, 505
  phylogenetic relationships, 442
Kinesis, cranial
  in birds, 403–408, 419, 425–427
  in caecilians, 282–285
  in reptiles, 346, 370–373, 375–
    376
Klinorhynchy, in mammals, 444
Kuehneosaurus, temporal fenestration
  of dermatocranium in, 364
Kuhneotherium
  auditory ossicles, 519
  phylogenetic relationships, 440
Kujdanowiaspis, cranial morphology
  of, fig. 5.5

Labeo bicolor, hyaline-cell cartilage
  in, fig. 3.12
Lacerta, cranial morphology and development in, 354–355, 372, 378
Lampetra
  cranial morphology, 141, figs. 4.4,
    4.5, 4.6
  phylogenetic relationships, 141
Lampreys
  and vertebrate origins, 26
  cranial morphology, 141–150
  ontogeny, 146–149
Lanthanotus, loss of upper temporal
  arcade in, 373
Larus argentatus, cranial kinesis in,
  fig. 8.7
Lateral line system, relation to dermatocranium, 53, 59, 63, 231, 234–
  235
Laterosphenoid, in reptiles, 353
Latimeria
  cranial morphology, 219–220, 239,
    241
  development, 242
Leiopelma, skull and hyobranchial
  morphology of, 313, 329, figs. 6.2,
  6.20
Lemur
  calcified cartilage, 99
  cranial morphology, figs. 9.22, 9.24

Lepidobatrachus, cranial morphology of, 328

Lepidosiren, cranial morphology of, 220, 234–235

Lepisosteus, exoskeleton of, 223

Leptictis
cranial morphology, 476, figs. 9.5, 9.8, 9.10, 9.11, 9.22
phylogenetic relationships, 441–442

Leptodactylus ocellatus, hyobranchial skeleton of, fig. 6.20

Leptorophus, phylogenetic relationships of, 256, fig. 6.1

Lepus, phylogenetic relationships of, 440

Lialis, cranial kinesis in, 375

Limnodromus
cranial kinesis, fig. 8.16
skull and jaw muscles, 424

Limnogale, auditory bulla of, fig. 9.24

Lingual skeleton, in cyclostomes, 134, 137, 145, 151

Liua shihi, cranial morphology of, 301

Locomotion, and vertebrate origins, 6

Longanellia scotica, reconstruction of, fig. 4.20

Lophius, skeletal histology in, 107, table 3.5

Lorius lory, skull and jaw muscles of, 421, fig. 8.13

Loxodonta, nasal cavities in, fig. 9.17

Lungmenshanaspis, cranial morphology of, 173, fig. 4.18

Macrocnemus, temporal fenestration of dermatocranium in, 363

Macroderma, cranial morphology of, fig. 9.6

Malerisaurus, temporal fenestration of dermatocranium in, 363

Manatis, auditory ossicles and ectotympanic in, fig. 9.33

Manis
cranial morphology, figs. 9.14, 9.22, 9.33
phylogenetic relationships, 441

Marmota, orbital region in, fig. 9.22

Masticatory apparatus, in mammals, 522–524

Mayomyzon
cranial morphology, 141, 149, fig. 4.7
phylogenetic relationships, 141

Megalobatrachus, adaptive zone of, 287

Mesodentine, in cephalaspid agnathans, 230

Metachirops. See *Philander*

Metamerism. *See* Segmentation

Metamorphosis
and vertebrate origins, 5
in lampreys, 149

Microcaecilia, microhabitat of, 268

Microsyops, phylogenetic relationships of, 442

Miguashaia, cranial morphology of, 231, 241

Mimia toombis, cranial morphology of, figs. 5.5, 5.6, 5.7, 5.8

Mineralization. *See* Calcification

Miniaturization
and evolution of snakes, 376
in anurans, 332–333
in lizards, 357, 373–375

Misgurnus, chondroid cartilage in, table 3.5

Moeritherium
cranial morphology, fig. 9.9
phylogenetic relationships, 442

Monodelphis, cranial morphology of, 483, 504, 512, figs. 9.4, 9.24

Monopeltis, secondary palate in, 370

Mordacia, phylogenetic relationships of, 141

Morganucodon
cranial morphology, 512, 517, 524, figs. 9.31, 9.32
phylogenetic relationships, 440

Mormyrops, exoskeleton of, 223

Morphogenesis, of dermal skeleton, 59

Morulius chrysophekadion, chondroid in, table 3.6

Moythomasia, cranial morphology of, 60, figs. 5.3, 5.10

Mucocartilage, in lampreys, 146–149, 168

Mus, phylogenetic relationships of, 441

Musculature, cranial
embryonic derivation of, 2–3, 16, 20, 45
in birds, 413–424, 427
in mammals, 522–524
in reptiles, 361–363, 371, 375

Myliobatis aquila, calcified cartilage in, 100

Myodomes, in osteichthyans, 220, 225, 232

Myotis
cranial morphology, 444, fig. 9.30
phylogenetic relationships, 440

Myrmecophaga, auditory ossicles and ectotympanic in, fig. 9.33

Myxine
chordoid cartilage, table 3.5
cranial morphology, 135, 140, figs. 4.2, 4.3
ontogeny, 140

Myxinikela siroka, cranial morphology of, 135, 140–141, fig. 4.3

Nandinia, auditory bulla of, 503, table 9.2, fig. 9.27

Nasal
basket, in hagfishes, 135
cartilages, in mammals, 444
septum, in mammals, 454
turbinals, in mammals, 448, 454–455, 477–483

Naso-hypophysial complex, of primitive craniates, 178–179

Natrix natrix, neurocranium of, figs. 7.4, 7.5

Necturus
dentition, 304
skull and plectral apparatus, 289, fig. 6.11–6.12

Neeyambaspis, phylogenetic relationships of, 173

Neoceratodus, cranial morphology and development of, 220, 234–236, fig. 5.6

Neomorph. *See* Novelty

Neomyxine, cranial morphology of, 135

Neopalatine, in neobatrachian anurans, 322

Neophema, skull and jaw muscles of, 422

Neoteny, in salamanders, 287, 289, 304

Neotis cafra, palate of, fig. 8.4

Nerodia rhombifera, cranial morphology of, fig. 7.5

Nerves, cranial
and head segmentation, 22–23, 45
foramina in actinopterygians, 214, 224–225, 240–241
foramina in birds, 399
foramina in mammals, 457–460, 471, 483, 490
in osteostracans, 165–167
See also Placodes, neurogenic

Neural crest
and the origin of vertebrates, 1–2, 5–7, 11, 14–18, 21
contribution to the vertebrate head, 13–18, 21, 24, 37, 41, 44–48, 148, 512

Neurocranium
and head segmentation, 41–42, 55–59
in birds, 394–402
in reptiles, 345–354
neural crest derivation, 42, 46–48
See also Braincase, Endocranium

Norselaspis, cranial morphology of, figs. 4.14, 4.15

Notabatrachus, phylogenetic relationships of, 310

Notaden, cranial morphology of, 328

Notharctus
cranial morphology, fig. 9.6
phylogenetic relationships, 441

Notochord, and evolution of the head, 9

Notophthalmus, skull and hyobranchial apparatus of, 297, 300, 306,
figs. 6.11–6.12
Notopterus, exoskeleton of, 223
Notoryctes
  auditory ossicles and ectotympanic,
  fig. 9.33
  phylogenetic relationships, 441
Novelty
  and origin of jaws, 178
  in bird skull, 418
  in lamprey skull, 143
  in lissamphibian skull, 322–323,
  333
  in mammal skull, 447, 468, 476
Nyctibius, cranial kinesis in, 406, fig.
  8.7

Occipital region, in mammals, 471–
  474
Okkelbergia, phylogenetic relationships of, 141
Onychodactylus japonicus, cranial
  morphology of, 302–303
Ophiacodon, phylogenetic relationships of, 440
Orbitotemporal region, in mammals,
  455–464, 490–495
Ornamentation, cranial, in birds, 410
Ornithoprion, mandibular rostrum of,
  208
Ornithorhynchus
  cranial morphology, 448, 454, 468,
  477, 483, 485, 489, figs. 9.20,
  9.33
  basicranial arterial circulation, 508,
  fig. 9.28
  phylogenetic relationships, 441
Orthagoriscus mola, bone marrow in,
  107
Orthosuchus, secondary palate in, fig.
  7.10
Orycteropus
  cranial morphology, figs. 9.15,
  9.22, 9.33
  phylogenetic relationships, 441

Oryctolagus, cranial morphology of,
  447, 456, fig. 9.33
Ossification
  and vertebrate origins, 8
  of anuran skull, 332–333
  of bird skull, 395–403
  of reptile skull, 345–360
  See also Hyperossification, Hypo-
    ossification, Osteoblasts,
    Osteoclasts
Osteichthyes, monophyly and phylogenetic relationships of, 217–218
Osteoblasts, and evolutionary origin
  of the skull, 110
Osteocephalus, cranial morphology
  of, 327
Osteoclasts, and evolutionary origin
  of the skull, 111
Osteostraci, cranial morphology of,
  161–169
Otic region, in mammals, 464–471
Ovis, braincase in, 485

Pachypleurosaurus edwardsi, dermatocranium of, fig. 7.7
Paedogenesis, and evolutionary origin
  of the skull, 12
Paedomorphosis
  and evolution of snakes, 375
  in anurans, 332–333
  in mammals, 503
  in lizards, 373–375
Palaeoherpeton, 57, fig. 2.8
Palaeopleurosaurus, temporal fenestration of dermatocranium in,
  364
Palaeospondylus, phylogenetic relationships of, 132
Palate
  in birds, 403, 411–412
  See also Secondary palate
Paleothyrus, sound-transmitting apparatus of, 356
Pan, absence of lamina transversalis
  posterior in, 448
Panderichthys, 53, 57, fig. 2.8

Paramyxine, cranial morphology of, 135

Paranasal sinuses, in mammals, 477–483

Pars canalicularis, in mammals, 468

Pelobates
atypical cartilage, table 3.5
cranial morphology, 322, figs. 6.18–6.19

Pelodytes, cranial morphology of, 321

Periophthalmus, mucoid chondroid in, table 3.6

Petaurus
auditory ossicles and ectotympanic in, fig. 9.33
phylogenetic relationships, 441

Petrolacosaurus, dermatocranium of, 362, 364, fig. 7.7

Petromyzon
cranial morphology, 141
phylogenetic relationships of, 141

Pharyngolepis, cranial morphology of, 159, fig. 4.12

Philander, auditory ossicles and ectotympanic in, fig. 9.33

Philomachus pugnax, cranial kinesis in, fig. 8.16

Phlebolepis, reconstruction and scale of, fig. 4.20

Phocoena, auditory ossicles and ectotympanic in, fig. 9.33

Phoeniculus, skull and jaw muscles of, 424

Phylogeny, of craniates, 133–135

Pionites leucogaster, skull and jaw muscles of, 421, fig. 8.13

Pipa
dentition, 329
skull and hyobranchial skeleton, 326, 331, figs. 6.18–6.19

Pipiscius
cranial morphology, 141, 150
phylogenetic relationships, 141, 150

Pituriaspida, cranial morphology of, 173–174

Pituriaspis, cranial morphology of, 173, fig. 4.19

Placodermi
classification, table 5.1
monophyly and phylogenetic relationships, 195–196

Placodes, neurogenic, 1–2, 11–12, 18

Planocephalosaurus, temporal fenestration of dermatocranium in, 364

Platycercus, skull and jaw muscles of, 422

Platyspiza. See *Camarhynchus*

Plectral apparatus, of lissamphibians, 262, 289, 315, 320

Plesiadapis
orbital region, 491
phylogenetic relationships, 442

Plesiochelys, orbitotemporal ossifications in, 351

Plesiolestes, phylogenetic relationships of, 442

Plethodon, cranial morphology of, 308, figs. 6.11–6.12

Pleurosaurus, temporal fenestration of dermatocranium in, 364

Plourdosteus canadensis, calcified cartilage in, 99

Pluvialis squatarola, schizorhinal nares in, fig. 8.15

Pneumatization, of bird skull, 408

Podarcis sicula, cranial development in, 372, 375

Podargus strigioides, cranial kinesis in, fig. 8.7

Poecilia sphenops, hyaline-cell chondroid in, 93, table 3.6

Polybranchiaspis liaojaoshanensis, cranial morphology of, fig. 4.17

Polypterus
exocranium, 223
phylogenetic relationships, 221

Poraspis, cranial morphology of, fig. 4.10

Pore-canal system, 230, 234

Powichthys, cranial morphology of, 231, 237–240

Predation, and vertebrate origins, 6, 10

Probainognathus, lower jaw of, fig. 9.31

Probosciger, skull and jaw muscles of, 421

Procavia, cranial morphology of, figs. 9.9, 9.15

Procolophon, tropibasic skull in, 375–376

Procynosuchus
  craniomandibular joint and masticatory apparatus in, 522, 524
  phylogenetic relationships, 440

Proganochelys, cranial morphology and kinesis in, 361, 372, fig. 7.9

Prolacerta, temporal fenestration of dermatocranium in, 363, 373

Propithecus verreauxi, calcified cartilage in, 99

*Proteus anguinus,*hyoid apparatus of, 306, fig. 6.13

Protopterus, exocranium of, 234–235

Protorosaurus, temporal fenestration of dermatocranium in, 363

Protosuchus, secondary palate of, 367

Psephotus, skull and jaw muscles in, 422

Pseudacris clarkii, hypo-ossification in, 322

Pseudemys. See *Chrysemys*

Pseudhymenochirus, cranial morphology of, 326, 329

Pseudogastromyzon myersi, lipohyaline-cell cartilage in, fig. 3.15

Pseudotriton, cranial morphology of, 303

Pseudotyphlops philippinus, effects of miniaturization in, fig. 7.13

Psittacula, skull and jaw muscles in, 421

Pteraspis. See *Errivaspis*

Pternohyla, cranial morphology of, 323

Pteropus, tympanic region of, fig. 9.13

Pterygolepsis, cranial morphology of, 159

Ptilocercus, auditory bulla of, table 9.2

Pycnosteus, dermal head armor in, 158, fig. 4.11

Pyrinestes, instraspecific variation in, 416

Python sebae, cranial morphology and kinesis in, 376, figs. 7.11, 7.14

Pyxicephalus, hyperossification in, 332

Quebecius, development of, 242

Ramphastos toco, cranial morphology of, fig. 8.3

Rana esculenta, cranial morphology of, fig. 6.17

Rattus, cranial morphology of, fig. 9.14

Recapitulation. *See* Heterochrony

Reichert's cartilage, in mammals, 503–504

Rhabdoderma, development of, 242

Rhampholeon, effects of miniaturization in, 357

Rhamphophryne, cranial morphology and hyperossification in, 309, 322, 326, figs. 6.18–6.19

Rhea, cranial development in, 395

Rheobatrachus, hypo-ossification in, 332

Rhinatrema
  dentition, 280
  microhabitat, 268, 282
  skull and hyobranchial skeleton, 281, fig. 6.8

Rhinolophus, cranial morphology of, fig. 9.14

Rhinophrynus, skull and hyobranchial skeleton of, 315, 328–329, figs. 6.18–6.19, 6.20

Rhinoplax vigil, casque of, 410

Rhyacrotriton
  phylogenetic relationships, fig. 6.9
  skull and hyobranchial morphology, 285, 297, 300, 303, 306, table 6.2A, fig. 6.13

Rhyncholepis, dermatocranium of, fig. 4.12

Rhynchops niger, cranial kinesis in, fig. 8.16

Rousettus, naso-palatine duct in, 447

Sacabambaspis
cranial morphology, 153–154
fossil record, 152
reconstruction, fig. 4.8

Salamandra
adaptive zone, 287
chondroid cartilage, table 3.5
skull and hyoid apparatus, 303, 306, 308, figs. 6.10, 6.13

Salamandrella keyserlingii, phylogenetic relationships of, fig. 6.9

Salamandrina, hyoid apparatus of, 308

Sanchaspis, cranial morphology of, 173, fig. 4.18

Sanzinia, orbitotemporal ossifications in, 353

Sarcopterygii, monophyly and phylogenetic relationships of, 230–231

Saurichthys, upper jaw of, 226

Scaphiopus, hyperossification in, 332

Schizorhiny, in birds, 424–425

Schoenfelderpeton, phylogenetic relationships of, 256, fig. 6.1

Sciurus
auditory ossicles and ectotympanic, fig. 9.33
phylogenetic relationships, 441

Sclerodus, cranial morphology of, 169

Scolecomorphus, skull and hyobranchial morphology of, 279, 283–284, figs. 6.6–6.7, 6.8

Scolenaspis, cranial morphology of, fig. 4.14

Scolopax rochussenii, skull and jaw muscles of, 409, 424, fig. 8.3

Scylacosaurus
cranial morphology, fig. 9.1
phylogenetic relationships of, 440

Scyllium, cranial segmentation and development in, 41, fig. 5.9

Secondary palate
in mammals, 444
in reptiles, 365–370

Segmentation, 18–25, 40–48. *See also* Dermatocranium, Somite formation, Somitomeres

Septomaxilla, in mammals, 455

Simosaurus, basicranium of, 350

Sinobius malanonychus, phylogenetic relationships of, fig. 6.9

Sinoconodon, phylogenetic relationships of, 440

Siren lacertina, cranial morphology of, 300, figs. 6.11–6.12

Skeletal tissues
chordoid and chondroid, 87–98
metaplasia of, 97
molecular basis of, 71
of anaspids, 159
of lampreys, 143, 146–149
See also Bone, Calcification, Cartilage, Cementum, Cosmine, Dentine, Enamel, Enameloid, Ganoine, Mucocartilage, Sutures, Tendon insertion structures

Skeleton
branchial. *See* Viscerocranium
dermal. *See* Dermatocranium, Exocranium, Exoskeleton
evolutionary origin, 7
neurocranial. *See* Braincase, Endocranium, Neurocranium
visceral. *See* Viscerocranium
See also Calcification, Skeletal tissues

Skull
base, in mammals, 460–464
origin of, 9
See also Skeleton

Solenodon
auditory bulla, 497
phylogenetic relationships, 441

Solnhofia parsoni, secondary palate in, fig. 7.9

Somite formation, and vertebrate origins, 12

Somitomeres, 3, 16, 20, 44–46, 178
Sorex, auditory bulla of, fig. 9.24
Spea, cranial morphology of, 327
Speonesydrion, cranial morphology of, 234, fig. 5.10
Sphenodon punctatus
  cranial development, 373
  neurocranium, 349, 353, 355, 376, fig. 7.4
  palate, 367–368, fig. 7.11
  temporal fenestration of dermatocranium, 362, 364, fig. 7.8
Splanchnocranium. *See* Viscerocranium
Squalus, head segmentation in, 41
Stapedial artery. *See* Basicranial arterial circulation
Stegokrotaphy. *See* Kinesis, cranial, in caecilians
Steneosaurus, secondary palate in, fig. 7.10
Sternoptyx, atypical cartilage in, table 3.5
Strigops habrobtilus, skull and jaw muscles of, 421, fig. 8.13
Strix nebulosa, cranial morphology and asymmetry in, 417, figs. 8.11, 8.12
Strunius, development of, 242
Struthio, postorbital process in, 402
Sturnella neglecta, cranial morphology of, fig. 8.14
Sturnus vulgaris, cranial morphology of, 424, fig. 8.14
Subarcuate fossa, in mammals, 468
Suncus, otic region in, 464
Sus, cranial morphology of, 472, fig. 9.18
Sutures, 104–106
Syngnathus, cartilage types in, table 3.5

Tachyglossus
  cranial morphology, 444, 468, 477, 483, 485, 489, 513–514, figs. 9.3, 9.13, 9.20, 9.24, 9.25, 9.33

  phylogenetic relationships, 440–441
  secondary cartilage, 525
Taeniopygia, coronoid in, 403
Talpa, cranial morphology of, 447, 456, 485
Tanichthys albonubes, hyaline-cell chondroid in, 93, table 3.6
Tanygnathus megalorynchos, skull and jaw muscles of, 421, fig. 8.13
Tanystropheus, temporal fenestration of dermatocranium in, 363
Tanytrachelos, temporal fenestration of dermatocranium in, 363
Taphozous, cranial morphology of, fig. 9.6
Tarsius, cranial morphology of, 448, 494–495, 503, fig. 9.23
Teeth. *See* Dentition
Tegmen tympani, in mammals, 468
Teleostomi
  classification, table 5.3
  monophyly and phylogenetic relationships, 213–215
Telmatobius
  dentition, 329
  hypo-ossification, 332
  plectral apparatus, 315, 320
Tendon insertion structures, 103
Tentacles, skeleton of, in hagfishes, 138–140
Terminal addition. *See* Hypermorphosis
Terrapene ornata, cranial morphology of, fig. 7.6
Tersomius, phylogenetic relationships of, 257
Tetrapleurodon, phylogenetic relationships of, 141
Thalattosaurus, temporal fenestration of dermatocranium in, 364
Thelodonti, cranial morphology of, 175
Thelodus, scale of, fig. 4.20
Thrinaxodon
  cranial morphology, 513, 522, 524, figs. 9.1, 9.31
  phylogenetic relationships, 440

Tinca tinca, mucoid chondroid in, table 3.6

Trachurus, chondroid cartilage in, table 3.5

Trachycephalus, cranial morphology of, 327

Traquairaspis, dermal head armor in, 158–159, fig. 4.11

Tremataspis, sclerotic ring and scleral ossifications of, fig. 4.15

Triadobatrachus, phylogenetic relationships of, 257, figs. 6.1, 6.14

Trichechus, cranial morphology of, 447, figs. 9.9, 9.15

Triprion, cranial morphology and hyperossification in, 322–323, 327, 332, fig. 6.18–6.19

Triturus, adaptive zone of, 287

Trogonophis, cranial morphology and effects of miniaturization in, 355, 370, fig. 7.13

Tupaia, cranial morphology of, 444–446, 448–449, 453, 456–457, 464–465, 490, 511, figs. 9.2, 9.12, 9.16

Tupinambis nigropunctatus, cranial morphology of, fig. 7.8

Turbinals. *See* Nasal turbinals

Turinia, cranial morphology of, fig. 4.20

Tylototriton, cranial morphology of, 300

Tympanic
cavity, in mammals, 470–471
membrane, in mammals, 510–522

Typhlonectes, skull and hyobranchial skeleton of, 302, figs. 6.6–6.7, 6.8

Typhlops, basicranium of, 349

Typhlosaurus
cranial morphology and effects of miniaturization in, 375, figs. 7.5, 7.13
sound-transmitting apparatus, 356

Tyto alba
adductor mandibulae externus muscle, 417
cranial morphology, figs. 8.11, 8.12

Uperoleia, cranial morphology of, 309

Uraeotyphlus narayani, cranial morphology of, figs. 6.6–6.7

Uranolophus, cranial morphology of, 231–232, 234, 236

Uria lomvia, cranial morphology of, fig. 8.2

Urogale, orbital region in, fig. 9.22

Ursus arctos, nasal cavities in, fig. 9.17

Varanosaurus acutirostris, dermatocranium of, fig. 7.7

Varanus salvator
cartilage development, 372
cranial morphology and kinesis, 371–372, figs. 7.11, 7.12

Velar skeleton, in cyclostomes, 136, 144–145, 151, 178

Vesperugo, paranasal sinuses in, 480

Viscerocranium
and head segmentation, 41–42, 47–48, 55–59
in acanthodians, 217
in actinopterygians, 225
in birds, 394–402
in chondrichthyans, 208–209
in crossopterygians, 241–242
in dipnoans, 236
in gnathostomes, 189–190
in hagfishes, 140
in lampreys, 143–146
in lissamphibians, 267, 280–281, 304–306, 329–331
in mammals, 474–477
in osteichthyans, 221
in placoderms, 199–203
in reptiles, 354–358
in sarcopterygians, 232
in teleostomes, 214–215
See also Amphistyly, Chondrocranium, Holostyly, Hyostyly

Xenacanthus, cranial morphology of, figs. 5.4, 5.5, 5.7

Xenopus
chordoid tissues, 89

Xenopus (*continued*)
  skull and hyobranchial skeleton,
    331, 326

Youngina capensis, dermatocranium
  of, fig. 7.7
Youngolepis, cranial morphology of,
  234, 237–241

Zenaspis, cranial morphology of, fig.
  4.13
Zygokrotaphy. *See* Kinesis, cranial, in
  caecilians
Zygomatic arch, in mammals, 460